The Physical Lincoln Sourcebook

By the author:

In Print:

      Zebra Cards: An Aid to Obscure Diagnosis

      The Astronaut Almanac: Volumes 1 and 2

      The Physical Lincoln

      The Physical Lincoln Sourcebook

On the Web:

      `www.doctorzebra.com`

      `www.expertmapper.com`

The Physical Lincoln Sourcebook

An Annotated Medical History
of
Abraham Lincoln and His Family

John G. Sotos, MD

Mt. Vernon, Virginia ▪ Mt. Vernon Book Systems
2008

Printing 1.1a

Mt. Vernon Book Systems
P.O. Box 21
Mt. Vernon, VA 22121

Visit us at:
www.physical-lincoln.com
www.doctorzebra.com
www.mtvernonbook.com

Printing 1.1a.   Year: 2008.   (Include printing in all citations.)

Please email comments to: contact2008@physical-lincoln.com
Kindly include the printing number.

Printed in the United States of America

This book was produced using Macintosh computers, the Python programming language, and the TeXShop front-end for the TeX typesetting system. TeX is a trademark of the American Mathematical Society. TeXShop is by Richard Koch and Dirk Olmes, and includes work by Gerben Wierda.

Library of Congress Control Number: 2008905220
ISBN 978-0-9818193-3-4

Contents

Figures

To my brother, George

and

To Hugh Rienhoff, who has helped at every stage

and

To my teachers in public schools,
in college and graduate classrooms,
and on the wards

In 1859 I was in the Supreme Court room in the [Illinois] State House. Lincoln was ... telling his yarns. A man, a farmer, said "Lincoln, why do you not write out your stories and put them in a book?"

Lincoln drew himself up, fixed his face, and said "Such a book would stink like a thousand privies."

– Henry E. Dummer*
[wilson p442]

One of the signs of obsession is an inability to tell the difference between what matters and what does not.

– Gore Vidal
[vidalA p691]

Introduction

This book collects and organizes physiological information about Abraham Lincoln and his family. Originally intended to aid in diagnosing the genetic cause of Lincoln's unusual height and unusual body build, I began assembling it after my initial diagnostic efforts failed, with the hope it might prove useful to those trying later.

The now-discarded introduction to an early draft of the book outlined potential utilities:

> *The Physical Lincoln Sourcebook* was primarily written for the person who will someday diagnose Lincoln correctly. This person will have two main needs.
>
> First, in making the diagnosis, he or she will take a clinical syndrome and look for its features in Lincoln's medical history. Today, that is no easy task. Despite the gargantuan body of writings about Lincoln, his detailed medical history has not been systematically recorded and analyzed.* Information about his blood relatives, important to any genetic hypothesis, is even more dispersed.
>
> Second, like any physician making a diagnosis, the person who someday diagnoses Lincoln inevitably must decide which statements to accept from their patient's history, and which to reject. With Lincoln as the patient, such decisions will require knowing the source and trustworthiness of each statement as a historian might assess them.
>
> To fill both these needs, I offer *The Physical Lincoln Sourcebook* – a sourcebook from which medical scholars can draw sound conclusions related to Lincoln's physiology. The book contains every statement related to Lincoln's body I have yet found. It slavishly provides the source for each statement and occasionally offers caveats about particular sources.
>
> Of course, I hope this book finds an audience larger than the one person who solves Lincoln's genetic puzzle. In writing about the medical history of American Presidents [aa106] [aa107], I have been continually amazed how the experience of illness can humanize even the most iconic historical figure. It's hard enough to be President of the United States during a civil war, but it's worse when you are chronically constipated and you have smallpox.

The book has already fulfilled its primary aim. The raw historical data in the *Sourcebook* proved indispensable in building the case that Lincoln had a hereditary cancer syndrome called multiple endocrine neoplasia type 2b (MEN2B). A companion book, *The Physical Lincoln*, details the events leading to the diagnosis and discusses evidence for and against MEN2B.

In fact, the *Sourcebook* was so useful while writing *The Physical Lincoln* that I decided to continue developing it. Many reasons prompted this:

- Anyone challenging the MEN2B diagnosis, or offering an alternate diagnosis, will need the *Sourcebook*'s data.

- Lincolnian medical mysteries remain (especially regarding Mary Lincoln).

- MEN2B is so rare, and detailed clinical histories today are so rare, that I believe Lincoln's history could potentially illuminate unrecognized features of MEN2B.

- Attempts to diagnose the ailments of historical figures vary widely in quality. I believe this book, teamed with its companion, offer a method worth emulating. The method merely copies the way generations of physicians have approached hospitalized patients.

- Scholars and teachers may find it a useful source of projects.

---

* [shutes] & [shutesE] come closest. [marx] & [bumgarnerB] are overviews. [kempfB] is unreadable.

The next two sections of the introduction explain the medical and historical approaches used in compiling this book.

Medical Approach

Abraham Lincoln's medical history is the centerpiece of the book. Physicians will immediately recognize its similarity to the standard "H&P" they learned to write in medical school.

An H&P ("history and physical") is the most thorough description a physician writes about a patient. Normally written when a patient is admitted to the hospital, an H&P always contains the same standard sub-sections arranged in the same standard order.

Lincoln's H&P, however, requires a modified structure because: (1) historical records, not living humans, provide its contents, and (2) it assumes that an undescribed genetic disorder is central to Lincoln's medical history. Thus, a structure containing the following sections has been adopted:

1. *Problem List* – As in standard H&Ps, this simple listing gathers all medical abnormalities encountered in Lincoln, no matter how insignificant. Classically, problems are listed in descending order of seriousness. Problems in Lincoln's blood relatives are not included unless pertinent to a problem of Lincoln himself.

2. *Family Trees* – These diagrams will help orient readers to the extended Lincoln family.

3. *Personal Histories* – Lincoln and all his first-degree relatives have histories in this book, limited in scope only by the information available. (A few, more distant relatives are aggregated in a single section at the end.) In general, each person's history begins with a table of contents, followed by a life chronology and by sub-sections that more or less correspond to organ systems. Physicians will recognize the sub-sections as comprising a "review of systems." Many of the sub-sections begin with introductory remarks highlighting key points related to that organ system. A few include ruminations on historical sources.

4. *Special Topics* – This section presents topics too large to fit nicely in the body of Lincoln's personal history.

5. *Bibliography and Personæ* – I want this book to help those first entering the Lincoln literature – certainly the case for physicians. The bibliography is, therefore, annotated. And, because an important and challenging task for novices is learning who-is-whom among countless Lincoln observers, short descriptions of selected observers are also provided.

Two sections of a traditional H&P are missing: the *Assessment* section and the *Plans* section. Obviously, no plans for Lincoln's medical management are needed. The Assessment section normally discusses items from the Problem List, in light of all the other evidence recorded in the H&P. It is where hypotheses are generated and diagnoses made. Aside from sprinkled editorial comments, this book omits the Assessment. *The Physical Lincoln* functions as the assessment section of Lincoln's H&P, addressing both medical and historical concerns. (It is also a significant component of the physical examination: much of the detailed photographic analysis in *The Physical Lincoln* is not repeated herein.)

What information should an H&P contain? In principle, the answer is: *everything* of even *potential* medical relevance to the subject. In practice, such records are never compiled because they would be too long. Virtually everything humans do, and virtually everything we might observe about each other, can, in some circumstance, be medically relevant. Ear lobes can matter. Handshakes can matter. How well one plays ball sports, specifically, can matter. Even the appearance of one's chairs can matter. Recall that the model for Sherlock Holmes was a physician.

Nevertheless, I have attempted to assemble such a record for two reasons: First, we cannot know which signs or symptoms may help establish a Lincoln diagnosis. The TGFβ signaling pathway is so extensive and so complicated that today's extraneous tidbit may be tomorrow's key finding. Or, as the English neurosurgeon Wilfred Trotter famously noted: "Disease often tells its secrets in a casual parenthesis" [aa122].

Second, the historical record is thin for many aspects of Lincoln's life. Where direct information is absent, the presence of multiple, congruent, indirect bits of information may allow reasonably certain conclusions.

The result is an H&P a medical student might write: unfiltered and over-detailed. I make no apologies for this. (I do admit, however, to becoming captivated by Lincoln, and to including *very occasional* anecdotes I would be hard-pressed to claim are medically informative, other than providing a fuller picture of the patient.)

Obviously, an H&P is not a traditional biography. It is a technical document, where prose style and narrative unity rank behind efficiency and clarity. Even so, the richest H&Ps chronicle a life and, because no human can be separated from their physical self, they do have a drama. I think readers will find that here.

Historical Approach

The prospect of writing about Lincoln – of hoping to say something *new* about him – was imposing in the extreme. I am very conscious of the thousands of extraordinarily bright, industrious, and tenacious people who have examined every aspect of the man's life and created a veritable Denali of literature.

Yet, there was an undeniable gap in the literature when it came to Lincoln's health. The last complete review was published in 1933 [shutes], the paleolithic era of molecular medicine. A 1960 review [marx] has no references, and more recent efforts [bumgarnerA] [bumgarnerB] are not based on primary sources. The only in-depth review of Lincoln and the Marfan sydrome was published a generation ago in the historical literature [borittA].

Some historians have consulted physicians before writing about Lincolnian health (e.g. [baker], [borittA]). Choreographing such consultations is tricky, however. Physicians must be supplied with information, but identifying and selecting the information to supply requires medical sophistication – a classic catch-22.

This book aims only to be useful. I have simply gathered statements, organized them in bins, and provided a thin layer of annotation to help readers start the difficult process of deciding what to trust and what to discard.

Filtering has been light. Scholars debate whether to fully trust William Herndon's statements (¶12) and have stopped debating whether to trust [ostendorfC]. But both appear in this book, with caveats, and with the understanding that proper filtering must occur at another level. Other traps for the researcher are identified, such as unauthentic handwriting samples (¶1578, ¶5148) and unauthentic footwear (¶1019).

Readers are strongly urged to consult original documents in all cases. Although I have assiduously tried to supply context for each statement, disagreement is possible. Furthermore, proofreading has been greatly complicated (and compromised) by the decision to preserve the exact spellings from source documents. ([wilson] did this, and it is the right decision.)

I have also tried to assign dates to each statement, although this is often impossible. In general, dateless statements are listed first in each section. Dated statements follow, in chronological order.

To help readers new to the Lincoln literature, each statement in the personal histories is marked as originating from a primary or secondary source. A primary source is defined as a written record that does not reference, implicitly or explicitly, another document as the source of information. Typical primary sources are letters, interview transcripts, and personal recollections. A secondary source is anything but a primary source.*

Assigning primary/secondary labels serves several purposes. First, it highlights the different roles played by primary and secondary sources. Primary sources contain the informational building blocks for the conclusions and syntheses made in secondary sources. Secondary sources "ratify" primary sources that have been accepted by the Lincoln community. Physicians, police officers, and journalists know that asking a question multiple times yields the most reliable story, so for dubious primary statements I have not hesitated to list multiple secondary sources.

Second, classifying sources highlights the traps inherent in secondary sources. For example, some secondary sources inflate meager primary sources into rich tapestries. (Carl Sandburg was a genius at this.) Because such over-generalizations may confuse readers who are new to the Lincoln literature, I identify them.

Third, it serves as a "things to do" list for the author. Ideally, all facts appearing in secondary sources should be traceable to a primary source. For now, I have recorded information from where I read it.

A great gathering of facts naturally tempts one to speculate, and I have not always resisted. The speculations can serve as a guide to the open issues in Lincoln's medical history.

The Lincoln community has very high standards for scholarship and completeness. Meeting both standards for the scope of material in *The Physical Lincoln Sourcebook* would take years. Delaying publication until then would deprive the community of what I believe is a valuable resource.

Thus, I have decided to strive for the highest scholarship standards, but will release the book earlier than Lincoln scholars of the past might have done. Typesetting on personal computers, combined with on-demand printing, make a staged release entirely feasible. An on-line index is planned.

Early release has the additional benefits of generating early feedback from the readership, and of involving the community in the continued evolution of the book. This allows more experimentation in the book and, compared to my solitary efforts, could actually accelerate progress toward completeness.

How to Read This Book

Each personal history is divided into organ systems (approximately) and each organ system is composed of one or more paragraphs. Each paragraph is numbered, to allow convenient reference to it. For example, "¶151" happens to refer to the paragraph containing Lincoln's self-description. (Paragraph numbers will not be consistent from edition to edition.)

Most paragraphs are *bulleted*. That is, they are prefixed by a symbol. The symbol characterizes the paragraph's contents, as described below. Sometimes the initial paragraph(s) of an organ system are not bulleted. These introductory paragraphs are editorializations not derived from the historical record. *Similarly, comments in this typeface are also editorializations.* Increasing indentation indicates a sub-paragraph.

Symbols characterize the contents of bulleted paragraphs as follows:

$\langle 1 \rangle$ indicates the paragraph's information derives from a primary source, as defined earlier.

$\langle \frac{1}{q} \rangle$ indicates a paragraph that quotes from a primary source, but the quote was read in a secondary source.

---

* Too late I realized that [herndon] is largely a secondary source. Fixing this error is a task for a later edition.

⟨2⟩ indicates a secondary source reporting a fact (vs. a quotation) – even if it documents the primary source.

⟨2⟩_c indicates a conclusion made in a secondary source, based on reasonably believable facts.

⟨S⟩ indicates speculation. This is similar to ⟨2⟩_c, but the reasoning and/or underlying facts are less certain.

⟨H⟩ indicates hearsay, i.e. the paragraph reports information of questionable validity.

[○] indicates a photograph is the basis for the paragraph's information. (The icon suggests a camera.)

⟨M⟩ indicates a miscellaneous, i.e. unclassified, source of information.

Here is an example: If I saw a phrase from Lincoln's 1859 self-description (¶151) quoted in a modern biography, the resulting paragraph in *The Physical Lincoln Sourcebook* would be ⟨1⟩_q. If I had seen the entire self-description in a scholarly collection of his writings, or in its original form, the paragraph would have been ⟨1⟩. If the biography said "Lincoln described himself as lean," the paragraph would be ⟨2⟩. And if the biography said "At 6'4" and 180 lbs., Lincoln must have been lean indeed," the paragraph would be ⟨2⟩_c.

Note that the ⟨1⟩ and ⟨2⟩ characterizations do not reflect the believability of the paragraph's information or source. For example, ⟨1⟩ would apply to an eyewitness account written immediately after an event. It would also apply to a statement made 60 years after the fact by the grandson of the eyewitness, who used to hear his aged grandfather tell the story. These sources have greatly different believabilities, but in both cases there is no further trail of references to pursue. Finally, if I, or others, thought the grandfather or grandson were not credible, the ⟨H⟩ rating would be applied.

While the dividing lines between these categories are not always sharp, in the overwhelming majority of cases, they work well. They can also help disambiguate the voice behind a quotation. Consider:

⟨1⟩_q Circa April 1864: "looked like a man worn and harassed with petty faultfinding and criticisms, until he had turned at bay, like an old stag pursued and hunted by a cowardly rabble of men and dogs" – Albert G. Riddle [donaldA p497]

⟨2⟩ Riddle had not seen Lincoln in 5 months and was "shocked by the change in his appearance." [donaldA p497]

In the first case, the ⟨1⟩_q indicates that Donald's book is quoting from something Albert Riddle wrote. Presumably, Donald has seen Riddle's document – the primary source. In the second case, the ⟨2⟩ indicates that Donald is the author of the language inside the quotation marks.

Other conventions used in the book:

- Square brackets around this typeface point to a reference from the bibliography section, e.g. [donaldA p497].
- Whenever "Lincoln" is used as an isolated name, it refers to President Abraham Lincoln.
- If a statement in a person's history has no explicit subject, the subject is that person.
- The symbol ±, as in "age 20±," means "approximately." By contrast, "age 20+" means "age 20 or higher."
- The symbol ∈ means, as in mathematics, that the current paragraph is a subset of another paragraph.
- The mis-spellings preserved in [wilson] and other references have been preserved here.
- Potential topics for scholarly projects are marked by ○○○ *Project:* and then described.

Acknowledgments

The *The Physical Lincoln Sourcebook* and *The Physical Lincoln* owe their existences to immensely helpful people, organizations, and technology.

People. My greatest thanks goes to those who read the entire manuscript of *The Physical Lincoln* and provided detailed, page by page comments: William Petros, Georgette Sotos, and George P. Sotos. Their improvements to the book cannot be underestimated, and my gratitude to them knows no bounds.

Drs Kevin Olden, Jeffrey Jones, and Hugh Rienhoff, Jr. read the entire manuscript and provided invaluable suggestions. Hugh has been my guide in all things TGFβ, but, more than that, has for 28 years been a fount of encouragement and a treasured friend. Olden I have learned to tolerate ... and thereby learned much else.

Many other physicians contributed their expertise in helpful discussions, for which I am grateful: David Walton, Thomas Traill, George A. Sotos, Mindy Shapiro, Chad Prodromos, John Mulliken, Neil Miller, Victor McKusick, Justin MacArthur, Richard Lange, Douglas Jabs, Tripp Heard, Henry Halperin, William Gottesman, Robert Gagel, Ronald Fishman, Charis Eng, Hal Dietz, Kevin Boylan, Kenneth Baughman, Douglas Ball, and Stephen Achuff. Dr. Lori Marion was my refraction-tutor. Please do not assume that these professionals endorse my conclusions!

Friends & family generously gave guidance, inspiration, and moral support: Carol & Rob Younge, Dr. James Weiss, Dr. Charles Wiener, Susan Weiner, Bruce Tognazzini, Dr. David Thiemann, Barbara Schroll, Marilyn Prodromos, Jacqueline Parker, Mike Morton, the Litt family, Dr. Paul Ladenson, Dr. Kathryn Hodge, Dr. David Herrington, Al Henning (and the Dartmouth Club of Silicon Valley), Judge Lauren Heard, Dr. Nicholas Fortuin, Doris Egan, John Catsis, David Brown, John Branscum, and Peter Blake.

To a greater extent than all these people realize, this book is a smorgasbord of their ideas (and restraints!). Many I know from Johns Hopkins, where the pervasive spirit of inquiry allows anyone to walk up to anyone else and begin a conversation, saying: "I've been working on this idea..."

The special roles of Richard Benson and James Mellon are discussed in *The Physical Lincoln*. Richard went above and beyond, graciously helping me understand how he did what he did, and explaining the subtleties of 19th century photography. For supplying images, I am grateful to Gabor Boritt, Eugene Knox III, Dr. Ronald Fishman, Dan Ostendorf (and family), and to Keya Morgan. Suzanne Walsh taught me the rudiments of graphics processing long ago; I wish she had taught me some of her artistic skill!

Professional advice from DeAnna Gibbons, Jonathan Baruch, and Richard Abate was much appreciated. Jason Emerson greatly helped my search for sources. Cindy VanHorn and Jane Gastineaux at the Lincoln Museum were unfailingly good-humored about my requests. Cindy, especially, helped in so many ways over a period of several months. Sue Cornacchia and Hallie Brooker of the U.S. Coast Guard Academy and Museum were nicer to me than I had any reason to expect. Carol Johnson at the Library of Congress went out of her way to answer my questions about Mary Lincoln photographs.

Heroically, George P. Sotos read a thick draft of *The Physical Lincoln Sourcebook*, cover to cover. That is a real example of parental love! He and my mother are the best parents imaginable; I owe everything to them.

Organizations. I am grateful for the services provided by ■ Stanford University Libraries ■ the Library of Congress ■ Palo Alto City Library ■ Lincoln Museum of Ft. Wayne, Indiana ■ National Portrait Gallery ■ San Francisco Public Library ■ Welch Medical Library and Eisenhower Library of the Johns Hopkins University ■ National Archives and Records Administration ■ Holt-Atherton Special Collections at the University of the Pacific Library ■ Georgetown University Library Special Collections ■ Waupaca Area Public Library (Wisconsin) ■ Lincoln Shrine and A.K. Smiley Public Library of Redlands, California ■ Abraham Lincoln Presidential Library and Museum of Springfield, Illinois ■ United States Coast

Guard Museum ▪ Medical Society of the State of New York ▪ Massachusetts Medical Society ▪ Smithsonian Institution.

Of these, Stanford University deserves special thanks for its policy of giving the community access to the vast majority of its libraries. My thanks to the staffs of the Green, Lane, SAL, art, SAL3, and Falconer libraries.

Technology. Software has played a huge role in the books. I am happy to say that the books were developed entirely with open-source software. To all who contributed to developing these systems, thank you. ▪ T$_E$X ▪ TeXShop ▪ the GIMP ▪ Python ▪ PIL ▪ Mediawiki ▪ Apache.

The Internet Archive (archive.org) and Google Books (books.google.com) are fantastic resources for anyone needing access to out-of-copyright books. I used both heavily, with gratitude at every download.

Finally. The errors in this book are mine alone – but if you don't tell me about them, they will be your errors in future editions. ☺

Abraham Lincoln's Medical Problem List

This section lists all of Lincoln's identified physical and medical abnormalities, no matter how trivial, plus pertinent data from selected relatives. A "?" indicates uncertainty.

Problems are grouped syndromically, rather than a traditional most-serious to least-serious ranking. This greatly simplifies what would otherwise be a long and ungainly list.

Skeletal and other dysmorphisms compatible with classic Marfan syndrome
1. Tall stature, long arms, long legs	¶322
2. Long thin hands, longish fingers (not classical arachnodactyly)	¶1448
3. Long thin feet, long great toes	¶921
4. Long thin neck	¶3039
5. Thin chest, stoop-shouldered, pectus excavatum	¶500
6. Tall forehead, tall mid-face	¶1641
7. High-pitched voice	¶3698
8. Mother: tall, thin-faced, high forehead	¶4744
9. Son #4: pubertal change to long, thin face	¶5368

Components of MEN2B
10. Large asymmetric lower lip; multiple lumps in upper and lower lips	¶2785
11. Surgical removal of cheek lump	¶1850
12. Large jaw	¶2807
13. Chronic constipation (? and "sick headache")	¶612
14. Left scleral (conjunctival) mass, right eyelid mass	¶778
15. Cutaneous masses (peri-oral, peri-nasal, nasolabial fold)	¶1657
16. Lifelong lack of body fat	¶391
17. Son #4: Large lower lip, lumpy lips	¶5460
18. Son #4: Wasting illness: pleural effusions, no fever, no pain, early death	¶5264
19. Son #3: Large lower lip, lumpy lips, tall, long lower body segment, early death	¶5679
20. Son #2: Asymmetric lower lip, tall, early death	¶3913
21. Mother: Early death, ? wasting illness	¶4055

Signs of muscle hyoptonia
22. Hypermobility in fingers and feet (flat feet)	
23. Spinal hypermobility (bending)	¶2244
24. "Lounging"	¶2967
25. Swinging gait	¶1070
26. Ptosis	¶899
27. Sad face	¶1757
28. Protruding ears	¶663
29. Skull asymmetries, possibly compatible with left deformational plagiocephaly	

Asymmetries of head
	¶267
30. Left ear displaced anteriorly and superiorly	
31. Chin displaced to right	
32. Other skull asymmetries probably compatible with left synostotic plagiocephaly	
33. Homely	¶1663
34. Intermittent left hypertropia; weak left superior oblique; right head tilt; diplopia	¶862

Pertinent negatives
35. No myopia; vision good until middle-age	¶782
36. No episodes of chest discomfort	
37. Only one episode of daytime somnolence	¶712
38. Great muscular strength	¶2826

Final months   ¶1203ff
39. Weight loss, temporal wasting
40. Syncope
41. Cold hands and feet
42. "Growing fatigue"
43. Headache
44. (? influenza-like) illness in March 1865   ¶1226

Findings of unclear significance
45. Prematurely aged skin: yellow, leathery, wrinkled   ¶3357
46. Asymmetric hands, feet, shoulders, gait, and ? chest   ¶267
47. Thin orbital plates   ¶3296
48. Flat-footed gait   ¶1053
49. Coarse hair   ¶1389
50. ? Poor sleep efficiency, ? parasomnia, ? snoring   ¶3417
51. Syncope and "sick headache" in 1861   ¶1884
52. Son #4: small jaw resolving in teens; large head; downsloped palpebrae   ¶5372
53. Son #4: learning disability   ¶5507

Infection
54. Smallpox (1863)   Special Topic §5
55. "Ague" (1830)   ¶2001
56. Every-other-day fever and chills (1835)   ¶2008
57. Probable lues (1835±)   Special Topic §2
58. ? Scarlet fever (1860)   ¶5748
59. Minor "indispositions" (presumed infectious)

Mental
60. Strong memory, strong verbal skills   ¶3062
61. Episode of low mood: bereavement and physical illness (1835)   ¶2695
62. Episode of low mood: possible depressive episode (1841)   Special Topic §3
63. Gloomy outlook
64. "Abstracted;" strong ability to concentrate   ¶2365

Trauma
65. Bullet wound to head   Special Topic §7
66. Head trauma and unconsciousness from horse-kick   ¶3568
67. Head trauma from robbery attempt   ¶3582
68. Head trauma from domestic violence   ¶3589
69. Hand trauma from handshaking   ¶1491
70. Hand trauma from axe   ¶1490
71. Wrist sprain from horse accident   ¶3602
72. History of "frozen feet"   ¶930
73. History of sunburn   ¶3372

Other
74. Exposure to elemental mercury (1835, 1860-1861)   ¶2287
75. Dental extractions, with complication   ¶2818
76. History of podiatric operation   ¶969
77. History of motion sickness (?)   ¶1271
78. History of food poisoning (?)   ¶640
79. History of gas toxicity (?)   ¶2286
80. Mild presbyopia   ¶801
81. Chin dimple   ¶1898

Family Trees

Three Lincoln family trees are provided: (1) his immediate family, (2) his paternal ancestors, and (3) his maternal family and step-family. In the scientific literature, [ranum] and [schwartzA] provide Lincoln family trees.

Immediate Family

The tree below shows Abraham Lincoln's parents, siblings, wife, children, and their age at death. A chapter in the present book is devoted to each named person shown.

Other Lincoln, Hanks, and Todd relatives are discussed starting in ¶5786. Lincoln's last direct descendant died in 1985. [beschloss] details the sordid end of the line. [neelyA] contains photographs of all Lincoln's descendants.

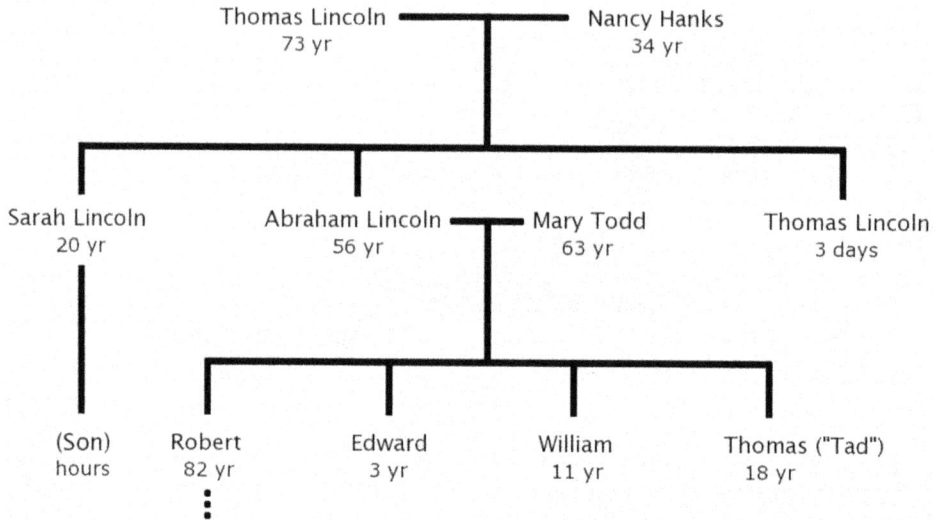

Figure 1

Selected Paternal Ancestors

The tree below, compiled from [montgomery] and [lincolnW], is incomplete, as only the last three generations show all Lincoln children. Furthermore, generation V's ordering has been adjusted to conserve space: Abraham was the eldest [lincolnW]. For some members, the states of their residence, or their descendants' residence, are listed in italics. Samuel Lincoln I-1 came to America (Salem, MA) in 1635 – just 15 years after the *Mayflower*.

It was long supposed that Abraham V-5 had a first wife, Mary Shipley, who was the mother of all persons in generation VI, except Thomas [lea p106] [tarbellEp226]. A thin thread of documentary evidence establishes Bathsheba as the mother of all in generation VI [lincolnW p202], a view unenthusiastically supported by [tarbellB p54]. Of note, [montgomery p291] still lists Mary Shipley as the first wife.

[ranum] provides interrupted and corrupted trees for descendants of Abraham V-5 and Bathsheba, and finds cases of type 5 spinocerebellar ataxia in this line (see ¶1025). Interruptions in these trees are filled by [lincolnW]. Members of generation VI, below, are not in birth order.

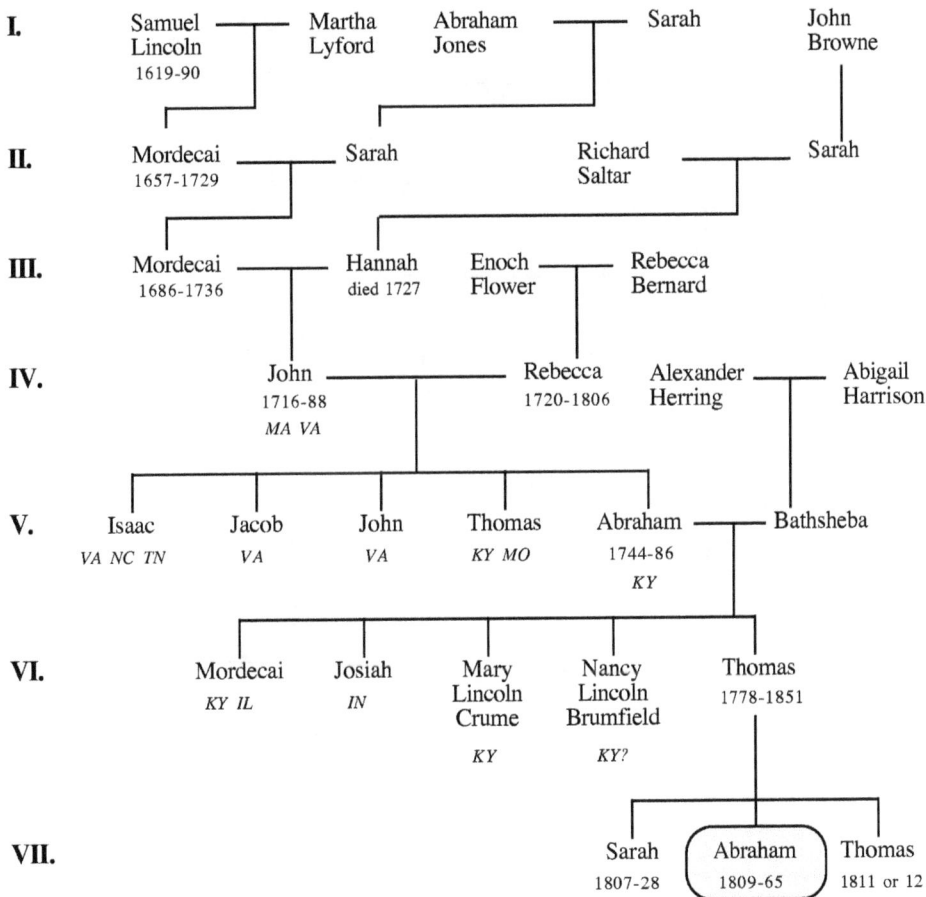

Figure 2

19

The maternal tree was compiled from the work of Paul H. Verduin [wilson pp779-783]. As [wilson p96n] notes, "The true family line of Nancy Hanks is much disputed. [We believe] the genealogy established by Paul Verduin ... is the best available."

Below, a solid dot indicates a union outside of marriage. Male X1 (from Virginia) and Male X2 (from Kentucky) have not been identified in the historical record. Note that there are two women named Nancy Hanks.

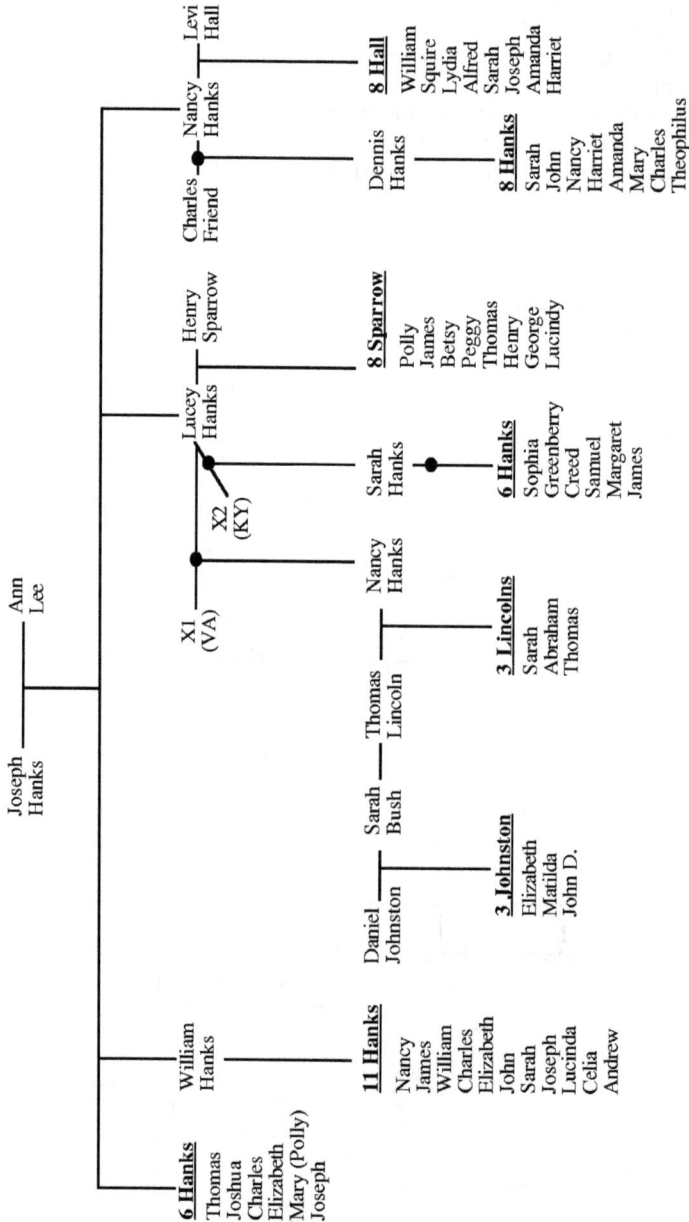

Joseph Hanks — Ann Lee

Charles Friend • Nancy Hanks — Levi Hall

Dennis Hanks

8 Hall
William
Squire
Lydia
Alfred
Sarah
Joseph
Amanda
Harriet

8 Hanks
Sarah
John
Nancy
Harriet
Amanda
Mary
Charles
Theophilus

Lucey Hanks — Henry Sparrow

8 Sparrow
Polly
James
Betsy
Peggy
Thomas
Henry
George
Lucindy

X1 (VA) • Lucey Hanks • X2 (KY)

Sarah Hanks • Greenberry Creed

6 Hanks
Sophia
Greenberry
Creed
Samuel
Margaret
James

Nancy Hanks — Thomas Lincoln

3 Lincolns
Sarah
Abraham
Thomas

Daniel Johnston — Sarah Bush

3 Johnston
Elizabeth
Matilda
John D.

William Hanks

11 Hanks
Nancy
James
William
Charles
Elizabeth
John
Sarah
Joseph
Lucinda
Celia
Andrew

6 Hanks
Thomas
Joshua
Charles
Elizabeth
Mary (Polly)
Joseph

Figure 3

Personal Histories

Prolog: Abraham Lincoln in 1861

In 1865 William Herndon described his former law partner in detail [herndonC pp356-359], *below. The Herndon-Weik biography of Lincoln reprints it, with some changes* [herndon pp471-472].

Abraham Lincoln was about six feet four inches high, and when he left this city was 51   1
years old, having good health and no gray hairs – or but few in his head. He was thin – tall –
wiry – sinewy, grisly – raw-boned man, thin through the breast to the back – and narrow
across the shoulders, standing he leaned forward – was what may be called stoop shouldered, inclining to the consumptive by build. His usual weight was about 160 pounds.
His organization – rather his structure functioned – that is, worked slowly. His blood had
to run a long distance from the heart to the tips of his frame, and his nerve force – mind
force had to travel through dry ground a long distance before the muscles & nerves were
obedient to his will. His structure – his build was loose and leathery. His body was shrunk
and shrivelled – having dark skin – dark hair – looking woe struck. The whole man – body
& mind worked slowly – creekingly, as if it wanted oiling. Physically he was a very – very
powerful man, lifting with ease 400 – or 600 pounds. His mind was like his body. His mind
worked slowly, but strongly.

When Mr. Lincoln walked he moved cautiously, but firmly, his long arms – his hands   2
on them hanging like giants hands, swung down by his side. He walked with even tread –
his toes – the inner sides of his feet were parallel, if not a little pigeontoed. He did not
walk cunningly – Indian like, but cautiously & firmly. In walking Mr. Lincoln put the whole
foot flat down on the ground at once, not landing on the heel. He lifted his foot all at
once – not lifting himself from the toes, and hence he had no spring or snap or get get
[sic] up to his walk. He had the economy of fall and lift of foot, though he had spring or
apparent ease of motion in his tread. Mr. Lincoln walked undulating up & down, catching
and pocketing tire – weariness & pain all up and down his person, preventing them from
special locations. The first opinion [of] a stranger or a man who did not observe closely
was that his walk implied – shrewdness – cunning – a tricky man, but his was the walk of
caution & firmness. Such is law. In sitting down on common chairs he was no taller than
ordinary men from the chair to the crown of his head. A marble placed on his knee would
roll hipward, down an inclined plane. His legs & arms were abnormally – unnaturally long,
& hence in undue proportions to the balance of his body. It was only when he stood up
that he loomed above other men.

Mr. Lincoln's head was long & tall from the base of the brain and from the eye brow –   3
the perceptive faculties. His head ran backward, his forehead rising as it ran back at a
low angle. ... The size of his hat, measured at the hatter's block was $7\,1/8$, his head being
from ear to ear $6\,1/2$ inches – and from the front to the back of the brain 8 inches. Thus
measured it was not below the medium size, it made rather large mass through the height
& length of it. Mr. Lincoln's forehead was narrow but high. His hair was dark – almost
black and lay floating where the fingers or the winds left it, piled up at random. His cheek
bones were high – sharp and prominent. His eyebrows heavy and jutting out. Mr. Lincoln's
jaws were long up curved and heavy. His nose was large – long and blunt, having the tip
glowing in red, and a little awry toward the right eye. His chin was long – sharp and up
curved. His eyebrows cropped out like a huge rock on the brow of a hill. His face was
long – sallow – cadaverous – shrunk – shrivelled – wrinkled, and dry, having here and there
a hair on the surface. His cheeks were leathery and flabby, falling in loose folds at places,
looking sorrowful and sad. Mr. Lincoln's ears were extremely large – and ran out almost at
right angles from his head – caused by heavy hats and partly by nature. His lower lip was
thick – material and hanging undercurved, while his chin reached for the lip up curved.
Mr. Lincoln's neck was neat and trim, his head being well balanced on it. There was the
lone mole on the right cheek and Adam's apple on his throat. ... He was not a pretty man
by any means – nor was he an ugly one; he was a homely man.

Lincoln, Abraham President

Chronology

Month	Year	Age	Home	Personal	Professional	4
February	1809	0	Kentucky	born		
?	1812	2	"	infant brother dies		
December	1816	7	Indiana			
October	1818	9	"	Mother dies		
December	1819	10	"	Step-mother arrives		
January	1828	18	"	sister Sarah dies		
March	1830	21	Macon Cty, Ill.			
July	1831	22	New Salem	leaves home		
April-July	1832	23			Militia: Black Hawk War	
August	1834	25	"		Elected to state legislature	
August	1835	26	"	Ann Rutledge dies		
April	1837	28	Springfield		Joins first law practice	
November	1842	33	"	weds Mary Todd	Retires from legislature	
August	1843	34	"	son #1 born (Robert)		
March	1846	37	"	son #2 born (Eddie)		
Dec.	1847	38	Washington		Serves in Congress	
March	1849	40	Springfield		Practices law	
February	1850	40	"	son Eddie dies		
December	1850	41	"	son #3 born (Willie)		
January	1851	41	"	Father dies		
April	1853	44	"	son #4 born (Tad)		
fall	1854	45	"		Re-enters politics	
Aug.-Oct.	1858	49	"		Lincoln-Douglas debates	
November	1860	51	"		Elected President	
March	1861	52	Washington		President	
February	1862	53	"	son Willie dies		

Chronology (continued)

April	1865	56	"		dies	
July	1871	–	–		son Tad dies	–
July	1882	–	–		wife Mary dies	–
July	1926	–	–		son Robert dies	–

Source = [fehrenbacherA pp835-852], [angle pp36-37]. More details in: Travel & Dwellings

⟨1⟩ The 1850 census lists Lincoln's age as 40. He was 41. [templeC] See ¶3968   5

Introduction & Sources

The following thoughts about Lincolnian information sources may help readers wish-   6
ing to begin their own research projects. The fundamental lesson is that there are no
easy answers. "In the Lincoln field above all others, debate can be endless" [borittD p9].

- The starting point for Lincoln scholars is always the biography written by his long-   7
  time law partner, William Herndon [herndon]. Herndon's biography is based on two
  main sources, totaling 10,000+ pages [hertz p23]:
  - ⟨-⟩ Information Herndon collected – By letter and by interview in the years after   8
    Lincoln's death, Herndon collected information from over 250 informants
    [wilson p x]. This material has been majestically collected and edited by Dou-
    glas Wilson and Rodney Davis [wilson].
  - ⟨-⟩ Herndon's own recollections and analyses – This mass of information is al-   9
    most as voluminous as his letter and interview corpus [wilson p vii]. Currently,
    the best source is [hertz].
  - ⟨-⟩ Even so, Herndon says "When I was around taking evidence soon after and   10
    long after Mr. Lincoln's death, *much, much* was told me which I did not re-
    duce to writing, but which, *much of which*, floats about in my memory. Time
    may have modified, altered, or changed what was told me. I rejected much
    which was told me, because what was told me was contrary to what I knew,
    contrary to my records, and contrary to nature; still, I now wish I had written
    it out..." [hertz p70]
  - ⟨2⟩ Herndon's in-person interviews yielded hurriedly-written notes that are best   11
    c   deciphered by imagining them as the answers to a series of questions posed
    by Herndon. [walsh p79]
- All Lincoln students must decide how much stock to place in Herndon's trove. The   12
  eminent and influential Lincoln scholar, James G. Randall, for example, regarded
  Herndon as an unreliable source [wilson p xxi]. Others view Herndon as a shrewd
  lawyer who manipulated people to say what he wanted them to say [randallC p356]
  [shenk p233]. Burlingame, however, makes extensive use of Herndon's materials [burl
  p xxiv]. All agree that Herndon has some problems, especially regarding testimony
  about Lincoln's paternity [wilson p xvi] (see ¶44), and the fact that Herndon filtered
  what people told him in interviews (because, at least, his transcription could not
  keep up with their talking) [wilson p xxi] [walsh p63]. Hertz notes that the consistency in Herndon's lectures from 1866 to 1891 helps disprove charges that "Herndon's memory played him false" [hertz p21]. Many of the more vicious personal attacks on Herndon resulted, in his own lifetime, from his controversial statements
  about Lincoln's religious views [hertz p23]. A more damning criticism comes from
  another lawyer in the Lincoln-Herndon law office: "With regard to second- and
  third-hand evidence, when presented by him, he could not refrain from drawing
  on his imagination for colouring to suit the conclusions already formed" [rankinA
  p90]. The problem for us is not so acute. A medical evaluation, in its first pass, in-
  volves the collection and organization of statements. Only in its second pass are

Introduction & Sources (continued)

untrustworthy or extraneous statements dropped from consideration. Because this volume is mostly performing a first-pass function, Herndon's information is herein included.

■ Actually, a younger man, Jesse Weik, did all of the writing for the Herndon biography [herndon], based on the information Herndon collected [hertz p440]. It is instructive to compare the writings of Herndon and Weik side-by-side. For example, Weik's general description of the physical Lincoln [herndon pp473-474] is *almost* the same one that Herndon used in a lecture 15 years earlier [herndonC pp356-360]. It is hard to know if differences are due to Weik's embellishment or Herndon's evolving knowledge.   13

■ Regardless of source, reminiscences cannot be trusted blindly. In particular, those set on paper decades after the fact are suspect [burl p xxiii] [wilson p xxi], as are those emanating from persons having an agenda (whether the agenda is apparent or not). Because a widespread hagiographic process started immediately upon Lincoln's shocking death (if not before), all reminiscences about him are suspect to some degree. As early as 30 years after Lincoln's presidency, "it had become all but impossible to permit the discussion of some of the information supplied by Lincoln's contemporaries" [hertz p4].   14

■ In addition to hagiography, the truth can also be clouded by the human tendency to magnify self-importance. For example, "Twenty-five different human beings asserted that they helped carry the body of Abraham Lincoln across the street from the theatre into the little house where he died. It is perfectly clear, to anyone who stops to think, that twenty-five people could not possibly get close enough to one man to join hands and carry him: yet all said they did, and their stories vary enormously. ... Maybe eyewitnesses are sometimes the worst witnesses..." – Bruce Catton [kunhardtB pp vi-vii] (Also: [kunhardtB p108])   15

■ Most perversely, even contemporaneous egoless documents cannot be blindly trusted. Consider the letters Lincoln "wrote" as President. One of his secretaries, John Hay, stated that Lincoln "wrote very few letters" as President. Instead, Hay wrote them and Lincoln "signed without reading them" [burl p78] [wilson p331]. Of note, Lincoln had a separate secretary for personal correspondence, W.O. Stoddard [evans pp299-300]. Few of Lincoln's letters as President bear on the present volume.   16

▣ The extensive photographic record of Lincoln (129 images spanning the 1840s to 1865) has been collected in several books, e.g. [mellon] [meserve] [hamilton] [ostendorfA] [kunhardtA] [lorant], of which [ostendorfA] is herein considered the reference standard. It is the only complete source. The best quality photographs, by far, are in [mellon].   17

    ▣ [ostendorfA] assigns each Lincoln photograph an identification number, called its "Ostendorf number" or "O-number." The numbers through 113 are in near-chronological order. Herein, we use a notation like [ostendorf #100] to refer to the photograph having Ostendorf number 100, for example.   18

    ▣ The "Meserve" identification scheme pre-dated the Ostendorf scheme. They are almost completely different. The Meserve scheme is rarely used now.   19

    ⟨2⟩ Harold Holzer showed that [ostendorf #130] is a version of another Lincoln photograph [burk p268].   20

▣ Photographs of Lincoln cannot always be accepted without question. Even with the crude photo-technology of his era, alteration of photographs was widespread and accepted [ostendorfA p256].   21

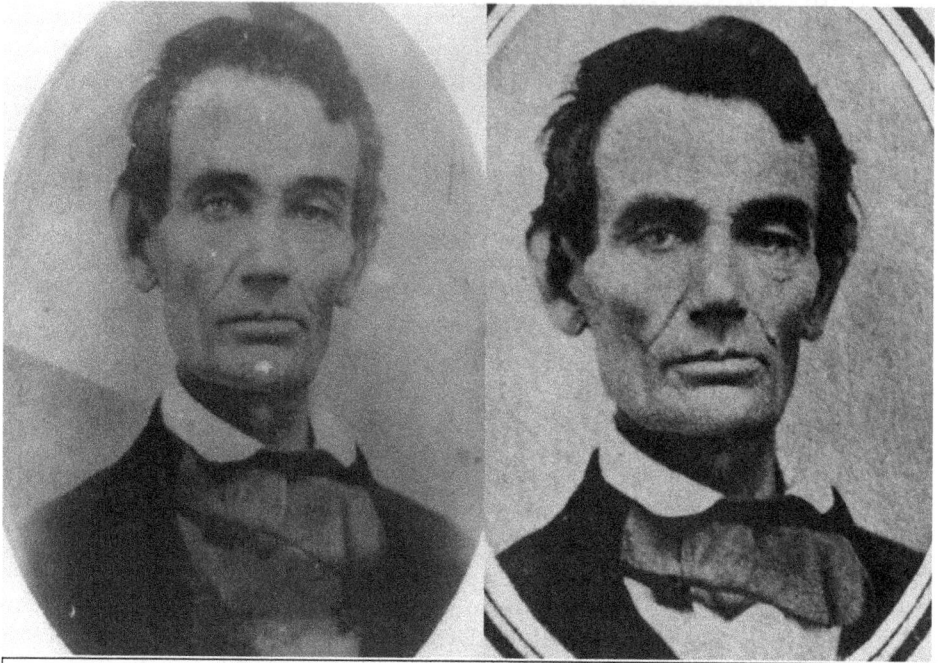

Figure 4. Distortion in Library of Congress print. Compared to the right-hand print, Lincoln's head is narrower in the left-hand print, even though these are two versions of the same 1858 exposure. For reasons unknown, this narrowing appears in the digital versions of several prints from the Library of Congress (¶27). Both images courtesy of the Library of Congress (LC-USZ62-2277, LC-USZ62-132820, respectively). Both are mirror-reversed as compared to reality (note the cheek mole).

Introduction & Sources (continued)

⟨2⟩ For example, the "Cooper Union" photograph ([ostendorf #17]) taken by Mathew Brady on Feb. 27, 1860 was "touched up to show him [Lincoln] smooth-cheeked" [kunhardtA p12]. It was widely distributed during that year's Presidential campaign [kunhardtA p12]. Lincoln said this photograph and the speech he made that day put him in the White House [ostendorfA p35]. — 22

⟨2⟩ [donaldA p238] calls the same image "a work of art." Brady "retouched the negative in order to correct Lincoln's left eye that seemed to be roving upward and eliminated harsh lines from his face to show an almost handsome, statesmanlike image." — 23

▣ Mary Lincoln was "mechanically added" to a photograph of Lincoln and Tad ([meserve #41]≈[ostendorf #93]). She and Lincoln were never photographed together [meserve p83]. — 24

▣ A "spirit photographer" generated an image of Mary being visited by her dead husband [kunhardtA p397]. — 25

⟨2⟩ "Brady had a special process for copying glass or collodion negatives so that the duplicate plate could not be distinguished from the original" [ostendorfA p165]. — 26

Introduction & Sources (continued)

◎ Another hazard of Lincoln photo-interpretation concerns several prints from the Library of Congress in which Lincoln appears to be vertically elongated, as in a funhouse mirror. See Fig. 4.   27

◎ More than 30 stereoscopic photographs of Lincoln had been discovered through 1960 [ostendorfB]. Eight of them, of varying quality, can be stereoscopically viewed in [zeller]. Although they provide little information beyond viewing of single images, seeing Lincoln in three dimensions is a jolting experience. ○○○ *Project:* Assemble high-resolution photographs into stereo pairs; the prints in [zeller] are of low resolution.   28

◎ In at least some studio photographs, a hidden iron support helped Lincoln steady his head during the camera exposures [meserve p4]. See [ostendorf #75] for a visible example [ostendorfA p140].   29

⟨2⟩ For the photographic record, we owe a debt to Lincoln himself. A visitor to Lincoln's home before the Presidency "saw Mrs. Lincoln come downstairs holding her apron full of photographs and saying to Mr. Lincoln, 'Father, I'm sick and tired of these. I'm going to throw them away.' And Mr. Lincoln said, 'Oh no, Mother, I wouldn't do that. Someone may want them some day." [meserve p24]   30

■ The `Head -- Casts` and `Hands -- Cast` sections describe casts made of Lincoln's head and hands.   31

⟨2⟩ "This was not a casual age and a chief executive was expected to expose only his face and, within limits, his hands to the pubic. Thus President Lincoln had remained perpetually hidden within his long-coated two-sizes-too-big black suit. Few people had seen even his lower extremities." [kunhardtB pp289-290] (See ¶522.)   32

■ The comments below are very insightful, and should be a warning against self-delusion to all who set out to "prove" something about Lincoln: 33

    ⟨2⟩c "For a century or more, generations of Americans were taught to be like Lincoln – forbearing, kind, principled, resolute – but what we've really wanted is for Lincoln to be like us, and this has never been truer than the present day." [ferguson p xiii]   34

    ⟨2⟩c "The mass of Herndon's research, flavorsome and evocative as it is, was shot through with inconsistencies and contradictions, touching on the most elementary matters. A biographer could pick and choose, according to his own principles of selection, and piece together any number of different Lincolns." [ferguson pp60-61]   35

⟨2⟩ Thompson's drug store, across from the Treasury building and later at 701 Fifteenth St. NW, filled the White House prescriptions. It operated from 1851 until at least the 1930s. Unfortunately, its drug records before 1890 were destroyed. [shutes p87]   36

Family History

■ Inherited traits: 37
    ⟨S⟩ [gordon] believes Lincoln's appearance derived from his mother.   38
    ⟨1⟩ "he was tall like his mother. Was 6 ft – 4 in in hight [sic]" – John Hanks [wilson p615]   39
    ⟨1⟩ Of Lincoln: "Mr L never said anything in My presents that I remember about which Side off his family he inherited his *Ways, Looks* or *thought*   he dose Not look like the Hanks family they are Sandy Complection Red Hair   40

Family History (continued)

& Freckel all but John Hanks I think & have allways thought he [sic] sound Judgment was from his Mothers side of the House" – Abner Ellis [wilson p210]

⟨1⟩ "Abraham took his disposition and Mental qualities from his Mother" – Dennis Hanks [wilson p598] *Of course, this was Hanks' side of the family!*　41

⟨1⟩ "Abraham L. inherited his fathers features rather than his mothers" – Harriet Chapman [wilson p646] *But, ¶4752 suggests Mrs. Chapman did not know Nancy Lincoln well.*　42

- Lincoln's paternity:　44
  ⟨1⟩ Local traditions identify another man as Abraham Lincoln's father [wilson pp613-615, 567, 571, 608, 611, 612, 613-615], whom Abraham resembled "in build, appearance & manners" [wilson p567].　45
  ⟨s⟩ Those traditions are today totally discounted [currentBk p28] [donaldA p605n]. Also see ¶5188.　46
  ⟨1⟩ But even Lincoln's long-time law partner could not fully dispel in his own mind the possibility that Abraham was not the son of Thomas Lincoln [hertz pp38, 63, 138-140, 146, 150, 170, 204, 205, 208, 223]. Herndon spent much energy researching that point [hertz pp 38, 42-43]. Herndon told Illinois governor Richard Oglesby, in 1887: "I had the materials out of which, by a lawyer's argument, that I could make it appear Lincoln was the lawful child of Thomas & Nancy" [wilson p637-639] also [wilson p635]. Elsewhere, Herndon says allegations that Enloe was Lincoln's father are not "borne out by good and sufficient evidence" [hertz p204 (also see p205)].　47
  ⟨s⟩ Lincoln supposedly resembled members of the Enlow (sometimes Enloe or Inloe) and Brownfield families [wilson pp673-674]　48
  ⟨1⟩ "yet I never Saw more striking resemblance that his picture & some of the Brownfield family" – E.R. Burba [wilson p240]　49
  ⟨1⟩ On many occasions, Herndon wrote that Thomas Lincoln had fought with Abraham Enloe, sometimes stating that Nancy was the cause, and that the Lincolns moved from Kentucky to Indiana to get Nancy away from Enloe. [hertz p94]　50
  ⟨1/q⟩ Ward Lamon also concluded that Thomas was not Lincoln's father. Two friends of Lincoln dissuaded Lamon from publishing this conclusion in [lamonL], yet admitted the evidence was "prima facie strong." [hertz p8]　51
  ⟨1/q⟩ May 1849: A letter reports Thomas describing Lincoln as a "Child that is of his own flush [sic] and blood" [randallC p116]　52
  ⟨2/c⟩ "Herndon himself wavered back and forth between belief and denial of the illegitimacy." [randallC p116]　53

⟨1⟩ "I cannot frame a genealogical tree of the Lincoln family for three generations, other than you find in your records." – William Herndon, 1870 [hertz p65]　54

- There were rumors Lincoln had children out of wedlock:　55
  ⟨1⟩ "i think that Mrs able Could aid you Considerabe she has a dauter that is thought to Be Lincolns Child thay favor very much" – J. Rowan Herndon [wilson p69] *The context clearly refers to Abraham (as opposed to Thomas).*　56
  ⟨1⟩ "Abe's son, which he had by Mrs Armstrong it was a joke – plagued Abe terribly" – James Tayor [wilson p482]　57

- Ethnicity and race: *These could be a political football even in the 19th century.*　58
  ⟨2⟩ "There were unfounded rumors that Lincoln was part Negro" in the 1860 campaign. [evans p173]　59

Family History (continued)

⟨1⟩ 1862: After denying the unreasonable petition of an old woman, Lincoln re-   60
marked "I'll be bound she has gone away believing that the worst pictures
of me in the Richmond press only lack truth in not being half black enough
and bad enough." [burl p85]

⟨1⟩ Upon Lincoln's death a member of the Cincinnati Synagogue announced: 61
"Brethren, the lamented Abraham Lincoln ... was supposed to be a descendant of Hebrew parentage. He said so in my presence, and indeed, he preserved numerous features of the Hebrew race in both countenance and character." [kunhardtB p240]

⟨S⟩ "The riddle of Lincoln's origin is possibly now soluble. I would search for a Vir-   62
ginia family that carries the stigma of this disease [Marfan syndrome] who were
probably neighbors to Joseph Hanks, Lincoln's great grandfather. If such a family
can be uncovered I believe Lincoln's maternal grandfather will be found among
them." [gordon] ○○○ *Project:* Population survey for Marfan-like disorders in the
Virginia region inhabited by Joseph Hanks.

Diagnoses

■ Proposed diagnoses to explain Lincoln's tallness and dysmorphic features: 63
⟨S⟩ Marfan syndrome [gordon] [schwartzA] [schwartzB]   64
⟨S⟩ MASS phenotype [marion]. *This is a mitral valve prolapse syndrome* [OMIM   65
entry 604308].
⟨S⟩ Stickler syndrome [herrmann]   66
⟨−⟩ [gordon] provides a very nice summary table of evidence for and against Mar-   67
fan syndrome.

■ Opinions on whether Lincoln had Marfan syndrome: 68
⟨S⟩ Did not have it [lattimerNY] (a physician)   69
⟨S⟩ Did not have it (historian and physician pair) [borittA]   70
⟨S⟩ Did not have it, but had something like it [marion] (a geneticist)   71
⟨S⟩ Unlikely he had it (Marfan specialist Harry Dietz) [ready]   72
⟨S⟩ 50:50 he had it [mckusickB] (Marfan specialist)   73
⟨S⟩ "Evidence is slim" he had it [donaldA p680n] (historian)   74
⟨S⟩ Uncritical acceptance: [durham], [templeC]   75

⟨S⟩ Calls to genetically test surviving samples of Lincoln's tissue for Marfan syndrome   76
were, after study in 1992 and 1999, not consummated [davidsonG] [micozzi] [ready]
[reilly].

⟨S⟩ Spinocerebellar ataxia, type 5 – see ⌈Gait⌉   77

■ Diagnoses of final months: 78
⟨S⟩ "a latent tuberculosis, which he feared, might have been gradually breaking   79
loose in his hard-muscled body during the war-harassed days in Washington
and might account in part for his haggard, ashen, pale face, his emaciation
and his fatigue." [shutes p74]
⟨S⟩ [schwartzB] proposed that advanced aortic regurgitation was slowly killing Lin-   80
coln. (See ¶1975.)
⟨S⟩ "fabulous health" [neelyL]   81

⟨2⟩ "Armchair post-postmortem [sic] diagnoses have been: endocrine disorders, hy-   82
pogonadism, tuberculosis, Marfan's syndrome, old depressed skull fracture with
neurological complications, heart failure and oedipus complex with other psychiatric abnormalities." [pearson]

Appearance

This sub-section is different from others. Several eyewitness descriptions of Lincoln cover multiple organ systems. As a rule, I send such descriptions to the chop shop: organ-specific phrases are extracted and filed in the proper sub-sections. In some cases, however, the descriptions cannot be pigeonholed into one of the standard sub-sections, and in other cases the unity of the full description is lost when divided.   83

Thus, this section preserves both unusual and cohesive descriptions of Lincoln. As such, it contains much information to refute what I call "the Lattimer school," which views Lincoln as merely a tall man [lattimerNY] [montgomeryJ]   84

⟨1⟩ See William Herndon's word portrait of Lincoln – it starts in ¶1. He painted other word portraits: 85

   ⟨1⟩ "You ask me if I ever saw in this great wild West many men of Lincoln's *type*, and to which I answer, *yes*. The first settlers of *central* and southern Illinois were men of that type. They came from the limestone regions of Virginia, Kentucky, Tennessee, etc., and were men of giant strength, physically fine, and and by nature were mentally strong. ... conditions made this class of men ... Limestone water, so scientists say, gave us big frames." – William Herndon [hertz p187] (Says, in [hertz p197], that he has seen a thousand men of Lincoln's type.) *Herndon's interpretation can be ignored. His general observation is probably accurate, unless it has been colored by his interpretation.*   86

   ⟨1⟩ "He was a great big, angular, strong man, limbs large and bony; he was tall and of a peculiar type." – William Herndon [hertz p195]   87

   ⟨1⟩ "his mind was tough, solid, knotty, gnarly, more or less like his body; he was angular in body ... he was a tall and big-boned man ... was not what is called muscular, but was sinewy, wiry." – Herndon [hertz p196]   88

   ⟨1⟩ "His eyebrows cropped out, like a huge jutting rock out of the brow of a hill; his face was long narrow, sallow and cadaverous, flesh shrunk, shriveled, wrinkled, and dry, having on his face a few hairs here and there; his cheeks were leathery and saffron-colored; his ears were large and ran out nearly at right angles from the sides of his head, caused by heavy hats ... and partly by nature; his lower lip was thick and on the top very red, hanging under-curved or downcurved, the red of his lips being a good sign of a tendency to consumption, if it was not on him, biting the life out of him; his neck was neat and trim and did not show much of the animal, though consumptives are quite passionate, goaty; his head was well balanced on his shoulders, his little grey eyes in the right place ... he was odd, angular, homely, but when those little grey eyes and face were lighted up by the inward soul on fires of emotion ... then it was that all those apparently ugly or homely features sprang into organs of beauty." – Herndon [kunhardtB p291]   89

   ⟨1⟩ "When standing erect he was six feet four inches high. He was lean in flesh and ungainly in figure. Aside from the sad, pained look due to habitual melancholy, his face had no characteristic or fixed expression. He was thin through the chest, and hence slightly stoop-shouldered. When he arose to address courts, juries, or crowds of people, his body inclined forward to a slight degree. At first he was very awkward, and it seemed a real labor to adjust himself to his surroundings. He struggled for a time under a feeling of apparent diffidence and sensitiveness, and these only added to his awkwardness, I have often seen and sympathized with Mr. Lincoln during these movements. When he began speaking, his voice was shrill, piping, and unpleasant. His manner, his attitude, his dark, yellow face, wrinkled   90

Appearance (continued)

and dry, his oddity of pose, his diffident movements – everything seemed to be against him, but only for a short time. After having arisen, he generally placed his hands behind him, the back of his left hand in the palm of his right, the thumb and fingers of his right hand clasped around the left arm at the wrist. ... [p. 332] ... He did not gesticulate as much with his hands as with his head. He used the latter frequently, throwing it with vim this way and that." [herndon pp331-332]

⟨2⟩ Agrees with: "Lincoln was exceptionally tall and painfully thin, with a melancholy physiognomy and sallow skin. [He] moved his arms and hands awkwardly, and looked like a jackknife folding up when he tried to bow." [donaldA pp214-215] describing Lincoln in 1858.   91

⟨1/q⟩ "Well, now, he looked just like any other baby, at fust – like red cherry pulp squeezed dry. An' he didn't improve none as he growed older. Abe never was much fur looks." – Dennis Hanks, recalling many decades after seeing the new-born Lincoln [kunhardtA p35]   92

⟨1/q⟩ "a tall, homely, loose-jointed man" – recollection of an Illinois attorney [burl p76]   93

⟨1⟩ 1831: "his external appearance was not prepossessing" – Dr. Jason Duncan [wilson p539]   94

⟨2⟩ About 1831: "... on an inclement day of winter, there was seen a rough uncouth youth of twenty one years of age plodding with awkward step his way from Beardstown to this place. ... His long arms protruded through the sleeves of a coat which scarcely reached beyond the elbow in one direction, or below the waist in the other. ... His large foot partially enveloped in a well worn pair of shoes, presented a singular contrast with his very small head surmounted by a sealskin cap." – clipping from the *Menard Axis*, Feb. 15, 1862 [wilson p24]   95

⟨2⟩ [randallC p362] identifies the author as John Hill, whom she calls "an anti-Lincoln man" and says did not know Lincoln in New Salem. *The tone of the article seems pro-Lincoln ("inspirational" [walsh p85]), not anti-Lincoln. Its account of the Ann Rutledge story (¶2695) probably fueled [randallC]'s ire. Hill's father was at one time in love with Rutledge, too [wilson p397] [walsh p27].*   97

⟨1/q⟩ 1832: "He was a very tall and gawky and rough-looking fellow then – his pantaloons didn't meet his shoes by six inches. But after he began speaking I became very much interested in him." – Stephen Logan [kunhardtB p272] [angle p50] (reprinting [nicolayC])   98

⟨1⟩ 1834: "Six feet and four inches high in his Stockings. Some Stoop Shouldered. his legs were long, feet large; arms long, longer than any man I ever knew, when standing Straiht, and letting his arms fall down his Sides, the points of his fingers would touch a point lower on his legs by nearly three inches than was usual with other persons. I was present when a number of persons measured the length of thire arms on thire legs, as here Stated, with that result. his arms were unusually long for his hight, and the droop of his shoulders also produced that result. His hands were large and bony, caused no doubt by hard labor when young. he was a good chopper. the axe then in use was a great clumsy tool, usually made by the country blacksmith, weighing about Six pounds, the handle being round and Strait, which made it very difficult to hold when chopping requiring a gripe as Strong as was necessary to wield a Blacksmiths Sledge Hammer. This and running barefoot when young among Stones, and Stumps, accounts for his large hands   99

Appearance (continued)

and feet." – Robert Wilson [wilson pp201-202] (Continues in ¶101) *It is quite reasonable to believe that a bone's development is influenced by its use.*

⟨-⟩ *Wilson was quite familiar with other tall men. He and Lincoln belonged
to the group of Illinois legislators from Sangamon County known as the
"long nine," whose collective height was supposedly 54 feet* [donaldA p60].   100
John Wentworth was six feet six inches tall.

⟨1⟩ 1834: "His eyes were a bluish brown, his face was long and very angular. when   101
at ease had nothing in his appearance that was marked or Striking, but when enlivened ... his countenance would brighten up the expression woul[d] light up not
in a flash. but rapidly the muscles of his face would begin to contract. Several
wrinkles would diverge from the inner corners of his eyes, and extend down and
diagonally across his nose, his eyes would Sparkle, all terminating in an unrestrained Laugh in which every one present willing or unwilling were compelled to
take part." – Robert Wilson [wilson p202] (preceded by ¶99)

⟨$\frac{1}{q}$⟩ About 1835: "Homely? Yes, I suppose he was, but I never thought of that then. I   102
remember his tall, lank, ungainly figure, and his big ears and mouth, but when he
talked one never thought of that." – Nancy Rutledge Prewitt [walsh p42]

■ Ungainly: (for "awkward," see ¶2907):   103
  ⟨$\frac{1}{q}$⟩ About 1835: "tall, lank, ungainly figure" – Nancy Rutledge Prewitt [walsh p42]   104
  (∈ ¶102)
  ⟨1⟩ 1836: "ungainly and poorly clothed man" [jayne p5]   105
  ⟨2⟩ Mid-1830s: "ungainly and angular" – Mary Owens (recalled by her son) [wil-   106
  son p610]
  ⟨1⟩ Pre-1861: "He was lean in flesh and ungainly in figure." [herndon p331] (∈ ¶90)   107
  ⟨$\frac{1}{q}$⟩ 1858: "Lincoln's tall, lank ungainly form..." – Carl Schurz [kunhardtA p108]   108
  ⟨1⟩ Oct. 13, 1858: "lank, ungainly body" – Carl Schurz [angle p243] (∈ ¶149)   109
  ⟨1⟩ Feb. 27, 1860: "He was tall, tall – oh, how tall! and so angular and awkward   110
  that I had, for an instant, a feeling of pity for so ungainly a man." – eyewitness [brooksA pp186-187] (∈ ¶156)
  ⟨1⟩ Generally considered to be "a plain ungainly man" [coffinA p169]   111
  ⟨1⟩ May 19, 1860: Formal ceremonies concluded, he "was no longer the ungainly   112
  schoolboy. The unnatural dignity... was laid aside." [coffinA p174]
  ⟨1⟩ 1860s: "I have heard it said that he was ungainly, that his step was awkward.   113
  He never impressed me as being awkward." [dana p173] (∈ ¶183)
  ⟨1⟩ About 1864: "he grew more and more cadaverous and ungainly month by   114
  month" [croffut] (∈ ¶196)
  ⟨$\frac{1}{q}$⟩ March 4, 1865: "tall and ungainly" – reporter Henry Watterson [shenk p173]   115
  ⟨1⟩ "He [Chauncey Depew] said he never could figure out why Mr. Lincoln had   116
  the reputation of being awkward and ungainly." – Marie de Montalvo [randallP
  box 15] (∈ ¶2942)
  ⟨1⟩ April 1865: "not a handsome man, and ungainly in his person" [porterD p296]   117
  ⟨2⟩ Also: [turner p xv]   118

■ Angular: 119
  ⟨1⟩ "a great big, angular, strong man" – William Herndon [hertz p195] (∈ ¶87)   120
  ⟨1⟩ "angular in body" – William Herndon [hertz p196] (∈ ¶88)   121
  ⟨$\frac{1}{q}$⟩ "odd, angular, homely" – William Herndon [kunhardtB p291] (∈ ¶89)   122
  ⟨1⟩ 1834: "his face was long and very angular" – Robert Wilson [wilson p202] (∈   123
  ¶101)

Appearance (continued)

⟨2⟩ Mid-1830s: "ungainly and angular" – Mary Owens (recalled by her son) [wilson p610]   124

⟨1⟩ 1847: "Tall, angular, and awkward" – Elihu Washburne [hunt p228]   126

⟨1⟩ 1848: "his tall, angular, bent form" – Henry Gardner [wilson p699] (∈ ¶138)   127

⟨1⟩ 1849: 'tall and angular frame" – Leonard Swett [wilson p732] (∈ ¶140)   128

⟨1⟩ Feb. 27, 1860: "oh, how tall! and so angular and awkward" – a witness [brooksA pp186-187] (∈ ¶156)   129

⟨1⟩ June 1860: "A tall, arrowy, angular gentleman" – Utica newspaper reporter [lincloreHDE] (∈ ¶159)   130

⟨1⟩ Spring 1862: "homely of face, large-boned, angular, and loosely put together" [bancroft] (∈ ¶182)   131

⟨1⟩ "stoops a little, is angular, a man of bony corners." – Daniel Voorhees [sandburgC v2p303] (∈ ¶184)   133

⟨1⟩ As President: "As he stood, his form was angular, with something of that straightness in its lines which is so peculiar in the figure of Dante by Flaxman." [sumnerA pp132-133](∈ ¶185)   134

⟨-⟩ "Angular" was also applied to Lincoln's mother's face. (See ¶4744.)   135

⟨1⟩ "He was a long, gawky, ugly, shapeless, man." – Joshua Speed [wilson p588]   136

⟨1⟩ [shastid]'s father, beginning as a child, knew Lincoln. "His earliest remembrance of   137
Lincoln was that of the long, gaunt, shambling, melancholy, kindly spoken shopkeeper." Lincoln would put "a long and angular but very kindly arm about the child," and would tell him a story. *It is unclear whether those adjectives come from Shastid the father or Shastid the son.*

⟨1⟩ 1848: "When he was announced [to speak], his tall, angular, bent form, and his   138
manifest awkwardness and low tone of voice, promised nothing interesting. But he soon warmed to his work." – Henry Gardner [wilson p699]

⟨1⟩ Spring 1849: Around daybreak, two men got into a stage coach that had arrived   139
in Terre Haute, IN: "We discovered that the entire back seat was occupied by a long, lank individual, whose head seemed to protrude from one end of the coach and his feet from the other. He was the sole occupant, and was sleeping soundly. Hammond slapped him familiarly on the shoulder, and asked him if he had chartered the stage for the day. The stranger, now wide awake, responded, 'Certainly not,' and at once took the front seat, politely surrendering to us the place of honor and comfort. We took in our travelling companion at a glance. A queer, oddlooking fellow he was... His very prominent features in repose seemed dull and expressionless. ..." – undated clipping from Terre Haute newspaper [wilson p641]

⟨1⟩ 1849: Leonard Swett saw Lincoln for the first time in a hotel room [wilson p772].   140
Swett knocked on the room's door and heard two voices say "Come in." He later remembered: "Imagine my surprise when the door opened to find two men undressed, or rather dressed for bed, engaged in a lively battle with pillows, tossing them at each other's heads. One, a low heavy-set man who leaned against the foot of the bed and puffed like a lizard, answered to the description of Judge Davis. The other was a man of tremendous stature; compared to Davis he looked as if he were eight feet tall. He was encased in a long, indescribable garment, yellow as saffron, which reached to his heels, and from beneath which protruded two of the largest feet I had, up to that time, been in the habit of seeing. This immense shirt, for shirt it must have been, looked as if it had been literally carved out of the original bolt of flannel of which it was made and the pieces joined together without reference to measurement or capacity. The only thing that kept it from slipping

Appearance (continued)

off the tall and angular frame it covered was the single button at the throat; and I confess to a succession of shudders when I thought of what might happen should that button by any mischance lose its hold. I cannot describe my sensations as this apparition, with modest announcement, 'My name is Lincoln,' strode across the room to shake my trembling hand. I will not say he reminded me of Satan, but he was certainly the ungodliest figure I had ever seen." [wilson p732]

⟨2⟩ Agrees with: [kunhardtB p287], which has considerably different phrasing.   141

⟨1/q⟩ Autumn 1854: After speaking to a crowd, J.B. Merwin hears calls for Lincoln.   142 "...turning, I saw, perhaps, the most singular specimen of a human being rising slowly, and unfolding his long arms and his long legs, exactly like the blades of a jack-knife. His hair was uncombed, his coat sleeves were inches shorter than his shirt sleeves, his trousers did not reach to his socks. First I thought there was some plan to perpetrate a 'joke' on the meeting, but in one minute, after the first accents of the pathetic voice were heard, the crowd hushed to a stillness..." [hobson p63]

⟨2⟩ 1857: "Tall, gaunt, and homely" [angle p177] reprinting Albert Woldman   143

⟨1⟩ 1858: "In his physical make-up Mr. Lincoln could not be said to be a man of   144 prepossessing personal appearance; but his splendid head and intellectual face made up in large measure for all his physical defects, if such they might be called. When intellectually aroused he forgot his embarrassment, his eyes kindled, and even in his manner he was irresistible." – Jonathan Birch [wilson p728]

⟨1⟩ 1858: "He had a lean, lank, indescribably gawky figure, and odd-featured, wrin-   145 kled, inexpressive, and altogether uncomely face. He used singularly awkward, almost absurd, up-and-down and sidewise movements of his body to give emphasis to his arguments. His voice was naturally good, but he frequently raised it to an unnatural pitch. ... It was really a ludicrous sight to see the grotesque figure holding frantically on to the heads of his supporters, with his legs dangling from their shoulders, and his pantaloons pulled up so as to expose his underwear almost to his knees." – journalist Henry Villard covering the Lincoln-Douglas debates [kunhardtA p108]

⟨1/q⟩ 1858, Lincoln-Douglas debate at Alton: "He rose from his seat, stretched his long,   146 bony limbs upward as if to get them into working order and stood like some solitary pine on a lonely summit." – Francis Grierson [meserve p2]

⟨1/q⟩ Summer 1858: "Mr. Lincoln in repose was ... a man of awkward and ungainly ap-   147 pearance, and exceedingly homely countenance. [A crowd met Lincoln when he arrived in Jacksonville, IL.] The enthusiasm of the multitude was great; but Mr. Lincoln's extremely homely face wore an expression of sadness. He rode in a carriage ... looking dust-begrimed and worn and weary; and though he frequently lifted his hat in recognition of the cheers of the crowds lining the streets, I saw no smile on his face, and he seemed to take no pleasure in the demonstrations of enthusiasm which his presence called forth. His clothes were very ill-fitting, and his long arms and hands protruded far through his coat sleeves, giving him a peculiarly uncouth appearance.... I had never before seen him when he appeared so homely; and I thought him about the ugliest man I had ever seen. There was nothing in his looks or manner that was prepossessing." – Rev. George C. Noyes [browneF pp289-290]

⟨1/q⟩ Aug. 1858: He "was as swarthy as an Indian, with wiry, jet-black hair, which was   148 usually in an unkempt condition. He wore no beard, and his face was almost

Appearance (continued)

grotesquely square, with high cheek bones. His eyes were bright, keen, and a luminous gray color, though his eyebrows were black like his hair. His figure was gaunt, slender and slightly bent. He was clad in a rusty-black Prince Albert coat with somewhat abbreviated sleeves. His black trousers, too, were so short that they gave an appearance of exaggerated size to his feet." – Martin P.S. Rindlaub [ostendorfA p19]

⟨1⟩ Oct. 13, 1858: "I must confess I was somewhat startled by his appearance. There he stood, overtopping by several inches all those surrounding him. Although measuring something over six feet myself, I had, standing quite near to him, to throw my head backward in order to look into his eyes. That swarthy face with its strong features, its deep furrows, and its benignant, melancholy eyes, is now familiar to every American. ... At that time is was clean-shaven, and looked even more haggard and careworn than later when it was framed in whiskers. ... His neck emerged, long and sinewy, from a white collar... His lank, ungainly body was clad in a rusty black dress coat with sleeves that should have been longer; but his arms appeared so long that the sleeves of a store coat could hardly be expected to cover them all the way down to the wrists. His black trousers, too, permitted a very full view of his large feet. ... I had seen, in Washington and in the West, several public men of rough appearance; but none whose looks seemed quite so uncouth, not to say grotesque, as Lincoln's." – Carl Schurz [angle p243]   149

⟨$\frac{1}{q}$⟩ 1859: "... lank, gaunt figure... he had a very pale, long face, big hands and feet, but the thing that impressed me most of all in regard to Abraham Lincoln was the extreme sadness of his eyes. Lincoln had the saddest eyes of any human being that I had ever seen." – John Widmer [shenk p155]   150

⟨1⟩ Dec. 1859: "If any personal description of me is thought desirable, it may be said, I am, in height, six feet, four inches, nearly; lean in flesh, weighing, on average, one hundred and eighty pounds; dark complexion, with coarse black hair, and grey eyes – no other marks or brands recollected." – Lincoln's self-description [baslerA v3p512] [donaldA p237] [arnold p15] *Actually, he had more than one "brand." See ¶1490 and ¶2275*   151

⟨1⟩ 1860: "Mr. Lincoln was the homeliest man I ever saw. His body seemed to me a huge skeleton in clothes. Tall as he was, his hands and feet looked out of proportion, so long and clumsy were they. Every movement was awkward in the extreme. He sat with one leg thrown over the other, and the pendant foot swung almost to the floor. ... He had a face that defied artistic skill to soften or idealize. ... It was capable of few expressions, but those were extremely striking. When in repose, his face was dull, heavy, and repellent. It brightened, like a lit lantern, when animated. His dull eyes would fairly sparkle with fun, or express as kindly a look as I ever saw, when moved by some matter of human interest." [piatt pp345-346].   152

⟨$\frac{1}{q}$⟩ 1860: "the long, ungainly figure, upon which hung clothes that ... evidently were the of an unskillful tailor; the clumsy hands ... the long, gaunt head capped by a shock of hair that seemed not to have been thoroughly brushed." – George H. Putnam [ostendorfA p57]   153

⟨$\frac{1}{q}$⟩ 1860: "His loose, tall frame is loosely thrown together. He is in every way large – brain included – and his countenance shows intellect, generosity, great good nature, and keen discrimination." – Gideon Welles [kunhardtB p65]   154

⟨2⟩ An anthropologist says: "Physically, Lincoln was one of the most distinctive Presidents in our history. His towering height alone might have been enough to draw   155

Appearance (continued)

attention to his physical presence. But this, combined with his extreme linearity, his unkempt appearance, his tousled hair and unusual face, focused extreme interest on his appearance. ... Consequently many of the newspaper accounts of his first visits to eastern cities and numerous memoirs of the period contain an undue emphasis on the appearance of the president from the Wild West." [shapiro]

⟨1⟩ Feb. 27, 1860, at Cooper Institute: "When Lincoln rose to speak, I was greatly disappointed. He was tall, tall – oh, how tall! and so angular and awkward that I had, for an instant, a feeling of pity for so ungainly a man. His clothes were black and ill-fitting, badly wrinkled – as if they had been jammed carelessly into a small trunk. His bushy head, with the stiff black hair thrown back, was balanced on a long and lean head-stalk, and when he raised his hands in an opening gesture I noticed that they were very large. He began in a very low tone of voice – as if he were used to speaking out-doors and was afraid of speaking too loud. ... But pretty soon he began to get into his subject; he straightened up and made regular and graceful gestures; his face lighted as with an inward fire; the whole man was transfigured. I forgot his clothes, his personal appearance, and his individual peculiarities. Presently, forgetting myself, I was on my feet with the rest, yelling like a wild Indian, cheering this wonderful man." – eyewitness account in [brooksA pp186-187] 156

⟨1⟩ May 19, 1860: "The lines upon his face, the large ears, sunken cheeks, enormous nose, shaggy hair, the deep-set eyes, sparkling with humor... [Few of us] had ever seen him before, but there was that about him which commanded instant admiration." [coffinA p173] 157

⟨1⟩ May 19, 1860: Being notified of his nomination by the convention's official party: "While Mr. Ashman spoke, Mr. Lincoln's form and features seemed to be immovable; his frame was slightly bent, and his face downcast and absolutely void of expression. It was evident that the voice which addressed him was receiving his exclusive attention. ... I contemplated his tall, spare, figure. [Ashman finishes talking] The bowed head rose as by an electric movement, the broad mouth, which had been so firmly drawn together, opened with a genial smile, and the eyes, that had been shaded, beamed with intelligence. [Lincoln responds] in a pleasant voice..." – William Kelley [riceA p258] 158

⟨1/q⟩ June 21, 1860: "A tall, arrowy, angular gentleman, with a profusion of wiry hair 'lying around loose' about his head, and a pair of eyes that seemed to say 'make yourself at home,' and a forehead remarkably broad and capacious, and arms that were somewhat too long for a statue of Apollo, made his appearance. The lips were full of character, the nose strongly aquiline, the cheek bones high and prominent, and the whole face indicative at once of goodness and resoluteness. In repose, it had something of rigidity, but when in play, it was one of the most eloquent I have ever seen. None of his pictures do him the slightest justice. ... After you have been five minutes in his company you cease to think that he is either homely or awkward." – Utica newspaper reporter [lincloreHDE] 159

⟨1/q⟩ Nov. 1860: "slouchy ungraceful ... round shouldered, leans forward (very much in his walk) is lean and ugly in every way" – Thomas Webster [randallC p163] 160

⟨1⟩ March 27, 1861: "Soon afterwards there entered, with a shambling, loose, irregular, almost unsteady gait, a tall, lank, lean man, considerably over six feet in height, with stooping shoulders, long pendulous arms, terminating in hands of extraordinary dimensions, which, however, were far exceeded in proportion by 161

Appearance (continued)

his feet. He was dressed in an ill-fitting, wrinkled suit of black, which put one in mind of an undertaker's uniform at a funeral; round his neck a rope of black silk was knotted in a large bulb, with flying ends projecting beyond the collar of his coat; his turned-down shirt-collar disclosed a sinewy muscular yellow neck, and above that, nestling in a great black mass of hair, bristling and compact like a ruff of mourning pins, rose the strange quaint face and head, covered with its thatch of wild, republican hair, of President Lincoln. The impression produced by the size of his extremities, and by his flapping and wide projecting ears, may be removed by the appearance of kindliness, sagacity, and the awkward bonhommie of his face; the mouth is absolutely prodigious; the lips, straggling and extending almost from one line of black beard to the other, are only kept in order by two deep furrows from the nostril to the chin; the nose itself – a prominent organ – stands out from the face, with an inquiring, anxious air, as though it were sniffing for some good thing in the wind; the eyes dark, full, and deeply set, are penetrating, but full of an expression which almost amounts to tenderness; and above them projects the shaggy brow, running into the small hard frontal space, the development of which can scarcely be estimated accurately, owing to the irregular flocks of thick hair carelessly brushed across it. One would say that, although the mouth was made to enjoy a joke, it could also utter the severest sentence which the head could dictate..." – William Howard Russell [russell pp37-38]

⟨2⟩ As President-Elect: "Visitors to his office often felt stunned by the sheer volume   163
of his words. He showered upon them opinions, ideas, and anecdotes concerning almost every subject in the world. ... What puzzled them most was his highly unpresidential habit of regaling guests with jokes and anecdotes. When telling these tales, his face lit up, and at the punch line his high-pitched laughter rang through the capitol. He might punctuate a story with a hearty slap on his thigh, and after a particularly good one he would rock with mirth, sometimes reaching out with his long arms to draw his knees almost up to his face. Lincoln liked puns, the more outrageous the better." [donaldA p259]

⟨1/q⟩ "Physio[logically] and Phrenologically the man was a [sort] of monstrosity. His   164
frame was large lo[ng, bony] and muscular – his head disprop[ortionately] small and shaped. He had large [square jaws] – large heavy nose, small lascivious mouth and Soft tender bluish eyes. I would say he was a cross between Venus and Hercules." – Elliott Herndon [wilson p459] (Also in [herndon p470n].)

⟨1⟩ "The mans mind partook [of] the incongruities of his body. He had no mind   166
[not] possessed by the most ordinary of [men]. It was simply the peculiarity of [his] mental, the odity [sic] of his physical and [qualit]ies of his heart that singled him out [from] the mass of men." – Elliott Herndon [wilson pp459-460]

⟨1⟩ "he was a tall, spare man, with large bones, and towering up to six feet and four   167
inches in height. He leaned forward, and stooped as he walked. He was very athletic, with long limbs, large hands and feet, and of great physical strength. There was no grace in his movements, but an expression of awkwardness, combined with force and vigor. ... His forehead was broad and high, his hair was rather stiff and coarse, and nearly black, his eye-brows heavy, his eyes dark grey, clear, very expressive, and varying with every mood ... at times with that almost superhuman sadness which it has been said is the sign and seal of those who are to be martyrs. His nose was large, clearly defined, and well shaped; his cheek bones high and projecting. His mouth was large..." [arnold p441]

■ Before the Presidency, appeared young for age: 168

Appearance (continued)

⟨$\frac{1}{q}$⟩ 1859 (age 50): so "exceedingly 'well preserved' that he would not be taken for more than thirty-eight." [burl p74] citing Cincinnati *Commercial*, Sept. 17   169

⟨$\frac{1}{q}$⟩ 1860 (age 51): "... he certainly has no appearance of being so old." [burl p74] citing [NYTribune - Nov. 10, 1860]   170

⟨2⟩ At the 1860 Republican nominating convention: "Only a few of the delegates had ever seen their candidate before, and they were startled by his appearance." [donaldA p251]   171

⟨1⟩ Feb. 1861; "He is a clever man, & *not* so *bad* looking as they say, while he is no great beauty. He is tall (6 f.4 in.) [sic] has a commanding figure; bows pretty well; is not stiff; has a pleasant face, is amiable & *determined*. ... We saw him on several occasions; near him three or four times, but did not seek any introduction to him." – George C. Shepard, 1861, typed transcript in [randallP box 15]. Original in Burton Historical Collection, Detroit Public Library   172

⟨1⟩ 1861 or later: "Abraham Lincoln was an unusually tall man, although he did not seem slender. He appeared to be as lean and his muscles as hard as a prize-fighter. He was obviously a very strong, powerful man, physically capable of immense endurance. His eyes slightly receded, were about normal in size and, according to my recollection gray in color – with no marked expression, except pensiveness and truthfulness. His head was large, both longitudinally and perpendicularly, with a tall and ample forehead. His hair was dark brown, without any tendency to baldness. His head, when he was in repose, drooped slightly forward, and his whole countenance was pensive to sadness." – Senator James Harlan (date of recollection unknown) [helmB p166] *A degree of hagiography has crept in with the description of "truthfulness" in the eyes.*   173

    ⟨1⟩ Harlan did not meet Lincoln until 1861 [helmB]   174

⟨$\frac{1}{q}$⟩ [currentBk p272] refers to a description of Lincoln by the *Liverpool Post* "in the midst of the war." *I do not have access to that description.*   175

⟨2⟩ "Lincoln could appear handsome at one time, homely at another. When his hair was too long or too short, when it shot out every which way like blown wheat or or stood up in spikes, Lincoln could look odd indeed. When his weak right eye wandered, or his beak of a nose was caught in sharp profile, or his thick lower lip hung down, when his hollow cheeks seemed sucked in more usual, when his massive jaw took on a mulish set, or sadness or melancholy deadened his eyes, then his visage was construed as heavy and unpleasant. People who knew him said that his face was impossible really to describe because it was forever changing expression. Its plasticity gave it a thousand different gradations and configurations, and even when the light was unflattering or the jutting eyebrows stood out, or the cheeks went hollow, it was only for a moment. Then, in another flash, any hint of oddness or lack of expression or looseness of skin or overabundance of jaw disappeared, and as the man warmed up and his sadness fled, his features revived and his countenance tuned radiant. Artists especially did not see homeliness in Lincoln's face." [kunhardtA p9]   176

⟨$\frac{1}{q}$⟩ As President: "Large head, with high crown of skull; thick, bushy hair; large and deep eye-caverns; heavy eyebrows; a large nose; large ears; large mouth; thin upper and somewhat thick under lip; very high and prominent cheekbones; cheeks thin and sunken; strongly developed jawbones; chin slightly upturned; a thin but sinewy neck, rather long; long arms; large hands; chest thin and narrow compared with his great height; legs of more than proportionate length, and large feet." – John Nicolay [meserve p5]   177

Appearance (continued)

⟨1⟩ 1862: "In lounged a tall, loose-jointed figure, of an exaggerated Yankee port 178
and demeanor, whom (as being about the homeliest man I ever saw, yet by no
means repulsive or disagreeable) it was impossible not to recognize as Uncle Abe.
... There is no describing his lengthy awkwardness, nor the uncouthness of his
movement ...[His] suit had adapted itself to the curves and angularities of his figure, and had grown to be the outer skin of the man. He had shabby slippers on his
feet. His hair was black, still unmixed with gray, stiff, somewhat bushy, and had
apparently been acquainted with neither the brush nor comb that morning.... His
complexion is dark and sallow ... he has thick black eyebrows and an impending
brow; his nose is large, and the lines about his mouth are very strongly defined.
The whole physiognomy is as coarse a one as you would meet..." [hawthorne pp309-
310]

⟨1⟩ March 1862±: "To say he is ugly is nothing: to add that his figure is grotesque is 179
to convey no adequate impression. Fancy a man six-foot high, and thin *out of*
proportion, with long bony arms and legs, which, somehow, seem to be always in
the way, with large rugged hands, which grasp you like a vice when shaking yours,
with a long scraggy neck, and a chest too narrow for the great arms hanging by its
side; add to this figure a head, cocoa-nut shaped and somewhat too small for such
a stature, covered with rough, uncombed and uncombable lank dark hair, that
stands out in every direction at once; a face furrowed, wrinkled, and indented,
as though it has been scarred by vitriol; a high narrow forehead; and, sunk deep
beneath bushy eyebrows, two bright, somewhat dreamy eyes, that seemed to gaze
through you without looking at you; a few irregular blotches of black bristly hair in
the place where beard and whiskers ought to grow; a close-set thin-lipped, stern
mouth, with two rows of large white teeth; and a nose and ears which have been
taken by mistake from a head of twice the size. Clothe this figure, then, in a long,
tight, badly-fitting suit of black, creased, soiled, and puckered up at every salient
point of the figure – and every point of this figure is salient – put on large, ill-fitting
boots, gloves too long for the long bony fingers, and a fluffy hat, covered to the top
with dusty puffy crape; and then add to all this an air of strength, physical as well
as moral, and a strange look of dignity coupled with all this grotesqueness, and
you will have the impression left upon me by Abraham Lincoln." [dicey v1pp220-221]
Dicey underestimates Lincoln's height. And how could he know the boots were
ill-fitting? ○○○ *Project:* Does the sparse beard have photo-confirmation at
this time?

⟨1⟩ Spring 1862: "The President had just come from a cabinet meeting and looked 182
worn and wearied. His hair stood up all over his head as though he had been
running his hands through it. [He looked] homely of face, large-boned, angular,
and loosely put together. [His eyes were] clear, calm, and honest, yet piercing
and searching... Cover the lower part of his face, and the expression of the upper
part was one of pathetic sadness... reverse the process and look upon the lower
half of his face, and the expression was humorous and kindly. He sat in his chair
loungingly, giving no evidence of his unusual height; a pair of short-shanked gold
spectacles sat low down upon his nose, the shanks catching the temples, and he
cold easily look over them if he so desired. [Later,] Mr. Lincoln (who had been
sunk down in his big chair up to this time) began to rise, and as I looked he went
up and up and up" [bancroft]

⟨1⟩ 1860s: "Mr. Lincoln's face was thin, and his features were large. His hair was 183
black, his eyebrows heavy, his forehead square and well developed. His complexion was dark and quite sallow. His smile was something most lovely. I have

39

Appearance (continued)

never seen a woman's smile that approached it in its engaging quality; nor have I ever seen another face which would light up as Mr. Lincoln's did when something touched his heart or amused him. I have heard it said that he was ungainly, that his step was awkward. He never impressed me as being awkward. In the first place, there was such a charm and beauty about his expression, such good humor and friendly spirit looking from his eyes, that when you were near him you never thought whether he was awkward or graceful; you thought of nothing except, What a kindly character this man has! Then, too, there was such shrewdness in his kindly features that one did not care to criticise him. His manner was always dignified, [start p174] and even if he had done an awkward thing the dignity of his character and manner would have made it seem graceful and becoming. The great quality of his appearance was benevolence and benignity: the wish to do somebody some good if he could." [dana pp173-174]

⟨1/q⟩ "Lincoln is lean and lathy; his long, dangling, rake-handle arms are strong as steel; he stoops a little, is angular, a man of bony corners. His awkwardness is all in his looks; in his movements he is quick, sure, and graceful. Even when he crosses his spiderlike legs or throws them over the arms of a chair he does it with a natural grace." – Daniel Voorhees, then-Representative of Indiana [sandburgC v2p303]   184

⟨1⟩ "In person he was tall and bony... As he stood, his form was angular, with something of that straightness in its lines which is so peculiar in the figure of Dante by Flaxman. His countenance had more of rugged strength than his person, and while in repose sometimes seemed sad; but it lighted up easily." [sumnerA pp132-133]   185

⟨1⟩ As President: "His old Illinois friends ... were sometimes shocked with the change in his appearance. They had known him at his home, and at the courts in Illinois, with a frame of iron and nerves of steel; as a man who hardly knew what illness was, ever genial and sparkling with frolic and fun, nearly always cheery and bright. Now, as the months of the war went slowly on, they saw the wrinkles on his face and forehead deepen into furrows, the laugh of old days was less frequent, and it did not seem to come from the heart. Anxiety, responsibility, care, thought, disasters, defeats, the injustice of friends, wore upon his giant frame. ... During these four years he had no respite, no holidays." [arnold pp453-454]   186

⟨S⟩ Decline in appearance as President generally ascribed to depression and overwork [dimsdale]   187

⟨1⟩ As President: "tall, homely form" – David Homer Bates [NYTimesTeleg]   188

⟨1⟩ As President: "stooping figure, dull eyes, care-worn face, and languid frame" [brooksR]. Brooks compares this to the "wiry" Lincoln of "earlier days" and also notes changes in Lincoln's mood.   189

⟨1⟩ As President: "President Lincoln's features are well known. People said that his face was ugly. He certainly had neither the figure nor features of the Apollo of Belvedere; but he never appeared ugly to me, for his face, beaming with boundless kindness and benevolence towards mankind, had the stamp of intellectual beauty. I could not look into it without feeling kindly towards him, and without tears starting to my eyes, for over the whole face was spread a melancholy tinge... President Lincoln's appearance was peculiar. There was in his face, besides kindness and melancholy, a sly humour flickering around the corners of his big mouth and his rather small and somewhat tired-looking eyes. He was tall and thin, with enormously long loose arms and big hands, and long legs ending with feet such as I never saw before; one of his shoes might have served Commodore Nutt as a   190

Appearance (continued)

boat. The manner in which he dressed made him appear even taller and thinner than he was, for the clothes he wore seemed to be transmitted to him by some still taller elder brother. In summer, when he wore a suit made of some light black stuff, he looked like a German village schoolmaster. He had very large ears standing oft a little, and when he was in a good humour I always expected him to flap with them like a good-natured elephant. Notwithstanding his peculiar figure, he did not appear ridiculous." – Agnes Elisabeth Winona Lelercq (Joy) prinzessin zu Salm-Salm [salmsalm p44]

⟨1/q⟩ Oct. 1, 1862: Lincoln "not only is the ugliest man I ever saw, but the most uncouth and gawky in his manners and appearance." – a soldier [donaldA p387] 191

⟨1/q⟩ 1864: "Mr. Lincoln stands six feet twelve in his socks.... His anatomy is composed mostly of bones, and when walking he resembles the offspring of a happy marriage between a derrick and a windmill. When speaking he reminds one of the old signal-telegraph that used to stand on Staten Island. His head is shaped something like a rutabago, and his complexion is that of a Saratoga trunk. His hands and feet are plenty large enough, and in society he has the air of having too many of them. The glove-makers have not yet had time to construct gloves that will fit him. In his habits he is by no means foppish, though he brushes his hair sometimes, and is said to wash.... A strict temperance man himself, he does not object to another man's being pretty drunk, especially when he is about to make a bargain with him. ... He can hardly be called handsome, though he is certainly much better looking since he had the small-pox." – from a mock biography in the 1864 campaign [meserve pp2-3] See ¶1892 for a facial pock-mark. 192

⟨1/q⟩ 1864: "The President looks thin and careworn. His form is bowed as by a crushing load; his flesh is wasted as by incessant solicitude; and his face is thin and furrowed and pale, as though it had become spiritualized by the vicarious pain which he endured in bearing on himself all the calamities of his country." – Rev. C.B. Crane [browneF p670] 193

⟨1⟩ Feb. 1864: "gaunt figure ... haggard-looking ... plain, awkward-looking" [carpenter pp18-19] 194

⟨1⟩ Early 1864: In Lincoln's office: "His hair was 'every way for Sunday.' It looked as though it was an abandoned stubble field. He had on slippers, and his vest was what was called 'going free.' He looked wearied, and when he sat down in a chair, looked as though every limb wanted to drop off his body." – Henry Beecher [riceA pp249-250] 195

⟨1⟩ About 1864: "I have never known so great a change to take place in any man's appearance as in Mr. Lincoln's during the three years following the day when I first saw him – March 4, 1861. He was never handsome, indeed, but he grew more and more cadaverous and ungainly month by month. The terrible labor which the war imposed prevented him from taking systematic exercise, and he became constantly more lean and sallow. He had a very dejected appearance, and ugly black rings appeared under his eyes. I well remember how weary and sad he looked at one" particular reception [croffut]. *But* [croffut] *also thought Lincoln was not as sad as he looked* – ¶2311. 196

⟨2⟩ "By 1865 Lincoln looks like a haggard old man, when only a few years before he looked healthy and vibrant." [burk p164] 197

⟨1⟩ Feb. 1865: "Mr. Lincoln, as I saw him every morning, in the carpet slippers he wore in the house and the black clothes no tailor could make really fit his gaunt, bony frame, was a homely enough figure." [crookA p14] [crookK] 198

41

Appearance (continued)

$\langle\frac{1}{q}\rangle$ March 1865: "very care-worn and fatigued appearance." [donaldA p572]   199

$\langle 1 \rangle$ April 1865: "He was very tall, but his bearing was almost peculiar; the habit of   200
carrying one shoulder higher than the other might at first sight make him seem
slightly deformed. He had also a defect common to many Americans – his shoulders were too sloping for his height. But his arms were strong and his complexion
sunburned, like that of a man who has spent his youth in the open air, exposed to
all inclemencies of the weather and to all hardships of manual labor; his gestures
were vigorous and supple, revealing great physical strength and an extraordinary
energy for resisting privation and fatigue. Nothing seemed to lend harmony the
decided lines of his face; yet his wide and high forehead, his gray-brown eyes
sunken under thick eyebrows, and as though encircled by deep and dark wrinkles, his nose straight and pronounced, his lips at the same time thick and delicate, together with the furrows that ran across his cheeks and chin, formed an
ensemble which, although strange, was certainly powerful." [chambrunA] (Cognate
in [chambrunB pp99-100].)

$\langle\frac{1}{q}\rangle$ John Hay remembered the President reading a humorous poem out loud, "seemingly unconscious that he with his short shirt hanging above his long legs and   201
setting out behind like tail feathers of an enormous ostrich was infinitely funnier
than anything in the book he was laughing at." [donaldA p429]

$\langle\frac{1}{q}\rangle$ An aristocratic army officer pronounced Lincoln "the ugliest man I ever put my   202
eyes on" but after conversing with him said he looked "much like a highly intellectual and benevolent Satyr." [donaldA p572]

$\langle 2 \rangle$ "He was a huge spare man, slightly stooping, who walked with the peculiar slow   203
woods-and-fields movement of the Western pioneer. ... A sculptor who made
most careful measurements and studies from photographs, tell us that, from a
sculptor's point of view, Lincoln's proportions were quite perfect." – Helen Nicolay [nicolayA p227]

$\langle\frac{1}{q}\rangle$ "President Lincoln was of unusual stature, six feet four inches, and of spare   204
muscular build; he had been in youth remarkably strong and skillful in athletic
games.... He had regular and prepossessing features, dark complexion, broad,
high forehead, prominent cheek bones, gray, deep-set eyes, and bushy, black
hair, turning to gray at the time of his death. Abstemious in his habits, he possessed great physical endurance. ... His patience was inexhaustible. He had naturally a most cheerful and sunny temper, was highly social and sympathetic, loved
pleasant conversation, wit, anecdote and laughter. Beneath this, however, ran an
under-current of sadness; he was occasionally subject to hours of deep silence
and introspection that approached a condition of trance. In manner he was simple, direct, void of the least affectation, and entirely free from awkwardness, oddity, or eccentricity. His mental qualities were a quick analytic perception, strong
logical powers, a tenacious memory, a liberal estimate and tolerance of the opinions of others, ready intuition of human nature; and perhaps his most valuable
faculty was rare ability to divest himself of all feeling or passion in weighing motives of persons or problems of state." – John Nicolay [browneF p736]

$\langle\frac{1}{q}\rangle$ April 9, 1865: "It was my first sight of Mr. Lincoln. He appeared somewhat younger   205
and more off-hand and vigorous than I should have expected[, having a] bright,
knowing, somewhat humorous look..." – a correspondent [browneF p697]

$\langle 1 \rangle$ April 14, 1865: "There was no waste or excess of material about his frame; nevertheless he was very strong and muscular. I remember that the last time I went   206

Appearance (continued)

to see him at the White House – the afternoon before he was killed – I found him in a side room with coat off and sleeves rolled up, washing his hands. He had finished his work for the day, and was going away. I noticed then the thinness of his arms, and how well developed, strong and active his muscles seemed to be. In fact, there was nothing flabby or feeble about Mr. Lincoln physically. He was a very quick man in his movements when he chose to be, and he had immense physical endurance. Night after night he would work late and hard without being wilted by it. And he always seemed as ready for the next day's work as though he had done nothing the day before." – Charles A. Dana [dana pp158-159]

⟨1⟩ April 14, 1865: Receiving a "cheering welcome" upon entering Ford's Theatre: "His face was perfectly stoical; his deep-set eyes gave him a pathetically sad appearance. The audience seemed to be enthusiastically cheerful, yet he looked peculiarly sorrowful, as he slowly walked with bowed head and drooping shoulders to the box. I was looking at him as he took his last walk." – Charles Leale, MD [lealeA p3]   207

⟨2⟩_c "To summarize these various descriptions of Lincoln, recorded by his contemporaries, an image emerges that is tall and thin, with unnaturally long loose arms and legs. The cartoonists of his day capitalized on these aberrations by showing Lincoln as an ape-like creature with his great arm spread measurements and bent by kyphosis. In addition he was loose-jointed, dolichocephalic and probably had a highly arched palate. He was flat footed, kyphotic, with large hands and feet, long stringy musculature and scant subcutaneous fat. His ears were large and malformed, his eyes small and deeply placed in his head. A chest deformity, prognathism and genu recurvatum is suggested in Herndon's description. These findings to me suggest the diagnosis of the Marfan syndrome." [gordon]   208

⟨2⟩ On his death-bed, Lincoln was disrobed. "The stunning surprise was that the President's body was the body of a much younger man and was unbelievably perfect. The beautiful proportions, the magnificent muscular development, and the clear, firm flesh were all the more astounding because the visible man had given no clue. Charlie Taft pointed out that there was not one ounce of fat on the entire frame. Charles Leale was something of a student of classical sculpture, and he remarked immediately that the President could have been the model for Michelangelo's Moses; he had the same massive grandeur." [kunhardtB p49]   209

⟨2⟩ "Dr. Leale also testifies to the fact that the President was without a single physical defect of any kind." [markens] *Taking this second-hand source at its word, this statement is demonstrably false, as Lincoln's facial skin had numerous masses (probably neuromata) and may have been marked from his bout of smallpox 17 months earlier – see ¶1892.*   210

⟨1⟩_q Naked on his deathbed, Lincoln was described as "smoothly muscled, well proportioned, lean, and strong" [flattman] *Is, I believe, quoting Curtis.*   211

■ See [Death Watch] and [Post-Mortem] for appearance while dying and dead, respectively.   212

⟨2⟩_c *Having read all the above, consider this criticism of George Barnard's statue of Lincoln in Cincinnati:* "Barnard's Lincoln is not only plain, but grotesque. We doubt the accuracy of the portrait. ... His pose is ungainly, the figure lacks dignity, and the huge hands crossed over the stomach suggest that all is not well with his digestion. The largeness of the hands and feet is unduly exaggerated." [NYTimes - 1917-08-26] *The lesson (from either T.S. Eliot or Woody Allen) is: "The people do not want too much reality."*   213

Arms

⟨1⟩ Lincoln described himself as "tall and long-armed" as a youth [wilson p662]   214

⟨2⟩ About age 17: "His feet and hands were large, arms and legs long and in striking   215
contrast with his slender trunk and small head." [herndon p35] (∈ ¶492) *Herndon
did not know Lincoln at age 17.*

⟨2⟩ In 1842 Lincoln admitted writing letters to the newspaper in Springfield, IL sat-   216
irizing the state auditor, James Shields. To uphold his honor, Shields challenged
Lincoln to a duel. Shields was a crack shot, but as the challengee, Lincoln had the
choice of weapons. He chose cow pies. Shields would not be deterred, however,
and eventually Lincoln chose to duel with cavalry broadswords. When Lincoln
and Shields met at the appointed place, Lincoln picked out a sword and, with his
remarkable height and long arms, began slashing at tree branches that the shorter
Shields could not reach. After this, an accomodation was reached and the duel
never took place. Although humorous in retrospect, the affair was deadly serious.
[gary pp9-10] *Unfortunately, other sources fail to mention the cow pies.* [randallC
p59] *says "the elaborate correspondence about the matter" has been preserved.*

  ⟨2⟩ Shields was 5 feet 9 inches tall. Lincoln later said "I did not intend to hurt   217
    Shields unless I did so clearly in self-defense. If it had been necessary, I could
    have split him from the crown of his head to the end of his backbone" [don-
    aldA p92]. Shields later became a Brigadier General and a U.S. Senator from
    Illinois, Missouri, and Minnesota.

  ⟨1⟩ Feb. 1865: Lincoln was asked a question about the Shields duel and replied: 219
    "If you desire my friendship you will never mention the circumstance again!"
    [carpenter p305]

    ⟨1⟩ [rossH pp127-129] also discusses the near-duel.   220

⟨$\frac{1}{q}$⟩ "Mr. Lincoln may not be as handsome a figure, but the people are perhaps not   221
aware that his heart is as large as his arms are long." – Mary Lincoln, comparing
him to Stephen Douglas [herndon p238]

- Asymmetry (Also see ¶302.):   222
    ⟨1⟩ "The collar of his coat on the right side had an unpleasant way of flying up   223
      whenever he raised his arm to gesticulate." [herndon p369]
    ⟨2⟩ "His left shoulder was higher than his right" [kunhardtA p321]   224

- Length: 225
    ⟨2⟩ About 1831: "His long arms protruded through the sleeves of a coat" – from   226
      Menard Axis, 1862 [wilson p24] (∈ ¶95)
    ⟨1⟩ 1834: "arms long, longer than any man I ever knew, when standing Straiht,   227
      and letting his arms fall down his Sides, the points of his fingers would touch
      a point lower on his legs by nearly three inches than was usual with other
      persons. I was present when a number of persons measured the length of
      thire arms on thire legs, as here Stated, with that result. his arms were un-
      usually long for his hight, and the droop of his shoulders also produced that
      result. " – Robert Wilson [wilson pp201-202] (∈ ¶99)
    ⟨1⟩ "long arms ... swung down by his side" [herndon p471] [herndonC] (∈ ¶2)   228
    ⟨1⟩ "His legs & arms were abnormally – unnaturally long, & hence in undue   229
      proportions to the balance of his body" [herndonC] (∈ ¶2)(Cognate in: [herndon
      p472].)
    ⟨1⟩ "limbs large and bony" – William Herndon [hertz p195] (∈ ¶87)   230

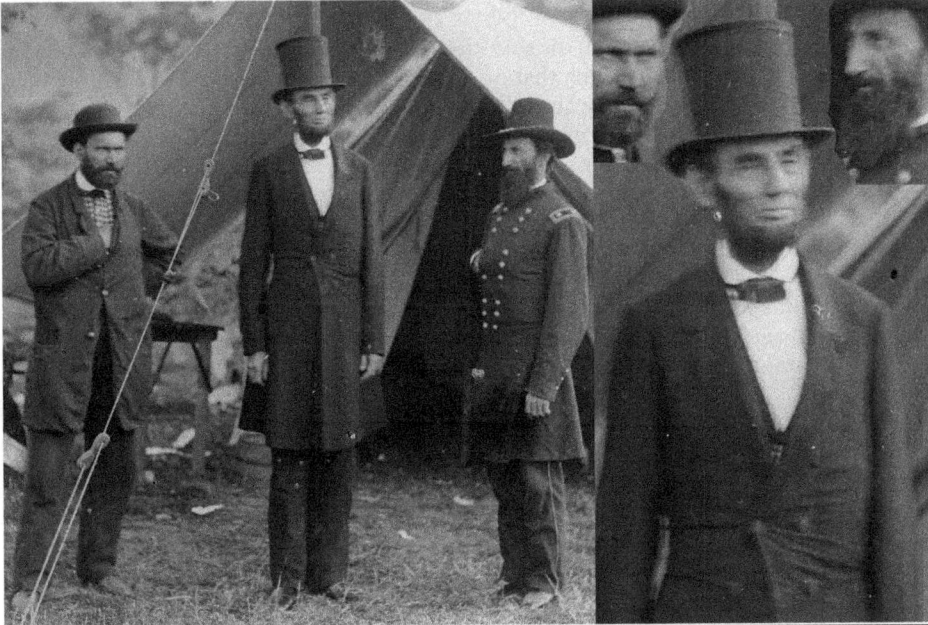

Figure 5. Lincoln at Antietam, about October 2, 1862, with detail in right panel. *Left panel:* Lincoln is flanked by Allan Pinkerton (to his right) and Major General John McClernand. The long length of Lincoln's arms is apparent. Lincoln does not have a John Wayne chest. His chest appears thin (especially in comparison to his hips) and his shoulders sag. Pinkerton's shoulders also fall forward, but his chest appears fuller than Lincoln's. Although Lincoln usually wore a too-large coat (see ¶32 ¶522), his coat does not look loose around the chest. His left shoulder, however, barely displaces the left sleeve outward (laterally), suggesting the coat is big in the shoulders. See ¶258ff for more findings in his photograph. *Photo credit:* [ostendorf #63], Library of Congress #LC-DIG-cwpb-04326.

Arms (continued)

⟨H⟩ In Indiana: Rejected by Susie Enlow because "my feet and hands were too big, and my legs and arms too long." [paulmier p26] 231

⟨1/q⟩ "He was fond of backing up against the wall and stretching out his arms to their fullest extent, and I never saw a man with so great a stretch." – Daniel Green Burner [templeB] Part of ¶2244 232

⟨1⟩ 1840s or 1850s: Attorney Lincoln "[stretches] out his long right arm and forefinger" at a trial witness [shastid]. *It is unclear if this is a second- or third-hand description.* 233

⟨1⟩ 1840s or 1850s: "a long and angular but very kindly arm" [shastid] (∈ ¶137) 234

⟨1⟩ 1847: "his long right arm extended towards the opposing counsel" – George Minier [wilson p708] (∈ ¶3715) 235

⟨1⟩ "long-armed, long-limbed" – Leonard Swett [riceA p464] 236

⟨1⟩ "long limbs, large hands and feet" [arnold p441] (∈ ¶167) 237

⟨1/q⟩ Autumn 1854: "a human being rising slowly, and unfolding his long arms and his long legs, exactly like the blades of a jack-knife.... his coat sleeves 239

Arms (continued)

were inches shorter than his shirt sleeves" – J.B. Merwin [hobson p63] (∈ ¶142)

⟨1⟩ 1855: "Why did you bring that d—-d long-armed ape here for?" – Stanton, 240
as overheard by Lincoln, according to Herndon [hertz p153]

⟨1/q⟩ "Where did that long-armed creature come from?" ... "Du Chaillu was a fool 241
to go all the way to Africa – he could have found the original gorilla in Springfield, Illinois." – big-city lawyer Edwin Stanton's assessment of small-town
lawyer Abraham Lincoln [kunhardtB p54]. Stanton is also recorded as calling
him a "giraffe" and a "long-armed baboon" [burl p98]. *Stanton later became
Lincoln's Secretary of War.*

⟨1/q⟩ Summer 1858: "His clothes were very ill-fitting, and his long arms and hands 242
protruded far through his coat sleeves, giving him a peculiarly uncouth appearance." – Rev. George C. Noyes [browneF p290] (∈ ¶147)

⟨1⟩ Oct. 13, 1858: "... sleeves that should have been longer; but his arms ap- 243
peared so long that the sleeves of a store coat could hardly be expected to
cover them all the way down to the wrists." – Carl Schurz [angle p243] (∈ ¶149)

⟨1/q⟩ 1858: "He swung his long arms sometimes in a very ungraceful manner" – 244
Carl Schurz [kunhardtA p110] (∈ ¶3719)

⟨1⟩ April 1860: Lincoln is speaking: "'... when I hear a man preach, I like to see 245
him act as if he were fighting bees!' And he extended his long arms, at the
same time suiting the action to the words." [volk]

⟨1/q⟩ June 21, 1860: "arms that were somewhat too long for a statue of Apollo" – 246
Utica newspaper reporter [lincloreHDE] (∈ ¶159)

⟨1/q⟩ During the Civil War Lincoln watched a regiment of Maine lumbermen and 247
remarked "I don't believe that there is a man in that regiment with longer
arms than mine." [rothschild p26]

⟨1⟩ 1861: "a long arm ... reached to my shoulder ... It was Mr. Lincoln" – "Nelson" 248
[wilson p642]. (∈ ¶3104)

⟨1⟩ March 1861: "long pendulous arms, terminating in hands of extraordinary 249
dimensions" – William Russell [russell pp37-38] (∈ ¶161)

⟨1/q⟩ "long arms" – John Nicolay [meserve p5] (∈ ¶177) 250
⟨1/q⟩ "enormously long loose arms" – Princess Salm-Salm [salmsalm] (∈ ¶190) 251
⟨1⟩ Spring 1862: "stretching out his long arm..." [bancroft] (∈ ¶182) 252
⟨1⟩ 1862: "long bony arms and legs, which, somehow, seem to be always in the 253
way" [dicey v1pp220-221] (∈ ¶179)

⟨1⟩ "long arms" – Schuyler Colfax [riceA p337] 254
⟨1⟩ As President: "enormously long loose arms" [salmsalm p144] (∈ ¶190) 255
⟨1⟩ Mar. 29, 1865: "waved a farewell with his long right arm" [porterH] 256
⟨1⟩ April 1865: "He stretched out his long right arm" [porterD p308] (∈ ¶2558) 257

🔲 Fig. 5 discusses length of arms and bulk of shoulders. Other notable aspects of 258
Fig. 5: (1) The left hemithorax appears more prominent despite Lincoln's right
foot being closer to the camera. Papers in an inside left pocket of the coat could
explain the prominence, however, [mckusickA p47] notes that asymmetric thorax
may be encountered in Marfan syndrome. See also ¶518. (2) Assuming the iliac
crests are the widest part of Lincoln's lower torso and that the bulge near the crook
of his right arm is the right crest, the photograph supports Herndon's statement
that Lincoln's height came from his legs (¶407). (3) The blurriness of Lincoln's face
(right panel) has been ascribed to him swaying during the long exposure needed
by cameras of that day (¶3144). Lincoln's face is blurrier than those of Pinkerton and McClernand (insets, at same magnification as Lincoln), but the double
image of the right side of Lincoln's white collar provides the clearest indication

Arms (continued)

of motion. A sway may have cardiovascular (¶1975) and/or neurological (¶3144) causes. (4) Lincoln's eyes are almost-closed slits, an appearance difficult to blame on a side-to-side sway. Bags appear to be under his eyes. Thus, the photograph fits a description written in mid-1863: "drooping eyelids, looking almost swollen [with] dark bags beneath the eyes" (∈ ¶1621). [ostendorfA p108] blames a blink for the eye appearance. (5) The head is tilted slightly to the right, a characteristic Lincoln pose. (6) Even accounting for the head tilt, the left eye appears to sit higher than the right (¶896), and the left eyebrow is clearly higher than the right. (7) Blubbery lower lip. (8) He is standing in his usual "toe even with toe" way (¶966).

⟨2⟩ Black hair on his arms [kunhardtA p321] 259

⟨1⟩ 1832: After leaving militia service, "thought of learning the black-smith trade" – Lincoln [baslerA v4p66] 260

⟨1⟩ Pre-presidential years: Of the game known as *fives*: "He loved this game ... Lincoln said – This game makes my shoulders feel well" – Charles Zane [wilson p492] See ¶2876 261

⟨2⟩ April 25, 1858: Lincoln donned a borrowed coat to sit for a photograph ([ostendorf #4]), then, according to a witness, was "overcome with merriment" when it "proved to be a bad misfit," leaving his arms sticking out "about a quarter of a yard." [ostendorfA p11] 262

🔲 Nov. 1863: [ostendorf #80] is said to show "Lincoln's powerful shoulders and arms" [ostendorfA p150]. 263

⟨1⟩ April 1865: "his arms were strong and ... his gestures were vigorous and supple, revealing great physical strength and an extraordinary energy for resisting privation and fatigue" [chambrunA] (∈ ¶200) 264

⟨1⟩ April 8, 1865: After an afternoon of shakings the hands of wounded soldiers: "I have shaken so many hands to-day that my arms ache tonight." – Lincoln [keckleyB p171] (∈ ¶1303) 265

⟨1⟩ April 14, 1865: Lincoln on his death-bed: "He had been stripped of his clothes. His large arms, which were occasionally exposed, were of a size which one would scarce have expected from his spare appearance." – Gideon Welles [kunhardtA p359] (∈ ¶552) 266

Asymmetry

Every part of Lincoln's body, for which data are available, was asymmetric: head, face, shoulders, fingers, chest (maybe), feet, and possibly even gait. 267

The older Lincoln literature is not surprised by this, seeing asymmetry as evidence of Marfan syndrome: 268
  ⟨-⟩ "Facial asymmetry is often described as part of this syndrome." [gordon] 269
  ⟨-⟩ "... numerous asymmetries in the Marfan syndrome..." [schwartzA] 270
  ⟨-⟩ "Asymmetric differences in growth and bilateral organs are not infrequent in the Marfan syndrome." [kempfB p4] 271

By contrast, the Marfan literature has little to say about asymmetry. Asymmetric pectus varieties may occur [mckusickA p47], but a Pubmed search and my questions to Marfan 272

Asymmetry (continued)

specialists disclosed no examples of more extensive asymmetry or pathophysiological hypotheses. Recently, however, the newly discovered Marfan-like disorder, Loeys-Dietz syndrome, provides one possible tie: craniosynostosis is part of this syndrome [aa67] [aa68] and an asymmetric skull is a cardinal sign of craniosynostosis.

More helpfully with respect to Lincoln, [kempfB p4] reminds us that asymmetries do not "permit the geneticist to attribute them entirely to genic determination." 273

Some degree of asymmetry exists in all persons, of course. Interestingly, a large body of research has identified facial symmetry as the dominant factor in physical attractiveness . Lincoln, of course, was frequently described as "homely" (¶1663ff and ¶1697ff), and his facial asymmetry has reportedly been noted by artists (¶290ff). The fact that asymmetry was noticed offers a guide to its severity: "While very few skulls are truly symmetrical, the asymmetry has to be extreme before it begins to affect the outward appearance of he face significantly" [aa89 p23]. Also, "A face has to show quite marked asymmetry before it becomes immediately noticeable to an observer " [aa89 p153]. 274

- Head & Face – views of [kempfB]: 275
  - ⟨S⟩ "Some recent medical observers have suggested that Lincoln's facial asymmetry developed possibly through habitually making voluntary efforts to correct a congenital strabismus. The marked difference in the muscular tonus of the two sides of his face seem to have been regarded superficially by most of his friends and biographers as an oddity of habitual expression." [kempfB p xvii] 276
  - ⟨2⟩$_c$ "asymmetrical differences in the growth of the bones of the right and left sides of his face ... subnormal neuromuscular tonus of the left side" [kempfB p4] 277
  - ⟨2⟩$_c$ "The left eye sets higher than the right. His left eyebrow is usually elevated more than the right to keep the upper lid retracted and the pupil of the left eye exposed. The tendency of the left eye to turn upward uncovered more of the white surface of the sclera below the iris, giving a slightly dull, weak, staring effect on that side, in strong disharmony with the more active right eye and face. The left eye in the best frontal photographs is shown definitely to be out of focus and turned reflexly slightly upward and outward." [kempfB p9] (See ¶880.) 278
  - ⟨2⟩ "The right side of the chin is is larger than the left." [kempfB p9] 279
  - ⟨2⟩ "His cheek bones were unusually high and prominent. The right was larger than the left, and the right orbital ridge and lower jaw were more heavily developed than the left, giving the whole face a decided morphological curve toward the right. This deformation becomes distinctly visible when the full face photographs are turned upside down. When the Volk mask is turned upside down, or viewed from below upward, the larger size of the face and the greater prominence of its lip, chin and lower jaw, and the greater depression of the face under the cheekbone, on the right side, is impressive." [lkempf p9] 280
  - ⟨S⟩ "All of these differences in facial muscle and bone development ... indicated to me that Lincoln had suffered a serious injury of his brain in childhood." [kempfB p9]. *Kempf next begins referring to the horse-kick incident; see §1a and ¶3568.* 281
  - ⟨2⟩ "The right side of Lincoln's face was animated and normally emotionally expressive, whereas the left side functioned more weakly, looked duller and strangely out of harmony." [kempfB p16] 282

Asymmetry (continued)

⟨S⟩ Prominence of right-sided activity when reading or thinking gave Lincoln a 283
perplexed look [kempfB p17]

⊡ Lincoln and/or his photographers seemed "to prefer the right side since 284
most photographs were taken from the right quarter or profile. Only a few
were taken from the left side or in front." [kempfB p17]

- Head & Face – views of [fishman]: 285
  ⟨1⟩ [fishman] performed laser-scanning on the 1865 cast of Lincoln's head (¶1914) 286
  to quantify areas of asymmetry in Lincoln's face. The superior orbital rims
  (i.e., brows) were the most asymmetric region, with the left appearing under-
  developed compared to the right.

  ⟨2⟩ [fishman] ascribes asymmetries in the lips, nose, and ears of the 1865 cast of 287
  c Lincoln's head (¶1914) to "extraneous" or "technical" factors associated with
  the casting. *This seems unlikely, as the same asymmetries are present in
  the 1860 cast (¶1905).*

  ⟨2⟩ Diagnosis: "craniofacial microsomia" [fishman] *This is a descriptive diagno-* 288
  c *sis, not an etiologic diagnosis.*

  ⟨S⟩ Lincoln's vertical eye deviation (Eyes -- Motor) could be due to asymmetry 289
  of the skull, affecting a nerve that controls eye movement [fishman].

- Head & Face – views of others: 290
  ⟨2⟩ "If one takes a paper and conceals one half of the Macomb face at a time 291
  c along a verticle [sic] line, there is an impression that is not easy to describe:
  not only the obvious fact of asymmetry which artists have noted, but different facets of the man's character which that asymmetry suggests." – J.G.
  Randall, manuscript page in [randallP box 15] *"Macomb face" probably refers
  to "the Macomb ambrotype" (ambrotype being an old photographic technique), [ostendorf #11], taken in Macomb, Illinois in August 1858.*

  ⟨2⟩ "his left eye was actually set higher than his right eye" [snyder] (∈ ¶896) 292

  ⟨2⟩ "Conant, who painted Lincoln in 1860, complains of his difficulties, faced as 293
  s he was by Lincoln's asymmetrical countenance." [gordon] *The complaint is
  not in* [conant].

  ⟨S⟩ Gutzon Borglum, the artist behind Mt. Rushmore, is reported to have said: 294
  "Lincoln laughed with the right side of his face and rippling all over it are delicate streams of humor, as from some freshening spring. They pour toward
  the right corner of his mouth where his laughter issued with a loud hearty
  guffaw. The left side is the side of melancholy and written all over it are the
  sufferings of a great, lonely soul." [lincloreBIG] *Given that Borglum was born
  after Lincoln died, his statement may contain considerable artistic license.*

  ⟨1⟩ Lincoln's spectacles had asymmetric frames [myers]. (See ¶920.) 295

- Head & Face – other references: 296
  ⟨-⟩ For asymmetry of lips, see ¶2785ff. 297
  ⟨-⟩ *The Physical Lincoln* uses photographs of Lincoln and his head casts to il- 298
  lustrate asymmetries in Lincoln's forehead, cheek bones, nose, lips, chin,
  ears, eye sockets, parietal region, and occiput. The famous full-face photograph, taken by Alexander Gardner in November 1863 ([ostendorf #77]), best
  demonstrates the asymmetry in his eyes and ears. Nothing in that photograph suggests that Lincoln's pose was asymmetric.

- Chest: 299
  ⊡ Figure 5 shows and discusses the more prominent left hemithorax. 300
  ⟨-⟩ The possibility that Lincoln had a pectus deformity is discussed in ¶501. 301

Asymmetry (continued)

- Shoulders: 302
  - ⟨1⟩ "The collar of his coat on the right side had an unpleasant way of flying up whenever he raised his arm to gesticulate." [herndon p369] 303
  - ⟨2⟩ "His left shoulder was higher than his right" [kunhardtA p321] (∈ ¶1078) 304
  - ⊡ Lincoln's left shoulder appears higher in several photographs, e.g. [ostendorf #77] as discussed in ¶298. 305
  - ⟨S⟩ Could a pectus have caused shoulder asymmetry? See ¶501 for discussion. 306
  - ⟨1⟩ Springfield years: Lincoln often had just one suspender working [wilson p452]. *Did this reflect a shoulder that was unable to keep a suspender in place?* 307
  - ⟨2⟩ "His coat always seemed rumpled and his cravat askew" [donaldH p28] 308
  - ⟨1⟩ April 1865: "the habit of carrying one shoulder higher than the other might at first sight make him seem slightly deformed" [chambrunA] (∈ ¶200) 309

- Fingers and hands: 310
  - ⟨1⟩ Anthropological measurements of Lincoln's hand casts were difficult (¶1525), but showed all fingers on the left hand were longer than on the right, except for the thumb. This was true even though the right hand was temporarily swollen when the cast was made (¶1517). In a right-handed person "it is unusual for the left hand to predominate in size. Nor am I able to account for this difference in the somewhat contrasting positions of the two hands. Probably the asymmetry, although unusual, was natural." [stewart] 311
  - ⊡ Hand asymmetry appears to present in a February 1864 photograph [ostendorf #91]. 312
  - ⟨2⟩c [kempfB p4] suggests that years of handling an axe could have produced asymmetric muscle development *(and bony development, if begun early enough in life?)*. He notes that, in a right-handed axe user, the left hand "carries more stress and does more work" than the right hand. 313

- ⊡ Feet: In the bootmaker's tracing of Lincoln's feet (¶1007), the resulting measurements of the two feet were "uneven." [kunhardtA p320] 314

- Gait: 315
  - ⟨2⟩ He led with his right shoulder when walking [kunhardtA p321] (See ¶1079.) 316

Blood

⟨2⟩ Blood type was "A." [davidsonG] citing 1950s(?) work by Col. Joseph Akeroyd of the US Army. 317

⟨2⟩ In Springfield: Lincoln bled after Mary struck him in the face for bringing home an unsatisfactory piece of meat for company – Jesse Dubois [wilson p692] (See ¶3593.) 318

⟨1⟩ July 27, 1848: "I never fainted from the loss of blood." – Lincoln [baslerA v1p511] *A facetious reference to battles with mosquitoes during his militia service.* 319

⟨1⟩ April 4, 1864: "Paler than ever his countenance..." [coffinA p187] (∈ ¶1294) 320

⟨1⟩ April 1865: A blood clot formed in the track made through Lincoln's brain by the bullet from the assassin's gun. [good p61] (Reprinted in Special Topic §7.) 321

Build – Adult

Classically, a person with Marfan syndrome has legs too long in comparison to the trunk. This tendency is quantified using the "upper segment/lower segment ratio" (US-LS ratio), as follows. The patient's height from the top of their head down to the pubic symphysis is divided by their height from the pubic symphysis down to the floor. A normal white adult has a US-LS ratio of about 0.93, meaning that the upper segment is somewhat shorter than the lower segment. Marfan patients have a US-LS ratio "in the vicinity of 0.85," indicating that their upper segment is relatively short. [mckusickA pp43-45]   **322**

Many observers describe Lincoln as long-legged. Unfortunately, no photographs permit estimation of his US-LS ratio, for two reasons. First, clothes obscure the location of the pubic symphysis, and, second, even if a photograph of the naked Lincoln existed, [mckusickA p45] warns: "The photograph in the nude on the measured grid cannot be relied on for more than a rough estimate of body proportions. Errors in estimating the site of the pubic symphysis and parallax make poor reproducibility and poor checks with direct measurements."   **323**

Could a non-standard approach quantify Lincoln's long-leggedness? For example, [kunhardtA p281] shows Lincoln standing with his hand on his hip. It is reasonable to assume the web of the thumb is at the top of the iliac crest because this is the most natural position for the hand and arm to assume. A figure in [mckusickA p49] shows a 1902 diagram of normal body proportions by age. In the adult drawing at far right, the top of the iliac crest is approximately 60% of the way from the floor to the top-of-head. One might use this as an analog to the US-LS ratio defined by the pubic symphysis and gauge Lincoln by it. There is no support for such an approach. (See ¶450.)   **324**

How much taller than average was Lincoln? Among the potential control populations, [stewart] cites: (1) Soldiers from LaRue County in Kentucky (where Lincoln was born) in the 1860s had an average height of 5-feet 8.2-inches. (2) In the 1920s, 727 white male Virginians and Tennesseeans, whose parents and grandparents on both sides were American-born, had an average height of 5-feet 8.6-inches, with a range from 60.5 to 76.0 inches.   **325**

- Also see individual skeletal segments: Head & Face , Arms , Hands , Legs , Feet , Chest & Shoulders .   **326**

⟨1⟩ A sculptor, writing to William Herndon, said Lincoln was "of good proportion." Herndon replied: "You will pardon me if I state that he was not of good proportion, was six feet four inches high in his sock feet, was thin, wiry, sinewy, not *muscular*, weighed from 160 to 180 pounds." [hertz p186]   **327**

⟨1⟩ Herndon clarified two weeks later: "When I said that Lincoln was not a man of good proportion, I compared him with others, the *general* man. ... Lincoln was a man of good proportions when we look at him alone and not by comparison with the *general* man, the great mass of men." [hertz p193]   **328**

⟨$\frac{1}{q}$⟩ 1864: "Mr. Lincoln's height was six feet three and three-quarter inches 'in his stocking-feet.' He stood up, one day, at the right of my large canvas, while I marked his exact height upon it." [carpenter p217]   **329**

⟨-⟩ *As in* [templeH], *this will be accepted as the definitive quantification of Lincoln's adult height.*   **330**

- Other quantitative assessments of Lincoln's adult height: **331**
  ⟨1⟩ Spring 1831: "his height was six feet four inches" – William Greene [wilson p17] Part of ¶394   **332**
  ⟨2⟩ In the latter part of 1831: "He was now six feet four inches high" [herndon p69]   **333**

Build – Adult (continued)

⟨2⟩ 1831: "six feet three or four inches in height" – William Herndon [moore p534]   334

⟨1/q⟩ Jan. 1, 1841: "emphatically a man of high standing, being about six feet four   335
in his stockings, slender, and loosely built" – Quincy *Whig* [shenk p263]

⟨1⟩ "When standing erect he was six feet four inches high." [herndon p331]   336

⟨1⟩ "six feet four inches high in his sock feet" – Herndon [hertz p186] (∈ ¶327)   337

⟨1⟩ "Mr. Lincoln was six feet four inches high." [herndon p471]   338

⟨1⟩ "six feet three and a-half inches tall" – Leonard Swett [riceA p464]   339

⟨1/q⟩ Sept. 22, 1848: "six feet at least in his stockings" – Boston *Daily Atlas* [randallC   340
p112]

⟨2⟩ Lincoln reviewed an 1860 campaign biography (by William Dean Howells)   341
and let stand the statement that he was 6 feet 3 inches tall [templeH].

⟨1⟩ See also ¶431. However, ¶432 has an erroneous result.   342

⟨1⟩ May 1860: After asking the governor of New York his height, Lincoln is asked   343
his. "Six feet four." [riceA p259]

⟨1⟩ 1862: "Fancy a man six-foot high, and thin *out of* proportion..." [dicey v1pp220-   344
221] (∈ ¶179)

⟨1/q⟩ April 17, 1864: "I am six feet four in my stockings" – Lincoln [kunhardtA p209]   345

⟨1⟩ "towering up to six feet and four inches in height" [arnold p441] (∈ ¶167)   346

⟨1⟩ 1865: "six feet four inches" [crookA p15] [crookK]   347

⟨1/q⟩ "When I get all the kinks out I am six feet four inches" – Lincoln to   348
Humphrey W. Carr [ostendorfA p118]

⟨2⟩ "He could go over 6 feet 4 if he drew himself up, which he loved to do when   349
challenging another tall man to a measure." [kunhardtA p321]

- Lincoln could apparently seem taller on occasion: 350

  ⟨1/q⟩ Herndon recalls an inflamed Lincoln in the courtroom: he "rose up to about   351
  9 f[eet] high" and then, "as with a thunderbolt," verbally undid a swindler.
  [burl p155]

  ⟨1⟩ "I once saw Mr. Lincoln look more than a man; he was inspired by the oc-   352
  casion. [Speaking to the jury] Lincoln loomed up, rose up to be about nine
  feet high, grew warm, then eloquent with feelings, then blasting as with a
  thunderbolt..." – William Herndon [hertz pp99-100]

  ⟨1⟩ 1832: "Lincoln remarked if any man thinks I am a coward let him test it,'   353
  rising to an unusual height. One of the Regiment made this reply to Mr Lincoln's last remarks – 'Lincoln – you are larger & heavier than we are.' ..." –
  William Greene [wilson pp18-19]

  ⟨1⟩ Pre-Presidency: As Lincoln warmed up in making a speech, "his figure   354
  seemed to expand" [arnold p90]

  ⟨1⟩ April 1865: Lincoln, angry: "his slouchy manner had disappeared ... and   355
  even his stature appeared increased." [porterD p307] (∈ ¶2558)

  ⟨2⟩ "It was once said that Lincoln looked seven feet tall when he spoke." [randallC   356
  p154]

  ⟨s⟩ *Possible explanation: Lincoln stood on his tip-toes to give emphasis.*   357
  Stopped this later in his career. See ¶3719.

⟨1/q⟩ After twice striking his head on a chandelier at a private home: "Well, that was an   358
awkward piece of business. You know we haven't got those things at our house."
[randallC p71]

⟨2⟩ His height scares Mary's younger half-sister. [randallC p93] probably referencing   359
[helmA]

- Weight: 360

Build – Adult (continued)

⟨1⟩ 1830: "when he left Indiana – weighed about 160" – David Turnham [wilson p121] (∈ ¶495)   361

⟨1⟩ "He was more fleshy in Indiana than Ever in Ills" – Sarah Bush Lincoln [wilson p108]   362

⟨1⟩ Spring 1831: "weighed 214" – William Greene [wilson p17] Part of ¶394   363

⟨1⟩ 1831-1832: "Mr Lincoln weighed when he & I Clk for Denton Offutt 214 lbs I have weighed him often" – William Greene [wilson p11]. Lincoln clerked for Offutt in the fall of 1831 and the winter of 1832 [wilson p9n]   364

⟨1⟩ 1831: "weighed two hundred and ten pounds" – Herndon [moore p534]   366

⟨1⟩ "[Herndon] says that Lincoln weighed 240 pounds when he lived in New Salem... The facts are that Lincoln never weighed over 175 pounds in his life." [rossH pp125-126] *Herndon said 210, not 240.*   368

⟨1⟩ December 1859: "I am... lean in flesh, weighing on average, one hundred and eighty pounds" – Lincoln [donaldA p237]. (∈ ¶431)   369

⟨1⟩ January 1861: "he had lost forty pounds in weight" since April 1860 [volk]. Part of ¶438.   370

⟨2⟩ He weighed 180 lbs in 1861, when he came to Washington, and by 1865 weighed 160 lb. [kunhardtA p321] *I have not seen a primary source for these data. Is there an assumption that Lincoln's weight was stable between December 1859 and March 1861?*   371

⟨2⟩ "His weight in maturity seems to have ranged from 160 to 180, the latter figure in his later days." [shapiro]   372

⟨1⟩ July 8, 1861: "He is a little thinner and paler than on the day of his inauguration" [stoddardB p14] (∈ ¶1140)   373

⟨1⟩ Oct. 21, 1861: Compared to May 1860, "The lines were deeper in the President's face... the cheeks more sunken." [coffinA p176]   374

⟨2⟩ Lincoln lost weight and was not eating well during the anxious times around the Seven Days' Battles in June 1862 [donaldA p358]. See ¶655   375

⟨2⟩ 1862 or later: "Always thin, he had now lost so much weight as to look cadaverous." [donaldH p43]   376

⟨$\frac{1}{q}$⟩ "I am growing thin as a shad (yea, worse – as thin as a shadder)" – note found in the front of John Hay's 1863 diary [hayB p53]. The same pun appears as a tellable story in [randallB p64].   377

⟨1⟩ About 1864: "I have never known so great a change to take place in any man's appearance as in Mr. Lincoln's during the three years following the day when I first saw him – March 4, 1861. ... he grew more and more cadaverous and ungainly month by month. ... he became constantly more lean and sallow." [croffut] (∈ ¶196)   379

⟨2⟩ Lincoln lost 35 pounds while in office [flattman]   380

⟨2⟩ 1865: "thirty-five pounds underweight" [bishop p37] citing no source   381

⟨$\frac{1}{q}$⟩ "looks thin and careworn ... his flesh is wasted as by incessant solicitude; and his face is thin and furrowed and pale" – Rev. C.B. Crane [browneF p670] (∈ ¶193)   382

⟨2⟩ "For some time he had been losing weight, and strangers now noted his thinness rather than his height." [donaldA p568]   383

⟨2⟩ "emaciated" at the end of the war [kunhardtB p290]   384

■ Undated weights, per William Herndon: 385

⟨1⟩ "His usual weight was about 160 pounds." (written 1865) [herndonC] (∈ ¶1)   386

⟨1⟩ "his usual weight being about one hundred and sixty or eighty pounds" (year unknown) [hertz p413]   387

53

Build – Adult (continued)

⟨1⟩ "His usual weight was one hundred and eighty pounds." [herndon p471]   388

⟨1⟩ "weighed from 160 to 180 pounds" (written 1887) [hertz p186] (∈ ¶327)   389

⟨-⟩ *Unfortunately, it is not clear when any of these applied.*   390

⟨2⟩ ? Lipodystrophy: "Charlie Taft pointed out that there was not one ounce of fat   391
on the entire frame." [kunhardtB p49] (∈ ¶209) *Taft was a physician who saw Lincoln naked on the autopsy table and death-bed. The many other references to Lincoln's leanness are compatible with a lipodystrophy.*

⟨1⟩ "Lincoln was tall and raw boned at 18." – Joseph Richardson [wilson p119]   392

⟨1⟩ "Mr L. at this time was about 22 years of age; appeared to be as tall as he ever   393
became, and slimmer than of late years" – James Short [wilson p72]

⟨1⟩ Spring 1831: "He was at that time well and firmly built: his thigs [sic] were as   394
perfect as a human being Could be. and weighed 214: his height was six feet four inches" – William Greene [wilson p17]

⟨1⟩ 1832: "tall and slender" [rossH p95] *Conflicts with ¶396.*   395

⟨1⟩ New Salem: "He was very stout" [rossH p122] *Conflicts with ¶395.*   396

⟨$\frac{1}{q}$⟩ About 1835: "I remember his tall, lank, ungainly figure" – Nancy Rutledge Prewitt   397
[walsh p42] (∈ ¶102)

⟨$\frac{1}{q}$⟩ While studying law: "He was so studious and absorbed in his applications at one   398
time, that his friends ... 'noticed that he was so emaciated we feared he might bring on mental derangement.' " [herndon p99]

⟨2⟩ "So intense was his application, and so absorbed was he in his study, that he   399
would pass his best friends without observing them, and some people said that Lincoln was going crazy with hard study." [arnold p40] (See ¶2370.)

⟨1⟩ New Salem: "I often imagine him Standing Six feet and upward pointing his long   400
bony finger at Old Bowling Green who was presiding in his Court" – Dr. Jason Duncan [wilson p541]

⟨1⟩ "He was careless of his dress, and his clothes, instead of fitting neatly ... hung   401
loosely on his giant frame." [herndon p332]

⟨$\frac{1}{q}$⟩ "His frame was large, long, bony and muscular" – Elliott Herndon, writing circa   402
the 1860s [herndon p470n]

⟨1⟩ "He was thin – tall – wiry – sinewy, grisly – raw-boned man, thin through the breast   403
to the back – and narrow across the shoulders, standing he leaned forward – was what may be called stoop shouldered, inclining to the consumptive by build. His usual weight was about 160 pounds. ... His structure – his build was loose and leathery. His body was shrunk and shrivelled..." [herndonC] (∈ ¶1)

⟨2⟩ Cognate in [herndon p471]: "He was thin, wiry, sinewy, raw-boned; thin through   404
the breast to the back, and narrow across the shoulders; standing he leaned forward – was what may be called stoop-shouldered, inclining to the consumptive by build. His usual weight was one hundred and eighty pounds. ... His structure was loose and leathery; his body was shrunk and shriveled." *Note difference in weight, presumably due to Jesse Weik.*

⟨1⟩ "He died at the age fifty-six years a sinewy tough iron-framed man; he had no   405
extra flesh on him, but was all nerve and sinew; he was not what is generally termed a muscular man, but a sinewy one and a very strong and glorious one." – William Herndon [hertz p440]

Build – Adult (continued)

⟨1⟩ "limbs large and bony; he was tall and of a peculiar type." – William Herndon [hertz p195] (∈ ¶87) 406

⟨1⟩ "In sitting down on common chairs he was no taller than ordinary men from the chair to the crown of his head. A marble placed on his knee would roll hipward, down an inclined plane. His legs & arms were abnormally – unnaturally long, & hence in undue proportions to the balance of his body. It was only when he stood up that he loomed above other men." [herndonC] (∈ ¶2) (Cognate in: [herndon p472].) 407

    ⊡ Photographs confirms this. (See *The Physical Lincoln*.) 410

    ⊡ An 1862 photograph [ostendorf #66] shows Lincoln and General George McClellan sitting on chairs in a tent. Lincoln's sitting height exceeds McClellan's by surprisingly little, considering their 9-to-10-inch difference in standing height. Lincoln is perhaps slouching in his chair, but he is closer to the camera than McClellan, and McClellan is bowed. 411

⟨2⟩ When laughing hard, "he would rock with mirth, sometimes reaching out with his long arms to draw his knees almost up to his face." [donaldA p259] 412

■ Undated qualitative assessments of height, no attempt made to be complete: 413
    ⟨1⟩ "long – tall & green" – Caleb Carman [wilson p373] 414
    ⟨1⟩ "long, gaunt" [shastid] (∈ ¶137) 415
    ⟨1⟩ "He was tall and thin ... The manner in which he dressed made him appear even taller and thinner than he was, for the clothes he wore seemed to be transmitted to him by some still taller elder brother." – Princess Salm-Salm [salmsalm] (∈ ¶190) 416

⟨1⟩ "Herculean frame" [herndon p490] (¶1127). "Herculean stature" [arnold p140]. 417

⟨1⟩ 1834: "Six feet and four inches high in his Stockings." – Robert Wilson [wilson pp201-202] (∈ ¶99) 418

⟨1/q⟩ 1848: "a very tall and thin figure" – *Boston Advertiser* [wilson p689] 419
    ⟨1⟩ some in the audience "were struck by his height, as he arose" – Edward Pierce [wilson p690] 420
    ⟨1/q⟩ "a capital specimen of a Sucker Whig, six feet at least in his stockings" – Edward Pierce [wilson p690] 421

⟨1/q⟩ 1849: "He would have been instantly recognized in any court room in the United States, as being a very tall specimen of that type of long, large-boned men produced in the northern part of the Mississippi valley, and exhibiting its most peculiar characteristics of the mountains of Virginia, Tennessee, Kentucky, and Illinois. He would have been instantly recognized as a Western man, and his stature, figure, dress, manner, voice, and accent indicated that he was from the Northwest." [arnold p83] *He seems to be saying that Lincoln was tall even for the long men of the northern Mississippi valley. The comment about "peculiar characteristics" escapes me.* 422

⟨1⟩ 1849: "tall and angular frame" – Leonard Swett [wilson p732] (∈ ¶140) 423

⟨1⟩ June 1858: "tall, gaunt figure" [volk] Part of ¶1096 424

⟨1/q⟩ Aug. 1858: "His figure was gaunt, slender and slightly bent." – Martin Rindlaub [ostendorfA p19] (∈ ¶148) 425

⟨1⟩ 1858: "He had a lean, lank, indescribably gawky figure" – Henry Villard [kunhardtA p108] (∈ ¶145) 426

55

Build – Adult (continued)

⟨$\frac{1}{q}$⟩ October 1858: Beside "Lincoln's tall, lank ungainly form, Douglas stood almost like a dwarf" – Carl Schurz, attending the sixth Lincoln-Douglas debate [kunhardtA p108]   427

⟨1⟩ 1858: Lincoln debating Douglas: "'Judge Douglas has,' he said, 'one great advantage of me in this contest. When he stands before his admiring friends, who gather in great numbers to hear him, they can easily see, with half an eye, all kinds of *fat offices* sprouting out of his fat and jocund face, and, indeed, from every part of his plump and well-rounded body. His appearance is therefore irresistibly attractive. His friends expect him to be President, and they expect their reward. But when I stand before the people, not the sharpest vision is able to detect in my lean and lank person, or in my sunken and hollow cheeks, *the faintest sign or promise* of an office. I am not a candidate for the Presidency, and hence there is no beauty in me that men should desire me.' The crowd were convulsed with laughter at this sally." [browneF p291]   428

⟨1⟩ "he was a tall, spare man, with large bones" [arnold p441] (∈ ¶167)   429

⟨$\frac{1}{q}$⟩ 1859: "lank, gaunt figure" – John Widmer [shenk p155] (∈ ¶150)   430

⟨1⟩ December 1859: "I am, in height, six feet, four inches, nearly; lean in flesh, weighing, on an average, one hundred and eighty pounds" – part of Lincoln's self-description [arnold p15] (∈ ¶151)   431

⟨1⟩ April 1860: "He stood up against the wall and I made a mark above his head, and then measured up to it from the floor, and said: 'You are just twelve inches taller than Judge Douglas, that is, just six feet one inch.'" [volk] *This height seems to be in error, and it would be surprising if Lincoln let the inaccuracy pass without remark. The accuracy of Volk's recollections are tarnished by this error. (Douglas was a foot shorter than Lincoln: 5'4"* [shenk p137].)   432

⟨$\frac{1}{q}$⟩ June 21, 1860: "tall, arrowy, angular" – Utica newspaper reporter [lincloreHDE] (∈ ¶159)   433

⟨$\frac{1}{q}$⟩ Nov. 1860: "lean and ugly in every way" – Thomas Webster [randallC p163] (∈ ¶160)   434

⟨$\frac{1}{q}$⟩ December 1860: "spare, bony, lean, and muscular" – Thomas D. Jones (sculpted Lincoln) [meserve p5]   435

⟨1⟩ 1860: "His body seemed to me a huge skeleton in clothes." [piatt p345] (∈ ¶152)   436

⟨$\frac{1}{q}$⟩ 1860: "the long, ungainly figure" – George H. Putnam [ostendorfA p57] (∈ ¶153)   437

⟨1⟩ January 1861: Sculptor Leonard Volk, who had made a bust of Lincoln in April 1860, visited Lincoln at home: "His little parlor was full of friends and politicians. He introduced me to them all, and remarked to me aside that, since he had sat to me [sic] for his bust, he had lost forty pounds in weight. This was easily perceptible, for the lines of his jaws were very sharply defined through the short beard which he was allowing to grow." [volk] *A 40-pound weight loss in 9 months is remarkable, but by no means impossible. As noted in the bibliography and ¶432, certain caveats attend* [volk].   438

  ⟨s⟩ "The loss of forty pounds of weight in six months is questionable, but there was enough to give Don Piatt his impression of 'a skeleton in clothes.'" [shutesE p129] (See ¶152 for Piatt.)   439

■ Feb. 1861: Lincoln travels by rail from Springfield to Washington, under constant heavy guard.   440

  ⟨1⟩ "he could not lay straight in his berth" – Allan Pinkerton [wilson p291]   441

Build – Adult (continued)

⟨1⟩ In Philadelphia (?) he walked "leaning upon my arm and stooping a consid-   442
erable for the purpose of disguising his hight" – Allan Pinkerton [wilson p323]

■ Testing his height against other tall men: 443
⟨2⟩ "A gambit he was frequently to employ in the White House" helped Lincoln   444
defuse tense situations: he would match his height against that of someone
else in the room [donaldA p251].

⟨1/q⟩ Lincoln liked to measure himself against other tall men. In doing so he   445
would stretch himself out "like India rubber." – Leonard Volk [kunhardtA p110]

⟨2⟩ Lincoln "rarely missed guessing the height of other men, even Tom Thumb,   446
who came just about to Lincoln's knee level." [kunhardtA p322] *Thumb was
3-feet 4-inches [randallC p287]. It is unlikely Lincoln's knees were that tall!*

⟨1⟩ May 19, 1860: Tests his height against one of the delegation notifying him of   447
his Presidential nomination. Both [coffinA p173] and [riceA p259] tell the story
first-hand, though slightly differently. (See ¶343.)

⟨2⟩ "He could go over 6 feet 4 if he drew himself up, which he loved to do when   448
challenging another tall man to a measure." [kunhardtA p321]

⟨1/q⟩ March 1861: "tall, lank, lean man, considerably over six feet in height, with stoop-   449
ing shoulders, long pendulous arms terminating in hands of extraordinary dimensions, which, however, were far exceeded in proportion by his feet" – William
Russell [russell pp37-38] (∈ ¶161)

☐ Photograph of Lincoln standing, with a hand presumably on hip, indicating a very   450
high position for his hip [kunhardtA p281]. [ostendorf #102]

⟨1⟩ As President: "In person he was tall and bony... As he stood, his form was angular...   451
His countenance had more of rugged strength than his person..." [sumnerA pp132-133]
(∈ ¶185)

⟨2⟩ "exceptionally tall and painfully thin" [donaldA p214].   452

⟨1/q⟩ October 1, 1862: Lincoln arrives at an Army camp in "a common ambulance, with   453
his long legs doubled up so that his knees almost struck his chin" – a soldier [don-
aldA p387]

⟨1⟩ 1862 or later: "When Mrs. Lincoln... was absent from home, the President would   454
appear to forget that food and drink were needed for his existence, unless he were
persistently followed up by some of the servants, or were finally reminded of his
needs by the actual pangs of hunger." [brooksC pp276-277] (∈ ¶657) *What's wrong
with waiting until pangs of hunger occur?*

⟨1⟩ Sept. 1863: "tall and lean... very tall" [harveyC] (∈ §6.2, §6.9)   455

⟨1⟩ Nov. 18, 1863: "He was looking very badly... thin" [cochrane] (∈ ¶2535)   456

⟨1⟩ Dec. 1863, during his bout of smallpox (see Special Topic §5): "Men of his habit of   457
body are not usually long-lived." [ChicagoTribune - Dec. 9, 1863] (∈ §5.76). *A fascinating
statement. What did the writer know?*

⟨2⟩ Dec. 1863: "Lincoln had scarcely recovered from his varioloid at this time and   458
Emilie thought he looked very ill but she merely replied, 'He seemed thinner than
I ever saw him.' " [randallC pp297-298] quoting Emilie Todd Helm *Emilie was Mary's
half-sister.*

⟨1/q⟩ 1864: "His frame was gaunt but sinewy" [carpenter p217]   459

⟨1⟩ 1865: ".... the black clothes no tailor could make really fit his gaunt, bony frame..."   460
[crookA p14] (∈ ¶198)

Build – Adult (continued)

⟨1⟩ March 1865: "tall and gaunt" [brooksC p238]   461

⟨1/q⟩ March 1865: Sailing to visit General Grant, Lincoln spent the first night aboard   462
ship (the *Malvern*) in a berth at least four inches too short for him. During the
next day Admiral Porter had it lengthened to 8 feet and said nothing. The next
morning Lincoln greeted him, smiling, and said: "A miracle happened last night;
I shrank six inches length..." [browneF pp687-688]

⟨1⟩ April 4, 1865: "tall, gaunt-looking man" [porterD p295]   463

⟨1⟩ April 1865: "He was very tall, but his bearing was almost peculiar..." [chambrunA] (∈   464
¶200)

⟨2⟩ Lincoln's death bed was 74 1/2 inches long [kunhardtB p97]. (See ¶553.) He was 75 3/4   465
inches long.

⟨2⟩ As his coffin passed through New York, his "cheeks seemed hollow and pitted" to   466
many [kunhardtB p240].

- Theories: 467
  ⟨S⟩ "Lincoln's height was wholly exceptional." He was about 7.5 inches taller   468
  than the 5 foot 8.5 inch average of a geographically-matched and time-
  matched control group. "Stature like this occurs once in about a thousand"
  in the control group. "Perhaps what Lincoln represents is a genetic make-up
  (apparently inherited from his mother) that was particularly responsive to
  the special environment in which he was born." "Even as late as the Civil
  War, the tallest men in the country came from Kentucky and Tennessee."
  Lincoln had a resemblance to this "Appalachian Mountain type" [shapiro],
  which Herndon noted, too.
  ⟨S⟩ Herndon wondered if limestone water gave big frames, "so scientists say"   469
  [shapiro]. He disclaimed theories about dietary pork and miasma [hertz p203].
  ⟨S⟩ "... indications of some thyroid dysfunction and possibly a slight postpuber-   470
  tal overactivity in the pituitary which might account for the disporportion-
  ately long legs and arms" – Dr. K.C. Wold [kempfB p6]

Build – Childhood

In Marfan syndrome, "The excess length is often demonstrable at birth and through-   471
out childhood and adolescence" [mckusickA p53]. Presumably this is true of MEN2B, too.
Both medical and historical confusion about Lincoln's childhood growth led [tripp] to
conclude, erroneously, that Lincoln underwent precocious (early) puberty. (See ¶683.)

⟨1⟩ On his day of birth: "he wuz the puniest, cryin'est little younster I ever saw" –   472
Dennis Hanks [wilson p726]

⟨2⟩ "He was a long, thin baby at birth, with unusually long arms and legs" [kempfB p5].   473
I know of no primary source for this statement.

⟨1/q⟩ "I ricollect how Tom joked about Abe's long legs when he was toddlin' round the   474
cabin. He growed out o' his clothes faster'n Nancy could make 'em. ... Abe never
give Nancy no trouble after he could walk excep' to keep him in clothes." – Dennis
Hanks [wilsonR pp21, 22]

⟨1/q⟩ "Physically, he was a stout, powerful boy, fat, round, plump, and well made as well   475
proportioned." – Dennis Hanks, recalling late in life [kunhardtA p36]

⟨2⟩ "There wasn't much to this boy at first. He was little and all spindle." [kunhardtA p36]   476

Build – Childhood (continued)

⟨2⟩ At age 7 was "tall and spidery" [kunhardtA p36]　477

⟨1⟩ "though very young, was large of his age" – Lincoln [baslerA v4p63]　478

　　⟨2⟩ [donaldA p25] applies this statement to Lincoln at age 8. *The source document*　479
　　offers no reason for this conclusion.

■ Ages 10-11:　480

　　⟨1⟩ Age 10±: "was a long tall dangling award drowl looking boy" [sic] – David　481
　　Turnham [wilson p120]

　　⟨1⟩ Age 10 or older: "He was then a slender well behaved quiet boy" – John Helm　482
　　[wilson p82]

　　⟨2⟩ "In his eleventh year he began that marvelous and rapid growth in stature　483
　　for which he was so widely noted in the Pigeon Creek settlement. 'As he
　　shot up,' says Turnham, 'he seemed to change in appearance and action.'
　　... Nature was a little abrupt in the case of Abraham Lincoln; she tossed him
　　from the nimbleness of boyhood to the gravity of manhood in a single night."
　　[herndon p25] *I don't buy this. The "shot up," "abrupt," and "single night"*
　　phrases appear to be literary inventions of William Herndon and/or his
　　co-author, Jesse Weik. Neither phrase appears in the record of David
　　Turnham's interview with Herndon. Herndon and Weik did not know
　　enough medicine to realize that puberty is only one reason for children to
　　grow rapidly. [tripp pp31-32] *makes the same error (¶683).*

⟨2⟩ Age 12: "The boy had limited energy because at about the age of twelve he began　485
growing so rapidly." [donaldA p33] (∈ ¶1109)

⟨1⟩ Age 15+: "Abe was a long – thin – leggy – gawky boy dried up & Shriveled" – Anna　486
Gentry [wilson p131]

■ Ages 16-17:　487

　　⟨1⟩ "When 16 years of age he was 6 feet high – he was somewhat bony & raw" –　488
　　Joseph Richardson [wilson p119]

　　⟨2⟩ At age 16 was 6 feet two inches tall and weighed about 160 lb. "One contem-　489
　　porary remembered he was so skinny that he had a spidery look. He grew so
　　fast that he was tired all the time." [donaldA p33].

　　⟨2⟩ "By the time he had reached his seventeenth year he had attained the phys-　490
　　ical proportions of a fullgrown man." [herndon p52]

　　⟨1⟩ "Lincoln was Large of his age – Say at 17 – he was 6 & 2 inches tall – weighed　491
　　about 160 pounds or a little more – he was Stout – withy-wirey" – Nathaniel
　　Grigsby [wilson p112]

　　⟨2⟩ Age 17: "He was now over six feet high and was growing at a tremendous　492
　　rate, for he added two inches more before the close of his seventeenth year,
　　thus reaching the limit of his stature. He weighed in the region of a hundred
　　and sixty pounds; was wiry, vigorous, and strong. His feet and hands were
　　large, arms and legs long and in striking contrast with his slender trunk and
　　small head." [herndon pp34-35]

⟨2⟩ Jan. 1828: "gaunt frame" – neighbor [shenk p14] citing [warrenY p82] *This is probably*　493
made up by Warren from ¶2438.

⟨2⟩ Uncertain age: "Abe was now becoming a man, and was ... already taller than any　494
man in the neighborhood." [lamonL p41] *Lamon did not know Lincoln at this time.*

⟨1⟩ 1830: "Abe was a long tall raw boned boy – odd and gawky – He had hardly at-　495
tained 6 ft - 4 in when he left Indiana – weighed about 160" – David Turnham
[wilson p121]

Build – Childhood (continued)

⟨1⟩ 1830±: "He was then, generally, a long awkward gawky looking boy." – Jesse   496
Dubois [nicolayO p30]

⟨1⟩ "A long tall bony lad" – Absolom Roby [wilson p132]   497

⟨1/q⟩ "he grew up to his present enormous height on our own good soil of Indiana." –   498
Lincoln, speaking in the third person, Sept. 1859 [warrenY p267] citing [baslerA v3p?463]

⟨2⟩ In Lincoln's "younger days:" "his father said he looked like he needed a carpenter's   499
plane put to him" [sandburgP v1p306] *Did Sandburg concoct these words?*

Chest & Shoulders

The major question related to Lincoln's chest have been: (1) Was the chest thin or ro-   500
bust? and (2) Was there a pectus deformity? Now a third should be added: (3) Was it
asymmetric?

The admiring comments from persons who saw Lincoln's chest unclothed (ante-   501
mortem ¶2849 and post-mortem ¶2939 ¶2940) are not indicative of either pectus ex-
cavatum or pectus carinatum. But neither do they rule it out. One wonders if the
combination of a mild pectus (of either type) plus well-defined muscles (owing to a
lack of body fat) could produce the appearance of a powerful chest.

- From [herndon]:   502
  - ⟨1⟩ About age 17: "His feet and hands were large, arms and legs long and in   503
    striking contrast with his slender trunk and small head." [herndon p35] (∈ ¶492)
    Herndon did not know Lincoln at age 17.
  - ⟨1⟩ "He was thin through the chest, and hence slightly stoop-shouldered." [hern-   504
    don p331]
  - ⟨1⟩ "His form expanded, and, notwithstanding the sunken breast, he rose up a   505
    splendid and imposing figure." [herndon p333]
  - ⟨1⟩ "thin through the breast to the back – and narrow across the shoulders,   506
    standing he leaned forward – was what may be called stoop shouldered, in-
    clining to the consumptive by build" [herndonC] (∈ ¶1) (Cognate in: [herndon
    p471].)
  - ⟨2/c⟩ "a chest deformity [is] suggested by Herndon's description" [gordon] citing ¶1   507
- Other descriptions: 508
  - ⟨1⟩ 1834: "his arms were unusually long for his hight, and the droop of his shoul-   509
    ders also produced that result. " – Robert Wilson [wilson pp201-202] (∈ ¶99)
  - ⟨1/q⟩ "chest thin and narrow compared with his great height" – John Nicolay   510
    [meserve p5] (∈ ¶177)
  - ⟨1⟩ 1862: "a chest too narrow for the great arms hanging by its side" [dicey v1pp220-   511
    221] (∈ ¶179)
  - ⊡ Lincoln's narrow chest is apparent in Figure 5.   512
  - ⟨2⟩ "shoulders too narrow and sloping for his height" [shutesE p215]   513
- ⊡ Best photograph of Lincoln's chest is Fig. 5.   514

⟨2⟩ 1857: As Lincoln, having removed his coat, argued the Duff Armstrong case: 515
"Soon one of his suspenders fell from a shoulder, but paying no attention to it,
he allowed it to hang during the rest of the speech." [angle p177] reprinting Albert
Woldman *Is this easy slippage a sign of narrow shoulders?*

⟨1⟩ April 1860: Sculptor Leonard Volk recalls: "[I] desired to represent his breast and   516
brawny shoulders, so he stripped off his coat, waistcoat, shirt, cravat, and collar,

Chest & Shoulders (continued)

threw them on a chair, pulled his undershirt down a short distance" and stood for about an hour. Lincoln returned moments after leaving Volk's studio, having forgotten to do up his undershirt, which was out-hanging below his coat. Volk helped re-dress him. [volk] ([rankinA pp375-376] finds fault with this story.)

⟨1⟩ April 1865: "his shoulders were too sloping for his height" [chambrunA] (∈ ¶200)   517

- Asymmetric features (also see ¶299 and ¶302):   518
  ⟨1⟩ "The collar of his coat on the right side had an unpleasant way of flying up   519
      whenever he raised his arm to gesticulate." [herndon p369]
  ⟨2⟩ "His left shoulder was higher than his right" [kunhardtA p321]   520
  ⟨○⟩ Figure 5 suggests Lincoln's left hemithorax is more prominent.   521

⟨○⟩ Possible effects of clothing on photographic appearance: 522
  ⟨2⟩ Lincoln's "long-coated black suit ... hung on him two sizes too big" [kunhardtA   523
      p322] (See ¶32.)
  ⟨2⟩ Lincoln usually wore a long-sleeved undershirt. [kunhardtA p321]   524

⟨2⟩c [lattimerNY] believes that pictures of Lincoln show "a perfectly well-rounded and   525
normal-looking chest and sternum area" and that this argues against Lincoln having pectus excavaturm.
  ⟨2⟩c "Photographs of the clothed man are unsatisfactory to prove whether he had   526
      a chest deformity. Different photographs give different impressions." [borittA]
  ⟨-⟩ *Notes: (a) there are no photos of Lincoln's chest unclothed, (b) clothes*   527
      can easily mask the presence of pectus excavatum, especially if mild, and
      (c) Fig. 5, is an example of a photograph showing a narrow chest.

- "Stoop:"   528
  ⟨1⟩ 1834: "Some Stoop Shouldered ... the droop of his shoulders" – Robert Wil-   529
      son [wilson pp201-202] (∈ ¶99)
  ⟨1⟩ Pre-1861: "slightly stoop-shouldered" [herndon p331] (∈ ¶90)   530
  ⟨1⟩ Pre-Presidency: "was what may be called stoop shouldered" [herndonC] [herndon   531
      p471] (∈ ¶1)
  ⟨1⟩ March 1861: "stooping shoulders" – William Russell [russell pp37-38] (∈ ¶161)   532
  ⟨1⟩ 1860s: "he stoops a little" – Daniel Voorhees [gordon] (∈ ¶184)   533
  ⟨1⟩ 1864: "inclined to stoop when he walked" [carpenter p217]   534
  ⟨1⟩q April 14, 1865: "he slowly walked with bowed head and drooping shoulders"   535
      [lealeA p3] (∈ ¶207)
  ⟨2⟩ "kyphotic" [gordon]   536
  ⟨-⟩ His mother (¶4779) and father (¶5094) were sometimes described as stoop-   537
      shouldered.

- Herndon thought Lincoln was predisposed to tuberculosis because of his chest's   538
  shape:
  ⟨1⟩ "thin through the breast to the back, and narrow across the shoulders ...   539
      was what may be called stoop-shouldered, inclining to the consumptive by
      build" [herndon p471]
  ⟨-⟩ *Although the idea that certain chest shapes predisposed to tuberculosis sur-*   540
      vived from the time of the ancient Greeks to the time of Lincoln, by the
      end of the 1800s the medical profession was abandoning this idea [osler
      p192]. By 1919, a tuberculosis textbook noted: "The so-called 'habitus ph-
      thisicus,' associated with a long, narrow, flat thorax with acute epigastric
      angle, sloping shoulders, and winged scapulae, and also with signs of de-
      fective nutrition, may be found in phthisis – but also without evidence of

Chest & Shoulders (continued)

the disease. Its occurrence amongst ordinary cases with definite lung tu-
berculosis is strikingly uncommon. ... The mere shape of the thorax is of
but little value to us in diagnosis; we shall note this and pass on" [aa96
pp20-21]

⟨2⟩ Black hair on his "back, narrow shoulders, chest" [kunhardtA p321]   542

⟨2⟩ As President: "His upper body still showed the remarkable muscle formation that   543
Leonard Volk had commented on in 1860" [kunhardtA p321] (See ¶2902)

Death Watch

This section covers the period when Lincoln was in the Peterson House, after being   544
shot. It gets short shrift because I am not very interested in the events surrounding
and following the shooting. From the moment the bullet entered Lincoln's skull, his
further (brief) existence as a physical organism had only one possible outcome. Lincoln's last hours do illuminate his earlier life in some ways, so this topic cannot be ignored completely, but I have made no attempt to consult the many writings by modern
traumatologists.

Other relevant sections: 545
⟨-⟩ Special Topic §7 reprints first-person accounts of the shooting and subse-   546
quent events. It also includes a reprint of the 1865 medical journal article
[taft] that described Lincoln's last hours.
⟨-⟩ Post-Mortem compiles information from the auopsy and other post-   547
mortem events.

⟨1⟩ Lincoln was moved to Peterson House, across the street from Ford's Theatre, and   548
"laid upon a bed in fifteen minutes from the time the shot was fired" [taft].

⟨2⟩ Eighty-four people [kunhardtB p108] came into the 19-by-17 foot [kunhardtB p48] death-   549
room during the night, many of them physicians (see ¶3222).

⟨2⟩ Lincoln lost blood and brain matter while being carried to the Peterson House.   550
"How much could never be measured," for it was ground into the muddy street.
[kunhardtB p47]

⟨2⟩$_c$ [lattimerAu] concludes that the bullet transected the lateral venous sinus (at the back   551
of the skull). He also notes that Drs Leale and Taft disagreed on which pupil was
dilated, and to what degree.

⟨$\frac{1}{q}$⟩ Lincoln on his death-bed: "The giant sufferer lay extended diagonally across the   552
bed, which was not long enough for him. He had been stripped of his clothes.
His large arms, which were occasionally exposed, were of a size which one would
scarce have expected from his spare appearance. His slow, full respiration lifted
the clothes with each breath that he took. His features were calm and striking. I
had never seen them appear to better advantage that for the first hour, perhaps,
that I was there. After that, his right eye began to swell and that part of his face
became discolored." [welles v2pp286-287]
⟨2⟩ He was too tall for the bed (¶465). Attempts to break off the end of the bed   553
failed [kunhardtB p47].

⟨2⟩ Lincoln's head was placed "on two overhanging pillows, which would soak up   555
blood for several hours at least before they could take no more. Then the red
puddle would begin to form on the worn Brussels carpet below." [kunhardtB p47]

Death Watch (continued)

⟨2⟩ "Hot water bottles were laid along the sides of the President's legs, which had grown cold to a point above the knees. Outsized mustard plasters were placed like clammy pies solidly over the entire upper surface of the body, from ankles to neck." Dr. Leale looked under a corner of the plaster, saw no pinkness of the skin, and ordered a stronger plaster and heated blankets. "Soon Mr. Lincoln lay between walls of bottles and under steaming layers of wool, and clinging to him as though a death mold ... was that hot yellow dough, enfolded in an assortment of cloths." [kunhardtB p49]   557

⟨2⟩ "Leale was annoyed when Dr. Taft tried brandy again, He didn't stop him, but as he said he knew would happen, the President almost strangled. Dr. Stone called for the same remedy later, with the same result." [kunhardtA p357]   558

⟨2⟩ "Dr. Barnes probed the wound" [kunhardtA p358]   559

⟨2⟩ When Senator Charles Sumner and Robert arrived, a physician told Sumner "He's dead." Sumner replied, "No, he isn't dead. Look at his face, he's breathing." When the physician replied "It will never be anything more than this," Robert broke down in tears. [kunhardtB p49] (See ¶4975 for a possibly different story.)   560

⟨2⟩ "snoring, jerky breathing" [kunhardtB p49]   561

⟨1⟩ After 11pm: "His face, lighted by a gas-jet, under which the bed had been moved, was pale and livid. His body already had the rigidity of death. At intervals only the still audible sound of his breathing could be faintly heard, and at intervals again it would be lost entirely." [chambrunA]   562

⟨2⟩ "At 11:30 p.m. a great protrusion of the President's right eye was noted, and for the next twenty minutes there was twitching on the left side of Lincoln's face." [kunhardtB p78]   563

⟨2⟩ "At five minutes before one o'clock he began making a struggling motion with his arms. His chest muscles stiffened, his breath held, and then finally exited as the spasm passed." [kunhardtB p78]   564

⟨1⟩ At about 3 a.m.: "breathing heavily and regularly" [dana p276]   565

⟨1⟩ Just after daylight: "The face of the dying had changed to a more ashy paleness. The dark patch around his right eye had spread. His breathing had become shorter and less labored. That dreadful sound had given place to a kind of wild gurgling. Occasionally for a few seconds it would entirely cease, and I would think that all was over. Then it would resume, and thus these intervals would continue, until at least, after a longer interval than any which had before taken place, the physician who was holding the President's hand whispered – 'This pulse has ceased breathing!' No change whatever took place in the expression of the dead." – a resident of the Peterson house [NYTimes - April 21, 1865]   566

⟨2⟩ Lincoln's breathing in his last moments: To some in the room it was "a deep snoring, a wild gurgling. To others, it had a musical quality, and Stanton likened it to an Aeolian harp. [Some watchers] heard not a sound." [kunhardtB p108]   567

⟨1/q⟩ "His stertorous breathing subsided a couple of minutes after seven o'clock. From then til the end only the gentle rise and fall of his bosom gave indication that life remained. The Surgeon General was near the head of the bed. Sometimes sitting on the edge, his finger on the pulse of the dying man. Occasionally he put his head down to catch the lessening beats of his heart. ... The first indication that   568

63

Death Watch (continued)

the dreaded end had come was at twenty-two minutes past seven, when the Surgeon General gently crossed the pulseless hands of Lincoln across the motionless breast and rose to his feet." – James Tanner [kunhardtA p359] [kunhardtB p80]

⟨2⟩ Rev. Gurley remembered the physician saying "He is gone; he is dead," followed by four or five minutes of absolute silence in the room, broken only by the loud ticking of watches in all the men's pockets [kunhardtB p80].   569

⟨2⟩ Four men claim to have been the one that put coins on Lincoln's eyes. [kunhardtB pp108-109]   570

⟨S⟩ "The mystery, if any, lies in the fact that he was not assassinated sooner than he was." [currentBk p277]   571

⟨S⟩ There is controversy over whose blood stained Mrs. Lincoln's clothing the night of her husband's shooting. "The account which pictures Mrs. Lincoln's dress as covered with blood is incorrect, since no blood flowed from the wound [in Lincoln's head] until the bearers started with the wounded man to the house across the street" [evans p186] citing: W.J. Ferguson. "Lincoln's Death." *Saturday Evening Post.* February 12, 1927.   572

⟨-⟩ *Major Rathbone, also in the Presidential box, had bled profusely after being stabbed by the assassin. See Special Topic §7.*   573

⟨-⟩ *Evans is wrong about the timing of the bleeding. Lincoln bled on Laura Keene's dress while still in the theater (¶3258). Even earlier, Dr. Leale found blood on Lincoln's shoulder just after removing Lincoln from his chair; Mary had been supporting his head, making it likely that blood did get on her clothing* [good pp59-62].   574

■ [eisenschimlC] appears to be on-topic, but should be approached with caution.   575

Diet & Digestion

What with all the references to his yellow skin, could he have had jaundice? Gilbert syndrome? Or a chronic hemolytic anemia causing jaundice? There is no record suggesting scleral icterus, even though there are lots of descriptions of his eyes, so one doubts he was jaundiced.   576

Medullary thyroid cancer (MTC) causes a secretory diarrhea. The historical record is silent on Lincoln's bowel habits in the White House, except that he stopped taking blue mass pills five months after becoming President because they "made him cross" [wilson p631]. [aa144] found, in sporadic MTC, that diarrhea occurred in less than half of patients with stage IV MTC.   577

Medications & Chemicals covers gastrointestinal remedies purchased by Lincoln's household.   578

⟨$\frac{1}{q}$⟩ Pre-1819: "Pore? We was all pore, them days, but the Lincolns was porer than anybody. ... It was all Tom could do to git his fambly enough to eat and to kiver 'em." – Dennis Hanks [wilsonR p21]   579

⟨2⟩ 1819: Lincoln's father left his children at home, under the care of Dennis Hanks, for six months while he searched for a second wife. Lincoln and his sister Sarah "had become almost nude for want of clothes and their stomachs became leathery from the want of food." – related in 1931 by the grandson of a Lincoln family friend [burl p95]   580

■ Favorites: 581

Diet & Digestion (continued)

⟨1⟩ "Mr L was very fond of honey. Whenever he went to S[hort]'s house he invariably asked his wife for some bread & honey. And he liked a great deal of bee bead [sic] in it." – James Short [wilson p90] *"Bee bread" is presumably honeycomb.* 582

⟨2⟩ fond of pears – Phineas Gurley [kunhardtB p72] (See ¶607.) 583

⟨1⟩ "fond of the Good things ... was fond of fruit Nuts" – J. Rowan Herndon [wilson p92] (∈ ¶595) 584

⟨1⟩ "He loved apples better than all Else – strong drink of Coffee – He loved oyesters" – Ward Hill Lamon [wilson p466] 585

⟨1⟩ "Was fond of Pop Corn I remember" – Abner Ellis [wilson p179] 586

- Appetite, pre-Presidency: 587

⟨1⟩ "Abe was a moderate Eater ... he Sat down & ate what was set before him, making no complaint: he seemed Careless about this." – Sarah Bush Lincoln [wilson p108] 588

⟨$\frac{1}{q}$⟩ 1820s-30s: "Abe was a moderate eater and I now have no remembrance of any special dish; he sat down and ate what was set before him, making no complaint. He seemed careless about this. I cooked his meals for nearly 15 years." – Sarah Bush Johnston Lincoln [bumgarnerB] 589

⟨1⟩ Lincoln's family: "thay took of A potato and ate them like apples" – Elizabeth Crawford [wilson p245] 590

⟨1⟩ "When Lincoln, Ab & I returned to the house from work, he would go to the Cupboard – Snatch up a piece of Corn bread – take down a book – Sit down on a chair – Cock his legs up as high as his head and read ... Abrm was a good hearty Eater – loved good Eating." – John Hanks [wilson p455] 591

⟨1⟩ 1830s: "the whole world knows Lincoln was a small feader" – William G. Greene [wilson p33] 592

⟨1⟩ "Mr Lincoln's habits were like himself odd & wholly irregular. He loved nothing and ate mechanically. I have seen him Sit down at the table and never unless recalled to his Senses, would he think of food. He was a peculiar man." – Elizabeth Todd Edwards [wilson p445] 594

⟨1⟩ "he was very fond of Eating and fond of the Good things But only & ordinary Eator Regular to his Meals But was fond of fruit Nuts" – J. Rowan Herndon [wilson p92] 595

⟨1⟩ "Mr Lincoln was what I Call a hearty eater and enjoyed a good meal of victuals as much as enny one I ever knew. I have often heard him say that he could eat corn cakes as fast as two women could make them. although his table at home was usually set very Sparingly." – Harriet Chapman [wilson p512] 596

⟨1⟩ "Was a fast eater, though not a very hearty one." – James Short [wilson p90] 597

⟨1⟩ 1830s: "Abe ate mechanically – very moderately – didn't seem to Care much what was Set before him – So it was clean." – Caleb Cannon, 1866 [wilson p374] 599

⟨1⟩ "He was a hearty Eater" – Ward Hill Lamon [wilson p466] (∈ ¶617) 600

⟨$\frac{1}{q}$⟩ Mary burned dinner (chicken) once because Lincoln arrived home late. Lincoln: "bring on the cinders and see how quickly they will disappear." [randallC p78] 601

⟨1⟩ Pre-Presidency: "he had a good but moderate appetite for food, and was satisfied with almost anything that would satisfy hunger, anything with which 'to fill up.'" – William Herndon [hertz p165] 602

⟨1⟩ "had a good appetite and good digestion, ate mechanically, never asking why such a thing was not on the table nor why it was on it, if so; he filled up and that is all; he never complained of bad food nor praised the good. ... [On the 603

Diet & Digestion (continued)

circuit] he never made any fuss about the food on the table; he ate and went about his business, though the food was 'cussed bad.' " – William Herndon [hertz p166]

⟨1⟩ "he could sit and think without rest or food longer than any man I ever saw." – William Herndon [hertz p196] — 604

⟨1⟩ "He had no expressed fondness for anything, and ate mechanically. I have seen him sit down at the table absorbed in thought, and never, unless recalled to his senses, would he think of food." [herndon p411] (∈ ¶1125) — 605

■ Available foods: — 606
  ⟨1⟩ Thomas Lincoln planted pear trees on the property where Abraham was born [wilson p56]. — 607
  ⟨1⟩ In Indiana: "The Honey Bee Luxuriated on the Prarie flowers and afforded in the Groves a large supply of wild honey" – Dennis Hanks [wilson p27] — 608
  ⟨-⟩ See ¶2081 for the Southern Indiana game animals hunted and eaten during Lincoln's time. — 609

⟨1⟩ 1830s: "eat his meals irregularly ... He was irregular in his habits of eating and Sleeping." – Joshua Speed [wilson p255] — 610

⟨1⟩ 1830s: [shastid] tells a story of Lincoln obliviously and voraciously eating the entire supply of quail placed on the table of a family he was visiting, leaving none for the family. — 611

■ Blue-mass pills and constipation: — 612
  ⟨1⟩ "What Stuart said was this 'Lincoln's digestion was organically defective so that the excreta escaped through skin pores instead of the bowels': and I 'advised him to take Blue Mass and he did take it before he went to Washington & for five months while he was President but when I went to Congress he told me he had quit because it made him cross.' " – Henry Whitney [wilson p631] — 613
  ⟨1⟩ "Stuart told me his liver did not secrete bile – that he had no natural evacuation of bowels &c. That was also a cause [of Lincoln's melancholy] but I beleive [sic] the former [prenatal influences per ¶2607] to be the principal one." – Henry Whitney [wilson p617] — 614
  ⟨2⟩ The quotations above are discussed by: [herndon p473], [shutes pp33-34], and [donaldA p164]. Mysteriously, [kunhardtA p322] quotes "peevish" instead of "cross." A redundant primary source: ¶2613. — 615
  ⟨1⟩ "Lincoln was a vegetable – His skin performed what other organs did for the [sic] He was sluggish – apathetic –" – John T. Stuart [wilson p482] — 616
  ⟨1⟩ "He was a hearty Eater – when hed had no passages he alwys had a sick head ache – Took Blue pills – blue Mass" [sic] – Ward Hill Lamon [wilson p466] — 617
  ⟨1⟩ "Blue-pills were the medicinal remedy which he affected most." [lamonL p475] — 618
  ⟨2⟩ Lincoln's "bowels were ... inactive. It was this that made him look so sad and depressed." – John T. Stuart [weik p112]. *This is Weik's re-wording of ¶614.* — 619
  ⟨2⟩ "Mr. Lincoln had an evacuation, a passage, about once a week, ate blue mass." – William Herndon [hertz p199] *This might be a primary observation.* — 620
  ⟨S⟩ Shutes concludes "Lincoln suffered from chronic constipation more or less all his life, which may explain his fondness for apples." [shutes p35] *I've not seen direct evidence to support the "all his life" claim.* — 621
  ⟨S⟩ A Dr. J.H. Kellogg accepts the opinion of Judge Stuart that "obstinate constipation and the frequent use of large doses of calomel" – which also contains — 622

Diet & Digestion (continued)

inorganic mercury – caused Lincoln's depression [evans p329]. *But see ¶2294 for calomel usage.*

⟨S⟩ [hirschhornC] asserts Lincoln took blue mass for longer than a few months and that melancholy was the indication. *I found no direct evidence for either claim. See ¶2421.* 623

⟨2⟩ Writing in the 1950s, [randallC pp67-68] says "sluggish liver" instead of "constipation." 624

⟨S⟩ [currentNY] and [vidalA] debate Lincoln's bowel habits. *Current's posturing is embarrassing. He seems unaware of the many references to Lincoln's constipation, referring only to the Herndon description (¶620). Current actually states: "Vidal would have us believe that every time Lincoln defecated he reported it to Herndon and Herndon kept a careful record of it."* 625

⟨-⟩ For mental effects, see ¶2419ff. Also see ¶2289ff. 626

- Drug store purchases from Corneau & Diller (also see Medications & Chemicals): 627
  ⟨2⟩c [turnerL] concludes that "The Lincolns *had* purchased carminatives often" and that one of the druggists may have remembered this. 628
  ⟨2⟩c "Remedies for stomach complaints seem to have been very popular with the Lincolns" [hickey] 629

- Poison laxative: 630
  ⟨1⟩ **Fiction:** "One of [the assassination] conspirators tried to poison Lincoln's laxative, which was made up at Thompson's drugstore; whether or not prescription clerk David Herold actually poisoned the medicine is not agreed upon" [vidalA pp691-692]. *This is fiction, literally: Vidal is describing a plot twist in his novel Lincoln. But it is based on a remarkable set of facts, described below.* 631
  ⟨2⟩ David Herold was indeed a co-conspirator in Lincoln's assassination [pitman]. Herold was found guilty, and hanged [kunhardtB]. Lincoln's medicines did indeed come from Thompson's drugstore (¶36). Herold did indeed work there are as a drug clerk [weichmann pp43-44]. After Lincoln's assassination, "There was talk around Washington that ... castor oil ordered from a pharmacy had arrived with deadly poison, but had had too queer a taste to be swallowed" [kunhardtB p5]. There was testimony of a failed plot by the assassin to poison Lincoln in Aug.-Nov. 1864 [pitman pp39-40] [weichmann pp42-44, 63-65]. No one knows if Herold was part of this poisoning plot [weichmann p44]. 632

⟨1⟩ 1832: "I can truly say I was often hungry." – Lincoln, remembering his militia service during the Black Hawk War [herndon p231] See ¶2099 633
  ⟨1⟩ Returning home after the war Lincoln and George Harrison were fed by two men: "... a feast on fish, corn bread, eggs, butter, and coffee ... Of these good things we ate almost immoderately, for it was the only warm meal we had made for several days" – Harrison [wilson p329] 634
  ⟨1⟩ Lincoln's fellow militiamen during the Black Hawk War remarked on the hunger they suffered [wilson pp 554, 556, and others]. 635

⟨1⟩ 1850s: "He never Complained of any food – nor beds – nor lodgings – He once Said at a table – "Well – in the absence of anything to Eat I will jump into this Cabbage." – David Davis [wilson p350] 636
  ⟨1⟩ "Lincoln didnt care what he ate – who who he ate with or where he slept or who he slept with." – Henry C. Whitney [wilson p648] 637

⟨1⟩ 1850s: "... the disregard he had of regular hours for his meal-time" was most noticeable when Mary was away from home. [rankinA p377] 638

Diet & Digestion (continued)

⟨1⟩ As President-elect: In their home the Lincolns served a meal to some campaign workers: "Supper was an old-fashioned mess of indigestion, composed mainly of cake, pies and chickens, the last evidently killed in the morning, to be eaten, as best they might, that evening." [piatt p345]   639

⟨1⟩ Early 1861: "One night every member of the family except the servants, was taken ill, physicians were hastily summoned, and for a time whisperings of 'Poison' were heard, but it proved to be only an over-indulgence in Potomac Shad, a new and tempting dish to western palates." [grimsley] *Potomac shad is a fish.*   640

> ⟨2⟩ The sewer-like "City Canal" (¶2059) flowed into the Potomac in those days [kunhardtB p113]. (See ¶3685.)   641

⟨2⟩ As President, "breakfast consisted of a boiled egg, toast, and coffee. Lunch could be as little as crackers and cheese, or a biscuit and milk, or grapes, or his favorite, a pear. Sometimes, when work piled up, leaving no time for lunch, Lincoln would eat an apple on his way over to the War Department and a second one on his way back. Dinner, taken between five and six o'clock, usually consisted of two courses; but ask Lincoln afterward what they had been and he was at a loss – he ate what was put before him without thinking, without savoring. His drink was water – Adam's ale he called it." [kunhardtA p322]   642

■ As President: 644

> ⟨1/q⟩ When Lincoln "lived in the country at the Soldiers' Home he would be up and dressed, eat his breakfast (which was extremely frugal, an egg, a piece of toast, coffee, etc.), and ride into Washington, all before 8 o'clock." – John Hay, 1866 [wilson p331]   645

> ⟨1⟩ "At noon the President took a little lunch – a biscuit, a glass of milk in winter, some fruit or grapes in summer. He dined at fr. 5 to 6. ... Before dinner was over, members and Senators would come back and take up the whole evening. ... He was very abstemious – ate less than any man I know." – John Hay, 1866 [wilson p331]   646

> ⟨1⟩ "was often summoned as early as five o'clock in the morning to the Cabinet Room and Mrs. Lincoln had repeatedly to send his coffee there, nor would he get his breakfast until nine or ten o'clock. But this soon began to tell upon even his iron constitution, and only repeated protests brought about any degree of regularity." Mary used various subterfuges to get the reluctant Lincoln to the breakfast table. [grimsley] *These observations apply to the first 6 months of Lincoln's Presidency, which included the Ft. Sumter crisis, because Grimsley was thereafter absent.*   647

> ⟨1/q⟩ When food brought to him, "he was often too busy or too abstracted to touch it" – unknown [randallC p303]   649

> ⟨1/q⟩ Mary asks helper Alice Johnstone "to make a dish of fricasseed chicken and small biscuits with thick cream gravy poured over it, all on one platter." Seeing the meal, Lincoln says "Oh, Mary, this is good. It seems like old times come back." Tad reported to Alice that Lincoln "ate three helps and more gravy than you and me and mother could" together. [randallC pp303-304]   650

> ⟨1/q⟩ "The President dines at six o'clock,, and often invites an intimate friend to take pot luck with him..." – Noah Brooks [randallC p286]. *Lincoln had few intimate friends.*   651

> ⟨1⟩ 1865: "...was a hearty eater. He never lost his taste for things a growing farmer's boy would like. He was particularly fond of bacon. Plentiful and   652

Diet & Digestion (continued)

wholesome food was one of the means by which he kept up his strength."
[crookA p15] [crookK]

⟨2⟩ Feb. 1862: Son Willie died on Thursday, Feb. 20 (see ¶2515ff). For the next one or 653
two Thursdays he gave himself over to grief and ate nothing. After some counsel-
ing, he announced "There shall be no more mourning Thursdays" [shutes p82].

⟨1⟩ April 19, 1862: "Another *Lincoln*. Dr. Bellows, apropos of something he said, ad- 654
vised him to take his meals at regular hours. His health was so important to the
country. Abe Lincoln *loquitur*, 'Well, I cannot take my vittles regular. I kind o' just
browze round.' " – George Templeton Strong [strong v3pp217-218]

⟨S⟩ [donaldA p358] says Lincoln had been losing weight around this time, and ex- 655
trapolates to: "He had lost weight because he felt under too much pressures
to eat meals at normal hours." *This extrapolation cannot be supported from
Strong's statement. Nothing is said about mental pressure, and no reason
for Lincoln's "browsing" is given. Given that Strong studiously omitted
Lincoln's "apropos"-causing remark, one might suspect it was an unbe-
coming reference to defecation. It seems like a stretch to say that an
irregular work schedule caused Lincoln's weight loss: he worked at home
and commanded a kitchen staff.*

⟨1⟩ 1862: Lincoln "sent us word that he was eating his breakfast, and would come as 656
soon as he could. His appetite, we were glad to think, must have been a pretty fair
one; for we waited about half an hour..." [hawthorne pp308-309]

⟨1⟩ 1862 or later: Lincoln was "never very attentive to the demands or the attractions 657
of the table. ... When Mrs. Lincoln... was absent from home, the President would
appear to forget that food and drink were needed for his existence, unless he were
persistently followed up by some of the servants, or were finally reminded of his
needs by the actual pangs of hunger. On one such occasion, I remember, he asked
me to come in and take breakfast with him, as he had some questions to ask. He
was evidently eating without noticing what he ate; and when I remarked that he
was different from most western men in his preference for milk for breakfast, he
said, eying his glass of milk with surprise, as if he had not before noticed what he
was drinking, 'Well, I do prefer coffee in the morning, but they don't seem to have
sent me in any.' " [brooksC pp276-277]

⟨2⟩ Mar. 24-25: Lincoln has an upset stomach for at least 24 hours while sailing to City 658
Point, VA. Seasickness and bad drinking water on-ship are suspected causes. Re-
fuses a drink of champagne, saying many people get "sea-sick ashore from drinking that very article" [porterH] (See ¶1261ff, ¶1272.)

⟨1⟩ July 1864 (probably): "I enjoy my rations, and sleep the sleep of the innocent." – 659
Lincoln [riceB p350]

■ March 23-25: Lincoln is unwell during river travel to City Point, VA. Ascribed to 660
the water aboard ship. Family may have been ill, too, on the 23rd. On the 25th,
however, Lincoln "does not look too well." See ¶1261.

⟨1⟩ April 4, 1865: Absent-mindedly eats "at least half a peck" of apples sitting in a bowl 661
on a table in front of him. [crookA p51]

⟨2⟩ April 14, 1865: Even after being called to dinner, Lincoln continues conversing 662
with two Illinois visitors, saying "I'd much rather swap stories than eat" [shenk p210].

Ears

The size and shape of the ears can be a feature of several disorders. For example, the ears project outwards in children with muscular hypotonia [aal p56]. The Beals syndrome [OMIM 121050] includes marfanoid habitus and crumpled-apearing ears, so it is a diagnostic consideration for Lincoln. No overt testimony suggests crumpled ears in any of the Lincolns, but in looking at his photographs, I have not been able to dispel the feeling that there is something unusual about their cartilaginous shape. 663

We should not be surprised that detailed word descriptions of Lincoln's ears are absent: "Ears are not normally important in recognition: identification done for the police using facial mapping have confirmed that, perhaps rather unexpectedly, no one ever really looks at ears provided that they are normal and complete" [aa89 p32]. (Lincoln was apparently not sensitive about his ears – see ¶1864.) 664

- Undated descriptions: 665
  - ⟨1⟩ "His ears were large, and ran out at almost at right angles from his head, caused partly by heavy hats and partly by nature." [herndon p472] 666
  - ⟨1/q⟩ "large ears" – John Nicolay [meserve p5] (∈ ¶177) 667
  - ⟨1/c⟩ As President: "He had very large ears standing off a little, and when he was in good humor I always expected him to flap with them like a good natured elephant." [salmsalm] (∈ ¶190) 668
  - ⟨1⟩ In Volk's 1860 cast of Lincoln's head, the ears are depicted "standing out less at right angles from the head than they did" [rankinA p373] (∈ ¶1938) 669
- ▢ Ironically, a profile photograph best suggests the degree to which his ears projected from his head: [ostendorf #80]. In this view, the front-back length of Lincoln's left ear is clearly very short, which implies that the ear is at a steep angle with respect to the camera. 670
- ▢ Stereo photographs in [zeller] confirm that Lincoln's ears stuck out from his head. A precise angle cannot be determined for either ear, but they seem to both be around 45 degrees. 671
- Modern physician assessments: 672
  - ⟨2⟩ "His ears were large and malformed." [gordon] 673
  - ⟨2/c⟩ "large, thick-lobed" [kempfB p5] 674
- ⟨1/q⟩ About 1835: "big ears" – Nancy Rutledge Prewitt [walsh p42] (∈ ¶102) 675
- ⟨1⟩ May 19, 1860: "the large ears..." [coffinA p173] (∈ ¶157) 676
- ⟨1/q⟩ March 1861: "flapping and wide projecting ears" – William Russell [russell pp37-38] (∈ ¶161) 677
- ⟨1⟩ 1862: "a nose and ears, which have been taken by mistake from a head of twice the size" [dicey v1pp220-221] (∈ ¶179) 678
- ▢ An 1865 photograph [ostendorf #118]) may show a downsloping crease in the lobe of Lincoln's left ear. The ear is out of focus. Interestingly, an 1846 photograph [ostendorf #1]) shows a left ear lobe having a downsloping "pinched in" appearance inferiorly. Thus, it is possible that the "crease" in the 1865 photo is just this pinched-in feature of Lincoln's ear lobes. 679
- ▢ Ears are asymmetrically positioned, vertically and horizontally. See ¶298. 680
- ▢ The length and breadth of the ears have been measured from casts of Lincoln's head [stewart] [shapiro]. The ears are tall. (See ¶1932.) 681
- ▢ Mass in the crura of the anti-helix of the right ear [ostendorf #2, 20, 35, 112, 113]. Best view is [ostendorf #35]. Alternatively, could merely be an unusual shape of the ear cartilage, i.e. a particularly prominent inferior branch of the crura. 682

Endocrine

Based on statements about Lincoln's height, [tripp pp31-32] claims that Lincoln underwent puberty at age 9. This thesis has several major problems: 683

⟨-⟩ Tripp assumes that a pubertal growth spurt caused Lincoln's tallness at age   684
10 (¶481), and does not consider that many other conditions, including Marfan syndrome (and presumably MEN2B) can produce tallness before puberty.

⟨-⟩ Tripp ignores evidence that Lincoln grew fast even as a toddler (¶474).   685

⟨-⟩ Tripp ignores evidence that puts Lincoln's pubertal growth spurt at age 16 or   686
17 (¶487).

⟨-⟩ Tripp treats William Herndon like a primary source, but Herndon did not   687
know Lincoln the youth. When [herndon p25] says Lincoln "shot up" in height at
age 10, this appears to have been a literary construction by Herndon's coauthor, Jesse Weik (¶483).

⟨-⟩ Tripp does not consider that other signs of puberty, e.g. shaving, would have   688
been readily apparent and would have provoked comment if they occurred
at age 9 or 10.

⟨2⟩ [tripp] argues that early puberty helps prove that Lincoln was homosexual.   689
_c_

⟨1⟩ "Tripp felt his date-of-puberty argument was the most-important 'smoking   690
gun' in the whole gay Lincoln arsenal." [nobile] commenting on [tripp]

■ Additional puberty data: 691

⟨2⟩ "Signs of puberty came early to 'Abram' in his eleventh year, according to   692
_c_ Herndon, but probably nearer his twelfth." [shutesE p23] *Seems to be uncritical
acceptance of* [herndon p25]. *See ¶483.*

⟨S⟩ Delayed puberty occurs in 43% of MEN2B [aa164]. *Fits rapid growth at age*   693
16 suggested by ¶487.

■ Cold tolerance: 694

⟨1⟩ Late Feb. 1865: Lincoln complains of persistently cold hands and feet – see   695
_q_ ¶1210.

⟨1⟩ Mar. 28, 1865, visiting Grant's headquarters: "It was a mild spring morning,   696
but he wore an overcoat" and stove-pipe hat [coffinA p179].

⟨2⟩ April 14, 1865: Watching the play in Ford's Theatre: "It was draughty in the   697
box. At a look from Mary, Mr. Lincoln rose from his seat and swung into
his overcoat" [helmB p257]. (The outside temperature had dropped 20 degrees
[kunhardtA p352].)

⟨-⟩ For another temperature-related episode, the "rum sweat," see ¶708.   698

⟨⊙⟩ Lincoln wore gloves while sitting in McClellan's tent at Antietam in Oct. 1862.   699
[ostendorf #66, 67]

⟨2⟩ April 4, 1865: Visits Richmond on a very warm day. Walks from waterfront to Con-   700
federate White House. Perspiration pours from him, even though he had removed
his coat. Finally sitting down, his first words are a request for water. *Some details
of this story suggest heat intolerance.* (See ¶1285.).

⟨1⟩ "He would nurse babies – do anything to accomodate any body" – Hannah Arm-   701
strong [wilson p526] *Unclear what this means. "Nurse" is obviously being used in
a non-lactating sense.*

Energy

This section was a bit of an experiment, meant to isolate references to low (and high) energy states. The experiment began too late to make it's coverage comprehensive. The General and General -- During Presidency sections contain relevant information.   702

⟨1⟩ "He was verry [sic] powerful physically ... I never heard Mr Lincoln complain of being fatigued   I think he was an utter stranger (in the early part of his life at least) to the feeling" – Joseph Gillespie [wilson p186]   703

⟨2⟩ Around his 16th year he was growing so fast that "he was tired all the time, and he showed a notable lack of enthusiasm for physical labor." [donaldA p33] (∈ ¶1109)   704

⟨1⟩ In late teens: "he was quick and moved with Energy: he never idled away his time" – Joseph Richardson [wilson p119]   705

⟨1⟩ "Lincoln was a vegetable – His skin performed what other organs did for the [sic] He was sluggish – apathetic –" – John T. Stuart [wilson p482] *This difficult-to-interpret sentence probably refers to Stuart's theories about Lincoln's constipation – see ¶612*   706

⟨1⟩ September 16-17, 1858: "Lincoln and I were at the Centralia Fair the day after the debate at Jonesboro – night came on and we were tired, having been on the fair ground all day – the train was due at mid-night – everything was full – I managed to get a chair for Lincoln in the Ills. Cen. R.R. Supt. office – but small politicians would intrude so that he could scarcely get a moments sleep – the train came and was filled instantly – I got a seat at the door for L. and myself; he was worn out and had to meet Douglas the next day at Charleston." – Henry C. Whitney [wilson p406]   707

⟨2⟩ October 13, 1858: After the sixth debate against Douglas (in Quincy, IL) Lincoln almost collapsed from exhaustion. Back at his boarding house, Lincoln worried he might have to withdraw from the campaign, as he was "mighty nigh petered out." The house's proprietress, Mrs. George P. Floyd, suggested a "rum sweat" as treatment. Lincoln proclaimed his abstinence, but once assured the rum was for external use only, "he was willing, in his extremity, to take a chance." He was therefore stripped, seated on a cane-bottomed chair, and covered in blankets. A pan of rum was lit, and placed under the chair. "This started a perspiration, after which he was put to bed and the sweating continued under more blankets and with the help of ginger tea. The next morning he appeared bright and early and feeling 'like a two year old,' vociferous with praise for Mrs. Floyd's treatment." Years later, as President, Lincoln encountered Mr. Floyd, saying: "I believe your wife saved my life.... Yes, I have taken that rum sweat that she prescribed for me many times and I have prescribed it for some of my friends. It has always been a dead shot." [shutes pp60-61]   708

    ⟨2⟩ This story has been called "doubtless apocryphal" [turnerL]   709
    ⟨⁻⟩ Original reference is probably [floyd].   710

⟨1⟩ Oct. 1858, after debate series with Douglas, Lincoln was "weary but not exhausted" [arnold p153]   711

⟨1⟩ April 1860: "He gave me on this day a long sitting of more than four hours, and when it concluded, went to our family apartment ... to look at a collection of photographs I had made ... in Rome and Florence. While sitting in the rocking-chair, he took my little son on his lap.... I held the photographs up and explained them to him, but I noticed a growing weariness, and his eyelids closed occasionally as   712

Energy (continued)

if he were sleepy, or were thinking of something besides Grecian and Roman statuary and architecture. Finally he said: 'These things must be very interesting to you, Mr. Volk, but the truth is I don't know much of history, and all I do know of it I have learned from law-books.' " [volk] *Although poor Lincoln was undoubtedly bored, boredom will not lead to sleep unless there is also a sleep debt.*

⟨2⟩ Lincoln while President-elect: 713

    ⟨2⟩ "Vigorous and athletic, he loped along in his countryman's gait at a pace that 714
tired out companions twenty years younger, and he bounded up stairways two or three steps at a time. His energy seemed inexhaustable." [donaldA p259] (See ¶1090.) *The data are too thin to allow a conclusion of inexhaustable energy.*

    ⟨1⟩ July 1860: At Lincoln's home: "Mr L. came tripping down the Stairs, as lively 715
as a young man of sixteen years of age – sliding his right hand on the bannister" – John Bliss [wilson p551]

    ⟨2⟩ After his election he held an open house each morning at the State Capitol 716
until he was "exhausted by the public" and trimmed it to 90 minutes a day. [kunhardtA p133]

    ⟨1⟩ At the State Capitol: "He appeared daily, except Sundays, between nine and 717
ten o clock, and held a reception till noon, to which all comers were admitted... At noon, he went home to dinner and reappeared at about two. Then his correspondence was given proper attention, and visitors of distinction were seen by special appointment... In the evening, old friends called at his home for the exchange of news and political views. At times, when important news was expected, he would go to the telegraph or newspaper offices after supper, and stay there till late. Altogether, probably no other President-elect was as approachable for everybody, at least during the first weeks of my stay. But he found in the end, as was to be expected, that this popular practice involved a good deal of fatigue, and that he needed more time for himself; and the hours he gave up to the public were gradually restricted." [villardM v1p142]

    ■ Feb. 1861: Lincoln travels by rail from Springfield to Washington, under constant 718
heavy guard. During at least one or two points in the trip he appeared fatigued. See ¶3474.

⟨2⟩_c "Lincoln worked harder than almost any other American President." [donaldA p310] 719

⟨1⟩_q April 1862, during Shiloh battle: "I called on Lincoln at eleven o'clock at night and 720
sat with him alone until after one o'clock in the morning. He was, as usual, worn out with the day's exacting duties." – A.K. McClure [angle p401]

⟨1⟩ Spring 1862: "had just come from a cabinet meeting and looked worn and wea- 721
ried" [bancroft] (∈ ¶182)

⟨1⟩ June 30, 1862: Secretary of War Stanton defers referring a matter to Lincoln that 722
evening, who has "gone to the country, very tired" [baslerA v5p295]

⟨2⟩ Aug. 1862: During the Second Battle of Bull Run (August 28-30, 1862) Lincoln was 723
"Exhausted from long hours spent in the telegraph office." [donaldA p371] Part of ¶2638

⟨1⟩ Spring 1863: From time to time he took a poor excuse for a vacation by visiting 724
the Army of the Potomac in the field [currentBk pp63-64]. On one visit, he seemed to be somewhat revived and rested. When a friend mentioned this, Lincoln replied:

Energy (continued)

"Well, yes, I do feel some better, I think; but, somehow, it don't appear to touch the tired spot, which can't be got at." [brooksR]

⟨2⟩ Brooks gives a different version of the remark in [angle p396].   725

⟨1⟩ "All familiar with him will remember the weary air which became habitual   726
during his last years. This was more of the mind that the body, and no rest
and recreation which he allowed himself could relieve it. As he sometimes
expressed it, the remedy 'seemed never to reach the *tired* spot.' " [carpenter
p217] *I am guessing Carpenter copied this from Brooks.*

⟨1⟩ "Speaking of the exhaustive demands upon him, which left him in no condition   727
for more important duties, he said, 'I sometimes fancy that every one of the numerous grist ground through here daily, from a Senator seeking a war with France
down to a poor woman after a place in the Treasury Department, darted at me
with thumb and finger, picked out their especial piece of my vitality, and carried
it off. When I get through with such a day's work, there is only one word which
can express my condition and that is – *flabbiness.*' " – Lincoln, quoted by [brooksR]

⟨2⟩ "The patient thoroughness he lavished on his appointments has inspired   728
many reminiscences. 'What's the matter?' a friend asked in alarm, coming
upon him sad and depressed. 'Have you bad news from the army?' 'No, it
isn't the army,' he replied with one of his weary, humorous smiles. 'It's the
post-office at Brownsville, Missouri.' " [angle p369] excerpting Helen Nicolay

⟨2⟩ June 1864: "Tired and sunburned" after visiting the troops at City Point, Virginia   729
(near Petersburg) for two days [donaldA p516]

⟨2⟩ Jan. 1, 1865: "The reception had been unusually well attended, and the President   730
was nearly overcome with fatigue." When seeing certain visitors, "he rallied from
his fatigue and gave them a hearty welcome." [browneF p677]

⟨2⟩ For a few days after his second inaugural Lincoln took to his bed, exhausted (see   731
¶1255). "He continued to be a physically powerful man, but he often felt terribly
tired." [donaldA p568]

⟨1/q⟩ April 1865: Visit to a military hospital, "although a labor of love, to him, fatigued   732
him very much." – Mary Lincoln [turner p217] (∈ ¶1312)

⟨2/c⟩ April 1865: "In early April every effort seemed to exhaust the President." [randallC   733
p339]

⟨2⟩ April 14, 1865: "But with all his lightness of spirit, Lincoln was still tired and worn-   734
out. He complained of it at the table but thought a good laugh at the comedy [at
Ford's Theatre] might help." [randallC p343]

Eyes

To simplify information retrieval, the sum-total description of his eyes is divided into   735
sections. Note: I have not tabulated the references to his eye-twinkle (e.g. [french p374]).

- For eyebrows, see [Hair]. For drooping eyelids, see ¶899ff.   736

⟨1⟩ As President: "His eyes slightly receded, were about normal in size and, according   737
to my recollection gray in color – with no marked expresssion, except pensiveness
and truthfulness." – Senator James Harlan [helmB p166] (∈ ¶173)

⟨1⟩ The only non-traumatic skull finding at autopsy was "orbital plates very thin" [lat-   738
timerAu].

Eyes (continued)

🔲 Lincoln's eyes *appear* to be narrowly spaced. The famous Alexander Gardner full-face photograph of Lincoln ([ostendorf #77], shows otherwise. It shows eyes spaced just under one eye-width apart, which is normal. Spacing of more than an eye-width is an informal definition for hypertelorism (wide spacing of the eyes) [aa1 pp62-63, 69]. (Lincoln's eyeglasses, however, provide some evidence for narrowly-separated eyes and allow measurement of inter-pupillary disrance ¶804.)   739

- Depth of seating: 740
  - ⟨1⟩ "His eyes slightly receded" – Senator James Harlan [helmB p166] (∈ ¶173)   741
  - ⟨1⟩ May 19, 1860: "the deep-set eyes..." [coffinA p173] (∈ ¶157)   742
  - ⟨1/q⟩ March 1861: "the eyes dark, full, and deeply set" – William Russell [russell pp37-38] (∈ ¶161)   743
  - ⟨1⟩ "large and deep eye-caverns" – John Nicolay [meserve p5] (∈ ¶177)   744
  - ⟨1⟩ "rather deep-set eyes" [conant] (∈ ¶834)   745
  - ⟨1⟩ Lincoln always sat on the east side of the long table in the middle of the Lincoln-Herndon law office. Herndon sat opposite him. "About one o'clock in the daytime the sun, especially in the summer, streamed through the western windows in our office and flooded Lincoln's face, so that I could see to the very back part of his eyes." – William Herndon [hertz p263] *The implication is that it was otherwise difficult to see to the back of Lincoln's eyes.*   746
  - ⟨2⟩ "... his eyes small and deeply placed in his head" [gordon]   747
  - ⟨1⟩ Nov. 18, 1863: "He was looking very badly... sunken-eyed" [cochrane] (∈ ¶2535)   748
  - ⟨1⟩ April 1865: "eyes sunken under thick eyebrows, and as though encircled by deep and dark wrinkles" [chambrunA] (∈ ¶200)   749

- Size: 750
  - ⟨1⟩ As President: "rather small and somewhat tired-looking eyes" [salmsalm p144] (∈ ¶190)   751
  - ⟨1⟩ As President: "were about normal in size" – Senator James Harlan [helmB p166] (∈ ¶173)   752

- Tears: 753
  - ⟨-⟩ *I did not carefully gather descriptions until late.*   754
  - ⟨1/q⟩ 1828: Upon learning his sister had died, "The tears trickled through his large fingers" – Captain J.W. Lamar [hobson p24] (∈ ¶2438)   755
  - ⟨1/q⟩ At age 38 Lincoln described his "old, withered, dry eyes" [burl p74] *This statement may have been made in a self-deprecating or poetic way, rather than being a strict medical report. See ¶1754.*   756
  - ⟨1⟩ April 1860: Before Leonard Volk casts Lincoln's head, a joke makes tears trickle down Lincoln's cheeks. Later, removing the plaster cast from his head – taking some hairs with it – "made his eyes water." [volk]   757
  - ⟨-⟩ See also: ¶1154, ¶2500, ¶2512, ¶2648.   758

- Expression: 759
  - ⟨1⟩ Oct. 13, 1858: "benignant, melancholy eyes" – Carl Schurz [angle p243] (∈ ¶149)   760
  - ⟨1/q⟩ 1859: "the thing that impressed me most of all in regard to Abraham Lincoln was the extreme sadness of his eyes. Lincoln had the saddest eyes of any human being that I had ever seen." – John Widmer [shenk p155] (∈ ¶150)   761
  - ⟨1⟩ May 19, 1860: "the deep-set eyes, sparkling with humor..." [coffinA p173] (∈ ¶157)   762
  - ⟨1/q⟩ June 21, 1860: "a pair of eyes that seemed to say 'make yourself at home' " – Utica newspaper reporter [lincloreHDE] (∈ ¶159)   763

Eyes (continued)

⟨1⟩ April 12, 1861: "deep, dark circles under his eyes and they were vacant." [stod-dardD p221]   764

⟨1⟩ Spring 1862: Eyes were "clear, calm, and honest, yet piercing and searching" [bancroft] (∈ ¶182)   765

⟨1⟩ "His eyes – surely the saddest and most solemn that ever looked on the wars of a sorrowing world" [riddle p330]   766

⟨1⟩ "his eyes dark grey, clear, very expressive, and varying with every mood ... at times with that almost superhuman sadness which it has been said is the sign and seal of those who are to be martyrs." [arnold p441] (∈ ¶167)   767

⟨1⟩ 1862: "bright, somewhat dreamy eyes, that seemed to gaze through you without looking at you" [dicey v1pp220-221] (∈ ¶179)   768

⟨1⟩ As President: "his rather small and somewhat tired-looking eyes" [salmsalm p144] (∈ ¶190)   769

⟨1⟩ Mid 1863: "drooping eyelids, looking almost swollen; the dark bags beneath the eyes; the deep marks about the large and expressive mouth." – Silas Burt [wilsonR p332] (∈ ¶1621)   770

   ⌐o⌐ See Figure 5.   771

■ Bags / rings under the eyes: 772

  ⟨1⟩ April 12, 1861: "deep, dark circles under his eyes and they were vacant." [stod-dardD p221]   773

  ⟨1⟩ Mid 1863: "the dark bags beneath the eyes" – Silas Burt [wilsonR p332] (∈ ¶770)   774

  ⟨1⟩ May 1864: "During the first week of the battles of the Wilderness he scarcely slept at all ... great black rings under his eyes" [carpenter p30] (∈ ¶2657)   775

  ⟨1⟩ About 1864: "ugly black rings appeared under his eyes" [croffut] (∈ ¶196)   776

  ⟨1⟩ April 1865: "gray-brown eyes sunken under thick eyebrows, and as though encircled by deep and dark wrinkles" [chambrunA] (∈ ¶200)   777

■ Masses: 778

  ⌐o⌐ Left eye: Several photographs give a hint – usually nothing more than that – of a white lesion bordering the iris at about the 7 o'clock position (i.e., infero-omedial). In most cases a magnifying glass is required to see it. See: [mellon pp11 (and 79), 19, 24, 26, 29, 31, 33, not 34, 39, not 45, 49, not 57, 73, 80, 81, 89, 103!, 134? but yes on 137, not 148-149, 157, not 159, 161?, 165, 174, not 175]. It is subtle to the point that its existence would be doubtful if it weren't visible in so many photographs. The best view of the lesion, by far, is [ostendorf #57] as printed in [mellon p103], which, when combined with the multiple other sightings, clearly establishes its existence.   779

  ⌐o⌐ Right upper eyelid: Lateral mass is best seen in Library of Congress print LC-USZ62-13016 of [ostendorf #77]. Also present in [mellon p47] and, less well, in [mellon pp4, 10]. Possible additional sightings: [mellon pp15, 66, 71]. Could be a conjunctival mass.   780

  ⌐o⌐ Left upper eyelid: Medial mass is best seen in the National Archives print 121-BA-6867 of [ostendorf #77]. Possibly seen in [mellon p148]. Could be a conjunctival mass.   781

Eyes – Acuity

Myopia is a hallmark of Marfan syndrome not associated with Loeys-Dietz syndrome [aa67].   782

■ For discussion of reading and headaches, see ¶1888ff.   783

Eyes – Acuity (continued)

⟨1⟩ March 1831: Guided a flatboat from Illinois to New Orleans. Having "a good pair of eyes and a good memory," he saw navigational hazards (e.g. "snags, sandbars, overhanging trees") and remembered them. This secured him a job as a steamboat pilot the next year. [rossH p110]   784

⟨1/q⟩ "I sold Abraham Lincoln his first pair of spectacles. It was about the time of the legislature in 1854, when he was a lawyer in Springfield. Some editor down there paid me $15.00 to make Mr. Lincoln a pair of gold spectacles; and those were the first he ever wore. When he was elected President I made him three pairs, one of gold and two of steel." – a Chicago oculist quoted in the [ChicagoTribune - 1883] "whom we have been unable to identify" [lincloreLFH]   785

⟨2⟩ Possible identities are Lewis Mauss, John Phillips, Isom T. Underwood. [lincloreLFH]   786

- The Bloomington eyeglasses: 787
  ⟨1⟩ "He bought his first pair of spectacles at a little shop in Bloomington in May '56 – gave 37 $^1/_2$ [cents] for them" – Henry Whitney [wilson p631].   788
  ⟨1/q⟩ He was 47 years old and "kinder" needed them [donaldA p191] (citing [whitney]).   789
  ⟨2⟩ A few weeks later he used eyeglasses while reading a speech [myers].   790

- The "Barrett" Chicago eyeglasses: 791
  ⟨1⟩ Two 1932 letters from famed Lincoln collector Oliver Barrett, now in [shutesP], relate to a pair of eyeglasses in his collection of Lincoln artifacts. Barrett describes taking the glasses to a Chicago optometrist, Almer Coe, "who examined the glasses and he wrote ... 'Plus 675 Sph. bi-convex O.K. ...' He said there was no question about the matter."   792
  ⟨2⟩ Barrett spectacles: "There is no proof that they were Lincoln's, or how or from whom [Barrett] obtained them." [shutesE p198]   794
  ⟨2⟩ [borittA] states that the authenticity of the high-diopter glasses is uncertain.   795
  ⟨2/c⟩ [shutes p65] says the strength of these glasses was far beyond the 2.5 diopters normal eyes need for reading past the age of 50.   796
  ⟨S⟩ [shutes p65] concludes that Lincoln had "a high degree of hyperopia" (farsightedness) that would have had been associated with symptomatic eyestrain.   797
  ⟨S⟩ "The glasses were apparently intended to aid him in reading small print, and were at least three times stronger than what he actually would have needed." [bumgarnerB]   798
  ⟨-⟩ [shutes p65] *and* [bumgarnerB] *assume the glasses were (a) Lincoln's, and (b) properly refracted. The contents of Lincoln's pockets on the night of his murder included two pairs of eyeglasses with a much different refraction. (See ¶801ff.)*   799
  ⟨2⟩ There is a pair of eyeglasses in the Chicago Historical Society having spherical powers of +6.50D. "We don't know when they were purchased or how long or if they were used by the President." [myers]. *Are these the Barrett glasses?*   800

- Ford's Theatre eyeglasses: 801
  ⟨2⟩ As Lincoln was dying, the contents of his pockets were sealed in a small box that was not opened until spring 1976. Inside were two pairs of eyeglasses (with cases) and a lens cleaner. They are shown in [myers].   802
  ⟨1⟩ Pair #1 "contained equal spherical lenses of +1.75D. Their front surfaces clocked +3.75D while their back surfaces clocked -2.5D. Lens dimensions were 26mm by 34mm and the BDL was 29mm. The nosebridge width was   803

Eyes – Acuity (continued)

18mm and the temples consisted of a front 80mm segment and a sliding posterior 75mm segment. The temples' hinges on both sides were loose although all screws were still tightly in place. ... The lens optical centers coincided with their geometrical centers. Engraved on the inside surface of the right temple was 'J. Philips,' presumably the manufacturer while on the inside portion of the posterior sliding temple was inscribed 'A. Lincoln, presented by Ward H. Lamon.' Their case was stamped 'Franklin & Company – Opticians – Washington, D.C.'" [myers]

⟨1⟩ Pair #2 "fold in the middle of the nosepiece so that they fit inside their silver case.... The temples are half-length. These are reading glasses, also, containing spherical +2.00D lenses 24mm by 33mm with front surface powers of +4.62D and back surface powers of -3.00. The DBL [distance between lenses] was 26mm, the width of the bridge 18mm and the length of the temples 46mm. Optical centers were at the geometrical centers and the PD [pupillary distance] was approximately 60mm; in keeping with the President's narrow face and close set eyes." [myers] (But see ¶739 for more on eye-spacing.)   804

⟨2⟩c "It appears President Lincoln required reading glasses of a power appropriate to his age of 56. The folding pair of +2.00 sphere O.U. were most likely the newer pair. Although my lens clock and lensometer were checked prior to the inspection the clock showed about 0.50D less power per lens than the lensometer. Since the latter's reading depends on the actual refractive action of the measured lens, while the former is based on measured curvature and an assumed index, it appears the lenses may have been made from glass having an index of refraction less than today's ophthalmic glass." [myers]   805

⟨1⟩ The collection of Louise Taper included a pair of Lincoln's reading glasses [ferguson p133]   806

- Any clinical analysis of Lincoln's visual acuity in later life must address the wide difference between the Chicago and Ford's Theatre eyeglasses.   807
  ⟨S⟩ [myers] cannot devise a physiological explanation. In the end he ignores the Chicago pair and concludes Lincoln "may have only required the reading glasses normal for a man of his age."   808

⟨1/q⟩ Fall 1856: James W. Somers remembers when Lincoln, "for the first time, used spectacles; apologizing to his audience, saying he was not as young as he used to be. This was, I think, in the fall of 1856." [lincloreLFH]   809

⟨1/q⟩ July 10, 1858: Giving a speech, Lincoln declines audience requests to read certain other remarks, saying: "Gentlemen reading from speeches is a very tedious business, particularly for an old man that has to put on spectacles, and the more so if the man be so tall that he has to bend over to the light." [lincloreLFH]   810

⟨1/q⟩ Aug. 21, 1858: As Lincoln prepares to read some remarks, a member of the audience at the first Lincoln-Douglas debate shouts: "Put on your specs." Lincoln's reply brought laughter: "Yes, sir, I am obliged to do so; I am no longer a young man." [lincloreLFH]   811

⟨2⟩ Feb. 1860: Lincoln: "Permit me to, fellow citizens, to read the tariff plank of the Chicago platform, or rather, to have it read in your hearing by someone who has younger eyes than I have." His secretary, John Nicolay, read the less-than-100-word passage. [lincloreLFH]   812

☐ May 9, 1860: The first photograph in which the cord to Lincoln's spectacles is clearly visible is [ostendorf #19] [ostendorfA p40]. The cord is also visible in [ostendorf #20   813

Eyes – Acuity (continued)

and 21], taken May 20, 1860 [ostendorfA p43]. There is no spectacle cord in [ostendorf #23], taken May 24, 1860 [ostendorfA p45].

⬚ "There is but one original photograph of Abraham Lincoln showing him wearing spectacles" [lincloreLFH]. It is [ostendorf #93]. *There are other photos, but they lack detail.*   814

⟨1⟩ Sept. 4, 1861, in the White House: "We ... looked at the opposite shores of the river through his glass, which he adjusted for me." [french p374] *Would be interesting to know French's visual acuity.*   815

⟨1⟩ Spring 1862, working in his office: "a pair of short-shanked gold spectacles sat low down upon his nose, the shanks catching the temples, and he cold easily look over them if he so desired." [bancroft] (∈ ¶182)   816

⟨1⟩ Feb. 1865: Lincoln sews with needle and thread, but [crookA p14] does not mention wear of eyeglasses.   817

⟨2⟩ Lincoln fired experimental weapons during the Civil War with impressive accuracy [lattimerNY]. *This implies his distant visual acuity was good – or better. It is not recorded whether he wore his spectacles while shooting.*   818

- Wearing reading glasses: 819
  ⟨2⟩ Mar. 4, 1861: while delivering his (first) inaugural address [kunhardtA p26]   820
  ⟨1⟩ Dec. 1864: wears reading spectacles [brooksC p299]   821
  ⟨2⟩ Mar. 4, 1865: wore steel-framed spectacles while delivering (second) inaugural address [shenk p173]   822

⟨2⟩ After he was shot, Lincoln's gold-rimmed eyeglasses were found in the street outside Ford's Theatre and thereafter taken to New Hampshire [kunhardtB p99]. *This seems unlikely, as it would be the third pair of eyeglasses Lincoln was carrying that night.*   823

Eyes – Color Of

It was once believed that "the sclerae may be impressively blue" in Marfan syndrome [mckusickA p56]. The more recent view is that blue sclerae are not associated with Marfan syndrome [aa67], while 40% of patients with Loeys-Dietz syndrome have blue sclerae [aa68].   824

Given the many descriptions of Lincoln's iris color, we can be confident that, had he possessed blue sclerae, someone would have noticed and written about it.   825

⟨1⟩ 1834: "His eyes were a bluish brown" – Robert Wilson [wilson p202] (∈ ¶101)   826

⟨1⟩ "His little gray eyes flashed in a face aglow with the fire of his profound thoughts" [herndon p333] Part of ¶1122   827

⟨$\frac{1}{q}$⟩ "soft, tender, bluish eyes" – Elliott Herndon [herndon p470n]   828

⟨1⟩ June 1858: "his beaming dark, dull eyes" [volk]   829

⟨$\frac{1}{q}$⟩ Aug. 1858: "His eyes were bright, keen, and a luminous gray color" – Martin Rindlaub [ostendorfA p19] (∈ ¶148)   830

⟨$\frac{1}{q}$⟩ March 1861: "the eyes dark, full, and deeply set" – William Russell [russell pp37-38] (∈ ¶161)   831

- Portrait painters' opinions: 832

Eyes – Color Of (continued)

⟨1⟩ 1864: "His eyes were blueish-gray in color, – always in deep shadow, however, from the upper lids, which were unusually heavy." [carpenter p218] **833**

⟨1⟩ "His bushy, overhanging brows caused a famous sculptor to speak of his rather deep-set eyes as 'dark.' But close observation revealed them a heavenly blue." [conant] **834**

⟨1⟩ Of Tad, Mary wrote, on Dec. 29, 1869: "His dark loving eyes – watching over me, remind me so much of his dearly beloved father's." [turner p32] **835**

⟨1/q⟩ "grey eyes" – part of Lincoln's self-description in December 1859 [donaldA p237] (∈ ¶151) **836**

⟨1⟩ "gray in color" – Senator James Harlan (date of recollection unknown) [helmB p166] Part of ¶173 **837**

⟨1⟩ April 4, 1865: "kind blue eyes over which the lids half drooped" [barnesB] (∈ ¶1286) **838**

⟨1⟩ April 1865: "gray-brown eyes" [chambrunA] (∈ ¶200) **839**

⟨1⟩ "I would say, that the eyes of Prest. Lincoln, were of blueish grey or rather greyish blue; for, without being *positive*, the blue ray was always visible." – Edward Dalton Marchant, 1866. Typewritten transcript is in [randallP box 15]. Original is perhaps in Library of Boston Athenaeum. **840**

⟨2⟩ "Lincoln's eyes were gray, and that color, and other dark hues, predominated in his family. In contrast, Marfan eyes are light" [borittA, citing: Ramsey MS, et al. The Marfan syndrome: a histopathologic study of ocular findings. Am J Ophthalmol. 1973; 76: 102-116]. *This claim about eye color in Marfan syndrome does not seem worth pursuing.* **841**

Eyes – Color Vision

The idea that Lincoln had defective color vision began with the speculation of [shastid] in 1929. Although Shastid was an "oculist," his speculation is based on (a) hopelessly indirect evidence, which he then mis-interprets, and (b) a profound misunderstanding of subnormal color vision. **842**

There is no way to rule out the possibility that Lincoln was one of the approximately 10% of men with sub-normal color vision. But I reject [shastid]'s speculation and conclude there is no evidence whatsoever that Lincoln's color vision was abnormal. **843**

⟨1⟩ [shastid] writes: "To my grandmother, who once wished to show him the flowers in her front yard, he said: 'I will look at your flowers, mother, but I really cannot understand what people see to admire in such things. I am somehow deficient.' " **844**

⟨S⟩ [shastid] continues: "From this I have often suspected that Lincoln was colorblind. He would often enough, in conversation and in public speeches, refer to the sunset, the flowers, and so on, but only, as it seemed, because these matters appeared beautiful to others." [shastid] *There is no support for a claim that sub-normal color vision prevents appreciation of beautiful flowers and sunsets. There have been color deficient painters and no one would deny that the black and white photographs of Ansel Adams are beautiful. The impact of color vision deficiencies on everyday perception is almost nil in pre-industrial societies. How else could one explain that color vision deficiencies were not described until John Dalton's writings in 1794 – about 4000 years after people started writing [aa58]?* **845**

⟨S⟩ [shutes pp70-71] is skeptical, saying: "It was Lincoln's habit to consider himself deficient in many ways, but it is probable that he meant esthetically and not **846**

Eyes – Color Vision (continued)

physiologically deficient." Shutes identifies [shastid] as the originator of the color vision theory.

- Other medical authors have picked up on [shastid]'s speculation: 847
  - ⟨2⟩ "There is also indirect evidence that Lincoln was colorblind." [adelson]   848
  - ⟨2⟩ "Lincoln was also color blind. He was unable to enjoy the sight of beautiful flowers or the colorful clothes that his wife wore." [bumgarnerA p95]   849
  - ⟨2⟩ "Lincoln also knew that he was color-blind, unable to enjoy the colorful blooms in the White House garden." [marx]   850

- Lincoln and flowers: 851
  - ⟨1⟩ "I don't care for flowers – have no natural or Educated taste for Such things" – ascribed to Lincoln, most likely in 1840s or 1850s, by Elizabeth Todd Edwards [wilson p445]   852
  - ⟨1⟩ "he did not it seems Care for Such things" – James Gourley [wilson p453]   853
  - ⟨1⟩ "I never knew him to make a garden, yet no one loved flowers better than he did." – Harriet Chapman [wilson p513]   854
  - ⟨-⟩ More about Lincoln and plants in ¶2052   855

⟨2⟩ Lincoln's color perception was sufficient for him to bestow the nickname "Old Blue-Nose Crawford" on a neighbor [shutes pp5-6]. (See ¶3158.)   856

⟨2⟩ Lincoln's description "of colors in the scene of an Indian massacre ... indicate that his perception of colors was not entirely deficient." [kempfB p14]   857

⟨1/q⟩ Lincoln notices that the posies in Mary's dress fabric matches her eyes. Mary writes her half-sister: "You see, Emilie, I am training my husband to see color. I do not think he knew pink from blue when I married him." [randallC pp83-84]   858

Eyes – Lens

Dislocation of the lenses (ectopia lentis) is a hallmark of Marfan syndrome not associated with Loeys-Dietz syndrome [aa67] or MEN2B.   859

⟨s⟩ Lattimer [lattimerNY] believes Lincoln's rough and tumble youth (which included a protracted period of unconsciousness after being kicked in the head by a horse – ¶3568) would certainly have lead to dislocation of the lens if Lincoln had Marfan syndrome. Lincoln also test-fired experimental weapons during the Civil War, which likely would have applied concussive jolts to his body [lattimerNY]. *Dislocation of the lens in Marfan syndrome is not associated with trauma* [aa74 p724].   860

⟨2⟩ [aa74 p708] says iridodonesis is linked with ectopia lentis. It is theoretically possible that an extraordinarily perceptive observer could, with the naked eye, see this in Lincoln, but of course it has not been recorded.   861

Eyes – Motor

Lincoln had three issues relating to the movement of his eyes and/or their appendages.   862
  - His left eye would intermittently turn upwards (i.e., an "intermittent left hypertropia"). Although well-documented in photographs, some scholars claim (untenably) that this is illusory (¶881ff).   863
  - Lincoln had rare, but definite, episodes of double vision (¶906ff).   864

Eyes – Motor (continued)

- Lincoln appeared to have intermittent ptosis (drooping of the eyelid) (¶899ff), usually, but not always, affecting the right eyelid. The explanation for this probably rests with Lincoln's generally low muscle tone (see `Muscle Energy`).   865

Much has been written about Lincoln's hypertropia. Based on the particulars of the double-vision events and the appearance of the hypertropia, [goldsteinJ] very reasonably concludes that Lincoln had impairment of the left superior oblique muscle (LSO). This implies damage to the trochlear nerve (cranial nerve IV). Trauma is the most common cause of trochlear nerve palsy – especially blunt frontal injury to the head [aa64 p424]. Thus, one reasonable explanation for Lincoln's misaligned eyes is the horse-kick that knocked him unconscious at age 9 (Special Topic §1). Lincoln's facial asymmetry is another very reasonable explanation. Over the years, the hypertropia has been explained in many ways (¶889ff).   866

Physicians have proposed several consequences of the hypertropia (¶884ff), some rather fantastic and some, like his habitual head tilt to the right (¶1827), quite sensible.   867

The pathophysiology of Lincoln's eye deviation and head tilt can be gleaned from [aa64 pp386-387, 407-409, 424-425, 581-583].   868

- Left hypertropia, observations: 869
  - ⟨1⟩ "... the left eye, from time to time, looked queer and then suddenly 'crossed,' i.e., turned up. ... my father told me this" – Thomas Shastid [shastid]   870
  - ⟨1⟩ At the climactic moment of a trial: "Lincoln rose, turned, and his left eye went up, as it often did in moments of excitement." [shastid]   871
  - ⟨S⟩ "Lincoln had been the victim of hyperphoria (a *tendency* of one eye upward) with, now and then, a momentary hypertropia (actual *turning* of one eye upward)." – [shastid]   872
  - ⟨1⟩ "... a peculiarity of one eye, the pupil of which had a tendency to turn or roll slightly toward the upper lid, whereas the other one maintained its normal position, equidistant between the upper and lower lids." – Herndon [shutes p67]   873
  - ⟨2⟩ 1858, during Lincoln-Douglas debates: "newspapermen wrote of his wildly rolling eye." [snyder]   874
  - ⟨2⟩ "his weak right [sic] eye wandered" [kunhardtA p9] (∈ ¶176)   875
  - ⟨⊙⟩ A "vertical strabismus of the left eye is apparent in a photograph [schwartzA] referring to one of [randallA p33 and facing p239]   876
  - ⟨⊙⟩ Photographs showing ocular misalignment: Nov. 25, 1860 [kunhardtA p12]   877
  - ⟨2⟩ Estimates "six or eight degrees of left hyperphoria" [mitchell]   878
  - ⟨2⟩ "left eye was directed upward 8 to 10 degrees" [snyder]   879
  - ⟨2⟩c "The left eye in the best frontal photographs is shown definitely to be out of focus and turned reflexly slightly upward and outward. This effect is due to the inferior oblique muscle of the eye being stronger than the weakened superior oblique which turns the eye inward and downward. Lincoln's right eye functioned normally and dominantly for general vision and reading." [kempfB p9] (See ¶278.)   880

- Left hypertropia, doubters: 881
  - ⟨S⟩ [shutes p71] thinks hypertropia more apparent than real, ie, due to sag of eyelid.   882
  - ⟨2⟩c [lattimerNY] calls Lincoln's ocular misalignment "occasional ... slight ... questionable."   883

Eyes – Motor (continued)

- Consequences of left hypertropia:　　　　　　　　　　　　　　　　　884
  - ⟨2⟩_c Caused Lincoln's habitual head tilt to the right (¶1827) – a "Bielschowsky 　885
    tilt." [goldsteinJ]
  - ⟨1⟩_q "The look of gloom and sadness so often noted in the many descriptions of 　886
    his countenance was more or less accentuated by" the ocular deviation. –
    Herndon [shutes p67]
  - ⟨s⟩ Hyperphoria and hypertropia yield "an intense form of eyestrain and is one 　887
    of the commonest causes of deep and protracted melancholy – the chronic
    inexpressible blues. Here, then, was the probable explanation of the well-
    known Lincolnian depression of spirits which lasted, off and on, until his
    death." [shastid] *I am not aware of any modern support for thinking hyper-
    phoria leads to depression, unless one believes a tenuous chain such as:
    hyperphoria leads to chronic eyestrain which leads to chronic headaches
    which leads to depression.*
  - ⟨2⟩_c "Lincoln's right eye was dominant and was always used for general vision 　888
    and no doubt entirely for reading. The tendency of the left eye to turn up-
    ward and outward produced more or less of an overlapping of visual images.
    The upward deviation of the left eye was certainly great enough to produce a
    lack of fusion of its image with that of the right eye. ... he reacted attentively
    to the image of the right eye and ignored that of the left eye." [snyder]

- Etiological hypotheses for left hypertropia:　　　　　　　　　　　　　889
  - ⟨s⟩ "may have been caused by an uncorrected refractive error and the use of the 　890
    eye" under poor illumination [mitchell] *I am unaware that lighting conditions
    lead to hyperphoria. Moreover, Lincoln's eyesight was apparently normal
    (i.e. without refractive error) until age 47. See* Eyes -- Acuity .
  - ⟨s⟩ The "'illusion' was due to a disturbance of the eyes, a complete relaxation of 　891
    the muscles that keep the two eyes together and enable them, in the normal
    state, to see everything single. This was a temporary condition due to the
    fatigue" associated with the election campaign [holt].
  - ⟨s⟩ [kempfB pp9-10] believes that the horse-kick to Lincoln's head as a child (Special 　892
    Topic §1) caused "permanent differences in the nervous tone of the ocular
    and facial muscles."
  - ⟨s⟩ [snyder] discusses Lincoln's many relatives with documented or suggested 　893
    ocular misalignment: Robert (¶4923), Willie (¶5724), and Dennis Hanks
    (¶5794). Robert's grandson also had strabismus (¶5809). *Lincoln had an
    enormous number of cousins who were at least as closely related as Den-
    nis Hanks.*
  - ⟨s⟩ Asymmetry of the skull, affecting the function of the left superior oblique 　894
    muscle that controls eye movement [fishman]. "Desagittalization" of the su-
    perior oblique has been seen in frontal plagiocephaly [fishman]. *This is the
    most reasonable theory.*

- Facial features of hypertropia:　　　　　　　　　　　　　　　　　895
  - ⟨2⟩ "His left eye was actually set higher than his right eye. ... his left eyebrow was 　896
    usually more elevated than the right. This it was felt, was possible the result
    of an effort to keep the upper lid retracted so the pupil of he left eye could be
    exposed. This tendency of the left eye to turn upward left more of the white
    surface of the sclera below the iris, and gave a slightly staring effect on that
    side in strange disharmony with the appearance of the right eye." [snyder]
  - ⟨2⟩_c "The corrugations of Lincoln's brow and the crow's-feet at the corners of his 　897

Eyes – Motor (continued)

eyes indicate that he habitually used auxilliary facial muscles to support the external muscles of the eyes in an attempt to obtain good vision" [snyder].

⟨2⟩ Feb. 27, 1860: Photographer Mathew Brady retouches an image [ostendorf #17] obtained this day "to correct Lincoln's left eye that seemed to be roving upward" [donaldA p238] (∈ ¶23)   898

■ Ptosis: 899
  ⟨-⟩ ○○○ *Project:* Tabulate photos showing right ptosis, left ptosis, and bilateral ptosis.   900
  ⟨2⟩ "drooping lids" [shutes p67]   901
  ⟨2⟩_c "Lincoln's froglike left eyelid, which sometimes imparted a look of cunning to his features" – [ostendorfA p93] commenting on [ostendorf #57]   902
  ⟨1⟩_q "the heavy eyelids give him a mark almost of genius" – Col. Theodore Lyman [ostendorfA p93]   903
  ⟨1⟩ April 4, 1865: "kind blue eyes over which the lids half drooped" [barnesB] (∈ ¶1286)   904
  ⟨2⟩_c "In some [photographic] portraits the lid of one eye is noticeably lower than the other." [meserve p26]   905

■ Double vision episodes: 906
  ⟨1⟩ "It was just after my election in 1860, when the news had been coming in thick and fast all day, and there had been a great 'Hurrah, boys!' so that I was well tired out, and went home to rest, throwing myself down on a lounge in my chamber. Opposite where I lay was a bureau, with a swinging-glass upon it ... and, looking in that glass, I saw myself reflected, nearly at full length; but my face, I noticed, had *two* separate and distinct images, the tip of the nose of one being about three inches from the tip of the other. I was a little bothered, perhaps startled, and got up and looked in the glass, but the illusion vanished. On lying down again I saw it a second time – plainer, if possible, than before; and then I noticed that one of the faces was a little paler, say five shades, than the other. I got up and the thing melted away, and I went off and, in the excitement of the hour, forgot all about it – nearly, but not quite, for the thing would once in a while come up, and give me a little pang, as though something uncomfortable had happened. When I went home I told my wife about it, and a few days after I tried the experiment again when [with a laugh], sure enough, the thing came again; but I never succeeded in bringing the ghost back after that, though I once tried very industriously to show it to my wife, who was worried about it somewhat. She thought it was 'a sign' that I was to be elected to a second term of office, and that the paleness of one of the faces was an omen that I should not see life through the last term." – Lincoln, as recalled by [brooksR] in 1865   907
  ⟨2⟩ Lincoln observed a "strange double image of himself which he told his secretary, John Hay, he saw reflected in a mirror just after his election in 1860" [herndon p352]   908
  ⟨2⟩ This incident is reprinted in many sources, e.g. [carpenter pp163-164], [lamonL pp476-477], [arnold p180 quoting Hay]   909

■ Thoughts of non-professionals regarding episodes of double vision: 910
  ⟨2⟩ Herndon thought this and other (non-ocular) incidents "strongly attest to his inclination to superstition" [herndon p352]   911
  ⟨2⟩ Mrs. Lincoln apparently told Dr. William Jayne (see ¶3180) this incident scared her. [shutes p71] citing [jayne]   912

Eyes – Motor (continued)

⟨2⟩ Mary thought the double image indicated a two-term presidency, but that the ghostly second image predicted death before the second term's end [kunhardtA p334].   913

- Thoughts of professionals regarding episodes of double vision: 914
  ⟨S⟩ Dr. Erastus Holt, in 1901, was the first to relate Lincoln's illusion to extraocular muscles. [shutes p69]   915
  ⟨S⟩ [shutes p71] believes the deviation is "simulated," due to sagging of the soft tissue inferior to the eye. "This gives the impression that the pupil or the iris of the left eye is higher than that of the right. ... If that deviation upward was a permanent error, it was so marked that one must wonder why Lincoln did not complain more often of seeing double. ... I am strongly inclined to the theory that the Lincoln 'squint' was more apparent than real, and that the sole incident of diplopia was the result of temporary excessive fatigue."   916
  ⟨S⟩ The diplopia episode has been "attributed to a hyperphoria or cyclophoria of Lincoln's external eye muscles, making that condition explain much of his physical laziness in youth and manhood and his fatigue during the Presidency, and claiming that Lincoln's habit of lounging was an instinctive search for a less tiring position for his eyes" – Ed. E. Maxey, MD as summarized by [shutes p70]. Reference, per [shutesP], is: June 1926 *Northwest Medicine* (Seattle): "The effect of impaired vision in Lincoln's personal habits." (For lounging, see ¶2967ff.)   917
  ⟨S⟩ "The incidents of double vision as seen in the mirror is [sic] not conclusive. Since the President reported that only his head appeared double, separated by only 'about three inches' and 'one of the faces was a little paler – say 5 shades – than the other,' this could have resulted from a local fault in the mirror itself or from a normal physiological diplopia." [myers]   919
  ⟨S⟩ [myers] continues: "The alleged hyperphoria should also be reexamined carefully to rule out a facial asymmetry." Myers notes that the right temple of the "Chicago eyeglasses" is higher than the left (cites picture on page 1252 of *Journal of the American Optometric Association*, October 1976) and himself demonstrated that Ford's Theatre pair #2, "when placed flat on a table, showed the right temple elevated 2mm above the left."   920

Feet

The main topics related to Lincoln's feet are: (1) their size, (2) their discomfort, and (3) the length of their big toes. The first is non-controversial: by all accounts, Lincoln's had large, if not enormous, feet (¶933 and ¶941).   921

The nature and extent of Lincoln's foot discomfort are unclear. Corns (¶969), flat feet (¶975), or even sequelae to cold injury (¶930) may be possible. Of these, flat feet (pes planus) have been linked to Marfan syndrome, and sometimes to MEN2B.   922

Lincoln's toes are another matter. A drawing of his feet (¶980), apparently made the day he died, shows over-long big toes of exactly the type seen in some persons with Marfan syndrome [mckusickA pp47&54]. The analysis of [borittB] dismisses this drawing. He claims that an 1864 tracing of Lincoln's feet, made by a bootmaker (¶1007), shows no signs of elongated great toes (¶1015). My analysis differs (¶985), noting that: (a) [borittB] has overlooked a confounding factor (Lincoln wore socks while his feet were traced); (b) the drawing is astonishingly canny; and (c) the only alternative explanation is modern forgery, but from what I can tell in [borittB], the drawing has excellent provenance.   923

Feet (continued)

Great toes of the Marfan type would make untenable any claim Lincoln was merely a 924
tall man, as they do not occur in the merely tall. They are an unequivocal sign of long
bone overgrowth.   Furthermore, they might explain Lincoln's peculiar gait. Specifically, long great toes, if they had a limited range of extensor motion, would compel
Lincoln to raise and lower his feet in exactly the flat-footed way Herndon describes
(¶1053). ○○○ *Project:* It would be revealing to see videos of the gait in persons with
overgrown great toes. (See ¶989.)

Secondary sources say Lincoln had trouble finding comfortable footwear (¶958). That 925
he engaged someone from New York City to make his boots (¶1007) would seem to
confirm this. Lincoln was spectacularly indifferent to his own attire (e.g. [kunhardtA p116]
[wilson p452]), making it very unlikely that vanity drove him to consult the New Yorker.
One wonders how overgrown halluces might have affected the shoe/foot interface or a
predisposition to corns.

- Barefoot youth: 927
  - ⟨1⟩ "He and I worked bare footed – grubbed it – plowed – mowed & cradled to- 928
    gether – plowed Corn" – John Hanks [wilson p455]
  - ⟨1⟩ In Illinois "boys went barefoot till 17 or 20 yrs of age in Sumer time" – George 929
    Miles [wilson p536]

⟨2⟩ 1830-31 "hard winter:" While crossing the frozen Sangamon (Illinois) River, his 930
feet were "badly frozen." Whether for that reason, or for the deep snow of that
winter which was still "famous" 100 years later, Lincoln was marooned for weeks
in the cabin of William Warnick and his family in Macon County, IL. Mrs. Warnick
treated Lincoln's feet by putting them in snow "to take out the frost-bite." [shutes
pp7-8]
  - ⟨2⟩ "he froze his feet by walking three wet miles from his home to the Warnicks" 931
    [shutesE p36]
  - ⟨S⟩ Shutes speculates that customary ointments such as goose-grease, skunk- 932
    oil, or rabbit-fat may also have been applied. [shutes p8]. *Skunk oil?! Really?*

- Size (quantitative): 933
  - ⟨2⟩ "They were size 14, as feet are measured today." [kunhardtA p321] 934
  - ⟨2⟩ "By modern measurement Mr. Lincoln would wear a size 14 shoe." [kunhardtB 935
    p291]
  - ⟨2⟩ "His feet were so large – size fourteen – that he had to have his boots specially 936
    made" [oatesM p34]. *"Had to" is a strong statement that I think goes beyond
    the data.*
  - ⟨2⟩ "18-inch boots" [ostendorfA p388], with no primary source reference 937
  - ⟨2⟩ Size 13 feet [borittB p1] with no primary reference. *This statement is likely* 938
    *based on measurements made from a tracing of Lincoln's feet. It is unclear,
    however, whether the tracing is an outline of Lincoln's feet, or an outline
    of his shoes. (See The Physical Lincoln.) Thus, this number cannot be
    accepted without reservation.*
  - ⟨2⟩ Using a pair of moccasin slippers at the Chicago Historical Society that are 939
    generally believed to be authentic Lincoln footwear [borittB p9], Paul Angle
    inserted sticks of varying length to determine that an 11-inch foot was the
    "most likely to have been comfortably accommodated in the left moccasin"
    [stewart].
  - ⟨2⟩ [stewart] quotes several other attempts to derive Lincoln's shoe size from ar- 940
    tifacts, but [borittB pp13-14] casts serious doubt on whether the artifacts are
    genuine. (See ¶1002.)

Feet (continued)

- Size (qualitative): 941
  - ⟨1⟩ As a youth, his large feet repelled at least one girl (¶2685) and maybe more (¶2682) 942
  - ⟨2⟩ At about age 17: "His feet and hands were large" [herndon p35] (∈ ¶503) 943
  - ⟨2⟩ About 1831: "His large foot partially enveloped in a well worn pair of shoes" – from *Menard Axis*, 1862 [wilson p24] (∈ ¶95) 944
  - ⟨1⟩ 1834: "his legs were long, feet large ... running barefoot when young among Stones, and Stumps, accounts for his large ... feet' – Robert Wilson [wilson pp201-202] (∈ ¶99) 945
  - ⟨1⟩ 1849: "two of the largest feet I had, up to that time, been in the habit of seeing" – Leonard Swett [wilson p732] (∈ ¶140) 946
  - ⟨1/q⟩ Aug. 1858: "His black trousers, too, were so short that they gave an appearance of exaggerated size to his feet." – Martin Rindlaub [ostendorfA p19] (∈ ¶148) 947
  - ⟨1⟩ Oct. 13, 1858: trousers allowed "a very full view of his large feet." – Carl Schurz [angle p243] (∈ ¶149) 948
  - ⟨1/q⟩ 1859: "big hands and feet" – John Widmer [shenk p155] (∈ ¶150) 949
  - ⟨1/q⟩ 1860: "Tall as he was, his hands and feet looked out of proportion, so long and clumsy were they." [piatt pp345-346] 950
  - ⟨1⟩ March 1861: "hands of extraordinary dimensions, which, however, were far exceeded in proportion by his feet" – William Russell [russell pp37-38] (∈ ¶161) 951
  - ⟨1⟩ "long limbs, large hands and feet" [arnold p441] (∈ ¶167) 952
  - ⟨1/q⟩ "large feet'" – John Nicolay [meserve p5] (∈ ¶177) 953
  - ⟨1/q⟩ "large hands and feet" – William Herndon [hertz p188] 954
  - ⟨1/q⟩ An exasperated Lincoln hurried a persistent, insulting caller's departure with "a large foot just behind him, suggesting to any naval constructor the idea of a propeller." [burl p162] 955
  - ⟨1/q⟩ "long legs ending with such feet as I never saw before; one of his shoes might have served Commodore Nutt as a boat" – Princess Salm-Salm [salmsalm] (∈ ¶190) 956
  - ⟨2⟩ "clown-like feet" [marion p91] 957
- Footwear habits: 958
  - ⟨-⟩ See `Feet -- Artifacts` for specific shoes. 959
  - ⟨2⟩ "Although as President his shoes were made to order for him, he never could find any pair of boots that was perfectly comfortable, and visitors to the White House more often than not reported him to be wearing old slippers." [kunhardtB p291] 960
  - ⟨2⟩ As President: "He would often wear his soft, low slippers instead of his boots, not only during breakfast, but while he worked as well – those backless slippers that made flip-flop sounds on the White House floors when he walked, a visiting relative reported. There were times he wore these slippers even when greeting guests, who were sometimes shocked. ... One Southern governor claimed Lincoln had received him in bare feet. ... Lincoln occasionally went without socks." [kunhardtA p321] 961
  - ⟨1⟩ 1862: "He had shabby slippers on his feet." [hawthorne pp309-310] (∈ ¶178) 962
  - ⟨1⟩ Dec. 1863: "his slippers were crushed down at the heels" [carrA pp242-253] 963
  - ⟨1⟩ Early 1864: In Lincoln's office: "He had on slippers" – Henry Beecher [riceA pp249-250] (∈ ¶195) 964
  - ⟨1⟩ 1865: "Mr. Lincoln, as I saw him every morning, in the carpet slippers he wore in the house..." [crookA p14] (∈ ¶198) 965

Feet (continued)

⟨1⟩ "He always stood squarely on his feet, toe even with toe; that is, he never put one foot before the other. He neither touched nor leaned on anything for support. He made but few changes in his positions and attitudes." [herndon p332] *Is this why he swayed in Fig. 5?* 966

⟨$\frac{1}{?}$⟩ "He never wore his shoes out at the heel and the toe more, as most men do, than at the middle of the sole; yet his gait was not altogether awkward, and there was manifest physical power in his step." [lamonL p470] (For discussion, see ¶1081.) 967

⟨$\frac{1}{q}$⟩ Late February 1865: Complains of cold feet – see ¶1210 968

- Corns (?) Bunions (?): 969
  - ⟨$\frac{1}{q}$⟩ Sept. 22, 1862: "Dr. Zacharie has operated on my feet with great success, and considerable addition to my comfort." – Lincoln [baslerA v5p436] [sandburgC p166] 970
  - ⊡ Sept. 23, 1862: A letter, signed by both Lincoln and his Secretary of State, William Seward, attests to Dr. Zacharie's skill with corns and bunions, as well as his high character [borittB p15]. *The text of the letter is not in Lincoln's hand. The letter does not say which, if any, of the signatories had corns or bunions. Thus, I do not believe this document establishes Lincoln's foot complaint(s).* 971
  - ⟨$\frac{1}{q}$⟩ Oct. 3, 1862: [NYHerald] humorously implies Lincoln was "troubled with corns" [baslerA v5p436] 972
  - ⟨2⟩ "aching corns and bunions" [kunhardtA p321] 973
  - ⟨2⟩ [shutesE p167] recounts numerous feet-related pokes at Lincoln, e.g. "unionism and bunionism." 974

- Pes planus: 975
  - ⟨1⟩ "had large hands and feet – foot flat" – William Herndon [hertz p188] 976
  - ⟨2⟩ "flat-footed … also slightly pigeon-toed." [kunhardtA p321] (See ¶992 for pigeon-toed.) 979

⊡ A drawing by Albert Berghaus shows Lincoln on his death bed, having very long great toes [kunhardtB pp46-47, 97-98, 291]. See *The Physical Lincoln*. 980
- ⟨2⟩ [schwartzC] made the original connection of these toes to Marfan syndrome. 981
- ⟨$\overset{c}{S}$⟩ Based on tracings of Lincoln's feet, [borittB] discounts the drawing (¶1015). I disagree (¶985). 982
- ⟨2⟩ Willie Clark, the bed's owner and a soldier in the Quartermaster's Department, described Lincoln's feet to artist Albert Berghaus [kunhardtB pp46-47, 97-98], apparently the day after Lincoln's death [swansonB]. Berghaus worked for *Frank Leslie's Illustrated Newspaper* [swansonB]. His drawing of Lincoln's death scene appears in the April 29, 1865 edition of that newspaper [purtle]. 983
- ⟨2⟩ "Lincoln's feet were long and narrow, with extraordinarily exaggerated big toes, the other four on each foot reducing markedly in size until a very small toe was reached." [kunhardtB p291] 984

⟨S⟩ There are several reasons to believe the Berghaus drawing of Lincoln's toes (¶980) reflects reality, as *The Physical Lincoln* discusses in detail: 985
- ⟨-⟩ *The provenance of the drawing appears superb (¶983). Tellingly,* [borittB] *does not question the drawing's source nor offer an alternate hypothesis on its source.* 986
- ⟨-⟩ *Skeptics must explain how a simple soldier in 1865 could invent a highly unusual new physical sign that would, 66 years later, be linked with <u>precisely</u> the as-yet-undiscovered disease thought 97 years later to afflict* 987

Feet (continued)

Lincoln. That is, Marfan syndrome was not described in the medical literature until 1896. Long big toes were not recognized as a sign of Marfan syndrome until 1931 [aa8] [mckusickA pp47&136]. And Marfan syndrome was not suspected in Lincoln until 1962 [gordon]. The Berghaus drawing was published in a book in 1965, with no mention of it being a recent find [kunhardtB pp46-47].

⟨-⟩ *The tracing of Lincoln's feet was made while he was wearing socks (¶1007). Just as a mitten obscures the outline of fingers, a sock may obscure the outline of toes. In particular, if the sock's fabric formed a straight line between the tip of the great toe and the tip of the fifth toe (those two structures serving as "support posts" for the free edge of the sock), and if the bootmaker did not aggressively try to hug the foot with his pencil, then the relatively great length of the big toe would be inapparent because the tip of the second toe would not affect the contour of the sock. One might assume the bootmaker was not aggressive with his pencil, because if his craft required a precise anatomical outline of the feet, he would have asked Lincoln to remove his socks.* 988

⟨-⟩ *Could Lincoln's peculiar flat-footed gait be a sign of overgrown halluces?* 989

⟨2⟩ 1858: Walks from the Danville, IL train depot to the home of Dr. William Fithian (116 Gilbert St.), with a crowd in tow. Goes upstairs, takes off his boots to relax, but the crowd insists on a speech. Unable to easily get his boots on over his swollen feet, he speaks from the window, at Fithian's suggestion, so the crowd could not tell his boots were off. [gary p58] 990

⟨1/q⟩ October 1858: "He sat in the room with his boots off, to relieve his very large feet from the pain occasioned by continuous standing; or, to put it in his own words: 'I like to give my feet a chance to breathe.' He ... sat tilted back in one chair with his feet upon another in perfect ease." – David Locke [riceA p441] 991

- Pigeon-toed: 992
  - ⊡ Oct. 1862: [ostendorf #67] shows Lincoln sitting "pigeon-toed" [ostendorfA p113]. 993
  - ⟨1⟩ "He was a little pigeon-toed" [lamonL p470] (∈ ¶1081) 994
  - ⟨2⟩ "slightly pigeon-toed." [kunhardtA p321] 995

⊡ It has been stated: "Many photographs show Lincoln's feet" [borittB p22] and "a distinguished Lincoln scholar dispatched to me photos of Lincoln's feet" [borittB p4]. *These are not photographs of Lincoln's naked feet.* 996

⟨1⟩ 1862: "large, ill-fitting boots" [dicey v1pp220-221] (∈ ¶179) *How would an observer know the boots were ill-fitting?* 997

⟨1⟩ March 1865: "I am sorry to say the President' socks had [two large] holes in them." [porterD pp284-285] 998

Feet – Artifacts

See ⟨Feet⟩. 999

The two major classes of artifacts related to Lincoln's feet are (a) footwear, and (b) tracings. [borittB] invaluably assesses the authenticity of artifacts in both classes. The genuine artifacts are important in evaluating whether Lincoln had overgrowth of bones in his big toes, as suggested by a drawing (¶980). 1000

Feet − Artifacts (continued)

○○○ *Project:* It is possible that wear patterns in the interior of Lincoln's footwear could show where the balls of his toes rested. An endoscopic, or perhaps, magnetic resonance, examination could yield such information non-destructively. ○○○ *Project:* The wear patterns on the soles of well-worn shoes could provide confirmation (or refutation) of Herndon's (¶1053) and Lamon's (¶1081) statements that Lincoln walked flat-footed. **1001**

⟨2⟩c In searching for authentic Lincoln footwear, [borittB p13] says: "I tracked numerous assertions about Lincoln footwear which turned out to be false." **1002**

 ⟨2⟩c Not-authentic: the "Clark boots" [borittB pp13-14] (See ¶1019.) **1003**
 ⟨2⟩c Authentic: a pair of moccasin slippers are at the Chicago Historical Society [borittB p9]. **1004**
 ⟨2⟩c Leaning toward non-authentic: a boot now at the Scholl College of Podiatric Medicine in Chicago [borittB p14] **1005**

⟨2⟩c According to [borittB pp4,7-8], non-authentic tracings of Lincoln's feet have been published in: (a) [lorant p220 but is actually p204], (b) *Dress and Care of the Feet* by Peter Kahler (published in several editions spanning at least 1882-1915), and (c) "A great man's feet" in *Philadelphia Press* newspaper, hand-dated 1882 (or possibly 1892 – date is indistinct) **1006**

⟨2⟩ Dec. 13, 1864: [borittB] concludes an extant, genuine tracing of Lincoln's feet was made on this day. **1007**

 ⟨2⟩ A bootmaker from Scranton, PA, Peter Kahler, "had the president stand in his socked feet on a sheet of plain brown paper, and traced with ink the outlines of his feet." [borittB p6] **1008**
 ⟨2⟩ An older source reports "Mr. Lincoln had stood on a piece of wrapping paper and himself drawn with a pencil around his own toes, insteps, and heels." [kunhardtB p49] **1009**
 ⟨2⟩ Kahler, later of New York, catered to customers with "interesting feet." [kunhardtB p49] **1010**
 ◻ The tracing is pictured in [borittB p16] and [kunhardtA p320] **1011**
 ⟨1⟩ The original tracing is now in the Special Collections of Gettysburg College [borittB p16] **1012**
 ⟨-⟩ [kunhardtA p320] *shows a pair of boots and implies they were made from the tracing. However, these are the "Clark boots" (see ¶1019) which may not be authentic.* **1013**
 ◻ The measurements of the two feet were "uneven." [kunhardtA p320] (See ¶314.) **1014**

⟨S⟩ From the Kahler tracing of Lincoln's stocking feet (¶1007), [borittB p9] concludes "we know now that Lincoln did not have arachnodactylic feet with elongated big toes." **1015**

 ⟨-⟩ *It is worth noting that* [borittB] *takes pains to question and establish the authenticity of footwear and tracings, but does not question the authenticity of the tracing or the circumstances of the tracing of Lincoln's feet.* **1016**
 ⟨-⟩ *The bigger problems with Boritt's conclusion are discussed in* The Physical Lincoln. **1017**
 ⟨1⟩ In stating "At times the great toes are elongated out of proportion to the others" the earliest reference cited by McKusick is 1931 [mckusickA pp47&54]. **1018**

⟨2⟩ Lincoln died in the Peterson House, in a room rented by one Willie Clark. Clark claimed to have ended up with Lincoln's boots, left behind after Lincoln's corpse was removed from the room. [kunhardtB pp49,97,104] [borittB pp13-14] **1019**

 ⟨2⟩c [borittB pp13-14] concludes these are **not** Lincoln's boots. **1020**

◯ The boots, shown in [kunhardtB p104] and [kunhardtA p320], have a squared-off toe.   1021

Gait

There is no doubt that Lincoln had an unusual gait. An embarrassingly thin reading   1022
of the historical record has been used to make the case that Lincoln was (and yet, was
not) ataxic, in order to support a diagnosis of spinocerebellar ataxia, type 5 (¶1025).
This theory has no merit.

Sorting out Lincoln's gait is no trivial matter. There are several factors that could have   1023
influenced his gait, and few data to help decide which are the most important: (1) Orthopedic considerations from his large great toes; (2) Orthopedic considerations if he
was asymmetric in his spine, pelvis, or legs, in the way he seemed to be asymmetric almost everywhere; (3) Muscular considerations from his generalized hypotonia;
(4) Considerations from peculiarities of muscle distribution or mass.

Special Topic §8 provides some of my early thinking on matters of gait. It predates the   1024
realization that muscular hypotonia may have been a significant factor.

⟨s⟩ Spinocerebellar ataxia type 5 (SCA5):   1025
   ⟨-⟩ Discussed at length in Special Topic §8.   1026
   ⟨-⟩ SCA5 is an autosomal dominant syndrome [OMIM entry 600224] known to   1027
   have afflicted more than 90 descendants of Lincoln's paternal grandparents
   [ranum]. In this kindred, the first symptom was gait disturbance, incoordination of the upper limbs, or slurred speech, generally occurring in the 3rd or
   4th decade of life and progressing for decades without shortening life. The
   oldest age at onset was 68. For Lincoln's grandparents, see ¶5811, ¶5816. For
   his paternal uncle and aunt who may have had the disease, see ¶5830, and
   ¶5786.
   ⟨s⟩ His odd gait has been ascribed to spinocerebellar ataxia type 5 [aa52] [ranum].   1028
   ⟨2⟩_c [nee] disagrees, but [hirschhornD] is favorable.   1029

⟨1⟩_q "His first steps were labored; he 'walked slowly, but surely,' a cousin remem-   1030
   bered." [kunhardtA p36]
   ⟨1⟩_q Instead of "walked" [donaldA p29] says "worked." *A completely different mean-*   1031
   ing! See ¶3321.

■ Distance: 1032
   ⟨2⟩ Latter 1820s: Walked more than 50 miles to Vincennes to buy a hunting rifle   1033
   [hobson p29].
   ⟨2⟩ In youth: "He walked thirty-four miles in one day, just on an errand, to please   1034
   himself, to hear a lawyer make a speech." [sandburgA p47]
   ⟨1⟩_q 1831±: Walked 6-8 miles and back to borrow a grammar book. – Mentor   1036
   Graham [walsh pp130, 166].
   ⟨1⟩ Spring 1832: Walked from New Salem to Beardstown to catch a steamboat   1037
   [rossH p111] *About 40 miles.*
   ⟨2⟩ Summer 1832: At the end of his militia service, his horse stolen, he (mostly)   1038
   walked from Black River, WI to Peoria, IL; then canoed to Havana, IL; then
   walked home to New Salem (over 60 miles in this last leg) [thomas pp56-57] *But*
   see ¶3632 for possible contradiction.
   ⟨2⟩ In New Salem: Walked 14 miles to Springfield to borrow a book, then back.   1040
   "It is said, he would often master thirty or forty pages of the new book on his
   way home." [arnold p40].

Gait (continued)

⟨1⟩ 1835 or later: Walked 2 1/2 miles to repay a 5-cent overcharge he made. –   1042
Allen Brooner [hobson p35]

⟨1⟩ Walked "13 or 16 miles" to work, sometimes 60 miles – Nathaniel Grigsby   1043
[wilson p114]

⟨1⟩ 1830s: As New Salem postmaster, when a highly anticipated letter was re-   1044
ceived "he would walk several miles, if necessary, to deliver it." [thomas pp66-67]

⟨1⟩ "After A Lincoln became law student he walked all way from Springfield to   1045
see his father" in Coles County, IL – George Balch [wilson p597] *Today this is a*
95-mile one-way drive.

⟨1⟩ ca. 1837-1841: Walks three miles to find a judge to sign papers. [rossH pp113-115]   1046

⟨2⟩ Feb. 9, 1864: Impatiently waiting for his carriage, Lincoln instead walks a   1047
mile to his appointment with a photographer. [ostendorfA p175] citing unpublished diary of Francis Carpenter

- Dancing: 1048

  ⟨1⟩ "I never saw him dance." – Daniel Burner, who lived with Lincoln in the   1049
  1830s [templeB]

  ⟨1⟩ "he cared little for dancing" [helmB p74]   1050

  ⟨1⟩ At an early meeting between Lincoln and Mary, he asked: "Miss Todd, I want   1051
  to dance with you the worst way." Her later comment: "And he certainly did."
  [helmB p74]

⟨1⟩ Running, pre-Presidency: Fleeing an incensed Mary: "Poor Abe, I can see him   1052
now running and crouching." – William Herndon [hertz p105]

- Gait descriptions - from Herndon: 1053

  ⟨1⟩ "When he walked he moved cautiously but firmly; his long arms and giant   1054
  hands swung down by his side. He walked with even tread, the inner sides
  of his feet being parallel. He put the whole foot flat down on the ground at
  once, not landing on the heel; he likewise lifted his foot all at once, not rising
  from the toe, and hence he had no spring to his walk. His walk was undu-
  latory – catching and pocketing tire, weariness, and pain, all up and down
  his person, and thus preventing them from locating. The first impression if
  a stranger, or a man who did not observe closely, was that his walk implied
  shrewdness and cunning – that he was a tricky man; but, in reality, it was the
  walk of caution and firmness." [herndon pp471-472] ((∈ ¶2), more or less)

  ⟨1/q⟩ "He walked like an Indian, with even tread, the inner sides of his feet being   1055
  parallel, betokening caution. He put the whole foot flat down on the ground,
  not landing on the heel; he likewise lifted it all at once, not rising from the
  toes; hence there was no spring to his step as he moved up and down the
  street." – Herndon [shutes pp41-42]

  ⟨1⟩ "He was a sad-looking man; his melancholy dripped from him as he walked."   1056
  [herndon p473]

  ⟨1/q⟩ Herndon called Lincoln's gait "stalking and stilting it" [kunhardtB p260]   1057

- Gait descriptions - other sources: 1058

  ⟨1/q⟩ In youth: "Abe'd come lopin' out on his long legs" – Dennis Hanks [wilsonR p27]   1059
  (∈ ¶2248)

  ⟨2⟩ "the long-striding, flat-footed, cautious manner of a plowman" [currentEB]   1060

  ⟨2⟩ About 1831: "on an inclement day of winter ... plodding with awkward step"   1061
  – from *Menard Axis*, 1862 [wilson p24] (∈ ¶95)

  ⟨1⟩ 1832: "The long strides of Lincoln..." – George Harrison [wilson p329]   1062

Gait (continued)

⟨$\frac{1}{q}$⟩ "He walked along with his hands behind him, gazing upward and noticing nobody." – 1909 recollection of William B. Thompson, who, as a boy, frequently encountered Lincoln on the Springfield streets [burl p58]   1063

⟨$\frac{1}{q}$⟩ "shambling" [shastid] (∈ ¶137)   1064

⟨1⟩ "He leaned forward, and stooped as he walked." [arnold p441] (∈ ¶167)   1065

⟨$\frac{1}{q}$⟩ Nov. 1860: "slouchy ungraceful ... round shouldered, leans forward (very much in his walk)" – Thomas Webster [randallC p163] (∈ ¶160)   1066

⟨1⟩ 1860s: "I have heard it said that he was ungainly, that his step was awkward. He never impressed me as being awkward." [dana p173] (∈ ¶183)   1067

⟨1⟩ March 1861: "a shambling, loose, irregular, almost unsteady gait" [russell pp37-38] (∈ ¶161) (See §8b!)   1068

⟨1⟩ July 18, 1861: Sees Lincoln on the street, "striding like a crane in a bulrush swamp" [russell pp428-429]   1069

⟨1⟩ Sept. 4, 1861: "the peculiar swinging gait that characterizes the old 'Rail splitter.'" [french p373]   1070

⟨$\frac{1}{q}$⟩ 1862 (Oct.-Nov.): A visitor to the greatly stressed President thought: "His introverted look and his half-staggering gait were like those of a man walking in sleep" – a visitor [donaldA p382].   1071

⟨1⟩ Summer 1863: "His step was slow and heavy" (while looking dejected) [keckleyB pp118-119] (∈ ¶2533)   1072

⟨1⟩ Sept. 8, 1863: "He was very tall and moved with a shuffling awkward motion." [harveyC] (∈ §6.9)   1073

⟨$\frac{1}{q}$⟩ 1864: "inclined to stoop when he walked" [carpenter p217]   1074

⟨1⟩ Summer 1864: "bowed and sorrow-laden ... he dropped himself heavily from step to step down to the ground." [browneF p670] (∈ ¶2538)   1075

⟨1⟩ April 14, 1865, in Ford's Theatre: "he looked peculiarly sorrowful, as he slowly walked with bowed head and drooping shoulders to the box. I was looking at him as he took his last walk." [lealeA p3] (∈ ¶207)   1076

⟨2⟩ Chauncey Depew said Lincoln "walked with dignity and sureness" – Marie de Montalvo, 1948 letter to J.G. Randall [randallP box 15] (∈ ¶2942)   1077

⟨2⟩ "His left shoulder was higher than his right [see ¶302] and his walk was undulating and slightly off balance, making him resemble, someone said, 'a mariner who had found his sea legs but had to admit there was a rough sea running" [kunhardtA p321].   1078

⟨$\frac{1}{q}$⟩ [Phineas Gurley], his pastor, said when Lincoln walked, he looked as if 'he was about to plunge forward, from his right shoulder, for he always walked, when he had anything in his hand, as if he was pushing something in front of him.'" [kunhardtA p321]   1079

⟨$\frac{1}{q}$⟩ Lincoln went from the War Department to the White House: "walking slowly, shoulders bent forward, hands folded behind his back" – John Widney [meserve p1]   1080

⟨$\frac{1}{?}$⟩ "'He did not walk cunningly, Indian-like, but cautiously and firmly.' His tread was even and strong. He was a little pigeon-toed; and this, with another peculiarity, made his walk very singular. He set his whole foot flat on the ground, and in turn lifted it all at once, not resting momentarily upon the toe as the foot rose, nor upon the heel as it fell. He never wore his shoes out at the heel and the toe more, as most men do, than at the middle of the sole; yet his gait was not altogether awkward, and there was manifest physical power in his step." [lamonL p470] *Part of this parrots, and part of this specifically*   1081

Gait (continued)

contradicts, Herndon's description of Lincoln's gait (¶1053). The source of the initial quotation is unclear.

⟨$\frac{1}{q}$⟩ "In walking, his gait is never brisk. He steps slowly and deliberately, almost always with his head inclined forward and his hands clasped behind his back." – eyewitness [shutesE p205] 1082

⟨2⟩ Lincoln "walked with the peculiar slow woods-and-fields movement of the Western pioneer" [nicolayA p227] (∈ ¶203) 1083

- Pace: 1084
  - ⟨1⟩ 1830s: "Whenever he walked with me, he would keep me in a trot all the time." – James Short [wilson p90] 1085
  - ⟨1⟩ June 1858: Difficult to keep up with [volk]. See ¶1096. 1086
  - ⟨$\frac{1}{q}$⟩ About 1859: "I well remember [my] first sight of him. He was striding along, holding little Tad, then about six years old, by the hand, who could with the greatest difficulty keep up with his father." – John Littlefield [angle p183] 1087
  - ⟨2⟩ 1860 (while President-elect): "he loped along in his countryman's gait at a pace that tired out companions twenty years younger" [donaldA p259] (∈ ¶714) 1088
  - ⟨1⟩ Mar. 28, 1865: "he walked slowly" [coffinA p180] 1089
- Stairs: 1090
  - ⟨1⟩ 1856: "he bounded up the stairs two steps at a time" – Henry Whitney [wilson p734] 1091
  - ⟨1⟩ Agrees with: "went up the stairs to the room three steps at a time" – Henry C. Whitney [wilson p407] 1092
  - ⟨1⟩ April 1860: "My studio was in the fifth story, and there were no elevators in those days, and I soon learned to distinguish his steps on the stairs, and am sure he frequently came up two, if not three, steps at a stride" [volk]. Echoed by ¶714. 1093

⟨$\frac{1}{q}$⟩ "Lincoln had a furtive way of stealing in on one, unheard, unperceived and unawares" – Henry C. Whitney [kunhardtA p81] [angle p170] 1094

⟨1⟩ Feb. 1861: "I thereupon waited and, while absorbed in a book , Lincoln came noiselessly in, and I was not aware of his presence until he actually stood before me." [whitney p494] 1095

⟨1⟩ June 1858: "On leaving the train, most of the passengers climbed over the fences and crossed the stubble-field, taking a short-cut to the grove, among them Mr. Lincoln, who stalked forward alone, taking immense strides, the before-mentioned carpet-bag and an umbrella in his hands, and his coat-skirts flying in the breeze. I managed to keep pretty close in the rear of the tall, gaunt figure, with the head craned forward, apparently much over the balance, like the Leaning Tower of Pisa, that was moving something like a hurricane across that rough stubble-field! He approached the rail-fence, sprang over it as nimbly as a boy of eighteen, and disappeared from my sight." [volk] 1096

⟨1⟩ 1858: On election night 1864, Lincoln told a story: "For such an awkward fellow, I am pretty surefooted. It used to take a pretty dextrous man to throw me. I remember, the evening of the day in 1858, that decided the contest for the Senate between Mr. Douglas and myself, was something like this, dark, rainy & gloomy. I had been reading the returns and had ascertained that we had lost the Legislature and started to go home. The path had been worn hog-backed & was slippering [sic]. My foot slipped from under me, knocking the other one out of the way, but I recovered myself & lit square, and I said to myself, 'It's a slip and not a fall.' " [hayD p244] 1097

Gait (continued)

⟨2⟩ Spring 1862: Lincoln visited the Army encampment at Aquia Creek, Virginia. General Irvin McDowell pointed out a bridge his men were building across a deep wide ravine. The bridge was a hundred feet above the water and only one plank wide at that time. Nevertheless, Lincoln exclaimed "Let us walk over" and led the way across without losing his balance. (Secretary of War Stanton became dizzy going across, and had to be helped by Admiral Dahlgren, who was himself rather giddy.) [donaldA p352]   1098

⟨$\frac{1}{q}$⟩ "He often said that he could think better after Breakfast – and better walking, than sitting, lying, or standing" – Joshua Speed [wilson p499] [herndon p420]   1099

⟨$\frac{1}{q}$⟩ Feb. 10, 1864: Lincoln runs with a "dog-trot" toward the burning White House stables, with guard Smith Stimmel trailing: "I struck out on the double-quick and went with him, keeping close to his side; but he took such long strides that his dog-trot was almost a dead run for me." [kunhardtA p235]   1100

  ⟨2⟩ Lincoln "leapt over a hedge and flung open the stable doors to get the animals out" [kunhardtB p297]. See ¶2537 for Lincoln's post-fire reaction.   1101

⟨2⟩ 1865 (probably): "He walked like a man whose feet hurt." [bishop p37] citing no source   1102

⟨2⟩ Lincoln carried a cane, but it was for self defense and at Mary's insistence. [kunhardtB p5]   1103

  ⟨2⟩ March 4, 1865: Carried a gold- or silver-headed walking-cane at second inaugural. [shenk p173]   1104

General

These observations about Lincoln's general state of health do not fit neatly into other categories. This section is restricted to the pre-Presidential years. See also General -- During Presidency and Energy .   1105

⟨2⟩ "When people talked about Lincoln, it was nearly always about one or more of these five things: (1) how long, tall, quick, strong, or awkward in looks he was; (2) how he told stories and jokes, how he was comical or pleasant or kindly; (3) how he could be silent, melancholy, sad; (4) how he was ready to learn and looking for chances to learn; (5) how he was ready to help a friend, a stranger, or even a dumb animal in distress." [sandburgP v1p200] *See ¶2397 for interesting remark on "ready to learn."*   1106

⟨1⟩ As a youth: "He was always in good health never was sick – had an Excellent Constitution" – Nathaniel Grigsby [wilson p113]   1107

⟨1⟩ "He always had good health – never was sick – was very careful of his person" – Sarah Bush Lincoln [wilson p108]   1108

⟨2⟩ "The boy had limited energy because at about the age of twelve he began growing so rapidly. By the time he was sixteen he had shot up to six feet, two inches tall, though he weighed only about one hundred and sixty pounds. One contemporary remembered he was so skinny that he had a spidery look. He grew so fast that he was tired all the time, and he showed a notable lack of enthusiasm for physical labor. 'Lincoln was lazy – a very lazy man,' Dennis Hanks concluded. ... The neighbors for whom he worked agreed that he was 'awful lazy,' and, as one remarked, 'he was no hand to pitch in at work like killing snakes.' " [donaldA p33]   1109

  ■ 1830s: 1110

General (continued)

⟨1⟩ "he was studious – so much so that he somewhat injured his health and constitution" – Mentor Graham [wilson p11] 1111

⟨1⟩ 1833: Learning law and surveying simultaneously: Lincoln "was so studious 1112
– took so little physical exercise – was so laborious in his studies that he became Emaciated & his best friends were afraid that he would craze himself
– make himself derange from his habits of study which were incessant." –
Henry McHenry [wilson p14]

⟨$\frac{1}{q}$⟩ After six weeks of hard study around 1833 (see ¶3334), Lincoln was "hol- 1113
low eyed and ill looking," prompting warnings from physician/friend Jason
Duncan (see ¶3168). [shutes pp12-13]

⟨$\frac{1}{q}$⟩ January 1841: In low spirits after a rift with Mary Todd (see ¶2746). Lincoln takes 1114
to bed. January 24: he appears "reduced and emaciated in appearance and seems
scarcely to possess strength enough to speak above a whisper." – James Conkling
[donaldA p88] [randallC p48]. *Can one become emaciated in a week? According* [shenk
pp58-59], *the answer is "yes" if your physician administers typical 19th century
treatments for mental disorders: bleeding, purging, fasting, blistering, etc.*

⟨1⟩ 1850s(?): Mary "was fearful about his health, which her brother-in-law, Dr. Wal- 1115
lace (¶3195) warned her to watch." [helmB p115]

⟨1⟩ Feb. 10, 1857: Received a note "yesterday, since which time I have been too unwell 1116
to notice it." – Lincoln [baslerA v2pp390-391]

⟨2⟩ August 1858, just before first debate with Douglas: "looked careworn and weary" 1117
– H.W. Beckwith [arnold p146]

⟨1⟩ August 1858 (Lincoln-Douglas debates): "Lincoln was then in the prime of life, of 1118
great physical and mental power" [arnold p118]

⟨$\frac{1}{q}$⟩ May 1860: "I found Mr. Lincoln sitting on a trunk, alone, at the end of the hall, 1119
with his head bowed down and leaning it upon his hand. 'I'm not very well,' he
said." – Lt. Governor Bross of Illinois, encountering Lincoln upon leaving the Republican convention in Decatur [shutes p74]

⟨$\frac{1}{q}$⟩ 1860 campaign: "He was care worn & more haggard & stooped than I ever saw 1120
him" [hirschhornC] citing [prattC p36, statement of W.H.L. Wallace]

⟨$\frac{1}{q}$⟩ Dec. 14, 1860: "The appearance of Mr. Lincoln has somewhat changed to the 1121
worse in the last week. He does not complain of any direct ailment but that he
looks more pale and care worn than heretofore is evident to the daily observer." –
Henry Villard [shutesE p128]

⟨1⟩ "His little gray eyes flashed in a face aglow with the fire of his profound thoughts; 1122
and his uneasy movements and diffident manner sunk themselves beneath the
wave of righteous indignation that came sweeping over him. Such was Lincoln
the orator." [herndon p333]

  ⟨1⟩ "About the year 1832 or 1833 Mr Lincoln made his first effort at public speak- 1123
  ing. ... he arose to speak his tall form towered above the little assembly. Both
  hands were thrust down deep in the pockets of his pantaloons. ... As he
  warmed with his subject his hands would forsake his pockets and would enforce his ideas with awkward gestures; but would very soon seek their easy
  resting place" – Robert Rutledge [wilson p384]

  ⟨1⟩ See also ¶3712 for more on Lincoln the orator. 1124

⟨1⟩ "His habits, like himself, were odd and wholly irregular. He would move around in 1125
a vague, abstracted way, as if unconscious of his own or anyone else's existence.

General (continued)

He had no expressed fondness for anything, and ate mechanically. I have seen him sit down at the table absorbed in thought, and never, unless recalled to his senses, would he think of food. But, however peculiar and secretive he may have seemed, he was anything but cold." [herndon p411]

⟨1⟩ In youth: "He was regular in his habits punctual in doing *any* thing was very systematic" – Mentor Graham [wilson p76]   1126

⟨1⟩ "The low and feeble circulation of his blood; his healthful irritability, which responded so slowly to the effects of stimuli; the strength of his herculean [sic] frame; his peculiar organism, conserving its force; his sublime patience; his wonderful endurance; his great hand and heart, saved this country from division, when division meant its irreparable ruin." [herndon p490]   1127

General – During Presidency

These observations about Lincoln's general health or general state of health do not fit neatly into other categories. This section is restricted to thePresidential years. See also General and Energy .   1128

- Pre-inauguration concerns about the pressures of the office: 1129
  ⟨1⟩ October 1860: "Among the many things said to Mr. Lincoln by his visitors there is nearly always an expressed hope that he will not be so unfortunate as were Harrison and Taylor, to be killed off by the cares of the Presidency – or as is sometimes hinted, by foul means. It is astonishing how the popular sympathy for Mr. Lincoln draws fearful forebodings from these two examples, which, after all, were only a natural coincidence. Not only do visitors mention the matter, but a great many letters have been written to Mr. Lincoln on the subject." – Lincoln's secretary (probably John Nicolay) [angle p289]   1130
  ⟨2⟩ After his election as President, the office seekers descended on him. "'Individuals, deputations, and delegations,' says one of Mr. Lincoln's biographers, 'from all quarters pressed in upon him in a manner that might have killed a man of less robust constitution.'" [herndon p379]   1131

⟨1⟩ Feb. 1861: " good health" when he moved to Washington [herndonC] [herndon p471] (∈ ¶1)   1132

⟨1⟩ "Took but little physical Exercise" – Ward Lamon [wilson p466] *In context, refers to Presidential years.*   1133

⟨2⟩ Early in Presidency: Mary "instituted the daily drive" and insisted Lincoln accompany her "as this was the only way in which she could induce him to take fresh air, which he so much needed." [grimsley]   1134
  ⟨-⟩ *At least until the 1920s, going out for a ride in a carriage (or automobile) was considered a form of exercise. (Presidents Taft and Wilson certainly believed so.)*   1136
  ⟨2⟩ "Lincoln's friends worried that he was confined to his office so much of the time and urged him to get fresh air and take exercise." [donaldH p31]   1137

⟨$\frac{1}{q}$⟩ March 1861: Lincoln looks "neglected and unkempt" – Gustave Koerner [meserve p1]   1138

⟨1⟩ April 12, 1861: "He was bent until he almost appeared to stoop... I was astonished, almost alarmed, for there were deep, dark circles under his eyes and they were vacant." [stoddardD p221]   1139

General – During Presidency (continued)

⟨1⟩ July 8, 1861: "President Lincoln, thus far, bears his load of responsibility wonderfully well. He is a little thinner and paler than on the day of his inauguration, and at times wears a wearied and harassed look..." – William Stoddard [stoddardB p14]   1140

⟨1⟩ Oct. 7, 1861: "The Overworked President: For a few weeks the President has been looking pale and careworn, as if the perpetual wear-and-tear of the load which presses upon him were becoming too much even for his iron frame and elastic mind." – William Stoddard [stoddardB p34]   1141

⟨$\frac{1}{q}$⟩ Feb. 22, 1862 (?): "The President's Illness: The serious illness of President Lincoln has created consternation and alarm in this city. [Several sentences review ailments of previous Presidents.] We now come down to our own time, and find Mr. Lincoln is sick, under the most suspicious circumstances. Whatever Old Abe's drawbacks, and weaknesses, he is regarded as an honest man, and this is enough to create him hosts of enemies. The wildest rumors are flying about the streets, and the above is the substance of the current gossip. – New York Sunday *Mercury* of Feb. 23, 1862, per transcript in [barbeeP - box 1 folder 51] *What was this illness? Did Barbee mis-type the date?*   1142

- April 1862:
  - ⟨1⟩ April 10, 1862: "sick and in bed," yet after dark was "comfortable and in very good spirits – having been out riding in the evening" – Orville Browning [browning p540] *By the next night, Browning is sick. Did he catch it from Lincoln?*   1144
  - ⟨1⟩ April 25, 1862: "He was alone and complaining of head ache." Browning talks and reads poetry with Lincoln for an hour and a half. [browning p542]   1145
  - ⟨1⟩ May 2, 1862: "He had the head ache and was not in his office" that night, but received Browning in the family room for an hour. [browning p543]   1146
  - ⟨-⟩ *It is unclear if this was one illness.*   1147

⟨2⟩ Spring 1862: "despite the grinding cares of his office, was in fine physical shape" [donaldA p352]   1148
  - ⟨-⟩ *Basis for this statement is uncertain. Donald tells the anecdote of crossing the plank bridge (see ¶1098) but one cannot infer good general health from good balance.*   1149

- Mid 1862:
  - ⟨1⟩ June 30, 1862: Lincoln goes "to the country very tired" – Edwin Stanton [baslerA v5p295] *This was during the Seven Days' Battles. "Country" may be the Soldiers' home.*   1151
  - ⟨2⟩ Was not sleeping according to Mary – had lost weight [donaldA p358] See ¶655   1152
  - ⟨2⟩ Circa 1862: "He was desperately exhausted. Always thin, he had now lost so much weight as to look cadaverous" [donaldH p43].   1153

⟨1⟩ July 15, 1862: "He looked weary, care-worn and troubled. I shook hands with him, and asked how he was. He said 'tolerably well' I remarked that I felt concerned about him – regretted that troubles crowded so heavily upon him, and feared his health was suffering. He held me by the hand, pressed it, and said in a very tender and touching tone – 'Browning I must die sometime,' I replied 'your fortunes are bound up with those of the Country, and disaster to one would be disaster to the other, and I hope you will do all all you can to preserve your health and life'. He looked very sad, and there was a cadence of deep sadness in his voice. We parted I believe both of us with tears in our eyes." [browning pp559-560]   1154

⟨2⟩ The approaching 1862 mid-term elections stressed the President.   1155

General – During Presidency (continued)

⟨1/q⟩ Appeared "literally bending under the weight of his burdens" [donaldA p382] 1156

⟨1/q⟩ "His introverted look and his half-staggering gait were like those of a man walking in sleep" – a visitor [donaldA p382] 1157

⟨1/q⟩ His face "revealed the ravages which care, anxiety, and overwork had wrought" – a visitor [donaldA p382] 1158

⟨2⟩ "Ordinarily the master of his emotions, he let his self-control slip at times" [donaldA p382] 1159

⟨1⟩ Nov. 1862: "My first thought, on arriving in Washington in 1862, was to see how far the President resembled the Lincoln of Illinois before the war. The change in his personal appearance was marked and sorrowful. ... His eyes were almost deathly in their gloomy depths, and on his visage was an air of profound sadness. His face was colorless and drawn, and newly grown whiskers added to the agedness of his appearance. When I had last seen him in Illinois, his face, although always sallow, wore a tinge of rosiness in the cheeks, but now it was pale and colorless." [brooksC p2] (Date is per [shenk p287].) 1160

⟨1⟩ Feb. 18, 1863: "He certainly is growing feeble. He wrote a note while I was present, and his hand trembled as I never saw it before, and he looked worn & haggard. I remarked that I should think he would feel glad when he could get some rest. He replied that it was a pretty hard life for him." [french p417]. 1161

  ⟨1⟩ French saw Lincoln writing a note to Attorney General Bates. It is in the National Archives (College Park) RG204 Record 460 [hirschhornC]. 1162

  ⟨2/c⟩ "Our own analysis of the handwriting suggests shakiness but no evidence of an intention tremor." [hirschhornC] 1163

■ June 1863: Short telegrams from Lincoln to Mary: 1164
  ⟨1⟩ June 11, 1863: "I am very well" [donaldH p84] 1165
  ⟨1⟩ June 15, 1863: "Tolerably well" [donaldH p84] 1166
  ⟨1⟩ June 24, 1863: "All well" [donaldH p103] 1167
  ⟨1⟩ June 29, 1863: "All well" [donaldH p103] 1168

⟨2⟩ Mid 1863 (before the Battle of Gettysburg): "drooping eyelids, looking almost swollen; the dark bags beneath the eyes; the deep marks about the large and expressive mouth" [wilsonR p332] (See Figure 5) 1169
  ⟨S⟩ Donald concludes "Under the enormous strain of worry [about the impending battle] the President's health began to suffer." [donaldA p446] 1170

■ Aug.-Sept. 1863: Short telegrams from Lincoln to Mary: 1171
  ⟨1⟩ Aug. 31, 1863: "All reasonably well" [donaldH p104] 1172
  ⟨1⟩ Sept. 3, 1863: "We are all well" [donaldH p90] 1173
  ⟨1⟩ Sept. 6, 1863: "All well" [donaldH p90] 1174

⟨1⟩ Sept. 7, 1863: "The springs of life are wearing away." – Lincoln. He was then asked if his great cares were injuring his health. "No," he replied, "not directly, perhaps." [harveyC p251] (§6.8 quotes at length.) 1175

■ Nov. 19-Dec. 28, 1863: Smallpox. See Special Topic §5. 1176
  ⟨1⟩ As late as Dec. 28 he was "steadily recovering his health and strength" [stoddardB p197] (∈ §5.92). 1177
  ⟨1⟩ "Men of his habit of body are not usually long-lived." [ChicagoTribune - Dec. 9, 1863] (∈ §5.76). 1178

⟨1⟩ Early 1864: "He looked wearied, and when he sat down in a chair, looked as though every limb wanted to drop off his body." – Henry Beecher [riceA pp249-250] (∈ ¶195) 1179

General – During Presidency (continued)

- Feb. 1864: — 1180
  - ⟨-⟩ *Unclear if this illness was the last throes of smallpox (see Special Topic §5).* — 1181
  - ⟨1⟩ Feb. 13, 1864: "I am unwell, even now, and shall be worse this afternoon." – Lincoln [baslerA v7p183] (∈ §5.103) — 1182
  - ⟨1⟩ Feb. 20, 1864: "The President is, a little better today" – Mary [turner p169]. (∈ §5.104) — 1183
  - ⟨2⟩ Feb. 23, 1864: Possibly still ill [kunhardtA p265]. (See §5.105.) — 1184
  - ⟨1⟩ No mention of this illness in near-daily diary entries of Feb. 12-29 in [welles v1pp521-533]. — 1185

⟨2⟩ Mar. 14, 1864: (**Error**) According to [shutes p87], Lincoln was in bed this day, met with the Cabinet in his bedroom, and attended to other important matters. Neither [welles v1pp540-541] nor [beale pp345-346] mention this, but exactly one year later [welles v2p257] does (See ¶1231.). *Given the lack of substantiating evidence, this event is, therefore, classified as an erroneous report.* — 1186

⟨2⟩ March 22, 1864: (**Error**) [porterH] incorrectly reports Lincoln visits City Point on this day, relating events of the 1865 visit (¶1261ff). — 1187

⟨1⟩ April 17, 1864: "The reports in a New-York Sunday paper of the perilous condition of the President's health, are fortunately without foundation at this writing." [NYTimes - April 18, 1864] — 1188

⟨1⟩ April 28, 1864: "I went that morning to take leave of the President. I had seen him but once before. I was pained, almost shocked, by the change in his looks and manner wrought during the intervening five months. He looked like a man worn and harassed with petty faultfinding and criticism, until he had turned at bay, like an old stag pursued and hunted by a cowardly rabble of men and dogs." [riddle p266] — 1189

⟨$\frac{1}{q}$⟩ June 20-23, 1864: Lincoln visits City Point, VA. The trip did "him good, physically, and strengthened him mentally." – Gideon Welles [donaldA p516] — 1190

⟨1⟩ April 28, 1864: "the goats and father are very well" – Lincoln telegram to Mary [donaldH p103] — 1191

⟨1⟩ Sept. 8, 1864: "All well, including Tad's pony and the goats" – Lincoln telegram to Mary [donaldH p105] — 1192

⟨1⟩ Sept. 11, 1864: "All well" – Lincoln telegram to Mary [donaldH p105] — 1193

⟨1⟩ Sept. 15, 1864: From a woman who pled her case at the White House: "The President sat behind a long table covered with green baize and had a worn and wary expression on his face. ... Thereupon he wrote a telegram and shuffled wearily across the room to the bell and sent it off. ... His lips relaxed into a gentle but weary smile..." – Elizabeth Morgan McElrath [shutesP: "A Rebel Woman's Visit to President Lincoln," on 4 typewritten pages in box 1, folder 1] (Precise date is from [baslerA v8p7].)) — 1194

⟨1⟩ Oct.± 1864: "The President lay on a sofa, apparently very weary." [stoddardD p339] — 1195

⟨1⟩ 1864: "Mrs. H. B. Stowe asked him 'what policy he proposed to pursue after the war.' With a mournful sort of laugh, he replied: 'After the war? I shall not be troubled about that. The war is killing me.'" [stoddardL pp408-409] ([randallC p333] supplies a different quote.) Henry Beecher [riceA p251] also supplies a different quote, and continues: "He had a presentiment that he would not live long, that he had put his whole life into the war, and that when it was over he would then collapse." — 1196

⟨1⟩ Dec. 1864: Accelerated decline begins about now, per editorial in New York *Daily Tribune* on Mar. 17, 1865, reprinted in §1e. (See ¶1257.) — 1197

General – During Presidency (continued)

- I read all 1865 entries (until April 15) in these diaries: [browning], [french], [miers] , and [welles]. Bates [beale] was then no longer Attorney General.   1198

⟨2⟩ Jan. 1, 1865: "Reception at White House 12-3. AL shook hands with 7000. In the very best of spirits and health." [barbeeP - box 2 folder 135] quoting or summarizing *National Republican* newspaper   1199

⟨2⟩ Jan. 10, 1865: "The President was in good spirits, and his countenance wore a peculiar expression, indicating that he is well satisfied with the progress of events just at present." [barbeeP - box 2 folder 135] quoting or summarizing *National Republican* newspaper   1200

⟨1⟩ Jan. 22, 1865: "The President appeared well and in excellent spirits and Mrs. Lincoln never appeared better." [french p463] (∈ ¶4423)   1201

⟨1⟩ Jan. 25, 1865: Lincoln is not taking calls, in the morning at least. [lincolnA - Schuyler Colfax to Lincoln]   1202

- February 6, 1865: Lincoln faints and is put to bed: 1203
  ⟨2⟩ The Attorney-General stormed in and made a provocative statement. "Lincoln jumped up and shouted back at him, 'If you think that I, of my own free will, will shed another drop of blood...' and then fainted and was put to bed. Dr. Stone ordered him kept there for an entire day and night, and with another warning insisted on more rest and shorter working hours." [shutes pp108-109]. *James Speed was then Attorney General.*   1204
  ⟨-⟩ *Depending on Lincoln's speech rate, he probably took from 4 to 7 seconds to utter his reply. Given the 7 second supply of oxygen in brain capillaries, this suggests an almost immediate halt to cerebral perfusion when Lincoln stood.*   1205
  ⟨S⟩ Writing decades later, Shutes [shutesE p172] calls this story "undocumented." Conceding "The story itself could be true," he doubts the date because such an incident would be improbable, coming just three days after a presumably restful escape to Hampton Roads, VA by boat. *Shutes' reasoning is dubious. "Rest" may have been immaterial.*   1206
  ⟨1⟩ Feb. 7: "The President, when I entered the room, was reading with much enjoyment certain portions of Petroleum V. Nasby to Dennison and Speed." [welles v2p238]   1207

⟨1⟩ Feb. 20, 1865: suspends White House public receptions "for the present" [miers v3] (citing Washington *Chronicle* of Feb. 19, 1865). At public reception on March 4, Lincoln shakes 6000 hands [miers v3p318].   1208

⟨1⟩ Feb. 23, 1865: "The President looked badly and felt badly – apparently more depressed than I have seen him since he became President." [browning pp7-8] *Lincoln and Browning were discussing an imminent hanging.*   1209

- Late Feb. 1865:   1210
  ⟨1⟩ "The last interview but one I had with him – was about ten days previous to his last inauguration ... [Speed sits in Lincoln's office while Lincoln hears, and grants, the impassioned pleas of two women. The women leave.] We were alone – I said to him – Lincoln with my knowledge of your nervous sensibility it is a wonder that such scenes as this dont kill you – I am said he very unwell – my feet & hands are always cold – I suppose I ought to be in bed – But things of that sort dont hurt me – For to tell you the truth – that scene which you witnessed is the only thing I have done to day which has given me any pleasure" – Joshua Speed, Jan. 12, 1866 letter to Herndon [wilson pp156-157]   1211

General – During Presidency (continued)

⟨1⟩ "The last time I saw him was about two weeks before his assassination. ...   1213
I went into his office about eleven o'clock. He looked jaded and weary. I
staid [sic] in the room until his hour for callers was over; he ordered the door
closed. [Lincoln hears, and grants, the pleas of two women. The women
leave.] We were then alone. He drew his chair to the fire and said 'Speed, I
am a little alarmed about myself; just feel my hand.' It was cold and clammy.
He pulled off his boots, and putting his feet to the fire, the heat made them
steam. I said overwork was producing nervousness. 'No,' said he, 'I am
not tired.' I said, 'Such a scene as I have just witnessed is enough to make
you nervous.' 'How much you are mistaken,' said he; 'I have made two people happy to-day...' " – Joshua Speed [speed pp26,28] See ⏍Heart & Circulation⏍.
*The timing is incorrect. Lincoln was visiting Grant in the field from March
23 to April 9. Thus, Speed could not have visited Lincoln in the White
House around April 1 ("about two weeks before his assassination").*

⟨-⟩ *Some details conflict in the two versions that came from Speed's pen.*   1214
Except for the date, it is not possible to tell which is more accurate.

⟨2⟩_c 1865: "He made a point of taking Mary and Tad on several little jaunts, ostensibly   1215
to inspect the armies, but in fact to secure a respite from his daily routine." [donaldH
p50]

- March 1865, around the March 4 inauguration: 1216
  ⟨1⟩ "Poor Mr. Lincoln is looking so broken-hearted, so completely worn out, I   1217
  fear he will not get through the next four years." – Mary Lincoln [kcckleyB p157]
  *Depending how one reads certain nuances in [keckleyB], this comment could
  have occurred as early as the November 1864 election.*
  ⟨2⟩ On the day of his second inauguration, March 4, Lincoln was "still unwell"   1218
  [kunhardtA p266].
  ⟨1/q⟩ "he was in mind, body, and nerves a very different man at the second inau-   1219
  guration from the one who had taken the oath in 1861. ... He aged with great
  rapidity." – John Hay [hayA] (∈ ¶2543)
  ⟨2⟩ "Those who observed Abraham Lincoln at the time of his first inaugural and   1220
  again saw him during the second inaugural ceremonies have testified to the
  great change which had occurred in his physical appearance. While it is accepted generally that the President wasted away during these four years until he was but a shadow of his old self, yet, he was almost without medical
  attention." [lincloreLHH]
  ⟨1⟩ March 4, 1865: Lincoln shakes about 5000 hands. His time for 100 hand-   1221
  shakes is measured on several occasions. The range is under 3 minutes to
  never over 5 minutes. [french p466]
  ⟨1/q⟩ Mar. 4: "look'd very much worn and tired" returning from inauguration cer-   1222
  emonies – Walt Whitman [luthin p593]
  ⟨2⟩ Mar. 6: Another inaugural ball. Stays 2-3 hours. [miers v3p318]   1223

⟨2⟩ Early March 1865: Mary buys $1000 worth of mourning goods [rossA pp246-247].   1224
*Possible explanations: (1) Mary realized, consciously or not, that Lincoln was
dying., (2) She thought son Robert, who was in the army, might die, and (3) It
was a shopping compulsion (Mary presumably had mourning clothes left over
from Willie's 1862 death).*

⟨2⟩ "Now and then, in the spring of 1865, he permitted a coachman to assist him in   1225
or out of his carriage. Lincoln was fifty-six; he looked old and sick. ... The Surgeon
General, Doctor Barnes, was worried about a nervous breakdown. The official

General – During Presidency (continued)

family began to speculate, for the first time, about what would happen to them and to the nation if he died. For a while, everyone including Mrs. Lincoln became solicitous of his health and his time. The police guards cleared the upstairs corridor of office seekers and favor seekers. His secretaries tried to hold the appointment calendar down, and his wife tried to coax him to take afternoon drives on sunny days. The attention was so pointed that even the President noticed it." [bishop p37] citing no references

- March 1865 illness: 1226
  - ⟨1⟩ Mar. 13: "Mr. Lincoln is reported quite sick to-day, and has denied himself to all visitors. The prayers of even those who have reviled him are offered for his continued health until the Vice President has recovered entirely from his 'incoherence.'" [NYHerald - Mar. 14, 1865] *Vice President Johnson had spoken almost incoherently at the March 4 inauguration (¶2676).* 1227
  - ⟨2⟩ Mar. 14: "Mr. Lincoln tried to arise from his bed and fell back. He could not summon the strength to get on his feet and Mrs. Lincoln, called from her bedroom, sent for Dr. Robert K. Stone, the family physician. He examined the President and came out of the bedroom announcing that the case was 'exhaustion, complete exhaustion.' Three hours later, the President held a Cabinet meeting in the bedroom. Word went out that his illness was influenza, and it was so reported in the press." [bishop pp37-38] 1228
  - ⟨1⟩ Mar. 14: "President Lincoln has been suffering with a severe attack of influenza for several days. He is confined to his bed to-day, and consequently not receiving visitors." [NYHerald - Mar. 15, 1865] [NYTimes - Mar. 15, 1865] (Almost identical sentence appears in [ChicagoTribune - Mar. 15, 1865].) 1229
  - ⟨1⟩ Mar. 14: "President Lincoln's health has been impaired for some days, he having been worn down with fatigue incident to the adjournment of Congress. He will be able to see visitors in a day or two." [NYTimes - Mar. 15, 1865] 1230
  - ⟨1⟩ Mar. 14: "The President was some indisposed and in bed, but not seriously ill. The members [of the Cabinet] met in his bedroom." [welles v2p257] 1231
  - ⟨1/q⟩ Mar. 14: "The President was forced to decline all interviews again today. Indisposition and the pressure of public business are his excuses." [NYTribune - Mar. 15, 1865] per written transcript in [barbeeP - box 2 folder 135] 1232
  - ⟨1⟩ Mar. 15: "The President, although suffering from weakness and fatigue, has received visitors to-day members of the Cabinet and Senators." [ChicagoTribune - Mar. 16, 1865] 1233
  - ⟨1⟩ Mar. 15: "The President has so far recovered as to be able to resume his official duties to-day. There were an army of applicants for all sorts of favors. The accumulation of three days. [sic]" [NYTimes - Mar. 16, 1865] 1234
  - ⟨2⟩ Mar. 15: "President has recovered from illness and is at his office today. He receives only his cabinet and others on urgent business." [miers v3p320] citing [WashingtonStar - Mar. 15, 1865] 1235
  - ⟨2⟩ Mar. 15: "...he was out of bed and in his office. He looked jaundiced and sick, and no appointments were made that day, but he worked at his desk." [bishop p38] 1236
  - ⟨1⟩ Mar. 15: "The health of Mr. Lincoln is so greatly improved that he was able to-day to give audience to a host of visitors ... and to accompany Mrs. Lincoln to the German opera this evening." [NYHerald - Mar. 16, 1865] 1237
  - ⟨1⟩ Mar. 15: Watching a play at Grover's Theater, Lincoln "sat in the rear of the box leaning his head against the partition paying no attention to the play and 1238

General – During Presidency (continued)

looking so worn and weary that it would not have been surprising had his soul and body separated that very night. When the curtain fell after the first act, turning to him, I said: 'Mr. President you are not apparently interested in the play.' 'Oh, no, Colonel,' he replied; 'I have not come for the play, but for the rest. I am hounded to death by office-seekers, who pursue me early and late, and it is simply to get two or three hours' relief that I am here.' After a slight pause he added: 'I wonder if we shall be tormented in heaven with them, as well as with bores and fools?' He then closed his eyes and I turned to the ladies." – James Grant Wilson [wilsonR pp424-425]

⟨$\frac{1}{q}$⟩ Mar. 15: "The President opened the doors of the White House again today and of course was ravished by a crowd of hungry office-seekers." [NYTribune - Mar. 16, 1865] per written transcript in [barbeeP - box 2 folder 135]   1239

⟨$\frac{1}{q}$⟩ Mar. 17: "President Lincoln's Health: Altho the President is yet quite feeble he is slowly gaining strength, and yesterday afternoon he took a short ride, appearing upon the avenue in his carriage, accompanied by his son, Master Tad. If the throngs of office seekers who are now here besetting hum upon every side would allow him to obtain a few days relaxation, he would doubtless speedily recover his usual health; but notwithstanding the President's indisposition and the fact that this is Cabinet day, the White House was again thronged this morning with parties eager to obtain an interview." [WashingtonStar - Mar. 17, 1865] per written transcript in [barbeeP - box 2 folder 135]   1240

⟨1⟩ Mar. 17: "The President, though still in feeble health, is annoyed by the pressure of importunate office seekers." [NYHerald - Mar. 18, 1865] (and New York *World* per [barbeeP - box 1 folder 51])   1241

⟨1⟩ Mar. 17: "Mr. Lincoln's health is improving under the influence of an enforced quiet by the rigid shutting out of all visitors, no matter under what pretence they demand an interview. It is truly lamentable to see the pertinacity with which many of these office-seeking cormorants literally demand the President's personal attention to their claims. the [sic] consideration of overtaxed energies and possible failing health, seems never to be thought of by them, and the President, contrary to his amiable character and desires, is obliged to enforce rules in regard to his time and business which he would be delighted to have people respect through their own sense of the delicacy of his position, and the vast amount of important public business constantly passing before him through the regular channels." [NYTimes - Mar. 18, 1865]   1242

⟨$\frac{1}{q}$⟩ Mar. 17: "Recovery of the President: Considerable uneasiness has been felt by the public, who were aware of the temporary confinement to his room of the President, lest his illness might prove serious and prolonged. We are gratified to be able to announce that he was not only able to be in his office during yesterday and the day before, but that he appeared in our streets yesterday afternoon, and was evidently much improved." – Washington *Chronicle* per typed transcript in [barbeeP - box 1 folder 51]   1243

⟨1⟩ Mar. 17: Long editorial on Lincoln's health in [NYTribune - Mar. 17, 1865]. See §1e.   1244

⟨$\frac{1}{q}$⟩ Mar. 17: Washington *Daily Times* quotes from the Mar. 16 *National Republican* per typewritten transcript in [barbeeP - box 1 folder 51]   1245

⟨$\frac{1}{q}$⟩ Mar. 17: "almost worn out" with a day of office seekers and documents – Henry Raymond [shutesE p177].   1246

⟨$\frac{1}{q}$⟩ Mar. 17 or 18: Lincoln presents a rebel flag to Indiana Governor (and future Vice President) Oliver Morton in a ceremony at the National Hotel. [WashingtonStar - Mar. 18, 1865] per written transcript in [barbeeP - box 2 folder 135]   1247

General – During Presidency (continued)

⟨1⟩ Mar. 20: "I am most happy to say, that my blessed Husband's health, has much improved." – Mary [turner p205] 1248

⟨1⟩ Mar. 21: Editorial in New York *Daily Tribune*, reprinted in §1f. 1249

⟨q/1⟩ Mar. 22: "President Lincoln's Tormentors - How to Stop Them" in [NYHerald - Mar. 22, 1865] per typed transcript in [barbeeP - box 1 folder 51] 1250

⟨q/1⟩ Mar. 22: "Mr. Lincoln's Health" in Rochester *Union and Advertiser* per typed transcript in [barbeeP - box 1 folder 51] 1251

⟨q/1⟩ Mar. 23: "A Day in the White House" in Baltimore *American* per transcript in [barbeeP - box 1 folder 51] 1252

⟨q/1⟩ Mar. 23: Washington *Daily Times* reprints "letter" from §1f and adds: "We heartily concur in this, and feel a double interest in the President's life, as his death would put one much less qualified than himself in the Executive office." [barbeeP - box 1 folder 51] 1253

⟨1⟩ Mar. 23, preparing for trip to City Point: "I cannot but devoutly hope, that change of air & rest may have a beneficial effect on my good Husband's health." – Mary [turner p209] 1254

⟨2⟩ March 1865: "Lincoln was so exhausted after the inauguration ceremonies that he took to his bed for a few days. There was nothing organically wrong. Despite his sedentary work, he continued to be a physically powerful man, but he often felt terribly tired. For some time he had been losing weight, and strangers now noted his thinness rather than his height. Though he was only fifty-six, observers at the second inauguration thought he looked very old. His photographs showed a face heavily lined, with sunken cheeks. ... For months [Mary] had been urging her husband to keep a lighter schedule." [donaldA p568] *Is this rationalization? Clearly it was more than exhaustion: it was organic illness.* 1255

⟨1⟩ March 22, 1865: An editorial in [ChicagoTribune - March 22, 1865] (full text in §1d) urges for "our really invalid President a month's furlough" because his "physical powers have been tested beyond their capacity of endurance, and that if this ordeal is to continue, his naturally strong constitution must at no distant date, give way." The editorial notes "his present worn and weakened condition" and observes "Many who saw him at his inauguration, where the opportunity for noting the change in his personal appearance was better than in his office or at the White House, were painfully impressed with his gaunt, skeleton-like appearance." The editorial identifies the mass of petitioners pressing upon Lincoln as the cause of his decline. "He needs at least a month's entire rest from his official duties, and thenceforward a systematic and enforced exemption from the vast and unprecedented pressure of calls, appeals, committees, &c." Amazingly, the editorial concludes such a furlough is practical because "Gen. Grant as Grand Marshal of the military operations at the front needs no watching. Secretary Stanton is at home in the War Department" and so on. *This is a wholly remarkable document. The editorialist clearly saw that Lincoln was, physically, in trouble. Urging a vacation was quite reasonable: given that that era had no effective medical treatments for wasting disease, a vacation would have worked just as well as anything else.* ○○○ *Project:* Did a major American newspaper at any other time urge a President to vacation for reasons of physical health? Harding? Franklin Roosevelt? Polk? Eisenhower? Wilson? 1256

⟨1⟩ Mar. 17: Editorial in New York *Daily Tribune*: "All who knew him in 1860 and have met him in 1865, must have observed his air of fatigue, exhaustion and languor – so different from his old hearty, careless, jovial manner. We are sure no good physician, who had seen him since last December, can 1257

General – During Presidency (continued)

have heard of his recent illness without feeling that this was what might and should have been expected" [barbeeP - box 2 folder 137] (Full text in §1e.) *This seems to date the start of Lincoln's accelerated decline to December 1864.*

⟨1⟩ Mar. 21: Editorial in New York *Daily Tribune* says Lincoln is dying: "The 1258 President is being killed by monstrous experiments on his patience and good nature... The office-seekers are not only killing the President; they are imperiling the life of the Nation. We urge the People to insist on their instant and thorough abatement." [barbeeP box 2 folder 135] (Full text in §1f.)

⟨1⟩ March 23, 1865: "The President has gone to the front, partly to get rid of the throng 1259 that is pressing upon him, though there are speculations of a different character. He makes his office much more laborious than he should. Does not generalize and takes upon himself questions that properly belong to the Departments, often causing derangement and irregularity. The more he yields, the greater the pressure upon him. It has now become such that he is compelled to flee. There is no doubt he is much worn down; besides he wishes the War terminated, and, to this end, that severe terms shall not be exacted of the Rebels." [welles v2p264] *This is the entire paragraph.*

⟨1⟩ "The President came down to City Point ... He came, in the first place, for 1260 rest; he looked much worn out with his responsibilities since I had last seen him, and needed the repose he sought." [porterD p281] *The "last time" was no earlier than 1862, probably mid-year* [porterD pp114-124].

■ March 23-24, 1865: Steaming from Washington to City Point, VA aboard the *River* 1261 *Queen.*

⟨2⟩ reason for the trip: "most of all, they needed rest" [donaldA p571]. "...both were 1262 breaking down; he physically, she [Mary] physically and mentally" [randallC p334].

⟨1⟩ March 23: Sailed in afternoon; retires about midnight; up later to check on 1263 Tad [crookA pp38-40]. According to Edwin Stanton, a "furious gale" came soon after Lincoln sailed [baslerA v8p374].

⟨1⟩ March 24: Morning: Rough water in Chesapeake Bay. Some aboard are sea-1264 sick. Lincoln appears on deck "looking very much rested. 'I'm feeling splendidly,' he said. 'Is breakfast ready?' He did full justice to the delicious fish when it was served." Calmer water in James River. Reached City Point after dark. [crookA p40]

⟨1⟩ Mar. 24, before 12:30 p.m., telegram from Ft. Monroe: "The President desires 1265 me to say he has just arrived at this point safely, and is now feeling well, having had a pretty fair passage." – C.B. Penrose [aa117 v46p96] (Online [baslerA v8p374] says [mistakenly] the telegram came from City Point.)

⟨1⟩ Mar. 24: "had been indisposed [the 24th] and attributed it to the drink-1266 ing water furnished the *Queen* at Washington; indeed we had stopped at Fortress Monroe [the 24th] and taken on a supply of fresh water in demi-johns, for Mr. Lincoln's special use." [barnesA]

⟨1⟩ Mar. 24: Lincoln requests water from Ft. Monroe [baslerA v8p374] 1268

⟨1⟩ Mar. 24, 9 p.m., telegram from City Point: "he has just arrived at this point 1269 safely, and both he and family are well, having entirely recovered from their indispositions of this morning." – C.B. Penrose [aa117 v46p97] *Lincoln was still ill. See below.*

⟨1⟩ Mar. 25: At City Point: "Arrived here, all safe about 9 A.M. yesterday." – Lin-1270 coln [baslerA v8p374] *No explanation is given for the discrepant arrival time.*

General – During Presidency (continued)

- March 24-April 2, 1865, at City Point: 1271

  ⟨1⟩ Mar. 24: "Upon arrival of the steam-boat at the wharf at City Point General 1272 Grant and several other members of his staff went aboard to welcome the Presidential party." Of Lincoln: "When asked how he was he said, 'I am not feeling very well. I got pretty badly shaken up on the bay coming down, and am not altogether over it yet.'" Champagne is offered as a seasickness remedy, but Lincoln declines. [porterH] (Note: [kunhardtA p242] dates the episode to June 21, 1864; [porterH] dates it to March 1864; [coffinB p489] gets it right.)

  ⟨1⟩ Mar. 25: "I reported to Mr. Lincoln early in the morning of the 25th, was in- 1273 vited to breakfast with the family... Mr. Lincoln, who was not looking well, had been indisposed the day before... After breakfast ... we all walked up to General Grant's headquarters..." [barnesA] *Suggests that Lincoln's illness lasted at least 24 hours.*

  ⟨2⟩ Mar. 25: "eats very little" at breakfast [miers v3p322]   1274

  ⟨1⟩ Mar. 25: Lincoln rides through a battlefield, seeing "great numbers of dead," 1275 wounded, and prisoners. Later, "Mr. Lincoln looked worn and haggard. He remarked that he had seen enough of the horrors of war..." Barnes tells him of a grievously wounded boy who died. "Mr. Lincoln's eyes filled with tears and his voice was choked with emotion." Lincoln "desired to rest on the *Queen* with his family," declines Grant's dinner invitation, and sees no one else that evening. [barnesA]

  ⟨1⟩ Mar. 26: "On reporting to Mr. Lincoln, I found him quite recovered from the 1276 fatigue and excitement of the day before." Reviewing Navy ships pass by, Lincoln waved his hat and "seemed as happy as a schoolboy." Riding to a military review, "was in high spirits, laughing and chatting." Mary Lincoln explodes in anger at the review. At 11pm, Lincoln, in the company of Mary, "seemed weary and greatly distressed" [barnesA] (See ¶2544.)

  ⟨1⟩ Mar. 27: Walks from the *Queen* to Grant's headquarters [barnesA]. In good spir- 1277 its [barnesB]; see ¶2546.

  ⟨1⟩ Mar. 28: "The President's Health Improving: The President has been in- 1278 dulging in riding on horseback, and his health has been considerably improved since he left Washington." [NYTimes - Mar. 29, 1865]

  ⟨2⟩ Mar. 28, 1865, visiting Grant's headquarters: "It was a mild spring morning, 1279 but he wore an overcoat" and stove-pipe hat [coffinA p179].

  ⟨1⟩ Makes excursions in James River on Admiral Porter's barge. Lincoln "said he 1280 should always look upon this time as the real holiday of his administration." [porterD p292]

  ⟨1⟩ Mar. 31: Lincoln "knew that Grant was to make a general attack on Peters- 1281 burg, and grew depressed." [crookB] *Crook thought the causes were the impending loss of life and the risk to Robert*

  ⟨2⟩ April 1: Walks deck most of the night. [miers v3p324] citing [crookB]   1282

  ⟨1⟩ April 2: "Tad & I are both well." – Lincoln, at City Point, VA [donaldH p112]   1283

  ⟨1⟩ April 3: "He was in high spirits, seemed not at all fatigued" [barnesB]   1284

- April 4, 1865: Visits Richmond. *This episode shows Lincoln's limited exercise* 1285 *tolerance. After a tense, slow, one-hour walk, during which he had to stop and rest, Lincoln is exhausted.*

  ⟨1⟩ After coming ashore at Rockett's landing, a crowd envelops Lincoln and his 1286 small party; "they were pushed, hustled, and elbowed along, without any regard to their persons" for "a half hour or more. The day was very warm, and as we progressed the street became thick with dust and smoke from the

General – During Presidency (continued)

smoldering ruins about us." A cavalry squad then appeared, and escorted the party to Jefferson Davis's house. In Davis' reception room, "Mr. Lincoln walked across the room to the easy chair and sank down in it. He was pale and haggard, and seemed utterly worn out with fatigue and the excitement of the past hour." At this "supreme moment [Lincoln's first words were] 'I wonder if I could get a drink of water.' He did not appeal to any particular person for it. I can see the tired look out of those kind blue eyes over which the lids half drooped; his voice was gentle and soft. There was no triumph in his gesture or attitude. He lay back in the chair like a tired man whose nerves had carried him beyond his strength. All he wanted was rest and a drink of water." [barnesB]

⟨2⟩ It was "a beautiful, warm day." Lincoln soon removed his long overcoat,   1287
which hung below his knees, but continued to wear his stovepipe hat. He frequently removed it to "wipe away big drops of perspiration on his forehead" [donaldA p576]. *Donald cites no primary source. Had Lincoln overdressed in the morning because of cold intolerance? Or did he want to present a dignified air to the citizens of Richmond? "Big drops" may be artistic license.*

⟨1/q⟩ "Our progress was very slow; we did not move a mile an hour [amidst the   1288
crowd]. It was a warm day, and the streets were dusty. ... The atmosphere was suffocating, but Mr. Lincoln could be seen plainly by every man, woman, and child, towering head and shoulders above that crowd; he overtopped every man there. He carried his hat in his hand, fanning his face, from which the perspiration was pouring. He looked as if he would have given his Presidency for a glass of water – I would have given my commission for half that." [porterD pp298-299]

⟨1/q⟩ "The procession moved at a rapid pace. The President manifested weariness,   1289
and halted for a moment near the railroad station on Broad Street. He was wearing his overcoat. The sun was shining from a cloudless sky." The cavalry squad rode to him. "The President lifted his own hat from his head, bowed [to an onlooker], wiped the gathering moisture from his eyes, and then the procession moved on" to Davis' house. The "party entered the building. Mr. Lincoln dropped wearily into a chair..." – Boston *Journal*, April 1865, quoted by [coffinB p506]

⟨1⟩ "We reached the base of Capitol Hill. The afternoon was warm, and the   1290
President desired to rest. The procession halted. The crowd had become so dense that it was difficult to advance. [After resting they go up the hill, with cavalrymen opening the way, and reach the rebel leader's mansion.] President Lincoln wearily ascended the steps, and by chance dropped into the very chair usually occupied [by the leader]. There was no sign of exultation, no elation of spirit, but, on the contrary, a look of unutterable weariness, as if his spirit, energy and animating force were utterly exhausted." [coffinA p186]

⟨1⟩ "The President manifested no signs of exultation. In Petersburg his counte-   1291
nance had been radiant and joyful, but at that moment it was one of indescribable sadness." [coffinB p506]

⟨2⟩ The distance walked was about two miles, uphill [ferguson p15].   1292

⟨2⟩ After lunch, "rides around in ambulance," with only one stop, before return-   1293
ing to ship. [miers v3p325]

⟨1⟩ "Later in the afternoon I saw President Lincoln riding through the streets...   1294
There was no smile upon his face. Paler than ever his countenance, deeper

General – During Presidency (continued)

than ever before the lines upon his forehead." [coffinA p187]

⟨1⟩ April 1865: "his gestures were vigorous and supple, revealing great physical   1295
strength and an extraordinary energy for resisting privation and fatigue" [chambrunA] (∈ ¶200)

⟨1⟩ April 8, 1865 (morning): "He was erect and buoyant, and it seemed to me that I   1296
have never seen him look so great and grand." – Elihu Washburne [riceB p120]

⟨1/q⟩ April 7 or 8, 1865: After several hours visiting hospitals, he was called to see an-   1297
other ward of troops. "The surgeon, who was thoroughly tired, and knew Mr. Lincoln must be, tried to dissuade him from going," but Lincoln went anyway. Afterwards, "The surgeon expressed the fear that the President's arm would be lamed with so much handshaking, saying it must certainly ache. Mr. Lincoln smiled, and saying something about his 'strong muscles,' stepped out at the open door, took up a very large, heavy axe which lay there by a log of wood, and chopped vigorously for a few moments, sending the chips flying in all directions; and then, pausing, he extended his right arm to its full length, holding the axe out horizontally, without its even quivering as he held it. Strong men who looked on – men accustomed to manual labor – could not hold the same axe in that position for a moment. Returning to the office, he took a glass of lemonade, for he would take no stronger beverage." [carpenter pp288-289] quoting the *New York Independent*.

  ⟨2⟩ This occurred on April 10 according to the *Independent*, as quoted by [carpenter   1298
p287], but [crookA p58], [donaldA p580], [pfanz p91], [browneF p694] all say Lincoln was back in Washington on April 9. Mary's April 11 letter (¶1312) gives April 7 as the hospital day, while [pfanz p84] [keckleyB p171] [barrett pp777-778] [chambrunA] [fisk p323] [sumnerA p133] all say April 8. Lincoln left City Point the morning of April 8 [barnesB]. He stopped at Fortress Monroe later that day, there visiting hospitals [coffinB p510].

  ⟨1⟩ "some of the surgeons told him that to attempt to shake hands with so many   1300
thousand men would be more than he ought to endure, but he overruled them, for he said he wanted to shake hands with the brave boys who had won the great victories. ... The President appeared to take great in it." [fisk p323] *Note that the wood-chopping demonstration is not mentioned.*

  ⟨2⟩ The surgeon was Edward S. Dalton. [shutes p99]   1301

  ⟨1⟩ "he passed through all the wards, stopping at bed after bed, till every man   1302
had touched his hand, and the whole five thousand of the camp had been treated with his friendly salutation." [anonA] (∈ ¶2191)

  ⟨1⟩ "He returned to the boat in the evening, with a tired, weary look. 'Mother,'   1303
he said to his wife, 'I have shaken so many hands to-day that my arms ache tonight. I almost wish I could go to bed now.' " – Lincoln [keckleyB p171]

  ⟨1⟩ Witnesses of the hospital tour, who do not mention the wood-chopping: 1304
[chambrunA] [fisk p323] [sumnerA p133]. Senator Harlan and [crookA p58] were probably witnesses, too.

▪ April 9, 1865:   1305

  ⟨2⟩ President returns in excellent health. *River Queen* arrives at 6 P.M. [miers   1306
v3p327] citing [WashingtonStar - April 10, 1865]

  ⟨1/q⟩ "Mr. Lincoln ... returned this afternoon ... musch stronger in body and soul   1307
than when he left." [NYTribune - Apr. 10, 1865] per typed transcript in [barbeeP - box 2 folder 135]

▪ April 10, 1865:   1308

General – During Presidency (continued)

⟨1⟩ "Called on the President, who returned last evening, looking well and feeling well." [welles v2p278]   1309

⟨1⟩ "On the morning after our return from City Point, I found the President already at his desk. 'Good morning, Crook. How do you feel?' I answered: 'First-rate, Mr. President. How are you?' 'I am well, but rather tired.' Then I noticed that he did, indeed, look tired. His worn face made me understand, more clearly than I had done before, what a strain the experiences at Petersburg and Richmond had been. Now that the excitement was over, the reaction allowed it to be seen." [crookA p60]   1310

⟨2⟩ "The visit to City Point rejuvenated Lincoln. Once he was away from the nagging pressures of Washington, his health returned." [donaldA p575]   1311

⟨1⟩ April 11, 1865: "I am happy to say that, Mr Lincoln is feeling much better to day, Friday's pilgrimage through the hospitals, although a labor of love, to him, fatigued him very much." – Mary [turner p217] *Friday was April 7. For details of visit, see ¶1297 and ¶2191.*   1312

⟨1⟩ April 12 (11?), 1865: Mary enters a White House room without knocking, after Lincoln had made a speech. "There was Mr. Lincoln, stretched at full length, resting on a large sofa from his oratorical efforts.... he rose impulsively... I did not stay too long, in order to let him rest" [chambrunB p93]   1313

⟨1⟩ April 13(?), 1865: "Mr Lincoln is indisposed with quite a severe headache, yet would be very much pleased to see you at the house, this evening." – Mary, to U.S. Grant [turner p219] *No date is on the letter. For reasons not given, [turner] assigns it to April 13. Contrariwise, [baslerA v8p589] and [miers v3p328] assign it to April 11.*   1314

⟨1⟩ April 13, 1865: "his eye had that expression of profound weariness and sadness which I never saw in other human eye [sic]" [field p321] (∈ ¶2563)   1315

⟨1⟩ April 14, 1865, late afternoon: "...was more depressed than I had ever seen him and his step unusually slow. ...earlier in the afternoon he had been extremely cheerful, even buoyant." [crookA p65] (∈ ¶2363)   1316

⟨1/q⟩ April 14, 1865: "at dinner he complained of being worn out with the incessant toils of the day, and proposed to go to the theatre and have a laugh over the Country Cousin. She says she discouraged going, on account of a bad headache, but he insisted that he must go, for if he stayed at home he would have no rest for he would be obliged to see company all the evening as usual. Finding that he had decided to go, she could not think of having him go without her, never having felt so unwilling to be away from him." – Anson Henry, writing five days later what Mary had told him [luthin pp629-630]   1317

⟨2⟩ At dinner: "looked cheerful, felt happy over the war's end, but spoke of a fatigued feeling. He believed that the theatre might do him some good." [luthin p629]   1318

⟨1⟩ April 14, 1865: Sitting in the drafty box in Ford's Theatre, Mary gives him "a look." Lincoln dons his overcoat [helmB p257]. (∈ ¶697)   1319

⟨1/q⟩ April 22, 1865: "When we last saw Mr. Lincoln, he looked so weary and haggard that he seemed unlikely to live out his term." – Horace Greeley [shutes p107]   1320

⟨1/q⟩ "When I last saw him, a few weeks before his death, I was struck by his haggard, care-fraught face, so different from the sunny, gladsome countenance he first brought from Illinois." – Horace Greeley [luthin p593]   1321

General – During Presidency (continued)

⟨2⟩ "His mind was like his body. His mind worked slowly, but strongly. Hence there *c* was very little bodily or mental wear and tear in him. This peculiarity in his construction gave him great advantage over other men in public life. No man in America – scarcely a man in the world – could have stood what Lincoln did in Washington and survived through more than one term of the Presidency." [herndon p472] *Weik appears to have added this phrase. It does not appear in the 1865 lecture by Herndon* [herndonC] *that forms the basis for this passage's surrounding material. It is possible, of course, that Herndon modified the lecture later.*   1322

⟨1⟩ "... there was something about him that made plain folks feel toward him a good *q* deal as a child feels toward his father." – Gilbert Finch [burl pp73-74]   1323

  ⟨S⟩ [burl pp73-91] is a chapter about this aspect of Lincoln – the "surrogate father." 1324
  ⟨-⟩ [burl] *does not suggest how Lincoln achieved this effect. Did his height or other aspects of his physical make-up contribute? No, says* [burl p75] *citing* [donaldB p129].   1325

Habits

■ Re: women, see ¶2216. Re: alcohol, see Habits -- Alcohol .   1326

⟨1⟩ "He had no vices – even as a young man" – Joshua Speed [wilson p499]   1327

■ Tobacco: 1328
  ⟨1⟩ "Lincoln never used tobacco in any form while I knew him." – Daniel Burner 1329
      [templeB]
  ⟨1⟩ "he did not in those days even smoke or chew Tobacco" – Abner Ellis [wilson 1330
  q p170] (∈ ¶1356)
  ⟨1⟩ Lincoln did not chew tobacco, smoke, or drink. [herndon p244]   1331
  ⟨1⟩ "I never heard him use a profain word ... or chew tobacco in my life" – Eliza- 1332
      beth Abell [wilson p557]
  ⟨2⟩ "never chewed or smoked tobacco" [kunhardtA p322]   1333

⟨1⟩ "He never played cards, nor drank, nor hunted" – James Short [wilson p73]   1334

⟨1⟩ "Never Swore an oath" – Geo. Glasscock [wilson p162] (∈ ¶1346)   1335

⟨1⟩ For his appointments with sculptor Leonard Volk: "He never failed to be on time." 1336
    [volk]. See Head -- Casts

Habits – Alcohol

⟨1⟩ "He never drank whiskey or other strong drink" – Sarah Bush Lincoln [wilson p108] 1337

⟨1⟩ Daniel Burner worked in the Lincoln & Berry store in New Salem in the early 1338
    1830s, where liquor was sold. Decades later he remembered: "Lincoln did not
    drink much. Only once in awhile did I see him take anything." Berry drank more.
    Lincoln once remarked to his partner: "Berry, if we had not been such good cus-
    tomers ourselves, our stock would have lasted longer." [templeB]

  ⟨S⟩ Of Lincoln's remark to Berry, [templeB] says: "Typical of Lincoln, he was at- 1339
      tempting to take some of the blame while pointing out the difficulty which
      had resulted because of Berry's drinking."
  ⟨1⟩ Burner further observed: "Drinking was not held in such low repute then as 1340
      now. Fact is, everybody indulged and liquor was kept in nearly every home
      and was set out when a visitor arrived. So we did not think Abe Lincoln was
      committing any great wrong when he sold whisky [sic]." [templeB]

Habits – Alcohol (continued)

- 1830s:
  - $\langle\frac{1}{q}\rangle$ "He never drank any intoxicating liquors – he did not even in those days smoke or chew tobacco." – A.Y. Ellis [herndon p96] — 1341 1342
  - $\langle 1 \rangle$ Lincoln did not chew tobacco, smoke, or drink. [herndon p244] — 1343
  - $\langle 1 \rangle$ "Sometimes he took his dram as Every body did at that time" – David Turnham [wilson p121] — 1344
  - $\langle 1 \rangle$ He "was in every respect a total abstainer." [herndon p392] — 1345
  - $\langle 1 \rangle$ According to Geo. W. Glasscock (a man Lincoln later pardoned), "Mr L in his younger days was a Man of good habits   he Says Mr L never drank a drop of Liquor to his Knowledge – Never Swore an oath had no desire for strange Woman" – Abner Ellis [wilson p162] — 1346
  - $\langle 1 \rangle$ 1830s: "I never knew him to take a drop of liquor – or get drunk" – Henry McHenry [wilson p15] — 1347
  - $\langle 1 \rangle$ 1830s: "I never Saw Mr Lincoln drink. he often told me he never drank, had no desire for the drink, nor the companionship of drinking men." – Robert Wilson [wilson p205] — 1348
  - $\langle 1 \rangle$ "He never was an intemperate lad: he did drink his dram as well as all others did, preachers & Christians included – *Lincoln was a temperate drinker.*" – Nathaniel Grigsby [wilson p112] — 1349
  - $\langle 1 \rangle$ "Abe once drank as all people here did at that time." – William Wood [wilson p123] — 1350
  - $\langle 1 \rangle$ "Never saw him under the influence of liquor – took his dram with me when he felt like it – not often" – Caleb Carman [wilson p373] — 1351
  - $\langle 1 \rangle$ "Drank his dram occasionally when he wanted it." – Caleb Carman [wilson p374] — 1352
  - $\langle 1 \rangle$ "I never heard him use a profain word drink a drop of spirits or chew tobacco in my life" – Elizabeth Abell [wilson p557] — 1353
  - $\langle 1 \rangle$ "He never played cards, nor drank, nor hunted" – James Short [wilson p73] — 1354
  - $\langle 1 \rangle$ "He never touched liquor of any kind.' – James Short [wilson p90] — 1355
  - $\langle 1 \rangle$ "Salem in those days was a hard place for a temperate young Man Like Mr Lincoln was and I have often wondered how he could be so extremely popular and and [sic] not drink and Carouse with them ... I am certain he never drank any intoxicating liquors he did not in those days even smoke or chew Tobacco" – Abner Ellis [wilson p170] — 1356
  - $\langle 1 \rangle$ "I never Saw him drink a drop of liquor" – Hannah Armstrong [wilson p526] — 1357
- $\langle\frac{1}{q}\rangle$ 1842: Lincoln says of alcohol: "In my judgment such of us as have never fallen victims have been spared more from the absence of appetite than from any mental or moral superiority over those who have." [herndon p206] — 1358
  - $\langle 1 \rangle$ The spirit of the times is well captured by the matter-of-fact statement from farmer Andrew Kirk: "Saturday was the universal day to go to Springfield & other villages to do business – get drunk and to fight." [wilson p603] — 1359
- Pre-presidency:
  - $\langle 1 \rangle$ "If Lincoln Ever drank it was as a medicine I think" – James Gourley [wilson p452] — 1360 1361
  - $\langle\frac{1}{q}\rangle$ "It is not true that he never drank a drop of whiskey in his life. Mr. Lincoln did sometimes take a horn. He played ball on the day of his nomination in Chicago with the boys and did drink beer two or three times during the day; he was nervous then, excited on that particular occasion, and drank to steady his nerves." – Herndon [bumgarnerB] (see ¶2504) — 1362

Habits – Alcohol (continued)

⟨1⟩ "Lincoln did drink when he thought that it would do him good; he was never 1363
seen under the influence of liquor more than once or twice in his younger
days when it, liquor, was quite in universal use." – William Herndon [hertz
p166]

⟨1⟩ "The fact that he was a total abstinence man was well known in Illinois." 1364
[stoddardD pp259, 260]

⟨1/q⟩ 1860: While seeking the Presidential nomination, Lincoln and Mary argued 1365
whether alcohol should be served to visitors in their home. Mary was for
it, Lincoln against. He wanted to serve only ice water. Donald implies Lincoln was courting temperance voters, but also quotes Lincoln's explanation:
"Having kept house sixteen years, and having never held the 'cup' to the lips
of my friends then, my judgment was that I should not, in my new position,
change my habit in this respect." [donaldA p251]

⟨1⟩ May 19, 1860: Emissaries of the Republication Party visit Lincoln at home to 1366
notify him formally that he is the Presidential nominee. Lincoln offers them
water only, saying: "I have no liquors in my house, and have never been in
the habit of entertaining my friends that way." [coffinA pp174-175]

⟨1⟩ "Lincoln has been often heard to say that 'I never drink much and am entitled 1367
to no credit therefor [sic], because I hate the stuff. ... It is unpleasant to me and
always makes me feel flabby and undone.' " – Herndon [hertz p165]

⟨2⟩ "His drink was water – Adam's ale he called it. When he was entertaining and wine 1369
was served, he would lift his glass and merely touch it to his lips, not because of
pledges from his early temperance days; he just didn't like the stuff or how it made
him feel." [kunhardtA p322]

⟨1/q⟩ "He drank nothing but water, not from principle but because he did not like wine 1370
or spirits." – John Hay, 1866 [herndon p416]

⟨H⟩ A "tradition" says that Lincoln was anti-liquor because of the influence of 1371
temperance advocate Dr. John Allen (see ¶3173) [shutes p19]

■ As President: 1372

⟨2⟩ "At least once in Washington, he drank a glass of champagne for his nerves, at 1373
a doctor's recommendation." [shenk p112] *As Congressman or as President?*

⟨1⟩ As good news about the battle of Ft. Donelson came to the War Department, 1374
"some fellow being jubilant cried out 'lets have a drink.' Lincoln said 'All
right bring in some water.' " – Dillard Donnohue [wilson p602]

⟨1/q⟩ June 1864: Lincoln, with an upset stomach, declines offered champagne, 1375
saying too many people get "seasick ashore from drinking that stuff" [kun-
hardtA p242]. (∈ ¶658)

⟨1⟩ April 4, 1865: Although very thirsty (¶1285), declines offered whiskey [crookA 1376
p55].

⟨2⟩ In the minutes and hours after being shot, Lincoln was given three sips of brandy 1377
(for medicinal reasons). Thus, the last drink ever to pass his lips was the drink
that he had all his life shunned. [kunhardtB p44]

Hair

■ Color: 1378

⟨1⟩ "dark hair." [herndon p471] 1379

⟨1⟩ Feb. 1861: "no gray hairs – or but few in his head" [herndonC] [herndon p471] (∈ 1380
¶1)

Hair (continued)

⟨1⟩ "his hair was dark, almost black" [herndon p472]   1381

⟨$\frac{1}{q}$⟩ 1860: "How they call him 'Old Abe' I do not see. You can hardly detect the   1382
presence of frost on his black hair." – [NYHerald] reporter [ostendorfA p52] (See
¶1756)

⟨1⟩ 1862: "His hair was black, still unmixed with gray" [hawthorne p310] (∈ ¶178)   1383

⟨1⟩ Sept. 1863: "his hair, well silvered, though the brown then predominated; his   1384
beard was more whitened." – Cordelia Harvey [harveyC] (∈ §6.2)

⟨1⟩ See ¶1387, ¶1400, ¶1419, ¶183   1385

■ Baldness: 1386

⟨1⟩ "His hair was dark brown, without any tendency to baldness." – Senator   1387
James Harlan (date of recollection unknown) [helmB p166] Part of ¶173

⌷ Nov. 1863: The photograph of Lincoln delivering the Gettysburg Address ([os-   1388
tendorf #81]) shows prominent bilateral temporal recession.

■ Texture and arrangement: 1389

⟨$\frac{1}{q}$⟩ 1830s: "fuzzy hair" – Erastus Wright [walsh p81]   1390

⟨$\frac{1}{q}$⟩ Feb. 1857: When sitting for a photograph ([ostendorf #2]), Lincon objected to   1391
having his hair combed, saying "The boys down in Sangamon would never
know me this way." Before the photo was taken he ran his fingers through
his hair and quipped "Now I've made a bird's nest of it again." [ostendorfA p13]

⟨$\frac{1}{q}$⟩ Lincoln said his hair "had a way of getting up as far as possible in the world."   1393
[ostendorfA p18] referring to [ostendorf #6]

⟨1⟩ "his hair was rather stiff and coarse, and nearly black" [arnold p441] (∈ ¶167)   1394

⟨$\frac{1}{q}$⟩ Aug. 1858: "wiry, jet-black hair, which was usually in an unkempt condition"   1395
– Martin Rindlaub [ostendorfA p19] (∈ ¶148)

⟨1⟩ Dec. 1859: "coarse black hair" – part of Lincoln's self-description [baslerA   1396
v3p512] (∈ ¶151)

⟨$\frac{1}{q}$⟩ "This coarse, rough hair of mine..." – Lincoln [ostendorfA p7]   1397

⟨1⟩ "... his hair ... lay floating where his fingers or the wind left it, piled up at   1398
random." [herndon p472]

⟨$\frac{1}{q}$⟩ Feb. 27, 1860: "His bushy head, with the stiff black hair thrown back" – anon.   1399
[brooksA p186] (∈ ¶156)

⟨1⟩ April 1860: "I found him in the United States District Court-room ... his feet   1400
on the edge of a table, one of his fingers thrust into his mouth, and his long,
dark hair standing out at every imaginable angle, apparently uncombed for
a week." [volk]

⟨$\frac{1}{q}$⟩ May 19, 1860: "shaggy hair..." [coffinA p173] (∈ ¶157)   1401

⟨$\frac{1}{q}$⟩ June 21, 1860: "a profusion of wiry hair 'lying around loose' about his head"   1402
– Utica newspaper reporter [lincloreHDE] (∈ ¶159)

⟨1⟩ March 1861: "strange quaint face and head, covered with its thatch of wild,   1403
republican hair" – William Russell [russell pp37-38] (∈ ¶161)

⟨1⟩ Spring 1862: "had just come from a cabinet meeting... His hair stood up all   1404
over his head as though he had been running his hands through it" [bancroft]
(∈ ¶182)

⟨1⟩ 1862: "rough, uncombed and uncombable lank dark hair, that stands out in   1405
every direction at once" [dicey v1pp220-221] (∈ ¶179)

⟨1⟩ 1862: "somewhat bushy, and had apparently been acquainted with neither   1406
the brush nor comb that morning" [hawthorne p310] (∈ ¶178)

⟨1⟩ As President: Lincoln asked to borrow a comb. He was handed a delicate   1407
one, made of shell. "He toyed with the comb. & said why this wont comb my

Hair (continued)

hair if you have such a thing as they comb a Horses tail with, I can do it: & laughed in his merry way" – LeGrand Cannon [wilson p680]

⟨1⟩ "thick, bushy hair" – John Nicolay [meserve p5] (∈ ¶177) 1408

⟨1⟩ Early 1864: "His hair was 'every way for Sunday.' It looked as though it was an abandoned stubble field." – Henry Beecher [riceA pp249-250] (∈ ¶195) 1409

⟨2⟩ Of Lincoln's hair: "when it shot out every which way like blown wheat or or stood up in spikes, Lincoln could look odd indeed" [kunhardtA p9] (∈ ¶176) 1410

- Part: 1411

  ⟨1⟩ Lincoln normally parted his hair on the left. [ostendorfA p177] 1412

  ⟨☐⟩ Feb. 9, 1864: Anthony Berger takes seven photographs of Lincoln ([ostendorf #88-94]), including those later used as the model for the one-cent coin and the $5 bill (both the 20th- and 21st-century versions). On this day, however, Lincoln's hair was parted on the right. On the back of a copy of [ostendorf #92], artist Francis Carpenter wrote: "From a negative made in 1864, by A. Berger ... This is the photographed engraved by J.C. Butre of New York, just after Mr. Lincoln's re-nomination. It was the basis after Mr. Lincoln's death of the portrait made by Marshall, and also the one made by Littlefield. In each engraving the parting of the hair was changed, to the *left side*, as Mr. Lincoln always wore it. His barber by mistake this day for some unaccountable reason, parted the hair on the President's *right side*, instead of his *left*." [ostendorfA p177] 1413

  ⟨-⟩ *It may not have been a mistake. Lincoln posed that day for profile photographs showing his right side. Perhaps he had planned ahead for such poses, and wanted the hair-part to be visible to the camera.* 1414

- Beard 1: 1415

  ⟨1⟩ Pre-beard: "His face was long – sallow – cadaverous – shrunk – shrivelled – wrinkled, and dry, having here and there a hair on the surface." [herndonC] (∈ ¶3) 1416

  ⟨1⟩ March 1861: "bristling and compact like a ruff of mourning pins"– William Russell [russell pp37-38] (∈ ¶161) 1418

  ⟨1⟩ 1862: " a few irregular blotches of black bristly hair in the place where beard and whiskers ought to grow" [dicey v1pp220-221] (∈ ¶179) 1419

- Beard 2: 1421

  ⟨1⟩ Eleven-year old Grace Bedell wrote Lincoln on Oct. 15, 1860, advising him to grow a beard "for your face is so thin." Lincoln carried her letter for years. [kunhardtA p13] 1422

  ⟨2⟩ Three days earlier New York City Republicans had advised Lincoln to "cultivate whiskers and wear standing collars" to improve his appearance. [kunhardtA p13] 1423

  ⟨2⟩ Lincoln met Bedell in 1861 and told her "See, I grew these whiskers for you, Grace" [kunhardtB p173]. 1424

  ⟨2⟩ One newspaper accused Lincoln of using an ointment to stimulate his beard growth [kunhardtA p13]. 1425

  ⟨S⟩ 1863, during his smallpox bout: "It is possible that the famous beard was shaved then due to a rash, and he was beardless for a short time" [gary p336]. See Special Topic §5. ○○○ *Project:* If his beard were shaved in late November 1863, they had regrown to full length by Jan. 8, 1864, as shown in several pictures taken that day. Is this enough time for regrowth? 1426

Hair (continued)

⟨2⟩ "The heavy beard softens the lines in his face, and makes him less gaunt."   1427
c
[ostendorfA p70] referring to [ostendorf #43]

⟨2⟩ Of Bedell: "To this dreadful young person ... was due the ill-designed hairy   1428
ornamentation which ... hid the really beautiful modelling of his jaw and
chin." – Lord Charnwood [randallC p161]

- Eyebrows: 1429
  ⟨-⟩ For bony brow, see ¶1834ff in ⌈Head & Face⌉.   1430
  ⟨1⟩ "eye-brows heavy" [arnold p441] (∈ ¶167)   1431
  ⟨1⟩ "bushy, overhanging brows" [conant] (∈ ¶834)   1432
  ⟨1⟩ "His eyebrows cropped out" – [herndonC] [kunhardtB p291] (∈ ¶3) (∈ ¶89)   1433
  ⟨1⟩ 1858: "his eyebrows were black like his hair." – Martin Rindlaub [ostendorfA   1434
  q
  p19] (∈ ¶148)
  ⟨1⟩ 1860s: "his eyebrows heavy" [dana p173] (∈ ¶183)   1435
  ⟨1⟩ 1860s: "heavy eyebrows" – John Nicolay [meserve p5] (∈ ¶177)   1436
  ⟨1⟩ 1862±: "bushy eyebrows" [dicey v1pp220-221] (∈ ¶179)   1437
  ⟨1⟩ 1862: "thick black eyebrows" [hawthorne pp309-310] (∈ ¶178)   1438
  ⟨1⟩ April 1865: "thick eyebrows" [chambrunA] (∈ ¶200)   1439
  ⟨2⟩ "jutting eyebrows" [kunhardtA p9] (∈ ¶176)   1440
  ⟨2⟩ "His left eyebrow is usually elevated more than the right" [kempfB p9] (∈ ¶278)   1441
  ⟨2⟩ "his left eyebrow was usually more elevated than the right" [snyder] (∈ ¶896)   1442
  ⟨2⟩ In death: "the eyebrows arched" [kunhardtB p95] (∈ ¶3300)   1443
- Body hair: 1444
  ⟨2⟩ extensive body hair [mearns]   1445
  ⟨2⟩ As President: "With his nightshirt off, black hair was revealed on his arms,   1446
  back, narrow shoulders, chest, and legs." [kunhardtA p321]

⟨1⟩ April 1865: Lincoln, angry: "his coarse hair stood on end" [porterD p308] (∈ ¶2558)   1447

Hands

"The rule of thumb for identification of arachnodactyly [is] longest digit at least 50%   1448
longer than the longest metacarpal" [mckusickA p116]. Like all rules of thumb, this is not
a rigid definition. It is also not possible to assess this accurately without an x-ray.

The visual impression of a hand results from two factors (at least): the bones of the   1449
hand and the muscles of the hand. For any given degree of long bone overgrowth in
the fingers, exuberant musculature will reduce the associated impression of arachnodactyly because the fingers won't seem so thin.

Certainly, years of axe-work and rail-splitting left Lincoln's hands well-muscled   1450
(¶1463). In today's softer society, it is unlikely that contemporary physicians have
seen patients with Marfan syndrome who performed the degree of manual (in the
strict sense of the word) labor that Lincoln did. Thus, the standards by which these
physicians judge arachnodactyly may be poorly calibrated to pre-industrial, mid-19th-
century hands. Even by standards of his own day, Lincoln's hand use may have been
extreme. He "was almost constantly handling" an axe from ages 8 to 23 (¶2832) and
probably did not give it up entirely until he became President: he was still chopping
his own wood while a Springfield lawyer (see ¶2830ff).

- See also: ⌈Hands -- Cast⌉, ⌈Handshaking⌉, ⌈Handwriting⌉.   1451

⟨1⟩ "After having arisen, he generally placed his hands behind him, the back of his   1452
left hand in the palm of his right, the thumb and fingers of his right hand clasped

Hands (continued)

around the left arm at the wrist." [herndon p331] *Is close to, but not quite, the Walker-Murdoch wrist sign in Marfan syndrome.*

⟨1/q⟩ Jan. 20, 1828, learning his sister had just died: "The tears trickled through his large fingers, and sobs shook his frame." – Captain J.W. Lamar [hobson p24] (∈ ¶2438)   1453

- Size: 1458
  - ⟨2⟩ About age 17: "His feet and hands were large, arms and legs long and in striking contrast with his slender trunk and small head." [herndon p35] (∈ ¶492) *Herndon did not know Lincoln at age 17.*   1459
  - ⟨1⟩ 1834: "His hands were large and bony, caused no doubt by hard labor when young. he was a good chopper. the axe then in use [required] a gripe as Strong as was necessary to wield a Blacksmiths Sledge Hammer. This ... accounts for his large hands." – Robert Wilson [wilson pp201-202] (∈ ¶99)   1460
  - ⟨1⟩ "giant hands" [herndon p471] Part of ¶1053   1461
  - ⟨1⟩ "large hands and feet" – William Herndon [hertz p188]   1462
  - ⟨2⟩ "huge hands, enlarged by years of plowing and splitting rails" [donaldH p28]   1463
  - ⟨H⟩ In Indiana: Rejected by Susie Enlow because "my feet and hands were too big, and my legs and arms too long." [paulmier p26]   1464
  - ⟨1/q⟩ Lincoln got upset when a butcher's son loosed his bulldog on another dog. "I shall never forget how big his fist looked as he shook it in the face of the butcher boy..." – a Springfielder [burl p159]   1465
  - ⟨1⟩ "long limbs, large hands and feet" [arnold p441] (∈ ¶167)   1466
  - ⟨1⟩ June 1858: "grasping my hand in both his large hands" [volk] (∈ ¶1537)   1467
  - ⟨1/q⟩ 1859: "big hands and feet" – John Widmer [shenk p155] (∈ ¶150)   1468
  - ⟨1⟩ Feb. 27, 1860, at Cooper Union: "when he raised his hands in an opening gesture I noticed that they were very large" – eyewitness [brooksA p186] (∈ ¶156)   1469
  - ⟨1⟩ 1860: "Tall as he was, his hands and feet looked out of proportion, so long and clumsy were they." [piatt pp345-346]   1470
  - ⟨1⟩ March 1861: "hands of extraordinary dimensions, which, however, were far exceeded in proportion by his feet" – William Russell [russell pp37-38] (∈ ¶161)   1471
  - ⟨1/q⟩ "large hands" – John Nicolay [meserve p5] (∈ ¶177)   1472
  - ⟨1⟩ 1862: "large rugged hands, which grasp you like a vice when shaking yours" [dicey v1pp220-221] (∈ ¶179)   1473
  - ⟨1/q⟩ "long bony hands, which grasp you like a vise" – eyewitness [shutesE p206]   1475
  - ⟨1/q⟩ "enormously long loose arms and big hands" – Princess Salm-Salm [salmsalm] (∈ ¶190)   1476
  - ⟨1/q⟩ Wearing white kid gloves gave "a rather ghastly effect on his large, bony hands" – Grace Greenwood [meserve p15]   1477
  - ⟨2⟩ Did not like kid gloves. "Once, holding up his hands encased in a new pair of these gloves, he said they looked like canvassed hams." [donaldH p29]   1478

- Some finger descriptions: 1479
  - ⟨1⟩ New Salem: "I often imagine him Standing Six feet and upward pointing his long bony finger at Old Bowling Green who was presiding in his Court" – Dr. Jason Duncan [wilson p541]   1480
  - ⟨1⟩ "... pointing his long, bony finger towards the venerable Parson Berry..." [rankinA p80]   1481
  - ⟨1⟩ 1840s or 1850s: Attorney Lincoln "[stretches] out his long right arm and forefinger" at a trial witness [shastid]. *It is unclear if this is a second- or third-hand description.*   1482

Hands (continued)

⟨2⟩ 1857: "he pointed a long forefinger at the page..." [angle p176] reprinting Albert Woldman   1483

⟨$\frac{1}{q}$⟩ 1862: "gloves too long for the long bony fingers" [dicey v1pp220-221] (∈ ¶179)   1484

⟨1⟩ Spring 1864: "long bony forefinger" [stoddardA p126] (∈ ¶3001)   1485

⟨1⟩ April 1865: "his lean forefinger" [porterD p308] (∈ ¶2558)   1486

- Fingerprints: See ¶3405.   1487

- For asymmetry of hands, see ¶310ff.   1488

- Trauma: 1489

  ⟨1⟩ June 1860: As Volk was readying to cast Lincoln's left hand, Lincoln said to   1490 him: "You have heard that they call me a railsplitter ... well, it is true that I did split rails, and one day while I was sharpening a wedge on a log, the ax [sic] glanced and nearly took my thumb off, and there is the scar, you see." [volk] *A linear scar over Lincoln's left forefinger is visible in* [ostendorf #91] *in* [mellon p157], *but not in other photographs of his left hand, all of which are less detailed.*

  ⊙ Feb. 1861: Right hand swollen after shaking many hands during pre-   1491 inaugural train trip from Illinois to Washington. [ostendorfA p80] (See ¶1547.)

  ⟨$\frac{1}{q}$⟩ Jan. 1, 1863: Mass handshaking impaired his handwriting. (See ¶1557ff.)   1492

  ⟨1⟩ April 1865: "I have shaken so many hands to-day that my arms ache to night.   1493 I almost wish that I could go to bed now." [keckleyB p171] (See ¶1303.)

⟨1⟩ In Springfield: "He did not gesticulate as much with his hands as with his head.   1494 He used the latter frequently, throwing it with vim this way and that." [herndon p332] Part of ¶90

⟨1⟩ In Springfield: "brawny-handed, with no superfluous flesh, toughened by labor   1495 in the open air, of perfect health, and his grip was like the grip of Hercules" – Leonard Swett [riceA p464]

⊙ Feb. 1860: The "Cooper Union" photograph [ostendorf #17] [kunhardtA p115] clearly vi-   1496 sualizes the length of Lincoln's fingers.

  ⊙ 1863: Another photo [ostendorf #79] [kunhardtA p309] shows his right thumb and   1497 index finger and his left ring finger *Is this a new sign of arachnodactyly? The thumb's tip ends proximal to the DIP joint when both the thumb and the DIP joint lie on a table surface.*

⟨$\frac{1}{q}$⟩ 1860: "clumsy hands" – George H. Putnam [ostendorfA p57] (∈ ¶153)   1498

⟨2⟩ Lincoln's hands as President: "All their coarseness, all the muscle flesh from his   1499 young years had vanished, and the very shape of his hands had changed. Now with the pen as their weapon, Lincoln's hands had actually turned graceful. But they were still strong, which was evident from his iron handshake or the firm double-handed greeting he favored so much." [kunhardtA p321] *The "pen" mention could imply that some of this description is metaphorical.*

  ⟨2⟩ "The hands of Abraham Lincoln in his thirties ... were still the hands of a   1500 farmer and a woodchopper – muscular, almost muscle bound from years of physical labor. The hands of Lincoln the President of the United States underwent a miraculous transformation, strangely parallel with the development of the man's mind and character. The coarse flesh vanished and the fingers appeared graceful and sensitive – hands refined by their habit of life, now turned to work with the pen, not the hoe and the ax [sic.' [kunhardtB p290]

  ⊙ Stereo-photograph in [zeller] shows prominent wrinkling of the skin on his   1501 left hand's finger II and, to a lesser degree, finger III in [ostendorf #69].

Hands (continued)

☐ About 1862, [ostendorf #61] shows the thinness of Lincoln's right wrist: it looks small sitting in the cuff of his shirt.   1502

⟨1⟩/q Late February 1865: Complains of cold hands – see ¶1210   1503

⟨2⟩ Chauncy Depew said Lincoln "handled objects with delicacy, used his hands gracefully and without wasting energy. He talked especially about Lincoln's beautiful hands." – Marie de Montalvo, 1948 letter to J.G. Randall [randallP box 15] (Part of ¶2942)   1504

- Gloves: 1505
    - ☐ Pictures of Lincoln's gloves: [kunhardtB pp102-103, 104]   1506
    - ⟨1⟩ 1861: Audibly bursts a glove while shaking hands [lamonR pp97-98]. (∈ ¶1556)   1507
    - ⟨1⟩ 1862: "gloves too long for the long bony fingers" [dicey v1pp220-221] (∈ ¶179)   1508
    - ☐ Oct. 3, 1862: [ostendorf #66] and [ostendorf #67] show Lincoln wearing gloves in Gen. McClellan's tent at Antietam. These are not kid gloves, and none of the many photographs taken that day suggest that the weather was cold.   1509
    - ⟨1⟩/q "The glove-makers have not yet had time to construct gloves that will fit him." [meserve pp2-3] (∈ ¶192) *Is part of a mock campaign biography, so cannot be considered reliable.*   1510
    - ⟨1⟩/q Wearing white kid gloves gave "a rather ghastly effect on his large, bony hands" – Grace Greenwood [meserve p15]   1511
    - ⟨2⟩ Did not like kid gloves. "Once, holding up his hands encased in a new pair of these gloves, he said they looked like canvassed hams." [donaldH p29]   1512
    - ⟨2⟩ Size 10 gloves [gordon]   1513

⟨1⟩/q "He may be President of the United States, but he has dirty fingernails" [seldes p245]. In 1927 Katherine Medill McCormick recalled that her mother used to say this – and several other disparaging things about the President – before sending her to play with the Lincoln children. McCormick's father, Joseph Medill, was a friend of Lincoln's. Lincoln was not alone in being an object of Mrs. Medill's scorn: she seemingly hated just about everyone and everything. [seldes p245]   1514

Hands – Cast

Leonard Volk, a sculptor, made casts of Lincoln's head and hands in June 1860. (See Head -- Casts.) He wrote about the experience twenty years later [volk].   1515

The hand casts both refute and support the possibility that Lincoln had Marfan syndrome.   1516

⟨1⟩ The night before the casting, Lincoln was officially notified of his nomination as the Republican candidate for President. A mass-handshaking followed. (See ¶1542.) In making the casts, Volk noticed: "The right hand appeared swollen as compared with the left, on account of excessive hand-shaking the evening before; this difference is distinctly shown in the cast." [volk]   1517

- Analysis of [micozzi]:   1518
    - ⟨1⟩ [micozzi] examined the casts and found the right hand appears larger than the left.   1519
    - ⟨2⟩ [micozzi] also says, without a reference citation, that the right hand "was so swollen and painful that Lincoln asked to hold a broomstick while the cast was setting because it was too painful to make a fist." *This account is not reflected in Volk's article* [volk]. *In fact, Volk says he was the one who wanted Lincoln to hold something in his right hand* [volk]. [micozzi] *also*   1520

Hands – Cast (continued)

errs in saying the casts were made in November 1860 (¶1912). Whether another source exists for Micozzi's statements is unknown to me.

⟨1⟩ Bartlett examined the hand casts in 1907. His summary: "They are large, long hands. The first phalanx of the middle finger is nearly half an inch longer than that of an ordinary hand. The bones are finely shaped, not unusually large, muscles thin, strongly defined in their own construction and in their relations, finger nails of good form and of ordinary length. The joints are very supple. Were it not for the length of the fingers, the shape of the nails, the resemblance of the knuckles and the movement of the muscles on the inside of the right hand, one would doubt it was the mate of the other. In contrast and variety of form, the left hand is as fine and original as is the mask; and both mask and hands are distinguished for exactitude of form." [schurz pp25-26]   1521

⟨-⟩ *The word "supple" perhaps had a different meaning in 1907 than it does now. Certainly it is not possible to assess movement around a joint from a plaster cast.*   1522

⟨1⟩ "There is an extra fullness of the back of the right hand, in spite of the firm grip on the object it holds, caused, Mr. Volk says, by shaking hands with several hundreds of people just before the cast was made." [schurz p26]   1523

⟨$\frac{1}{q}$⟩ Another sculptor: "The skin folds on the back of the left hand show very prominently. One might question why the skin folds are not as noticeable on on the back of the right hand but they would be if in the same position as the left. I have tried holding a stick and bending my wrist in the position of that of Lincoln's and and I find that the skin becomes stretched. This accounts for the difference which you may notice." – Avarel Fairbanks, circa 1942 [purtle] *The handshaking-induced swelling of the right hand (¶1517) may also have contributed.*   1524

- Anthropological measurements, by [stewart]:   1525
  ⟨2⟩ Anthropologist made measurements of Lincoln's hands from the cast, and concluded they were long and narrow. [schwartzA] cites [stewart]   1526
  ⟨2⟩ The anthropologist also found that Lincoln's left hand was longer than his right, and that this asymmetry could not be attributed solely to the difference in position of the two hands.   1527
  ⟨2⟩ Left thumb is more than 10mm shorter than the right thumb, and is the shortest of all 10 digits [schwartzA] perhaps citing the anthropologist.   1528
  ⟨-⟩ *See ¶310 for more about hand [a]symmetry.*   1529

- Evidence against Marfan syndrome from the cast: 1530
  ⟨2⟩ [lattimerNY] finds "thick bones and powerful musculature of a big strong man with normally proportioned hands, rather than the excessively slender bones and excessively long thumbs of someone with the classical Marfan syndrome."   1531
  ⟨2⟩ [lattimerNY] disputes the claim that the cast of Lincoln's hands show the left as larger than the right.   1532
  ⟨2⟩ [lattimerNY] claims the anthropologist did not say the hand bones were disproportionately long or slender for a man of Lincoln's height.   1533

☐ [lattimerNY] helpfully juxtaposes the cast of Lincoln's left hand with the left hand of a normal 6-foot- 4-inch man. Lattimer comments on their similar appearance, but does not mention that Lincoln's fingers are clearly longer and clearly thinner than the normal man's, and that Lincoln's hand is longer with less musculature in the thenar and hypothenar eminences.   1534

Handshaking

Handshaking is a signal act of politics. For many years the White House opened its 1535 doors every New Year's Day, allowing (almost) anyone to come in and shake the President's hand. Many chief executives sustained injury after literally thousands of repetitive motions ensued. Others carefully developed their handshaking technique to minimize wear and tear.

⟨1⟩ 1850s: "his grip was like the grip of Hercules" – Leonard Swett [riceA p464] (∈ ¶1495)   1536

■ Leonard Volk shook hands with Lincoln at least three times, all of them in a one-   1537
on-one setting (i.e., not a mass handshaking ceremony):
  ⟨1⟩ June 1858: "He saluted me with his natural cordiality, grasping my hand in   1538
  both his large hands with a vice-like [sic] grip." [volk]
  ⟨1⟩ April 1860: "recognizing me at once with his usual grip of both hands." [volk]   1539
  ⟨1⟩ June 1860: "Those two great hands took both of mine with a grasp never to   1540
  be forgotten. ... I thought my hands were in a fair way of being crushed." [volk]

⟨1⟩ "hearty grasp of the hand" [arnold p442]   1541

⟨1⟩ June 1860: Lincoln performed a mass-handshaking after being officially notified   1542
of his nomination as Republican candidate for President. The notifying committee had arrived in Springfield by special train. The train included "a large number of people, two or three hundred of whom carried rails on their shoulders. ... The evening was beautiful and clear, and the entire population was astir. ... The bonfires blazed brightly, and especially in front of that prim-looking white house on Eighth street. The committee and the vast crowd following passed in at the front door, and made their exit through the kitchen door at the rear, Mr. Lincoln giving them all a hearty shake of the hand as they passed him in the parlor." [volk]
  ⟨-⟩ *From this description it is difficult to tell if Lincoln shook hands with*   1543
  only the train passengers, or with the entire town. Other eye-witness
  descriptions no doubt exist.
  ⟨1⟩ The next morning Lincoln's right hand was swollen, and it was in this state   1544
  that the cast of his hands was made. [volk] See ¶1517.

⟨1/q⟩ June 21, 1860: Lincoln "extended his hand, and gave mine a grasp such as only a   1545
warm-hearted man knows how to give." – Utica newspaper reporter [lincloreHDE]

⟨1/q⟩ 1860: Lincoln "came and *shook hands* (ouch!)" – Carl Schurz writing to his wife   1546
[randallC p164]

■ Feb. 1861: Prodigious handshaking as Lincoln travels to Washington to assume   1547
the Presidency.
  ⟨2⟩ Lincoln's limbs became stiff according to journalist Henry Villard [kunhardtA   1548
  p6]
  ⊡ Six photographs of Lincoln taken on Feb. 23, 1861 [ostendorf #50-53] all show the   1549
  right hand partially hidden and partially closed.
  ⟨2⟩ [kunhardtA p24] claims the images show "a right hand swollen from shaking so   1550
  many hands on the trip east." *This seems to be a supposition, rather than*
  a first-hand report.

■ As President: 1551
  ⟨2⟩ By the end of formal White House evening functions, "his own hands were   1552
  usually raw with blisters" [donaldH p45]
  ⟨1⟩ 1862: "large rugged hands, which grasp you like a vice when shaking yours"   1553
  [dicey v1pp220-221] (∈ ¶179)

Handshaking (continued)

⟨2⟩ "Iron handshake [and] the firm double-handed greeting he favored so much" [kunhardtA p321] (Part of ¶1499)   1554

⟨1⟩ During an evening reception of incessant handshaking, Lincoln was asked if this was more fatiguing than his work in the office. "Oh, no – no. Of course, this is tiresome physically; but I am pretty strong, and it rests me, after all, for here no man asks me for what I can't give him!" [croffut]   1555

⟨1⟩ 1861: At a reception "he had on a tight-fitting pair of white kids, which he had with difficulty got on." He greeted an old Illinois friend "with a genuine Sangamon County shake, which resulted in bursting his white kid glove with an audible sound. Then, raising his brawny hand up before him, looking at it with an indescribable expression, he said ... 'Well, my old friend, this is a general bustification...' " [lamonR pp97-98]   1556

⟨2⟩ Jan. 1, 1863: "Lincoln shook hands with everyone in a cordial but businesslike manner, which reminded some observers of a farmer sawing wood." He shook hands until noon. [donaldA p407]   1557

⟨$\frac{1}{q}$⟩ Lincoln then went to sign the Emancipation Proclamation. He twice picked up his pen then put it down, saying "I have been shaking hands since nine o'clock this morning, and my right arm is almost paralyzed. If my name ever goes into history, it will be for this act, and my whole soul is in it. If my hand trembles when I sign the Proclamation, all who examine the document hereafter will say, 'He hesitated.' " [boller p143]   1558

⟨$\frac{1}{q}$⟩ [kunhardtA p226] cites a story by John Forney in the *Washington Chronicle* as the source of this quote.   1559

⟨$\frac{1}{q}$⟩ [donaldA p407] supplies a different, possibly more reliable, Lincoln monolog: "Now, this signature is one that will be closely examined, and if they find my hand trembled, they will say 'he had some compunctions.' But, any way, it is going to be done!"   1560

⟨2⟩ "For all the care he took, his signature was noticeably uneven and infirm" [currentBk pp214&228]   1561

☐ Signature appears in: [sandburgC p177]   1562

⟨2⟩ Interestingly, he signed "Abraham Lincoln" instead of his usual "A. Lincoln" [currentBk p214]   1563

⟨1⟩ March 4, 1865: Lincoln shakes about 5000 hands. His time for 100 handshakes is measured on several occasions. The range is under 3 minutes to never over 5 minutes. [french p466]   1564

⟨2⟩ After the second inauguration, had blisters on all four fingers of his right hand as a result of handshaking – per Phineas Gurley [kunhardtB p72]   1565

⟨1⟩ April 7, 1865: Arms ache after an afternoon of shakings the hands of wounded soldiers [keckleyB p171]. (See ¶1303.)   1566

⟨1⟩ April 8: "his warm hand-clasp" [barnesB]   1567

⟨$\frac{1}{q}$⟩ "long bony hands, which grasp you like a vise" – eyewitness [shutesE p206]   1568

Handwriting

I had expected that someone would have cataloged all known samples of Lincoln's handwriting, but no such reference seems to exist. People who sell Lincoln autographs   1569

Handwriting (continued)

tell me that there are thousands and thousands of his notes in existence, mostly uninteresting official documents such as commissions. The 8-volume size of [baslerA] testifies to the volume of Lincoln's correspondence.

I have not made a study of Lincoln's handwriting, but it would not surprise me if it 1570
degraded over time for a variety of reasons. As late as 1864, however, Lincoln could
still hand-write beautifully when called upon (¶1587). ○○○ *Project:* Quantitative
analysis of the "control" evident in Lincoln's handwriting over time.

⟨2⟩ Lincoln's handwriting "remained precise and admirable, all through his life." [lat- 1571
timerNY] *There were at least a few exceptions, as noted in this section.*

- Youth: 1572
  ⟨1⟩ 1820s or 1830s: "Abraham was the best penman in the Neighborhood." – 1573
  Joseph Richardson [wilson p473]
  ⟨2⟩ During his brief formal schooling, Lincoln was "a good penman" [angle p25] 1574
  (reprinting [bartonB]). Part of ¶3326.
  ▣ Signatures as old as 1823 survive [lorant (1941 edition)] 1575
  ⟨1⟩ March 1826: "he wrote a clear, neat, legible hand, which is instantly and 1576
  easily recognized as his by those familiar with Lincoln's handwriting when
  President." [arnold p25]

⟨2⟩ "Lincoln wrote very, very slowly, dipping his pen in the inkwell and waiting long 1577
periods before using it." [kunhardtB p298]

⟨2⟩ March 6, 1833: A signature of this date on a permit to sell liquor is thought to be 1578
that of his partner, William F. Berry [angle p54]

⟨2⟩ Jan. 22, 1841: Lincoln's handwriting changed in mid-document as he started writ- 1579
ing about his mental state. He "pressed harder on the page" and the writing became smaller [shenk p62]

⟨1⟩ Oct. 10, 1860: Lincoln writes good news to Herndon. "The handwriting of the 1580
note was a little tremulous, showing that Lincoln was excited and nervous when
he wrote it." [herndon p376]
  ⟨2⟩ The note itself is lost. Only Herndon's transcription exists. [hirschhornC] 1581

- Jan. 1, 1863: After three hours of non-stop handshaking, Lincoln went to sign 1582
  the momentous Emancipation Proclamation. He worried his overworked hand
  would produce a wavering signature that might be interpreted as a wavering com-
  mitment to the Proclamation. See ¶1557

⟨1⟩ Feb. 18, 1863: "He wrote a note while I was present, and his hand trembled as I 1583
never saw it before" [french p417]. (∈ ¶1161)
  ⟨2⟩ Handwriting is shaky but shows no evidence of intention tremor [hirschhornC]. 1584
  c (See ¶1161ff.)

▣ Nov. 27, 1863: Lincoln pens a note saying that, because of illness, he cannot meet 1585
the Cabinet. He had smallpox (see Special Topic §5).
  ⟨2⟩ "This is a most interesting autograph, written on a card in an unsteady hand 1586
  c and with an atypical signature of a quite sick President." [baslerB p211]. *The
  card is in the Lincoln Museum in Ft. Wayne.*

▣ March 1864: Lincoln pens a copy of the Gettysburg Address for the Baltimore San- 1587
itary Fair [nicolayG]. The penmanship is excellent.

Handwriting (continued)

◯ April 10, 1865: Sample of Lincoln's handwriting in [sandburgC p198] is not up to its usual quality. Neither tremulousness nor ataxia are suggested. It looks more like carelessness. ⟨1588⟩

⟨1⟩ "Lincoln never made an error in his writing. ... He never scratched out or erased a word." –Civil War telegraph operator (1926 recollection) [NYTimesTeleg] ⟨1589⟩

⟨1⟩ "To read Lincoln's letters in holograph is revelatory; the writing changes dramatically with his mood." [vidalA pp703-704] ⟨1590⟩

Head & Face

"It is the common wonder of all men, how among so many millions of faces, there should be none alike." – Sir Thomas Browne [aa89 p10] ⟨1591⟩

Dolichocephaly, high-arched palate, long narrow face, and prognathism are part of the Marfan phenotype [mckusickA p47]. ⟨1592⟩

The thickness of facial tissues reflects, to some degree, a person's degree of adiposity. This is relevant to tracking Lincoln's weight loss. When comparing emaciated and normal American whites, the difference in facial tissue thickness is most pronounced in: mid-philtrum (3.75mm), mental eminence (4.25mm), inferior malar (4.75mm), lateral orbit (5mm), midway on the zygomatic arch (4.25mm), supraglenoid (4.25mm), gonion (7mm), cheek area (6mm+) [aa89 p26,27] ⟨1593⟩

Literature on the natural history of untreated craniosyntostosis is limited [aa26] [aa38] and will probably never grow. ⟨1594⟩

See also: Head -- Casts , Ears , Eyes , Mouth , Asymmetry , Post-Mortem . ⟨1595⟩

For beard, see ¶1415 and ¶1421 in Hair section. For eyebrows, see ¶1429 in Hair . ⟨1596⟩

⟨S⟩ "No American, I suppose, can look at the face of Lincoln with a completely fresh eye." [shapiro] ⟨1597⟩

⟨1⟩ Pre-Presidency: "Mr. Lincoln's head was long & tall from the base of the brain and from the eye brow – the perceptive faculties. His head ran backward, his forehead rising as it ran back at a low angle. ... The size of his hat, measured at the hatter's block was $7\frac{1}{8}$, his head being from ear to ear $6\frac{1}{2}$ inches – and from the front to the back of the brain 8 inches. Thus measured it was not below the medium size, it made rather large mass through the height & length of it. Mr. Lincoln's forehead was narrow but high. His hair was dark – almost black and lay floating where the fingers or the winds left it, piled up at random. His cheek bones were high – sharp and prominent. His eyebrows heavy and jutting out. Mr. Lincoln's jaws were long up curved and heavy. His nose was large – long and blunt, having the tip glowing in red, and a little awry toward the right eye. His chin was long – sharp and up curved. His eyebrows cropped out like a huge rock on the brow of a hill. His face was long – sallow – cadaverous – shrunk – shrivelled – wrinkled, and dry, having here and there a hair on the surface. His cheeks were leathery and flabby, falling in loose folds at places, looking sorrowful and sad. Mr. Lincoln's ears were extremely large – and ran out almost at right angles from his head – caused by heavy hats and partly by nature. His lower lip was thick – material and hanging undercurved, while his chin reached for the lip up curved. Mr. Lincoln's neck was neat and trim, his head being well balanced on it. There was the lone mole on the right cheek and Adam's apple on his throat." [herndonC] (∈ ¶3) ⟨1598⟩

Head & Face (continued)

⟨1⟩ Cognate in [herndon p472]: Herndon's less flattering phrases of 1865 are softened or removed.   1599

■ General head appearance: 1600

[⊙] "Bright lighting softens his features" (example: [ostendorf #18]) [ostendorfA p50]   1601

[⊙] "Subdued light makes his face rugged" (example: [ostendorf #32]). [ostendorfA p51]   1602

⟨1/q⟩ "Large head, with high crown of skull; thick, bushy hair; large and deep eye-caverns; heavy eyebrows; a large nose; large ears; large mouth; thin upper and somewhat thick under lip; very high and prominent cheekbones; cheeks thin and sunken; strongly developed jawbones; chin slightly upturned" – John Nicolay [meserve p5] (∈ ¶177)   1603

⟨1/q⟩ "... his head small and disproportionately shaped. He had large, square jaws; large, heavy nose; small lascivious mouth" – Elliott Herndon [herndon p470n]   1604

⟨1/q⟩ "The plainest looking man in Springfield" – one of Mary's sisters [randallC p15]   1605

[⊙] "There is a peculiar curve of the lower lip, the lone mole on the right cheek, and a pose of the head so essentially Lincolnian; no other artist has ever caught it." – William Herndon, apparently referring to [ostendorf #26] [ostendorfA p46]   1606

⟨1⟩ "his cheek bones high and projecting" [arnold p441] (∈ ¶167)   1607

⟨1/q⟩ Aug. 1858: "his face was almost grotesquely square, with high cheek bones." – Martin Rindlaub [ostendorfA p19] (∈ ¶148)   1608

⟨1/q⟩ 1858: "No complete idea of the irregularity of the profile of his features can be had from his pictures. ... In the courtroom, while waiting for the Armstrong case to be called for trial, I studied his face for two full hours. ... His forehead protruded beyond his eyes more than two inches and retreated rapidly, about 25 degrees from the perpendicular. ... From the front his eyes looked very deep-set and sunken, by reason of this abnormal extension of the frontal bone." – Judge Abram Bergen [ostendorfA p105]   1609

⟨1⟩ March 1859: "His face was not handsome, to be sure, but at any time there was a great deal of expression in it.... This morning was evidently a thoughtful one and his expression varied from minute to minute, all the while being cloudy. [Lincoln reads a letter silently.] His face at first grew darker and the deep wrinkles in his forehead grew deeper.... Then, if you can imagine how a dark lighthouse looks when its calcium light is suddenly kindled, you may get an idea of the change which came into the face of Abraham Lincoln. All the great soul within him had been kindled to red heat, if not to white, and his eyes shone until he shut them.... I did not disturb Mr. Lincoln or try to speak to him." [stoddardD pp206-207]   1610

⟨1/q⟩ June 21, 1860: "forehead remarkably broad and capacious ... the cheek bones high and prominent" – Utica newspaper reporter [lincloreHDE] (∈ ¶159)   1611

⟨1⟩ Aug.-Sept. 1860: "My notion of his features had been gained solely from the unskilled work of the photographers of the period, in which harsh lighting and inflexible pose served to accentuate the deep, repellent lines of his face, giving it an expression easily mistaken for coarseness ... But as he talked animatedly, I saw a totally different countenance, and I admitted to myself his frequent smile was peculiarly attractive. I determined to secure that expression in my portrait." – Alban Conant [conant]   1613

⟨1⟩ "He looked up with his peculiar smile and eye-twinkle..." [french p374]   1614

⟨1⟩ 1860s: "Mr. Lincoln's face was thin, and his features were large. ... his forehead square and well developed" [dana p173] (∈ ¶183)   1615

⟨1/q⟩ March 1861: "plain, ploughed face" – Henry Adams [angle p337]   1616

Head & Face (continued)

⟨1⟩ Oct. 21, 1861: Compared to May 1860, "The lines were deeper in the President's face... the cheeks more sunken. They were lines of care and anxiety." [coffinA p176]   1617

⟨1⟩ 1862: "a head, cocoa-nut shaped and somewhat too small for such a stature, covered with rough, uncombed and uncombable lank dark hair, that stands out in every direction at once; a face furrowed, wrinkled, and indented, as though it has been scarred by vitriol; a high narrow forehead; and, sunk deep beneath bushy eyebrows" [dicey v1pp220-221] (∈ ¶179)   1618

⟨1⟩ 1862: " The whole physiognomy is as coarse a one as you would meet" [hawthorne p310] (∈ ¶178)   1619

⟨1/q⟩ Nov. 1863: A 15-year old boy hid under the platform from which Lincoln delivered the Gettysburg address and was able to see, through cracks between the planks, the "deep lines, the wrinkled brow, the deep-set brooding eyes" of Lincoln's face [kunhardtA p312].   1620

⟨1⟩ 1863: "The drooping eyelids, looking almost swollen; the dark bags beneath the eyes; the deep marks about the large and expressive mouth; the flaccid muscles of the jaws, were all so majestically pitiful..." – Col. Silas Burt [wilsonR p332]   1621

⟨1⟩ Sept. 1863: "His face was peculiar; bone, nerve, vein, and muscle were all so plainly seen" [harveyC] (∈ §6.2) *Suggests thin, translucent skin.*   1622

⟨1⟩ As President: "His countenance had more of rugged strength than his person" [sumnerA pp132-133]   1623

⟨1⟩ April 1865: "Nothing seemed to lend harmony the decided lines of his face; yet [certain facial features] formed an *ensemble* which, although strange, was certainly powerful" [chambrunA] (∈ ¶200)   1624

⟨2/c⟩ "unusual face" [shapiro]   1625

■ Size: 1626

⟨2⟩ About age 17: "His feet and hands were large, arms and legs long and in striking contrast with his slender trunk and small head." [herndon p35] (∈ ¶492) *Herndon did not know Lincoln at age 17.*   1627

⟨1⟩ "The size of his hat measured at the hatter's block was seven and one-eighth, his head being, from ear to ear, six and one-half inches, and from the front to the back of the brain eight inches. Thus measured it was not below medium size." [herndon p472]   1628

⟨2⟩ About 1831: "His large foot ... presented a singular contrast with his very small head" – from *Menard Axis*, 1862 [wilson p24] (Part of ¶95)   1629

⟨1⟩ "His head was large, both longitudinally and perpendicularly, with a tall and ample forehead" – Senator James Harlan [helmB p166] Part of ¶173   1630

⟨2⟩ "large head" [kempfB p4]   1631

⟨1⟩ "I was most startled by the smallness of the head. ... this vulpine little face seems strangely vulnerable. The cheeks are sunken in. The nose is sharper than in the photographs, and the lines about the wide mouth are deep. With eyes shut, he looks to be a small man, in rehearsal for death." [vidalA p702], looking at the 1865 casting of Lincoln's head (See ¶1914.)   1632

⟨2/c⟩ His hat size of 7 1/4 [sic] "is smaller than usual for a man of six feet, four inches in height." [lattimerNY] *No supporting data cited.*   1633

⟨1⟩ "large bony face" – James Miner [ostendorfA p139] (∈ ¶1795)   1634

⟨1/q⟩ "Large head, with high crown of skull" – John Nicolay [meserve p5] (∈ ¶177)   1635

⟨1/q⟩ "... his head small and disproportionately shaped" – Elliott Herndon [herndon p470n] (∈ ¶1604)   1636

Head & Face (continued)

⟨1⟩ Aug. 1858: "his face was almost grotesquely square, with high cheek bones." — Martin Rindlaub [ostendorfA p19] (∈ ¶148) 1637

⟨1⟩ 1860s: "Mr. Lincoln's face was thin, and his features were large. ... his forehead square and well developed" [dana p173] (∈ ¶183) 1638

⟨1⟩ 1862: "a head, cocoa-nut shaped and somewhat too small for such a stature" [dicey v1pp220-221] (∈ ¶179) 1639

⟨2⟩ "dolichocephalic" [gordon] 1640

- Shape: 1641

  ⟨1⟩ "Mr. Lincoln's head was long, and tall from the base of the brain and from the eyebrows. His head ran backwards, his forehead rising as it ran back at a low angle. ... His forehead was narrow but high." [herndon p472] 1642

  ⟨2⟩ Anthropological measurements by [shapiro] show that Herndon was wrong about Lincoln's forehead being narrow. [shutesE pp204, 207] 1643

  ⟨2⟩c "head... judged from the life masks made of him, was not abnormally elongated" [lattimerNY] 1644

  ⟨1⟩q 1859: "he had a very pale, long face" – John Widmer [shenk p155] (∈ ¶150) 1645

  ⟨1⟩q 1860: "the long, gaunt head" – George H. Putnam [ostendorfA p57] (∈ ¶153) 1646

  ⟨2⟩c "The forehead is wide, high and bulges slightly in the middle. There is an unusual depression in the Volk mask with a palpable edge near the midline above the left eye. I have examined the Mills mask and found a similar depression in its forehead." [kempfB pp8-9] 1647

  ⟨1⟩ "His forehead was broad and high" [arnold p441] (∈ ¶167) 1648

  ⟨1⟩ April 1865: "his wide and high forehead" [chambrunA] (∈ ¶200) 1649

- Anthropological analysis, based on the 1865 life-mask: 1650

  ⟨2⟩c "Perhaps one of the most distinctive features of Lincoln's face was its great breadth, emphasized by the jutting arch of his cheek bones. The actual width of the face is distinctly greater than the norm of these 'Old Americans' of Hrdlicka [a control group]. It falls indeed, near its upper limit. ... The lateral projection of the cheek bones was so prominent it made the cheek below it look hollow by comparison, thus giving the 'cadaverous' look so frequently noticed." [shapiro] 1651

  ⟨2⟩c "The hollow, sunken cheek appearance was further emphasized by the enormous width of Lincoln's jaw at the angle just below and forward of the ear lobe. This – the bigonial width – measures 126 millimeters and lies at the very extreme of variation found in the Old American faces. The bony structure of the face was thus wide, both at the cheek bones and particularly the corners of the lower jaw – two elevated ridges with the intervening cheek valley between them. These peculiarities account for the frequently mentioned angularity and prominence of the bony structure of Lincoln's face observed by so many of his contemporaries." [shapiro] 1652

  ⟨2⟩c "Among the racial strains to be found in Lincoln's geography, one could match these dimensions easily only among the Indians." [shapiro] 1653

  ⟨2⟩c Disagrees with Herndon's description of Lincoln's forehead as "narrow," calling it instead broad, tall, and with a distinct slope. [shapiro] 1654

  ⟨2⟩c "Lincoln's face was long in absolute dimension... But its length lay largely in the mid-facial region, and particularly in the nasal area. The chin was not especially deep from the mouth down." [shapiro] 1655

  ⟨-⟩ See also: nose (¶1862) 1656

- Mole(s): 1657

Head & Face (continued)

⟨1⟩ "the lone mole on the right cheek" [herndonC] [herndon p472] (∈ ¶1606) (∈ ¶3) 1658

⟨2⟩_c "A mole on the right side of his face near the mouth is seen in all his full-face photographs." [meserve p26] 1659

🔲 The "mole" is not visible in the oldest known photograph of Lincoln ([ostendorf #1], taken about 1846), but this may be due to technical factors such as motion and poor focus. 1660

⟨2⟩_c The mass visible in the left nasolabial fold in the 1860 head cast (¶1905) is an artifact [stewart]. 1661

⟨2⟩_c "Three genetic moles, one on the right side and two on the left side of the face..." Of the left-sided moles, "one lies on the cheek above the crease where it turns backward from the upper lip, and the other lies lower down on the side of the face, in back of the crease, after it joins the mouth muscle-cheek muscle crease [sic]." Some symmetry among the moles is noted. [kempfB p5] 1662

- Lincoln's ugliness 1: 1663
  ⟨1⟩ In youth: "so awful homely" [burl p124] (∈ ¶2686) 1664
  ⟨1⟩ April 1829: "I saw Lincoln at my father-in-law's two days after [my] marriage. He was not a good looking young man." – Elizabeth Grigsby, remembering 70 years later [hobson p26] 1665
  ⟨1⟩_q About 1835: "Homely? Yes, I suppose he was, but I never thought of that then." – Nancy Rutledge Prewitt [walsh p42] (∈ ¶102) 1666
  ⟨1⟩_q "Mr. Lincoln may not be as handsome a figure, but the people are perhaps not aware that his heart is as large as his arms are long." – Mary Todd Lincoln, comparing him to Stephen A. Douglas [herndon p238] 1667
  ⟨1⟩_q About 1847: "not pretty" – Mary [randallC p91] 1668
  ⟨1⟩ "He was not a pretty man by any means, nor was he was an ugly one; he was a homely man, careless of his looks, plain-looking and plain-acting." [herndon p472-473] 1669
  ⟨1⟩ "he was homely, awkward, diffident" [arnold p46] 1670
  ⟨1⟩_q "Who in the hell are those two ugly men?" – stranger's remark, seeing Lincoln sitting next to Archibald Williams [angle p30, from beveridge] 1671
  ⟨1⟩ 1858: "odd-featured, wrinkled, inexpressive, and altogether uncomely face" – Henry Villard [kunhardtA p108] (Part of ¶145) 1673
  ⟨1⟩ March 1859: "His face was not handsome, to be sure" [stoddardD p206] (∈ ¶1610) 1674
  ⟨1⟩ "His face is certainly ugly, but not repulsive; on the contrary, the good humor, generosity and intellect beaming from it, makes the eye love to linger there until you almost fancy him good-looking." – [foster p221] 1675
  ⟨1⟩_q 1860: "His features are not handsome" – "a biographer" [meserve p4] (Part of ¶2806) 1676
  ⟨1⟩ May 19, 1860: His smile "lighting up every homely feature" on his face [coffinA p173] 1677
  ⟨1⟩_q June 21, 1860: "After you have been five minutes in his company you cease to think that he is either homely or awkward." – Utica newspaper reporter [lincloreHDE] (∈ ¶159) 1678
  ⟨1⟩_q Nov. 1860: "lean and ugly in every way" – Thomas Webster [randallC p163] (∈ ¶160) 1679
  ⟨1⟩_q Feb. 1861: "Mr. Lincoln is very homely" – Allan Pinkerton [wilson p291] 1680
  ⟨1⟩_q Fall 1861: "The Pres. is not half so ugly as he is generally represented." – a soldier [randallC p205] 1681
  ⟨1⟩ Spring 1862: "homely of face, large-boned, angular, and loosely put together" [bancroft] (∈ ¶182) 1682

Head & Face (continued)

⟨1⟩ 1862: "To say he is ugly is nothing: to add that his figure is grotesque is to convey no adequate impression." [dicey v1pp220-221] (∈ ¶179) 1683

⟨1⟩ "He's not an ugly man – but is a good looking man – What do you call him ugly? I don't" – a visitor, charmed by Lincoln [wilson p462] 1684

⟨1⟩ As President: "People said that his face was ugly. He certainly had neither the figure nor features of the Apollo of Belvedere; but he never appeared ugly to me, for his face, beaming with boundless kindness and benevolence towards mankind, had the stamp of intellectual beauty." [salmsalm p144] (∈ ¶190) 1685

⟨$\frac{1}{q}$⟩ "the neighbors told me that I would find that Mr. Lincoln was an ugly man, when he is really the handsomest man I ever saw in my life." – a woman, immediately after Lincoln commutes her son's death sentence [riceA p341] 1686

⟨$\frac{2}{c}$⟩ "Lincoln could appear handsome at one time, homely at another." [kunhardtA p9] (Part of ¶176) See ¶1601ff for effects of lighting. 1687

⟨2⟩ "All the synonyms which harmonize with such words as homely, ugly, repulsive, etc. have been used to describe his countenance by some writers." [lincloreBIG] 1688

⟨$\frac{2}{c}$⟩ "... a consensus ... among those who knew Lincoln that his ugliness disappeared when he spoke." [burk p229] 1689

⟨1⟩ As President: "tall, homely form" – David Homer Bates [NYTimesTeleg] (See ¶188.) 1690

⟨$\frac{1}{q}$⟩ 1860: "He is said to be a homely man; I do not think so." – painter John Henry Brown [ostendorfA p62] 1691

⟨$\frac{1}{q}$⟩ 1861: "His face was a pleasant surprise... I remember thinking how much better-looking he was than I had anticipated, and wondering that anyone should consider him ugly." – John M. Winchell of the *New York Times* [ostendorfA p71] 1692

⟨2⟩ "Lincoln was in fact a homely man with simple tastes, indifferent to personal comfort." [donaldA p215] 1693

⟨1⟩ About 1864: "He was never handsome, indeed, but he grew more and more cadaverous and ungainly month by month." [croffut] (∈ ¶196) 1694

⟨1⟩ 1865: "... was a homely enough figure..." [crookA p14] [crookK] (∈ ¶198) 1695

⟨1⟩ April 1865: "not a handsome man, and ungainly in his person" [porterD p296] 1696

■ Lincoln's ugliness 2: 1697

⟨1⟩ "The first time I saw Mr. Lincoln I thought him the homeliest man I had ever seen." [carrA p252] (∈ ¶1812) 1698

⟨$\frac{1}{q}$⟩ 1858: "I thought him about the ugliest man I had ever seen." – Rev. George C. Noyes [browneF p290] (∈ ¶147) 1699

⟨1⟩ 1860: "Mr. Lincoln was the homeliest man I ever saw." [piatt pp345-346] (∈ ¶152) 1700

⟨1⟩ 1862: "about the homeliest man I ever saw, yet by no means repulsive or disagreeable" [hawthorne p309] (∈ ¶178) 1701

⟨$\frac{1}{q}$⟩ Oct. 1, 1862: Lincoln "not only is the ugliest man I ever saw, but the most uncouth and gawky in his manners and appearance." – a soldier [donaldA p387] 1702

⟨$\frac{1}{q}$⟩ Early 1865: "the ugliest man I have ever put my eyes on" – Colonel Theodore Lyman [meserve p15] 1703

⟨$\frac{1}{q}$⟩ About 1858: "I am the homeliest man in the State of Illinois." – Lincoln [ostendorfA p29] (∈ ¶1716) 1704

■ Lincoln's ugliness 3 (his self-view): 1705

⟨$\frac{1}{q}$⟩ "my homely face" [kunhardtA p8] 1706

⟨$\frac{2}{q}$⟩ Lincoln told jokes about ugliness, e.g., woman to a man: "Well, for the land's sake, you are the homeliest man I ever saw!" Man: "Yes ma'am, but I can't 1707

Head & Face (continued)

help that." Woman: "No, I suppose not, but you might stay at home." [meserve p3]

⟨1/q⟩ After being called two-faced in a debate: "I leave it to my audience. If I had another face, do you think I'd wear this one?" [kunhardtA p8]   1708

⟨1/q⟩ "I was once accosted ... by a stranger who said 'Excuse me, sir, but I have an article in my possession which belongs to you.' 'How is that?' I asked, considerably astonished. The stranger took a jackknife from his pocket. 'This knife,' said he, 'was placed in my hands some years ago, with the injunction that I was to keep it until I found a man *uglier* than myself. Allow me *now* to say, sir, that I think *you* are fairly entitled to the property.' " [kunhardtA p8]   1709

⟨2⟩ "I don't know why you boys want such a homely face." – Lincoln, when urged to have a photograph [ostendorfA p7]   1710

⟨1⟩ "A yarn is told of him..." Lincoln was splitting rails with "Collar open" when a man came up and pointed a gun at him. "Says Lincoln   What do you mean, the man replied that he had promised to shoot the first man who was uglier than himself." Looking at the man's face, Lincoln said "If I am uglier then you, then blaze away" – Samuel Haycraft [wilson p85]   1711

⟨2⟩ "On repeated occasions he remarked to some woman or to an audience, 'In the matter of looks I have the advantage,' meaning that they had to look at him while he couldn't see himself." [meserve p3] [welles v1p528]   1712

⟨1/q⟩ A man in Dayton, Ohio began painting a portrait of Lincoln, who said to him: "Keep on. You may make a good one, but never a pretty one." [meserve p3]   1713

⟨2⟩ Lincoln told a story of being approached by a man who said: "I promised long ago that if I ever met a man uglier than myself I would hand him this pistol and tell him to shoot me." Lincoln's reply: "Well, if I am uglier than you are, for God's sake, go ahead and shoot." [meserve p4]   1714

⟨1/q⟩ 1858: "Nobody has ever expected me to be President. In my poor lean, lank face nobody has ever seen any cabbages were sprouting out." – Lincoln self-description, before growing his beard [meserve p3] [currentBk p4] [sumnerA p135]   1715

⟨1/q⟩ About 1858: "I cannot see why all you artists want a likeness of me unless it is because I am the homeliest man in the State of Illinois." – Lincoln [ostendorfA p29]   1716

⟨1/q⟩ May 1860: Referring to [ostendorf #28], "That picture gives a very fair representation of my homely face." – Lincoln [ostendorfA p48]   1717

⟨1⟩ Dec. 3, 1863: Ill with smallpox, Lincoln jokes "There is one consolation about the matter, doctor, it cannot in the least disfigure me!" [ChicagoTribune - Dec. 8, 1863, p2] *He was wrong – see ¶1892.*   1718

⟨1⟩ Feb. 1864: "Do you think, Mr. Carpenter, that you can make a handsome picture of *me?*" – Lincoln to portrait painter Francis Carpenter [carpenter p19]   1719

⟨1/q⟩ Secretary of War Edwin Stanton, frustrated with Lincoln, exclaimed "We've got to get rid of that baboon in the White House." Lincoln was told of the insult and responded: "Insult? insult? That is no insult. It is an expression of opinion. And what troubles me most about it is the fact that Stanton said it, and Stanton is usually right." [ostendorfA p217]   1720

⟨1/q⟩ "If I have one vice, it is not being able to say no! Thank God for not making me a woman, but if He had, I suppose He would have made me just as ugly as He did, and no one would ever have tempted me." – Lincoln to General Elbert Viele [ostendorfA p217]   1721

⟨1⟩ As President, while sitting for a painting: "... as he was glancing at his letters, he burst into a hearty laugh, and exclaimed: 'As a painter, Mr. Healy, you shall   1722

Head & Face (continued)

be a judge between this unknown correspondent and me. She complains of my ugliness. It is allowed to be ugly in this world, but not as ugly as I am. She wishes me to put on false whiskers, to hide my horrible lantern jaws. Will you paint me with false whiskers? No? I thought not.' " [healy pp69-70]

⟨1/q⟩ Explaining his homeliness: "When I was two months old I was the handsomest child in Kentucky, but my Negro nurse swapped me off for another boy, just to please a friend who was going down the river, whose child was rather plain-looking." [ostendorfA p216]   1723

- Lines and wrinkling: 1724

⟨1/q⟩ "His face and forehead were wrinkled even in his youth. They deepened in age, 'as streams their channels deeper wear.' " – Joshua Speed [ostendorfA p23]   1725

⟨1/?⟩ Lincoln looked like: "An honest old lawyer, with a face half Roman, half Indian, wasted by climate, scarred by a life's struggle." – London journalist [ostendorfA p51]   1726

⊡ 1846±: The vertical furrow in his right cheek is already visible in [ostendorf #1].   1727

⟨1⟩ 1858: "wrinkled" – Henry Villard [kunhardtA p108] (Part of ¶145)   1728

⟨1⟩ Oct. 13, 1858: "That swarthy face with its ... its deep furrows..." – Carl Schurz [angle p243] (∈ ¶149)   1729

⟨1⟩ Mar. 1859: As he read, "the deep wrinkles in his forehead grew deeper" [stoddardD p206] (∈ ¶1610)   1730

⟨1/q⟩ Sept. 17, 1859: "The face had a battered and bronzed look... and an expression of sadness." – Moncure D. Conway [ostendorfA p31]   1731

⟨2⟩ Feb. 27, 1860: Lincoln sits for a photograph. Mathew Brady's retouching "eliminated harsh lines from his face to show an almost handsome, statesmanlike image" [donaldA p238] (Part of ¶23.)   1732

⟨1⟩ May 19, 1860: "The lines upon his face..." [coffinA p173] (∈ ¶157)   1733

⟨1/q⟩ 1860: "There are so many hard lines in his face that it becomes a mask to the inner man." – painter John Henry Brown [ostendorfA p62]   1734

⟨1⟩ 1860: "He had a face that defied artistic skill to soften or idealize" [piatt p346] (∈ ¶152)   1735

⊡ Referring to a photograph: "The 1860. one that was from the 'Century' magazine picture was taken: you will observe that the wrinkles are considerably smoothed out of it, but I think they are the best that are available." – Henry Whitney [wilson p621] *He seems to be suggesting something was done to minimize the appearance of the wrinkles.*   1736

⟨1⟩ March 1861: "two deep furrows from the nostril to the chin" – William Russell [russell pp37-38] (∈ ¶161)   1737

⟨1⟩ 1862: "the lines about his mouth are very strongly defined" [hawthorne p310] (∈ ¶178)   1738

⟨1⟩ Mid 1863: "deep marks about the large and expressive mouth." – Silas Burt [wilsonR p332] (∈ ¶1621)   1739

⟨1⟩ Sept. 6, 1863: "deep lines of thought and care were around his mouth and eyes" [harveyC] (∈ petFirst)   1740

⟨2⟩ circa 1864: "Even though his face was lined with sudden age, still it glowed." [kunhardtA p3-6]   1741

⟨1⟩ April 3, 1865: "Perhaps I was mistaken, but the lines upon his face seemed far deeper than I had ever seen them before." [coffinA p182]   1742

⟨1⟩ April 4, 1865: "deeper than ever before the lines upon his forehead" [coffinA p187] (∈ ¶1294)   1743

Head & Face (continued)

⟨1⟩ April 1865: "the furrows that ran across his cheeks and chin" [chambrunA] (∈ ¶200) — 1744

⟨1/q⟩ "The deep careworn lines about his rugged face told of trouble or melancholy of far older standing than any late misfortune could have occasioned." – contemporary observation [burl p106] — 1745

⟨2/c⟩ [kempfB p4] concludes that the pattern of Lincoln's mid- and lower-facial creases is unusual, yet names cousins (on both sides of the family) who have similar creases. — 1746

⟨2⟩ "Deep creases over the forehead and at the outside corners of the eyes and around the mouth..." [kempfB p6] — 1747

⟨-⟩ For brow corrugations and crow's-feet, as related to eyes, see ¶897 — 1748

⟨1⟩ Looking at 1865 cast, "the lines about the wide mouth are deep" [vidalA p702] (∈ ¶1632) — 1749

- "Old Abe:" — 1750

⟨2⟩ In his 20s, "the deep pink in his cheeks abruptly blanched and the new young man began to be called Old Abe" [kunhardtB p291]. — 1751

⟨1⟩ 1854: "Although he was but forty-five, he was alluded to in popular parlance as 'old Mr. Lincoln' ... Mr. Lincoln was asked how long they had been calling him old. Said he: 'Oh, they have been at that trick many years. They commenced it when I was scarcely thirty.' It seemed to amuse him." – Lawrence Weldon [riceA pp197-198] — 1752

⟨2⟩ Elihu Washburne heard Lincoln called Old Abe in July 1847 and "ever afterwards called him 'Old Abe.'" [hunt p228] — 1753

⟨2⟩ The term "Old Abe" was applied to Lincoln as early as age 38, and at age 39 Lincoln wrote "I suppose I am now one of the old men." [burl p74] — 1754

⟨1/q⟩ July 10, 1858: Lincoln calls himself "an old man" [lincloreLFH] (∈ ¶810) — 1755

⟨1/q⟩ 1860: "There is no appearance of age about the man. How they call him 'Old Abe' I do not see." – [NYHerald] reporter [ostendorfA p52] (See ¶1382) — 1756

- Expression: — 1757

⟨-⟩ For lability of expression, see ¶2333ff. — 1758

⟨1⟩ "I can now see Lincoln, his image before me; it is a sad beseeching look. I feel sad." – William Herndon, 20+ years after last seeing Lincoln alive [hertz p117] — 1759

⟨1⟩ "Aside from the sad, pained look due to habitual melancholy, his face had no characteristic or fixed expression." [herndon p331] — 1760

⟨S⟩ [mitchell] speculates that Lincoln's sorrowful expression was enhanced by facial lines resulting from his ocular misalignment (see ¶1837). — 1761

⟨1⟩ About 1815: "Some of 'em said Abe went mopin' round, and had spells like his father; but then they war mistak'n about him, just like they war about Thomas. Abe did n't have spells. It was just the way his face 'peared when he was sober and thinkin' like and a-studyin', what he allus did when he could get a book; and it did set everybody a-wonderin' to see how much he knowed, and he not mor'n seven." – a Kentucky neighbor [browneR v1p83] — 1762

⟨1/q⟩ About 1840: Watching Lincoln talk to women at a party "the face of L. was occasionally distorted into a grin" – James Conkling [randallC p13] — 1763

⟨1/q⟩ 1848±: "a far-away, absent minded look, scarcely to be classed as sad, yet falling little short of it" – Presley Edwards. Seeing Lincoln again, in 1851, Edwards thought the look had intensified. [shenk p108] — 1764

Head & Face (continued)

⟨1⟩ "His very prominent features in repose seemed dull and expressionless." [wilson p641] (∈ ¶139)   1765

⟨1/q⟩ 1849, after serving in Congress: "That Star gazing thinking Look, as if Looking at vacancy, he also Contracted them in Washington or Soon after he Came home" – Abner Ellis [wilson p500]   1766

⟨1/q⟩ 1854 or later: "more than once I remember waking up early in the morning to find him sitting before the fire, his mind apparently concentrated on some subject, with the saddest expression I have ever seen in a human being's eyes." – Lawrence Weldon [hirschhornC] *Weldon says Lincoln habitually awakened earlier than other lawyers: ¶3459.*   1767

⟨1/q⟩ 1858: When a telling story "his facial expression was so irresistibly comic that the bystanders generally exploded in laughter before he reached what he called the 'nub' of it." – Horace White [angle p233]   1768

⟨1/q⟩ Oct. 4, 1854: "It was a marked face, but so overspread with sadness..." – Horace White [shenk p132]   1769

⟨1⟩ 1858 and later: "I never saw a more thoughtful face, I never saw a more dignified face, I never saw so sad a face. ... his was the saddest face I ever looked upon." – David Locke [riceA pp442, 443]   1770

⟨1/q⟩ Summer 1858: Campaigning against Douglas: "He rode in a carriage ... looking dust-begrimed and worn and weary; and though he frequently lifted his hat in recognition of the cheers of the crowds lining the streets, I saw no smile on his face, and he seemed to take no pleasure in the demonstrations of enthusiasm which his presence called forth." – Rev. George C. Noyes [browneF p290]   1771

⟨1⟩ Oct. 13, 1858: face "looked even more haggard and careworn than later when it was framed in whiskers" – Carl Schurz [angle p243] (∈ ¶149)   1772

⟨1⟩ March 1859: "His face was not handsome, to be sure, but at any time there was a great deal of expression in it" [stoddardD p206] (∈ ¶1610)   1773

⟨1⟩ March 1861: "the eyes dark, full, and deeply set, are penetrating, but full of an expression which almost amounts to tenderness" – William Russell [russell pp37-38] (∈ ¶161)   1774

⟨1/q⟩ 1860: In reviewing Alban Jasper Conant's painting of Lincoln, Mary says "That is excellent, that is the way he looks when he has his friends about him." [randallC p162]   1775

⟨1⟩ As President: "I could not look into it without feeling kindly towards him, and without tears starting to my eyes, for over the whole face was spread a melancholy tinge. ... There was in his face, besides kindness and melancholy, a sly humour flickering around the corners of his big mouth and his rather small and somewhat tired-looking eyes." [salmsalm p144] (∈ ¶190)   1776

⟨1⟩ March 1862±: "There was a look of depression about his face, which, I am told by those who see him daily, was habitual to him, even before the then recent death of his child... You cannot look upon his worn, bilious, anxious countenance, and believe it to be that of a happy man." [dicey v1pp221-222]   1777

⟨1⟩ Spring 1862: "Cover the lower part of his face, and the expression of the upper part was one of pathetic sadness... reverse the process and look upon the lower half of his face, and the expression was humorous and kindly." [bancroft] (∈ ¶182)   1778

⟨1⟩ Sept. 7, 1863: "After a moment he said, 'Well,' with a peculiar contortion of face I never saw in anybody else." [harveyC] (∈ §6.5)   1779

Head & Face (continued)

⟨1⟩ Sept. 7, 1863: "a more than mortal anguish rested on his face" [harveyC] (∈ §6.8) 1780

⟨1⟩ Nov. 18, 1863: "sad face" [cochrane] (∈ ¶2535) 1781

⟨1⟩ 1864: "In repose, it was the saddest face I ever knew. There were days when I could scarcely look into it without crying." [carpenter p30] 1782

⟨1⟩ About 1864: "He had a very dejected appearance, and ugly black rings appeared under his eyes. I well remember how weary and sad he looked at one" particular reception. [croffut] (∈ ¶196) 1783

⟨1⟩ May 1864: Contemplating the Battle of the Wilderness: "his dark features contracted still more with gloom; and as he looked up, I thought his face the saddest one I had ever seen." – Schuyler Colfax [riceA p337] 1784

⟨1⟩ Summer 1864: "But his face! – oh, the pathos of it! – haggard, drawn into fixed lines of unutterable sadness, with a look of loneliness, as of a soul whose depth of sorrow and bitterness no human sympathy could ever reach. ... The impression I carried away was that I had seen, not so much the President of the United States, as *the saddest man in the world*." [browneF p670] (∈ ¶2538) 1785

⟨1⟩ Aug. 12, 1864: "Lincoln's dark brown face, with the deep cut lines, the eyes, & c., always to me with a latent sadness in the expression ... [Once, as he rode by,] I saw the President in the face fully ... his look, though abstracted, happen'd to be directed steadily in my eye. He bow'd and smiled, but far beneath his smile I noticed well the expression I have alluded to." – Walt Whitman [riceB p414] 1786

⟨1⟩ 1865: "the expression of Mr. Lincoln's face was always sad when he was quiet" ... "was such a sad looking man usually, it seemed good to have him happy." [crookA pp13,18-19] [crookK] 1787

⟨2⟩ Mar. 1865: "His rugged and strongly marked features, lately so deeply furrowed with care, anxiety, over-work, and responsibility, were now full of hope and confidence." [arnold p420] 1788

⟨1⟩ Mar. 23, 1865: "All the sadness of his face came out now when he was quiet." [crookA p39] 1789

⟨2⟩ General William T. Sherman recalled that, at rest or listening, Lincoln sat with his arms hanging as if lifeless and his face dull; he would light up when he talked. [currentBk p248] 1790

⟨1⟩ April 14, 1865: Receiving a "cheering welcome" upon entering Ford's Theatre: "His face was perfectly stoical; his deep-set eyes gave him a pathetically sad appearance. The audience seemed to be enthusiastically cheerful, yet he looked peculiarly sorrowful..." [lealeA p3] (∈ ¶207) 1791

⟨1⟩ April 14, 1865, comatose: "His features were calm and striking. I had never seen them appear to better advantage" [welles v2p287] (∈ ¶552) *Lincoln was supine, so his muscles sagged in a different direction!* 1792

⟨2⟩ "In repose, Lincoln's face had a cold, chiseled look." [shenk p117] 1793

⟨1⟩ "That serious, far-away look" – John Nicolay [ostendorfA p84] 1794

⟨1⟩ "His large bony face when in repose was unspeakably sad and as unreadable as that of a sphinx, his eyes were as expressionless as those of a dead fish; but when he smiled or laughed at one of his own stories of that of another then everything about him changed; his figure became alert, a lightning change came over his countenance, his eyes scintillated and I thought he had the most expressive features I had ever seen on the face of a man." – James Miner [ostendorfA p139] 1795

Head & Face (continued)

⟨2⟩ "Whenever Lincoln posed, a dark melancholy settled over his features." [ostendorfA p139] · 1796

⟨1⟩ Post-mortem: "The face was the same as in life. Death had not changed the kindly countenance in any line. There was upon it the same sad look that it had worn always, though not so intensely sad as it had been in life. ... The face had a expression of absolute content... I had seen the expression on his living face only a few times, when, after a great calamity, he had come to a great victory. It was the look of a worn man suddenly relieved." – David Locke [riceA pp452-453] (See also: ¶3241 and ¶3307.) · 1797

- Change with emotion: · 1798
  ⟨-⟩ For lability of expression, see ¶2333ff. · 1799
  ⟨2⟩_c A brief article, "The countenance of Abraham Lincoln" [lincloreBIG] (1937), emphasizes the remarkable transformation that his face underwent when engaged with other people. See also ¶176. · 1800
  ⟨2⟩ "He was a practiced actor and an individual artist in the use of his face. ... It was an experienced comedian's face." [meserve p4] · 1801
  ⟨1⟩ March 1859: "... his expression varied from minute to minute, all the while being cloudy. [Lincoln reads a letter silently.] His face at first grew darker and the deep wrinkles in his forehead grew deeper.... Then, if you can imagine how a dark lighthouse looks when its calcium light is suddenly kindled, you may get an idea of the change which came into the face of Abraham Lincoln.... I did not disturb Mr. Lincoln or try to speak to him." [stoddardD pp206-207] (∈ ¶1610) · 1802
  ⟨1⟩_q 1860: "His features are not handsome, but extremely mobile; his mouth particularly so. He has the faculty of contorting that feature to provoke uproarious merriment. Good humor gleams in his eye and lurks in the corner of his mouth." – "a biographer" [meserve p4] · 1803
  ⟨1⟩ 1860: Of Lincoln's face: "It was capable of few expressions, but those were extremely striking. When in repose, his face was dull, heavy, and repellent. It brightened, like a lit lantern, when animated. His dull eyes would fairly sparkle with fun, or express as kindly a look as I ever saw, when moved by some matter of human interest." [piatt pp345-346] (∈ ¶152) · 1804
  ⟨1⟩_q June 21, 1860: "... the whole face indicative at once of goodness and resoluteness. In repose, it had something of rigidity, but when in play, it was one of the most eloquent I have ever seen. None of his pictures do him the slightest justice." – Utica newspaper reporter [lincloreHDE] (∈ ¶159) · 1805
  ⟨1⟩ 1860s: "nor have I ever seen another face which would light up as Mr. Lincoln's did when something touched his heart or amused him." [dana p173] (∈ ¶183) · 1806
  ⟨1⟩_q October 1, 1862: Lincoln arrives at an Army camp in a common ambulance, "grinning out of the windows like a baboon" – a soldier [donaldA p387] · 1807
  ⟨1⟩ Sept. 6, 1863: "the most curious, comical face in the world" [harveyC] (∈ §6.4) · 1808
  ⟨1⟩ Sept. 7, 1863: "While I was speaking the expression of Mr. Lincoln's face had changed many times. He had never taken his eye from me. Now every muscle in his face seemed to contract, and then suddenly expand." [harveyC] (∈ §6.6) · 1809
  ⟨1⟩ "inexpressive" – Henry Villard [kunhardtA p108] (Part of ¶145) · 1810
  ⟨1⟩ Of a photo: "It represents him with no more expression than a post & yet it is just as he would look when sitting for a photo & putting on his most serious look, as though he had been just sentenced to death. The trouble was that · 1811

135

Head & Face (continued)

this photographer did not have the *gumption* to stir him up & make him look animated. There was more difference between Lincoln dull & Lincoln animated, in facial expressions, than I ever saw *in any other human being.*" – Horace White [wilson p698]

⟨1⟩ "The first time I saw Mr. Lincoln I thought him the homeliest man I had ever seen. Afterwards, when I had seen his face light up in conversation, I really came to regard him as a handsome man." [carrA p252]   1812

⟨1⟩ "He was odd, but when that gray eye and that face and those features were lit up by the inward soul in fires of emotion, then it was that all those apparently ugly features sprang into organs of beauty or disappeared in the sea of inspiration that often flooded his face. Sometimes it appeared as if Lincoln's soul was fresh from its Creator." [herndon p475]   1813

⟨-⟩ See ¶2333ff for the rapid changes in Lincoln's apparent mood.   1814

- Color and texture: 1815
  ⟨-⟩ *Comments about Lincoln's general skin tone are in* [Skin] *¶3376ff. Comments about his facial skin tone are here.*   1816

  ⟨1⟩ "his dark, yellow face, wrinkled and dry." [herndon p331] Part of ¶90   1817
  ⟨1⟩ Oct. 13, 1858: "swarthy face" – Carl Schurz [angle p243] (∈ ¶149)   1818
  ⟨1⟩q 1859: "he had a very pale, long face" – John Widmer [shenk p155] (∈ ¶150)   1819
  ⟨1⟩q Sept. 17, 1859: "The face had a battered and bronzed look... and an expression of sadness." – Moncure D. Conway [ostendorfA p31]   1820
  ⟨1⟩ "his face was long narrow, sallow and cadaverous ... his cheeks were leathery and saffron-colored" – Herndon [kunhardtB p291] (∈ ¶89)   1821
  ⟨1⟩ Pre-Presidency: "His face was long – sallow – cadaverous – shrunk – shrivelled – wrinkled, and dry" [herndonC] (∈ ¶3)   1822
  ⟨1⟩ 1863, after Battle of Chancellorsville: "his face, usually sallow, was ashen in hue" – Noah Brooks [brooksC pp57-58] (∈ ¶2644)   1824
  ⟨1⟩q "the flesh was coarse, pimply, dry, hard, harsh, wrinkled, saffron-brown with no blood seemingly in it" – Herndon [shutesE p205]   1825
  ⟨1⟩ "I still think that he had a fine network of nerve under the coarse flesh." – William Herndon [hertz p203]   1826

- Movement and position, including head tilt: 1827
  ⟨1⟩ In Springfield: "He did not gesticulate as much with his hands as with his head. He used the latter frequently, throwing it with vim this way and that." [herndon p332] Part of ¶90   1828
  ⟨1⟩ "His head, when he was in repose, drooped slightly forward." – Senator James Harlan [helmB p166] Part of ¶173   1829
  ⟨1⟩q "Will was the true picture of Mr. Lincoln, in every way, even to carrying his head slightly inclined toward his left shoulder." – Springfield neighbor [burl p66] citing [NYHerald - May 26, 1861] *Given Lincoln's left hyperphoria, one would expect tilt toward the right shoulder. See ¶1827.*   1830
  ⊡ Many photographs show Lincoln with head tilted to his right.   1831
  ⊡ There is one non-posed pictures of Lincoln reading. It shows him with head tilted to the right, wearing spectacles, reading his second inaugural address [ostendorf #108]. ([ostendorf #109] probably shows the same, but is too blurry to be useful.) (In [ostendorf #93], a posed photograph, Lincoln is looking at a picture book, not reading a Bible as is often supposed.)   1832
  ⟨2⟩c' Lincoln's habitual head tilt to the right, diagnosed as a Bielschowsky tilt by [goldsteinJ], is consistent with his left hypertropia. [aa64 pp407-409] explains the physiology of the Bielschowsky tilt.   1833

Head & Face (continued)

- Brow: 1834
  - ⟨-⟩ For eyebrows, see ¶1429ff in ⌐Hair⌐. 1835
  - ⟨2⟩ "jutting eyebrows" [kunhardtA p9] (Part of ¶176) 1836
  - ⟨S⟩ "One of the most common symptoms observed in those who suffer from het- 1837 erophoria is the corrugation of the brow and its resulting 'crow-foot,' which does so much to lend the human face an expression of sorrow. ... a hyper- phoria of several degrees would lend its mite to make the marks of sorrow more eloquent and expressive." [mitchell] (Agrees with [snyder].)
  - ⟨1⟩ March 1861: "the shaggy brow, running into the small hard frontal space, the 1838 development of which can scarcely be estimated accurately, owing to the irregular flocks of thick hair carelessly brushed across it" – William Russell [russell pp37-38] (∈ ¶161)
  - ⟨1⟩ 1862: "thick black eyebrows and an impending brow" [hawthorne p310] (∈ ¶178) 1839
  - ⟨-⟩ Also see ¶1429ff. 1840
  - ⟨2⟩c "The corrugations of Lincoln's brow and the crow's-feet at the corners of his 1841 eyes indicate that he habitually used auxilliary facial muscles to support the external muscles of the eyes in an attempt to obtain good vision" [snyder].

- Cheeks & thinness: 1842
  - ⟨1⟩ 1858: "my sunken and hollow cheeks" – Lincoln, perhaps exaggerating for 1843 comic effect [browneF p291] (∈ ¶428)
  - ⟨2⟩ "hollow cheeks" [kunhardtA p9] (Part of ¶176) 1844
  - ⟨1⟩ April 1860: "the cheek-bones were higher than the jaws at the lobe of the 1845 ear" [volk] Part of ¶1905
  - ⟨1⟩ May 19, 1860: "sunken cheeks..." [coffinA p173] (∈ ¶157) 1846
  - ⟨1⟩q cheeks were 'leathery and flabby, falling in loose folds at places, looking sor- 1847 rowful and sad" – William Herndon [herndonC] (∈ ¶3)
  - ⟨1⟩q "my poor lean, lank face" – Lincoln's self-description, before growing his 1848 beard [meserve p3] [currentBk p4] [sumnerA p135] (∈ ¶1715)
  - ⟨1⟩ Looking at 1865 cast, "The cheeks are sunken in" [vidalA p702] (∈ ¶1632) 1849
- ⟨2⟩ In Springfield, presumably: Dr. Merryman (¶3183) was "known to have surgically 1850 removed a 'lump' from Lincoln's cheek." [pearson]

- Nose: 1851
  - ⟨1⟩ "large – long and blunt, having the tip glowing in red, and a little awry toward 1852 the right eye" [herndonC] (∈ ¶3)
  - ⟨1⟩q "a large nose" – John Nicolay [meserve p5] (∈ ¶177) 1853
  - ⟨1⟩ "His nose was large, clearly defined, and well shaped" [arnold p441] (∈ ¶167) 1854
  - ⟨1⟩ May 19, 1860: "enormous nose..." [coffinA p173] (∈ ¶157) 1855
  - ⟨1⟩q June 21, 1860: "the nose strongly aquiline" – Utica newspaper reporter [lin- 1856 cloreHDE] (∈ ¶159)
  - ⟨1⟩ March 1861: "a prominent organ – stands out from the face" – William Rus- 1857 sell [russell pp37-38] (∈ ¶161)
  - ⟨1⟩q Fall 1861: "his nose is rather long but he is rather *long* himself, so it is a Ne- 1858 cessity to keep the proportion complete." – a soldier [randallC p205]
  - ⟨1⟩ 1862: "a nose and ears, which have been taken by mistake from a head of 1859 twice the size" [dicey v1pp220-221] (∈ ¶179)
  - ⟨1⟩ 1862: "his nose is large" [hawthorne p310] (∈ ¶178) 1860
  - ⟨2⟩ "his beak of a nose" [kunhardtA p9] (Part of ¶176) 1861
  - ⟨2⟩c "The nose is long, but this length no doubt was in part the result of the 1862 marked linearity of growth so evident in Lincoln's whole conformation. The

Head & Face (continued)

marked length of the nose gives its moderate width almost the appearance of narrowness." [shapiro]

⟨2⟩ When Lincoln laughed, the tip of his nose moved, per Philip Hone (1780-1851) [vidalA p702]   1863

⟨2⟩ "His nose was not relatively oversized, but it looked large because of his thin   1864
ᶜ face. The nostrils did not extend as far into the tip of the nose as in most people, which made the end look heavy. Lincoln was said, when young, to have been somewhat sensitive about his nose, but not about his ears." [kempfB p5] (See ¶664.)

⟨1⟩ April 1865: Lincoln, angry: "his nostrils dilated like those of an excited racehorse" [porterD p308] (∈ ¶2558)   1865

⟨1⟩ Looking at 1865 cast, "The nose is sharper than in the photographs" [vidalA   1866
p702] (∈ ¶1632)

[○] The length and breadth of the nose has been measured from casts of Lincoln's head [stewart] [shapiro]. It is long, but not especially wide. (See ¶1932.)   1867

■ Lips: See ¶2785ff in [Mouth].   1868

⟨1⟩ March 1861: "strange quaint face and head" – William Russell [russell pp37-38] (∈   1869
q ¶161)

[○] 1861: [ostendorf #44] "reveals more of the back of Lincoln's head than any other portrait." [ostendorfA p71]   1870

■ Head trauma – also see [Trauma]:   1871
⟨1⟩ See ¶3568 and §1a for the loss of consciousness episode that followed a   1872
horse-kick to the head [herndon pp51-52]

⟨2⟩ During a race to see which team could husk corn the fastest, "the young Lincoln taunted a member of the opposition so badly that the aggrieved man hurled a rocklike corn nub that created an ugly gash above Lincoln's eye. [burl p149]   1873

⟨1⟩ "I hit him with an Ear of Corn once – cut him over the Eye – he got mad – My   1874
mother whipt me severely as she should have done" – Green Taylor [wilson p130]

⟨2⟩ 1828: After being attacked during a New Orleans trip (¶3582ff), "received   1876
a scar which he carried with him to his grave" – Ward Lamon [shutesE p197] (Presumably a head scar)

⟨1⟩ Before 1860: Mary struck Lincoln on the head with a piece of wood, cutting   1877
his nose – see ¶3589 – Margaret Ryan [wilson p597]

⟨1⟩ See Special Topic §7 for fatal gunshot wound to head   1878
⟨2⟩ On his deathbed, physicians found "two small scars on his scalp well hidden   1879
among the black locks." [kunhardtB p49]

■ Headaches: 1880
⟨1⟩ Headaches associated with constipation. See ¶617.   1881
⟨2⟩ "Before his presidential years, there is only one record of a specific complaint   1882
ᶜ of headache (with sore throat)." [shutesE p106] *Probably ¶5748, when Willie had scarlet fever.*

⟨S⟩ [shutesE p106] assumes that headache was present whenever Lincoln described   1883
himself as "unwell." *The assumption does not seem warranted.*

⟨1⟩ March 30, 1861: Recently "had keeled over with sick headache for the first   1884
q time in years." [shenk p285]. (∈ ¶2627) *Phrasing suggests previous episodes. Called a migraine headache by [donaldA p289], but see ¶2628 for caveats.*

Head & Face (continued)

Abraham

⟨1⟩ April 25, 1862: "He was alone and complaining of head ache." [browning p542] 1885
(∈ ¶1145)

⟨1⟩ May 2, 1862: "He had the head ache and was not in his office" that night, but 1886
received Browning in the family room for an hour. [browning p543]

⟨1⟩ April 13, 1865: severe headache [turner p219]. See ¶1314. 1887

■ Headaches related to reading and/or eyeglasses: 1888

⟨-⟩ *I'm skeptical because I've not found descriptions of such headaches in* 1889
primary sources.

⟨2⟩ "The glasses were apparently intended to aid him in reading small print, and 1890
were at least three times stronger than what he actually would have needed.
This may explain why Lincoln often suffered from severe headaches after
long periods of reading." [bumgarnerB] (See ¶791.)

⟨2⟩ "Reading tended to produce severe eyestrain ... with the sequelae of 1891
headache, nausea, indigestion, chills, mental distraction and gloominess"
[kempf p13]. *Kemp ascribes the eyestrain to Lincoln's oculomotor problems*
– see Eyes -- Motor .

■ Smallpox scarring: 1892

⟨1⟩ As Lincoln recovered: "His face is slightly marked" [ChicagoTribune - Dec. 11, 1863]. 1893
See Special Topic §5 entry for Dec. 6, 1863.

⊙ Photographs taken after Lincoln's smallpox episode of Nov.-Dec. 1863 show 1894
a dark spot on the right side of the tip of his nose. See [ostendorf #90, 116, 118] as
printed in [mellon]. Library of Congress image LC-USZ61-1938 shows the spot
particularly well.

⊙ Counter-evidence: The [mellon p49] print of [ostendorf #15] shows a beardless Lin- 1895
coln with a discoloration of the right tip of his nose. No other pre-smallpox
photograph shows it well. It may also be present in [mellon p81] = [ostendorf #42].

⟨S⟩ Certain technical features of 1860s photography also factor into assess- 1896
ment's of Lincoln's skin. See §5e and *The Physical Lincoln*.

⟨S⟩ ○○○ *Project:* If Lincoln had an abnormality of the elastin or collagen in 1897
his skin, how would development of pockmarks be affected?

■ Chin dimple [OMIM 119000]: 1898

⟨2⟩ Lincoln's beard obscured the dimple in his chin "but his old friends and 1899
most especially his barber remembered it well" [kunhardtB p288]. His barber
was William Florville [kunhardtB pp274-275].

⊙ In descending order of obviousness, the chin dimple is visible in [ostendorf #1, 1900
6, and 8].

⊙ Robert (¶4951) and Tad (¶5369) also had a chin dimple. 1901

⟨$\frac{1}{q}$⟩ The only non-traumatic skull finding at autopsy was "orbital plates very thin" [lat- 1902
timerAu].

Head – Casts

Casts of Lincoln's head were made twice. The first, on March 31, 1860 [lincloreBDA], was 1903
by Leonard W. Volk, who also cast his hands [volk]; see Hands -- Cast . The second, in
February 1865, was by Clark Mills [borittA] [hayA] [kunhardtB p80] [shapiro]. They are readily
distinguished: Lincoln is bearded in 1865, but not in 1860.

Lincoln's asymmetric skull, coupled with his hat size and the remarks of many eyewit- 1904
nesses that his head seemed too small for his body, means that mild craniosynostosis
cannot be ruled out.

Head – Casts (continued)

- Some technical details about the 1860 Volk cast: 1905
  - ⟨1⟩ Volk wrote that Lincoln wanted to go the barber before having the cast. "I 1906 requested him not to let the barber cut it too short, and said I would rather he leave it as it was; but to this he would not consent." [volk]
  - ⟨2⟩ Quills in Lincoln's nostrils permitted breathing. Holes were left for the eyes. 1907 Lincoln sat upright in a chair for about an hour. [kunhardtA p119]
  - ⟨1⟩ "It was about an hour before the the mold was ready to be removed, and 1908 being all in one piece, with both ears perfectly taken, it clung pretty hard, as the cheek-bones were higher than the jaws at the lobe of the ear. He bent his head low and took hold of the mold, and gradually worked it off without breaking or injury; it hurt a little, as a few hairs of the tender temples pulled out with the plaster and made his eyes water." [volk]
  - ⟨2⟩ Apparently Volk cast only a life mask, as [lincloreBDA] states that Volk made an 1909 "idealized head" from the mask and gave it a "luxurious growth of hair." *I am not sure of this interpretation. Profile views of the cast* [randallP] *show that it was not so extensive that it couldn't have been removed in one piece from Lincoln's head.*
  - ⟨2⟩ Volk also took measurements of Lincoln's head and neck [lincloreBDA] *The* 1910 *reference is not clear whether the measurements were from life, or from the life-mask, or both, or neither.*
  - ⟨1⟩ Within nine months of sitting for the cast, Lincoln's weight dropped 40 1911 pounds. See ¶438. [volk]
  - ⟨2⟩ [micozzi] says the first head casting was in November 1860. *This, like ¶1520,* 1912 *is an error.*
  - ⟨2⟩ "The fact that there are no eyes in the sockets and no hair on the front part 1913 of the scalp has led people to call this cast a death mask." [lincloreBDA]

- Some technical details about the 1865 Mills cast: 1914
  - ⟨2⟩ "The circumstances surrounding the making of the second face mold are 1915 unknown." [stewart] *Stewart then quotes an eyewitness account of Mills making a cast in 1845. Unless a primary source was discovered after* [stewart] *was published in 1953, I suspect that the accounts below are merely echoes of Stewart's 1845 account.*
  - ⟨2⟩ "The sculptor Clark Mills made the plaster mask in about fifteen minutes, 1916 one-fourth of the time Volk had required in 1860. Mills first put a tight cap over Lincoln's hair, then spread wet plaster over his entire face and greased whiskers. He left only the nostrils open." [ostendorfA p232]
  - ⟨2⟩ Straws were inserted into Lincoln's nose to allow breathing. [kunhardtB p80] 1917
  - ⟨2⟩ "In working off the plaster it broke into bits, but Mills artfully fitted the pieces 1918 into a whole." [kunhardtB p80] [kunhardtB p80]
  - ⟨S⟩ [stewart] is not certain that a cast was actually taken of the part of Lincoln's 1919 head covered by hair. "If a head cast actually was taken, Lincoln's coarse and unruly hair night have imparted a lumpy effect to the cast and Mills might have been forced to modify the surface. Also, whether he reduced the diameters of the head beyond the surface of the compacted hair there is no sure way of telling."

- Cast instances: 1920
  - ⟨1/q⟩ 1860 cast: A copy in the Armed Forces Institute of Pathology was made from 1921 a copy owned by Thomas Starr (once President of the Lincoln Club of Detroit) which, in turn, was made from Volk's original mold [purtle]. Hand casts,

Head – Casts (continued)

too.

⟨2⟩ 1860 cast: "The casts of Lincoln's face and hands made by Volk are in the 1922
National Museum in Washington" [purtle]. *I suspect these are the casts in
the National Portrait Gallery.*

⟨1⟩ 1860 and 1865 casts: Masks in the National Portrait Gallery in Washington, 1923
on public display (Jan. 2007), alongside hand casts.

⟨1⟩ 1860 cast: The Zeta Psi fraternity at the University of Illinois possessed a 1924
mask in 1940, at least [randallP box 17]. However, photographs in [randallP box
17] seem to show two different masks: one with seams and one without.

⟨2⟩ 1865 mask: "After the death of Cark Mills in 1883 his sons parted with two 1925
or three copies of the Lincoln mask, one (two?) going to Colonel Hay (1886),
and another to the U.S. National Musem (1889). The sequence of the gifts
does not necessarily indicate the sequence of manufacture." [stewart]

⟨2⟩ 1865 bronze mask: "This replica of Lincoln remained in the hands of Mr. 1926
Mills' sons until 1886 when it came into the possession of Mr. John Hay...
Apparently it was cast in both plaster and bronze. The only bronze in exis-
tence ... belongs to Clarence Hay..." [shapiro]

⟨1⟩ 1865 bronze mask: As of May 2007 a bronze-looking mask is in the Smithso- 1927
nian "Castle" building, perhaps not on public display [personal observation].

⟨2⟩ 1865 plaster mask: "About three years after John Hay acquired the masks, an- 1928
other plaster copy drawn from the same molds was presented to the Smithsonian Institution." [shapiro]

- John Hay describes his impressions of the two head casts: 1929
  ⟨1⟩ "The first is of a man of fifty-one, and young for his years. The face has a 1930
  clean, firm outline; it is free from fat, but the muscles are hard and full; the
  large mobile mouth is ready to speak, to shout, or laugh; the bold, curved
  nose is broad and substantial, with spreading nostrils; it is a face full of life,
  of energy, of vivid aspiration." [hayA]
  ⟨1⟩ "The other is so sad and peaceful in its infinite repose that the famous sculp- 1931
  tor Augustus Saint-Gaudens insisted, when he first saw it, that it was a death-
  mask. The lines are set, as if the living face, like the copy, had been in bronze;
  the nose is thin, and lengthened by the emaciation of the cheeks; the mouth
  is fixed like that of an archaic statue; a look as of one on whom sorrow and
  care had done their worst without victory is on all the features; the whole expression is of unspeakable sadness and all-sufficing strength. Yet, the peace
  is not the dreadful peace of death; it is the peace that passeth understanding." [hayA]

⟨1⟩ Measurements by anthropologist [stewart]. All results in millimeters, except for 1932
cephalic index:

Measurement	1860 Mask	1865 Mask
Total face height (menton-crinion)	194	?
Lower face height (menton-nasion)	122	?
Face breadth (bizygomatic)	148	?
Nose height	54	56
Nose breadth	38	38
Mouth breadth	55	59
External ocular width	102?	102
Ear length (right)	77?	78?
Ear length (left)	78	?

Head – Casts (continued)

Ear breadth (right)	43	46?
Ear breadth (left)	30	37?
Head measurements		
Maximum length from glabella		210
Maximum breadth (above ears)		170
Head height (position of poria and bregma estimated)		165
Circumference (as for hat)		573
Arc between ear openings over bregma		370
Cephalic index		81.0

⟨2⟩ [stewart] defines each of the measurements in a book: "Stewart TD. *Hrdlička's Practical Anthropometry*. 4th ed. Philadelphia." 1933

⟨1⟩ [stewart] has an important list of of caveats related to these measurements, e.g. measurements on a living face are guided by the feel of the underlying bone, which is, of course, unavailable in a cast. See ¶1919 for issues related to the scalp region of the Mills cast. 1934

⟨1⟩ The measurements in the table translate to a hat size of $7\,1/4$ to $7\,3/8$, and a front to back distance of $8\,1/4$ inches. Herndon quoted hat size as $7\,1/8$, ear-to-ear distance as $6\,1/2$ inches, and front to back of brain as 8 inches [herndonC] (∈ ¶3). 1935

⟨2⟩ Wikipedia says that a cephalic index of 81 is solidly in the "brachycephalic" range for a man, meaning the head is short in relation to its width. 1936

⟨2⟩ John Nicolay and John Hay measured the 1865 cast [stewart]. The ear to ear distance was $6\,3/4$ inches, the distance "from the front to the back of the brain" was $7\,3/4$ inches, and the estimated hat size was $7\,1/4$ or $7\,3/8$. 1937

⟨1⟩ 1860 cast: "The short hair in Volk's mask of Lincoln with the ears standing out less at right angles from the head than they did, are the only serious defects noticed by those who say him daily during his residence in Springfield." [rankinA p373] 1938

🔲 1860 cast: Right side shows a prominent vertical crease in the cheek [kunhardtA p118] 1939

⟨2/c⟩ 1860 cast: Although it shows masses in both the right and left nasolabial folds, [stewart] says the left mass is an artifact. 1940

⟨1/q⟩ 1860 cast: "I have seen many reproductions of the Volk mask and hands but in none, before [these], have I seen such details. ... The wrinkles and even the texture of the quality of Lincoln's face were particularly noticeable." – sculptor Avarel Fairbanks, circa 1942 [purtle] 1941

■ Putative skull fracture from horse-kick (see ¶3568 and §1a): 1942

  ⟨2/c⟩ "The sharp depression in the forehead above the left eye with a definitely palpable edge ... shows where his skull had been fractured..." [kempfB pp9-10] 1943

  ⟨2/c⟩ "I am unable to detect anything in the copies of the Volk and Mills masks in the National Museum that I would interpret as evidence of fracture" [stewart]. 1944

  ⟨2/c⟩ [fishman] does not find [kempfB]'s forehead depression. "However, a furrow in the left side of the glabella is visible on the 1865 mask. This ... is most likely related to the way the plaster mold was removed." [fishman] *dismisses Lincoln's ear asymmetry similarly, but this is probably incorrect. See The Physical Lincoln.* 1945

  🔲 There is a depression in the right brow line in the 1860 mask. 1946

■ 1865 life mask: 1947
  🔲 1865 life mask shown in [dimsdale] shows an asymmetric skull. 1948

142

Head – Casts (continued)

⟨-⟩ See ¶1632 for impressions of [vidalA p702]; and ¶1931 for Augustus Saint-   1949
Gaudens and for Hay.

⟨2⟩ "Because of the sunken eyes and cadaverous cheeks [it] is often mistaken for   1951
a death mask." [ostendorfA p232]

Hearing

There is no mention in historical sources of Lincoln asking persons to repeat them-   1952
selves or of missing words.

⟨1⟩ July 3, 1861: After being denied entry to Lincoln's office, Orville Browning leaves,   1953
but a few minutes later "the secretary came down an said the President had heard
my voice and wanted to see me." – [browning p475] *The geography is not explicit,
but it appears Lincoln could hear well enough through doors or around corners.*

Heart & Circulation

Peripheral vasoconstriction was noted in two instances: (a) Joshua Speed's description   1954
of Lincoln's cold, clammy hand and the closeness with which Lincoln put his feet to the
fire (¶1210), and (b) the coolness of Lincoln's extremities as he lay dying (¶557). Differential diagnosis: (1) catecholamine excess, as in pheochromocytoma, (2) heart failure (perhaps caused by dilated cardiomyopathy resulting from pheochromocytoma),
(3) ? expected part of head wound. Note: (i) Aortic regurgitation would be expected to
produce the opposite – vasodilation – at least until final decompendation. (ii) A man
with MEN2B who lived into his 50s undiagnosed had a large fleshy plethoric face [aa159].

Re: aortic dissection: Lincoln had a Cushing reflex whenever oozing from his head   1955
wound was obstructed. Yet, even with the very high blood pressures that accompany
the Cushing reflex, his aorta did not tear and lead to death by exsanguination. (It must
be admitted that most dissections do not cause quick death.)

- Vascular coloration and reactivity: 1956
  - ⟨2⟩ In his 20s, "the deep pink in his cheeks abruptly blanched and the new young   1957
    man began to be called Old Abe" [kunhardtB p291].
  - ⟨1⟩ 1831: "florid complexion" – Herndon [moore p534]   1958
  - ⟨1/q⟩ Lincoln's nose: "having the tip glowing in red" – William Herndon [donaldA   1959
    p115]
  - ⟨1/q⟩ Lincoln could become angry such that "his face turned lurid with majestic   1960
    and terrifying wrath" – Henry Whitney [burl p148] *This may or may not refer
    to facial redness.*
  - ⟨1/q⟩ During the Black Hawk War, some of the men in Lincoln's company de-   1961
    nounced him as a coward. Lincoln became "swarthy with resolution and
    rage" [thomas p55]
  - ⟨1⟩ 1857: Blushed with embarrassment when he unintentionally interrupted   1962
    a public reading with "a sudden and explosive guffaw.'" [herndon p479] See
    ¶2498.
  - ⟨1⟩ "He was pale and his spirits seemed deeply moved" as he began to deliver a   1963
    courtroom argument. – Joshua Speed [wilson p589]
  - ⟨1⟩ Spring 1860: At the Decatur Republican Convention: "Mr Lincoln rose bow-   1964
    ing and blushing" [wilson p463]
  - ⟨1⟩ 1860: Turned pale and trembled on the day he was nominated for President   1965
    – see ¶2506

Heart & Circulation (continued)

⟨1⟩ 1860s: When asked about his 1842 duel (¶216), "Mr Lincoln, with flushed face, replied..." – Mary [turner p299]   1966

⟨1/q⟩ Feb. 11, 1861, leaving Springfield: His "face was pale" and he was almost unable to speak – Henry Villard [shenk p171]   1967

⟨2⟩ As President: pale when apologizing for short-temperedness the day before [NYTimes - Aug. 22, 1869]   1968

⟨1/q⟩ July 1861: When an Army doctor criticized Lincoln's attire, "A little red spot of hectic red burned for a moment on his cheeks." [burl p206] [hirschhornC]   1969

⟨1⟩ Oct. 21, 1861: Lincoln's face is "pale and wan" after learning a close friend has been killed in combat. [riceB pp176-177] (∈ ¶2512)   1970

⟨1⟩ After Battle of Chancellorsville, spring 1863: "his face, usually sallow, was ashen in hue" – Noah Brooks [brooksC pp57-58] (∈ ¶2644)   1971

⟨1⟩ Sept. 7, 1863, perturbed: "I had noticed the veins in his face filling full within a few moments, and one vein across his forehead was as large as my little finger, and it gave him a frightful look. ... He was very pale." [harveyC] (∈ §6.7)   1972

⟨1⟩ Sept. 9, 1863, after a compliment: "He colored a little and laughed most heartily." [harveyC] (∈ §6.11)   1973

⟨2⟩ [shutes p102] speaks of Lincoln's "habitual low blood pressure." *No data supports this. Measurement of blood pressure in the 1860s was neither routinely done nor routinely possible. Perhaps* [shutes] *interpreted Lincoln's faintings as low blood pressure.*   1974

- Cardiac pulsation – photograph 1:   1975
  - ▣ A November 1863 photograph [ostendorf #78] shows Lincoln sitting with legs crossed and with the toe of one boot out of focus. After seeing the picture and the out-of-focus toe, Lincoln established that when he sat with legs crossed his foot moved in concert with his heart beat.   1976
  - ⟨1⟩ Looking at the photograph, Lincoln said: " 'I can understand why that foot should be so enormous [in the picture]. It's a big foot anyway, and it is near the focus of the instrument. But why is the outline of it so indistinct and blurred? I am confident I did not move it.' [Noah] Brooks suggested that the throbbing of the arteries may have caused an imperceptible motion. The President crossed his legs and watched his foot. 'That's it! That's it!' he exclaimed. 'Now that's very curious, isn't it?' " [ostendorfA p147]   1977
  - ⟨S⟩ Schwartz [schwartzB] has taken this as a sign of aortic regurgitation.   1978
  - ⟨S⟩ Lattimer [lattimerNY] thinks the toe was out of focus because it was significantly closer to the camera than the rest of Lincoln's body; he dismisses the fact that Lincoln confirmed his foot moved.   1979
  - ⟨-⟩ *Movement of the foot, when seated with legs crossed, may be observed in persons with a normal cardiovascular system (e.g., the author). It should also be recalled that photographic exposure times were on the order of several seconds during Lincoln's time.*   1980
  - ⟨-⟩ *The photograph was taken about 10 days before Lincoln became symptomatic with smallpox. The circulation can become hyperdynamic early in infection and lead to bounding pulses, but ten days is probably too early before symptoms to have resulted in circulatory changes.*   1981

- Cardiac pulsation – photograph 2:   1982
  - ▣ A photograph of Lincoln standing, without support, shows his face blurred – compatible with side-to-side movement (¶3144, Fig. 5).   1983

Heart & Circulation (continued)

⟨-⟩ *The de Musset sign of severe aortic regurgitation causes pulsatile head*   1984
movement, but this is described as nodding [aa3 p249]. *However, the photograph possibly shows Lincoln's hands to be blurry, which would suggest Lincoln's entire body was moving. Although I have not seen total-body movement described in aortic regurgitation, the existence of the ballistocardiogram proves that even persons with normal aortic valves have some body movement derived from cardiac contraction. Such body movement would not be expected to be from side-to-side, however, unless the heart were rotated horizontally. Horizontal rotation would be unlikely in a tall, thin-chested man like Lincoln. Moreover, head swaying is described as a sign of a different valvular malfunction: severe tricuspid regurgitation* [aa3 p388]. *Thus, I do not believe this photograph can be interpreted as supporting an aortic valve leak.*

⟨-⟩ *Non-cardiovascular causes of Lincoln's movement are discussed in* ¶*3057.*   1985

- Cardiac pulsation – photograph 3:   1986

    ⊙ ○○○ *Project:* Is it true that in photographs of Lincoln's second inaugural,   1987
his image is less sharp than the people around him, as if he were moving?

- Cardiac pulsations – discussion: 1988

    ⟨-⟩ *If Lincoln had had aortic regurgitation so severe as to cause heart failure*   1989
and cardiac cachexia (the hypothesis of [schwartzB]*), then at some point in his illness he would have had bounding pulses in his carotid arteries. This would have had two sartorial effects* [aa49]: *(a) wearing tight collars would have been uncomfortable, and (b) his bowties would have bobbed. Neither has been recorded in Lincoln.* ○○○ *Project: Review Lincoln photographs to see if his neckwear changed over time.*

    ⟨-⟩ *Cold extremities (*¶*1210) are at odds with aortic regurgitation, where vasodilation is the usual mode of circulatory compensation – until the final stages.*   1990

    ⟨H⟩ Some have named the leg-bobbing phenomenon "the Lincoln sign" [kroen] or   1992
"Lincoln-Brooks sign" [schwartzB] of aortic regurgitation. *This practice should be vigorously resisted. The Physical Lincoln confidently concludes that Lincoln did not have aortic regurgitation.*

⟨1⟩ July 27, 1848: "I never fainted from the loss of blood." – Lincoln [baslerA v1p511] *A*   1993
facetious reference to battles with mosquitoes during his militia service.

⟨2⟩ March 30, 1861: Recently "had keeled over with sick headache for the first time   1994
in years." [shenk p285]. (∈ ¶2627) *Phrasing suggests previous episodes. Called a migraine headache by* [donaldA p289], *but see* ¶*2628 for caveats.*

⟨1⟩ Sept. 1863: "His face was peculiar; bone, nerve, vein, and muscle were all so   1995
plainly seen" [harveyC] (∈ §6.2) *Suggests thin, translucent skin.*

⊙ Jan. 8, 1864: [ostendorf #85] shows a prominent left temporal vein.   1996

⟨2⟩ Feb. 6, 1865: Faints after standing up quickly and angrily. He is then put to bed.   1997
[shutes pp108-109]. See ¶1203.

⟨1/q⟩ Late February 1865: "I am very unwell now; my feet and hands of late seem to be   1998
always cold, and I ought perhaps to be in bed." – Lincoln (See ¶1210.)

⟨1/q⟩ March 4, 1865: The sun broke through the overcast just as Lincoln took the oath   1999
of office. The next day Lincoln remarked: "Did you notice that sunburst? It made my heart jump." [browneF p680] *If accepted as literally true, then it says something about the chronotropic responsiveness of Lincoln's heart.*

Height

See ⌊ Build -- Adult ⌋ and ⌊ Build -- Childhood ⌋.

2000

Infection

- March 1830, after Lincoln's extended family had just settled in Macon Country, Illinois: 2001

  ⟨$\frac{1}{q}$⟩ "In the autumn all hands were greatly afflicted with ague and fever, to which they had not been used, and by which they were greatly discouraged, so much so that they determined on leaving the country." – Lincoln [angle p37] *Interestingly, this implies that Lincoln knew about acquired resistance to infection.*   2002

  ⟨$\frac{1}{q}$⟩ "we had fever an' ager turrible" – Dennis Hanks [wilsonR p30]   2003

  ⟨2⟩ "All that fall, members of the group had suffered from chills and fever. To combat the ague and its malaise, they had purchased quantities of 'barks' at James Renshaw's store in Decatur. 'Barks' was a mixture of whiskey and Peruvian bark. Abe, himself, had no need for ague remedies. This was a year of marvelous vigor and expenditure of energy for him." [shutes p8]   2004

  ⟨-⟩ *Peruvian bark was, in 1830, a 200-year-old remedy for malaria. It was made from "Cinchona" trees that grew in Peru and contained, as active ingredient, quinine. Quinine is, in fact, an effective anti-malarial drug, and the discovery of the "fever bark tree" is one of the most important events in the history of western medicine (the Peruvians having discovered it long before). In 1830s Illinois, however, "quinine was then a new, expensive extract of cinchona; most people on the frontier had to stay with the common cinchona bark" [shutesE p46].*   2005

  ⟨-⟩ *Because infectious diseases were so dangerous in the pre-antibiotic era, and because Peruvian bark was the only effective anti-infective medicine known in Lincoln's time, it was common for people to take it whenever they developed a fever, regardless of the fever's apparent cause. Thus, without more clinical information, it is not possible to say the Lincoln family had malaria at this time. Certainly, however, malaria was a common problem in that place and era.*   2006

  ⟨-⟩ *It is not clear from Shutes' wording whether Lincoln took the bark or not.*   2007

- Summer 1835:   2008

  ⟨-⟩ §1b reprints extensive primary material.   2009

  ⟨1⟩ Lincoln had "chills and fever on alternate days" for over a month. He took "heroic doses of Peruvian bark, boneset tea, jalap and calomel." ("Peruvian bark" is explained in ¶2005). His course was complicated by grief over the death of his friend/fiancee Ann Rutledge (see ¶2695). Lincoln had been ill before she died. Under the direction of Dr. John Allen (see ¶3173), he was nursed at the home of Bowling Green, being "discharged" only after he had been three weeks without a fever. [rankinA pp72-87]   2010

  ⟨-⟩ *A regular, every-other day pattern of fever suggests malaria, specifically the vivax or ovale type of disease. Most likely, Lincoln had the vivax type, as the ovale type is native to West Africa, not the United States [aa24 p1478]. (Conceivably, however, West African slaves could have brought the ovale parasite to Illinois in their blood.) Lincoln's 1835 illness may have been a primary infection or reactivation of an earlier infection (e.g., the possible 1830 infection: ¶2001).*   2012

  ⟨1⟩ William Herndon disputes the presence of malaria: "These people were not touched by 'the malaria' nor dwarfed by the 'miasma.' " [hertz p157] *His dis-*   2013

Infection (continued)

agreement arises, in part, because this contradicts his own theories of Lincoln's gloominess [hertz pp 157, 163-164].

⟨2⟩ Ann Rutledge died on Aug. 25 [rankinA p73]. Lincoln was, at least partially, back at work as the town's postmaster by Sept. 22 [shutesE p47]. By Sept. 24 he was performing surveyor work [donaldA p57]. — 2014

⟨s⟩ For Lincoln's psychological reaction, see ¶2695. — 2015

- Lincoln and syphilis – part 1: — 2016
    ⟨-⟩ See Special Topic §2 for complete details about Lincoln and syphilis. — 2017
    ⟨1⟩ "When I was in Greencastle in 1887 I said to you that Lincoln had, *when a* — 2018 *mere boy,* the syphilis, and now let me explain the matter in full, which I have never done before. About the year 1835-36 Mr. Lincoln went to Beardstown and during a devilish passion had connection with a girl and caught the disease. Lincoln told me this..." – Herndon [hertz p259]
    ⟨2⟩ "Herndon wrote that Lincoln had related this to him in an unguarded mo- — 2019 ment, and that afterwards he (Herndon) had written it down. In his letter to Weik Herndon wrote that when Lincoln moved to Springfield and began rooming with Joshua Speed, the disease presumably persisted. Lincoln, not trusting he local physicians, wrote about his problem to Dr. Daniel L. Drake." [bumgarnerB] citing [hertz p259]. Also see [hertz p233] and ¶2467.
    ⟨s⟩ "The story makes one wonder whether Herndon ever told the truth about — 2020 what Lincoln said to him. There is absolutely no reason to believe that Lincoln, a man of rugged health, father of a normal family, ever contracted what was in his time an incurable and devastating malady." [currentBk p36] *This argument, which reflects an incomplete understanding of syphilis, reduces the probability that Lincoln had syphilis, but does not rule it out.*
    ⟨1⟩ "Lincoln wrote a letter (a long one which he read to me) to Dr Drake of — 2021 Cincinnati descriptive of his case. Its date would be in Decer 40 or early in January 41 – I think he must have informed Dr Drake of his early love for Miss Rutledge – as there was a part of the letter which he would not read. ... I remember Dr Drakes reply – which was that he would not undertake to priscribe for him without a personal interview." – Joshua Speed [wilson p431]
    ⟨2⟩c [bumgarnerB] reviews Douglas Wilson's argument that Herndon was genuine in — 2022 his belief Lincoln had syphilis. Wilson also notes that Lincoln may have been mistaken in his diagnosis, as dread of syphilis was common in that era. *I am not convinced by this argument. See §2e.*

- Lincoln and syphilis – part 2: — 2023
    ⟨1⟩q Herndon thought Lincoln's children may have been affected: "Poor boys, — 2024 they are dead now and gone! I should like to know one thing and that is: What caused the death of these children? I have an opinion which I shall never state to anyone." [hirschhorn] citing [hertz p128] See §2f.
    ⟨2⟩c "...none of the Lincoln sons showed signs of congenital syphilis (although — 2025 one-third of children born in the primary or secondary stages of a mother's infection and more than 90 percent born later remain free of syphilis)." [hirschhorn]
    ⟨2⟩c Congenital syphilis is transmitted from mother to child. Based on the infec- — 2026 tivity of syphilis over time and a review of Lincoln's chronology, [hirschhorn] concludes "It would be well beyond the expected range for him to infect Mary Lincoln after their November 1842 marriage, unless a primary infection occurred later than 1836." *Robert was born exactly nine months after the Lincolns wed.*

Infection (continued)

⟨2⟩ 1848: Congressman Lincoln opposes the Mexican-American war and asks if the   2027
spot where the war-starting attack occurred was American or Mexican soil. This
leads to satirical articles from political opponents saying Lincoln had "spotted
fever." [angle pp138-139]

⟨1⟩ July 4, 1860: Willie "has just had a hard and tedious spell of scarlet-fever and he   2028
is not yet beyond all danger. I have a head-ache and a sore throat upon me now,
inducing me to suspect that I have an inferior type of the same thing." – Lincoln
writing to Dr. Anson Henry (see ¶3180) [baslerA v4p82]

⟨1⟩ Commenting about the unhealthiness of Washington, [stoddardA p124] says "The   2029
President has had only the smallpox, but he was well seasoned before he came"
to Washington.

⟨2⟩ November 1863: Having delivering the Gettysburg address, Lincoln returned to   2030
Washington with a headache and, probably, a fever. This proved to be smallpox,
and he was semi-quarantined for 3 weeks. Special Topic §5 reviews this illness in
excruciating detail.

   ⟨2⟩ Tad had been recently ill with "scarlatina" (¶5395). Some speculate that this   2031
was actually smallpox, which was then transmitted to Lincoln [lincloreLHH].
Conventional wisdom finds no evidence Lincoln was previously vaccinated,
but I am not so sure. See §5e.

   ⟨2⟩ "The Stoddard account of Lincoln's attack of smallpox goes into much detail,   2034
both from the clinical standpoint and as to the measures of control which
were undertaken" [evans pp140-141]. *Clinical detail is thin.* [stoddardA pp107-109]
is reprinted in §5d.

   ⟨2⟩ [goldman] questions the conventional wisdom that Lincoln's illness was mild.   2035
*I agree. §5e concludes that Lincoln's course was typical for "ordinary
smallpox."*

   ⟨1⟩ Sequelae: Into December, Mary's half-sister Emilie thought Lincoln looked   2036
"very ill" and "thinner that I ever saw him" [randallC pp297-298]

   ⟨1⟩ Sequelae: Lincoln's face was "slightly marked" by the pox. See Special   2037
Topic §5, entry for Dec. 6, and ¶1892.

   ⟨1⟩ Ida Tarbell did not know Lincoln had smallpox. [shutesP: Letter of June 28, 1928 from   2038
her]. Shutes notes: "A dear old lady – must have forgotten much."

Infection – Exposures

Careful medical histories in the 21st century record situations where exposure to dis-   2039
ease could occur. Given the health practices of his day, recording potential disease
exposures for Lincoln would nearly require recording his entire life! Nevertheless, certain elements of Lincoln's are recorded below, to provide specifics and to provide a
more general picture of 19th century life.

Lincoln must certainly have been exposed to some of the foci listed in the analogous   2040
section for Mary (¶4283ff).

⟨2⟩ 1814: "Many persons in and around Elizabethtown [Kentucky] had died of a dis-   2041
ease which the people called the 'cold plague,'" including the husband of Sally
Bush Johnston [lamonL p29]

  ■ 1832: War exposures: 2042
   ⟨2⟩ Lincoln escaped the cholera epidemic associated with the Black Hawk War   2043
[shutes p92]

Infection – Exposures (continued)

⟨1⟩ One of Lincoln's fellow militiamen recalled "there was but one rain during the whole time that I was out from home in the army; at that time there was also quite a storm of wind .. we got a thorough drenching" – George Harrison [wilson p556] But see ¶2149.   2044

⟨2⟩ 1837: Springfield had less than 1500 people and lacked sewers and paved streets. Hogs "wallowed freely about town, rooting out garbage. ... The notorious quagmire of mud after a rain or a melt could keep Springfielders inside their houses for days at a time." [kunhardtA p52]   2045

⟨1/q⟩ August 31, 1851: "We have had no cholera here for about two weeks." – Lincoln [carman]   2046

⟨1/q⟩ January 14, 1854: "On account of illness in his family, Mr. Lincoln was not present" at a speaking engagement In Springfield. – *Illinois Journal* as cited by [shutes p61]   2047

    ⟨S⟩ About this time Lincoln took Robert to Terre Haute, IN for madstone treatment after a dog-bite – see ¶4953   2048

⟨1⟩ Oct. 2, 1854: The Lincoln household purchases "cholera mix" from a local drugstore [hickey]. (On Aug. 12, 1854 the Essex County *Republican*, a weekly newspaper in upstate New York, prints a warning that "cholera mix" should not be used when cholera occurs.)   2049

- Lincoln-Herndon law office: 2050
  - ⟨1/q⟩ John Littlefield started cleaning up the office soon after he arrived there to study law. "Mr. Lincoln had been in Congress and had the usual amount of seeds to distribute to the farmers. ... In my efforts to clean up, I found that some of the seeds had sprouted in the dirt that had collected in the office." [angle p184]   2051

- Plants: 2052
  - ⟨1⟩ Lists of plants growing near Lincoln's Indiana home are listed in: [wilson pp104, 228, 248, 252, 260-261, 261, 335]   2053
  - ⟨1⟩ "Lincoln never planted any trees –: he did plant Some rose bushes once in front of his house ... He once – for a year or So had a garden & worked in it" – James Gourley [wilson p452]   2054
  - ⟨1⟩ "Mr nor Mrs Lincoln loved the beautiful – I have planted flowers in their front yard myself to hide nakedness – ugliness &c. &c. have done it often – and often – Mrs. L never planted trees – Roses – never made a garden, at least not more than once or twice" – Frances Todd Wallace [wilson p486]   2055

⟨2⟩ On the circuit, "Tavern food was plentiful, but often poorly cooked with poor sanitary conditions." [gary p7] *See Herndon's comment about the "cussed bad" food (¶603).*   2056

- In the White House: 2057
  - ⟨2⟩ "As ordered by Buchanan, the luxury of running water had been installed during the spring with porcelain sinks in most rooms providing cold, polluted Potomac River water. The house was near the smelly Washington Canal, sewerage outlets, and waste dumps that produced unsanitary and unpleasant smells and conditions" [gary pp332-333].   2058
  - ⟨2⟩ Lincoln's White House office overlooked the "City Canal" flowing on its stagnant way into the Potomac River. [kunhardtB p112] (See ¶640)   2059
  - ⟨1/q⟩ The smell of the City Canal and nearby swamps that reached the White House was like "twenty thousand drowned cats" – John Hay [beschloss p97]   2060

Infection – Exposures (continued)

⟨-⟩ See ¶3685ff for more about the Canal and Washington.   2061

⟨1⟩ 1865: The east side of the White House "beyond the extension... was a row of   2062
outhouses... Back and east were the kitchen-garden and the stable" [crookA]
[crookK] *Fecal contamination of food?*

⟨1⟩ Nov. 1862: It was so cold at the Soldiers Home (the out of town retreat from the   2063
White House) that two guests of the Lincolns wanted to move to the White House
[donaldH p83]

⟨2⟩ "Mrs. Lincoln was always so solicitous about his going out without a muffler or   2064
something about his throat" [shutes p74].

   ⟨S⟩ [shutes p74] suggests this indicates "Lincoln must have been subject to more or   2065
less trouble" with throat infections.

Infection – Exposures (to animals)

Animals are a potential source of infectious disease. Of course, animal exposure was   2066
far more common in the 19th century than now, so it is probably not possible (and
probably not that helpful) to extensively catalog Lincoln's animal encounters. There is
an entire book about Lincoln and animals, which the author has not consulted: *Lincoln's Animal Friends: Incidents About Abraham Lincoln and Animals, Woven into
an Intimate Story of His Life*, by Ruth Painter Randall and illustrated by Louis Darling
(Boston: Little, Brown, 1958; 152pp).

- Wild animals: 2067

  ⟨1/q⟩ 1818±: Gave his sister a baby raccoon and a turtle, trying to cheer her up   2068
  after their mother died. [wilsonR p24]

  ⟨2⟩ The Lincoln homestead in Indiana was cleared in an unbroken forest.   2069
  Thomas has to cut out a trail his family could follow. Lincoln mentioned
  the presence of bears, panthers, wild turkeys. The family ate deer and bear
  meat. [donaldA p25]

  ⟨1⟩ "When we landed in Indiana in 1817 I think there were lots of bears – deer –   2070
  turkeys – ate them as meat ... Could track bears – wolves – horses – cattle" –
  Dennis Hanks [wilson p104]

  ⟨1⟩ Of Indiana: "When first my father settled here, / 'Twas then the frontier   2071
  line: / The panther's scream, filled night with fear / And bears preyed on
  the swine." – Lincoln [baslerA v1p387]

  ⟨2⟩ In Indiana: "The dense forest around him abounded in every form of feath-   2072
  ered game" and deer [angle p18] (reprinting Nicolay & Hay)

  ⟨1/q⟩ Learned to write with a pen made from a buzzard's quill. [donaldA p29]   2073

  ⟨2⟩ Ate quail [shastid]. (See ¶611.)   2074

  ⟨1⟩ land terrapins [wilson p109], snakes [wilson p335]   2075

  ⟨1⟩ Indiana: "Bar Deer Turkyes and Coon wilecats and other things and frogs"   2076
  [wilson p252]

  ⟨1⟩ Bears [wilson p228]   2077

  ⟨1⟩ Lincoln placed back into their nest two little birds that had been blown from   2078
  it by a storm [wilson p590]

  ⟨1⟩ Birds common in the Indiana region where Lincoln lived: "Humming Bird,   2079
  Blue Bird, Robins, Blue Jay: Wood-Pecker: Quail (a species of the Pheasant
  – usually hunted & bagged as *game*) Pheasants: Meadow Larks: Red Bird:;
  Thrush: Owl: Night Hawk: Chicken Hawk: Whip-poor-will: Ground Rob-
  bins: English Snipe: Crane (water-fowl), Turkey Buzzard: Crows: Black Birds:

Infection – Exposures (to animals) (continued)

Wild & Tame Pigeons: Wood-cocks: Turtle Doves: Wren; Rain Crow; Swallows: Martins; Cat Birds, King Fishers (Water fowls)." – J.W. Wartmann [wilson p392]

⟨1⟩ Fish common in the Indiana region where Lincoln lived: "Cat Fish –. 2 Kinds, Blue & Mud: Buffalo: Yellow White and Grey fin Perch: Carp: Bass (not many); Toothed Herring; Skip-Jacks; Black-fin Suckers. Pike (more in the *White* than Ohio River): Gar-fish; Shovel fish; Sturgeons, Minnows (very small –, usually used as bait for larger fish); Sun fish: Eels: *Soft-Shell Turtles*" – J.W. Wartmann [wilson p392] **2080**

⟨1⟩ Game common in the Indiana region where Lincoln lived: Deer: Squirrels: Rabbits: Coons: Wild Turkies: Wild Ducks: Oppossum: (Musk-rats, Otter, Panthers, Wild Cats Catamounts Red & grey foxes and a few Bear were in this Co, in Lincoln's day, and were hunted as *game*, but, with the exception of the Bear, were never eaten). Coon hunts at nights was, & still is, a favorite sport for boys & young men. The game usually hunted for eating purposes was, in L's day, & still is, Deer, Squirrels, Rabbits. Wild Turkies. Wild Ducks & Pheasants & Quails & *'Possums* I, myself, have known persons to have little other meat to Eat during the fall & winter than, Deer, Squirrels, Wild Turkies & 'possum & rabbits: The kinds of game I have named is common all through Southern Indiana." – J.W. Wartmann [wilson p392] **2081**

⟨2⟩ A man from New York sent President Lincoln a live "American Eagle the bird of our land" which had lost a foot in a trap. [donaldH p32] **2082**

- Hunting and fishing: **2083**
  ⟨1⟩ 1818: "A few days before the completion of his eigth year, in the absence of his father, a flock of wild turkeys approached the new log-cabin, and A. with a rifle gun, standing inside, shot through a crack, and killed one of them. He has never since pulled a trigger on any larger game." – Lincoln [baslerA v4p63] Also: [wilson p229] *A psychoanalyst's weird view of this episode is reprinted in* [shenk p239]. **2084**
  ⟨1⟩ In Indiana, shot deer, "although Abe was not so fond of a gun as I was" – David Turnham [wilson p217] **2085**
  ⟨1⟩ "On one occasion ran a Groun hog in a hole in the rocks – we worked some 4 or 5 hours in trying to git him out." Lincoln eventually got it. – John Duncan [wilson p557] **2086**
  ⟨1⟩ While a boy in Indiana: "worked all one day trying to dig som kind of a 'varmint' out of the ground" – Charles Friend [wilson p676]. Also: [wilson pp234-235] **2087**
  ⟨1⟩ Early 1830s: "hunting squirrels with a gun" – Henry McHenry [wilson p14] **2088**
  ⟨1⟩ "Lincoln did not do much hunting – sometimes we went Coon hunting & turkey hunting of nights" – Nathaniel Grigsby [wilson p113] **2089**
  ⟨1⟩ "He loved fishing & hunted Some – not a great deal" – David Turnham [wilson p121] **2090**
  ⟨1⟩ "had a fondness for fishing and hunting with his dog & Axe when his dog would run a Rabbit in a hollow tree he would chop it out" – E.R. Burba [wilson p241] **2091**
  ⟨1⟩ "he would slipe out of a Knight after the old man had Gon to Bed and take a hunt But thay took the fist along thay Caut a Coon and skind him and then streched it over the Litle Dog and soad him up and turned him Loos and put the other Dogs on the track" – J. Rowan Herndon [wilson p51] **2092**
  ⟨1⟩ "He never played cards, nor drank, nor hunted" – James Short [wilson p73] **2093**

Infection – Exposures (to animals) (continued)

⟨1⟩ Indiana years: "The farm is on Knob Creek – Abe used to go with me down the branch to shoot fish in puddles & holes washed by the water – killed a fawn – Abe was tickled to death" – Dennis Hanks [wilson p103]   2094

⟨1⟩ "We were Excellent bow shots – a squirrel couldnt Escape unless he got in his hole and then if Abe took the notion he would pull him or it out of his hole" – Dennis Hanks [wilson p105]   2095

⟨1⟩ "Abe loved Shakespear but not fishing – still Kelso would draw Abe: they used to sit on the back of the river and quote Shakespear" – Caleb Carman [wilson p374] (Kelso was John A. Kelso, "a School Master." [wilson p374])   2096

⟨1⟩ "L & my self always stopt at Hobbitts on the Kickapoo: here we Enjoyed ourselves much – read – went fishing &c." – John T. Stuart [wilson p519]   2097

⟨1⟩ As President: "Mr. Lincoln was anything but a crack shot. I later learned from Hill Lamon that he never had been." [stoddardD p249] (See ¶2527 and ¶3839.)   2098

■ Insects and vermin: 2099

⟨2⟩ Springfield: Lincoln home had no fly screens. [randallC p76]   2100

⟨1⟩q In 1848, Lincoln compared his experience in the 1832 Black Hawk War to the military record of Presidential candidate General Lewis Cass: "If he saw any live fighting Indians, it was more than I did, but I had a good many bloody struggles with the mosquitoes; and, although I never fainted from loss of blood, I can truly say I was often hungry." [herndon p231]   2101

⟨1⟩q 1858: Almost loses his cool trying to sleep in a bedbug-infested room. [browneF pp294-296] See §1c. On Sept. 6, 1859 the Lincoln household bought a bottle of "Dead Shot" to combat bedbugs [hickey] [shutes p57].   2102

⟨1⟩ Lincoln typically reclined on a horsehair sofa when visiting the telegraph office during the Civil War. "One day while we were all seriously attentive to our task, he arose abruptly and, knocking a bug from his collar, said: 'Boys, I have been very fond of that old lounge, but I will have to discard it now that it has become a little buggy.' " – David Homer Bates [NYTimesTeleg]   2103

⟨2⟩ 1861: White House was rat infested [donaldH p23]   2104

⟨2⟩ Insects were in the White House, "buzzing about the room and butting their heads against the window panes" – John Nicolay [beschlossB p97]   2105

■ Domestic animals: 2106

⟨2⟩ Was devoted to a pet pig in childhood. His father killed it. [burl p40]   2107

⟨H⟩ As a child, set a dog's broken leg. [paulmier pp22-25]   2108

⟨1⟩ Jumped into an icy river to rescue a dog, taking it "in his long & strong arms" – Jesse Dubois, 1888 recollection [wilson p718]   2109

⟨1⟩ As a child (?age15): "had a pet cat that would follow him to the spring" – Matilda Johnston Hall Moore [wilson p109]   2110

⟨1⟩ Freed a "mired down" hog on the prarie [wilson p262]   2111

⟨1⟩ "[I] Don't think Mr L. was much attached to Cats & dog – one reason" may have been the dog that bit Lincoln's son Bob, prompting Lincoln to seek out a mad stone; see ¶4953. – Frances Todd Wallace [wilson p485]   2112

⟨1⟩ Saved a baby pig being eaten by its mother [wilson p424]   2113

⟨1⟩ In Springfield: "fed & milked his own Cow" – James Gourley [wilson p453] Also: [wilson p616]. The 1855 Illinois census records that Lincoln owned $200 worth of livestock [templeC].   2114

⟨2⟩ Lincoln groomed his own horse and cleaned his own stable [burl p37]   2115

⟨2⟩ "Lincoln allowed his boys, Willie and Tad, to have all the pets they wished, and the result was a family menagerie of cats, turtles, white rats, frogs, chicks, dogs, and a talking crow." [ostendorfA p32]   2116

Infection – Exposures (to animals) (continued)

⟨2⟩ Helped Tad raise his kitten and train his dog [donaldA p428].   2117

⟨1⟩ "He did love Tadds Catt – less Tadds goats" – Ward Hill Lamon [wilson p466]   2118

⟨2⟩ Lincoln's "little dog Jip ... was never absent from the Presidential lunch. He   2119
was always in Mr. Lincoln's lap to claim his portion first, and was caressed
and petted by him through the whole meal." [boyden p82]

⟨2⟩ Milk cows were at the White House [burl p275]   2120

⟨1⟩ A front page article in the *New York Dispatch* on April 24, 1864, entitled   2121
"Very dangerous illness of the President's dog," was satire and had nothing
to do with any real animal. Photostat in: [randallP box 72]

⟨1⟩ Late March 1865: Plays with three orphaned kittens in the telegraph hut at   2122
City Point [porterD pp286-287]

- Farm animals: 2124

  ⟨1⟩ In Kentucky (probably): "The Lincolns had a cow and calf, milk and butter"   2125
  – Christopher Graham [tarbellE p235]

  ⟨1⟩ "got hogs in Ky – took them to Indiana – bears got among them – scared   2126
  them" – Dennis Hanks [wilson p104]

  ⟨1⟩ Indiana years: the family had some sheep [wilson p102]   2127

  ⟨1⟩ 1830: Lincoln drove a team of oxen when the family moved from Indiana   2128
  to Illinois [baslerA v4p64] [wilson p718]. Two borrowed horses were part of the
  caravan [angle p17].

  ⟨1⟩ Ox team used by militia – see ¶2149.   2130

  ⟨1⟩ Chickens, for food. [riceB p345]. See ¶639.   2131

- Industrial animals: 2132

  ⟨1⟩ Occasionally worked killing hogs in early adulthood [wilson pp130, 44, 457]   2133

  ⟨1⟩ March 1831: "The ludicrous incident of sewing up the hogs eyes:" A man   2134
  named Offutt "bought thirty odd large fat live hogs, but found difficulty in
  driving them from where [he] purchased them to the boat, and thereupon
  conceived the whim that he could sew up their eyes and drive them where
  he pleased. No sooner thought of than decided, he put his hands, including
  A. [Lincoln] at the job, which they completed – all but the driving. In their
  blind condition they could not be driven out of the lot or field they were in.
  This expedient failing, they were tied and hauled on carts to the boat." –
  Lincoln [baslerA v4p65]

  ⟨2⟩ Sperm whale oil was used to light houses [kunhardtB p275], including some in   2135
  Washington when Lincoln was a Congressman. There, at parties, one person
  recalled "wax and stearine candles ... used to send down showers of sperma-
  ceti on our shoulders" [angle p135]

  ⟨1⟩ In Indiana: "Hogs and Venison hams was a Legal tender and Coon Skins all   2136
  so" – Dennis Hanks [wilson p154]

  ⟨2⟩ 1837 Springfield: "hogs wallowed freely about town, rooting out garbage"   2137
  [kunhardtA p52] (part of ¶2045).

- Other cats: 2138

  ⟨1⟩ In childhood "had a pet cat that would follow him to the spring" – Matilda   2139
  Johnston Moore [wilson p109]

  ⟨1⟩ In New Salem: two pet cats, Jane and Sarah [wilson p504]   2140

  ⟨1⟩ Uncertain time, 1834-1860: "Lincoln I think had no dog – had Cats" – James   2141
  Gourley [wilson p453]

  ⟨1⟩ 1844: Staying at someone else's home, Lincoln gets up in the middle of the   2142
  night to attend to a mewing cat [wilson p128]

Infection – Exposures (to animals) (continued)

⟨2⟩ April 1862: Watching Lincoln use a White House fork to feed a cat sitting on a chair next to him (Lincoln) at dinner, Mary asked a guest at the table "Don't you think it is shameful for Mr. Lincoln to feed tabby with a gold fork?" Lincoln replied: "If the gold fork was good enough for Buchanan I think it is good enough for Tabby" and continued feeding the cat [burl p274]   2143

⟨1⟩ "Was fond of cats – would take one & turn it on its back & talk to it for half an hour at a time." – James Short [wilson p91]   2144

■ Horses: 2145

⟨-⟩ *Cataloging Lincoln's exposures to horses is like cataloging someone's exposure to automobiles today.*   2146

⟨2⟩ 1816: Two borrowed horses were part of the caravan that moved the Lincolns from Kentucky to Indiana [angle p17].   2147

⟨1⟩ 1832: Horses and men both suffered from hunger in the Black Hawk War: "Bill Clary had 2 ox 2 yoke each teams – The ox teams did more good than a thousand horses: they could go through mud & mire – slosh & rain and do well – not so with horses. ... The horses gave out – wore literally out – no grass – no nothing - too early for grass – in May – cold up there. The horses were jaded." – Royal Clary [wilson p372] *Inconsistent with statement that there was but one rain during militia service ¶2044*   2149

⟨1⟩ Circa 1832: "As a regular means of support during this time, he 'stood' a stallion for a farmer living near to New Salem, and is said to have attended to the business pretty well." – *Menard Axis*, Feb. 15, 1862 [wilson p24]   2151

⟨1⟩ Early 1830s: "Berry and Lincoln owned a horse in partnership" – Henry McHenry [wilson p534]   2152

⟨1⟩ A superstition of the time: "horse breathing on a child would cause hooping Cough" [wilson p536]   2153

⟨2⟩ 1837: When Lincoln moved to Springfield, he rode in on a borrowed horse [angle p89]   2154

⟨1⟩ "In 1837 during visit Abrah L. represented neighbor Rogers in Coles Co before Justice and got possession of mare. 1860 during visit to step mother before going to Wash. [illegible] John Rogers came over and bought same mare" – George Balch [wilson p597]. This horse was "Old Trim" [wilson p594]   2155

⟨1⟩ Lincoln owned a horse in March 1837 [burl p97]   2156
⟨2⟩ Lincoln's horses included: Old Tom (his first circuit horse), Old Buck (about 1850-1855), and Old Robin (also known as Old Bob) [ostendorfA p32].   2157

⟨1⟩ In Springfield: "Kept his own horse – fed & curried it ... He loved his Horse well." – James Gourley [wilson p453]   2158

⟨2⟩ Lincoln's horse in Springfield was "Old Bob" (to distinguish him from son Robert). He had a "sway back and rounded belly" and was kept in the carriage house behind the Lincoln home, along with a cow, hay, grain, and a two-seat buggy. Before leaving for Washington to serve as President, Lincoln gave the horse to a friend. Old Bob survived Lincoln, and marched in Lincoln's funeral procession in Springfield [kunhardtB pp245,264-266], in the "choice position" immediately following the hearse[kunhardtA p385]   2159

🖳 Photographs of Old Bob: [kunhardtA pp81, 385] [kunhardtB pp264-265])   2160

⟨1⟩ Other horses: 1832: "a sprightly animal owned by John T. Stewart [sic]" [wilson p329]   2161

⟨1⟩ Other mentions of a horse owned or used by Lincoln: [wilson ppp 436, 437, 590, 720]   2162

Infection – Exposures (to animals) (continued)

⟨2⟩ As Lincoln rode in a carriage to the White House after his first inaugura- 2163
tion, his horse-mounted guards "were ordered to spur their animals with
pretended clumsiness so that there would be constant, unpredictable movement, and any weapon firing at the head of the new Chief Magistrate would
be apt merely to drill a hole in a horse's stomach." [kunhardtB p6] *Unusual
benefits can result from exposure to animals!*

⟨2⟩ His favorite horse while President was branded *U.S.* [kunhardtA p131]. His fa- 2164
vorite horse was named "Old Abe" [beschlossB p98]; this was the horse he was
riding during the Aug. 1864 near-shooting (¶3603).

⟨1⟩ Mar. 1865: "was a good horseman." While visiting Grant, rode the horse 2165
"Cincinnati." [porterH]

■ There are accounts (but no photographs) of Lincoln riding a horse: 2166

⟨1⟩ June 1858: "While Douglas was speaking, Mr. Lincoln suddenly re-appeared 2167
in the crowd, mounted upon a fine, spirited horse." [volk]

⟨1⟩ Nov. 1863: He rode a horse to the ceremonies at Gettysburg Cemetery. "Be- 2168
fore he reached the grounds he was bent forward, his arms swinging, his
body limp, and his whole frame swaying from side to side. He had become
so absorbed in thought that he took little heed of his surroundings, and was
riding just as he did over the circuit in Illinois" [carrB p39]. *Perhaps he was
not feeling well. See Special Topic §5.*

⟨1⟩ Nov. 19, 1863: "was mounted on a beautiful chestnut bay horse" [cochrane] 2169

⟨2⟩ Riding General Grant's large bay horse in 1864, "he managed the horse well" 2170
[donaldA p515]

⟨1⟩ "He was passionately fond of fine Horses" – Ward Hill Lamon [wilson p466] 2171

⟨1⟩ Mar. 26, 1865: "rode with some ease... with very long stirrup leathers, length- 2172
ened to their extreme to suit his extraordinarily long limbs." [barnesA]

⟨1⟩ 1865: "was a good horseman, but always rather an ungainly sight on horse- 2174
back" [crookA p42]

⟨2⟩ Lincoln's dog in Springfield was Fido. A "small nondescript yellow dog," he was 2175
accustomed to receiving tastes from persons at the dining table. Lincoln would
let him carry parcels in his mouth home from the market. Fido was given to a
friend as the Lincolns left Springfield and survived his former master. [kunhardtA
pp136-137] and [kunhardtB pp266-269] show a photograph of Fido. [ostendorfA p33] shows
three photos.

⟨1⟩_q Late 1863: Fido "is a live and Kicking doing well" – William Florville, from 2176
Springfield [randallC p137]

⟨2⟩ When Lincoln left Springfield in 1861, he knew "every man, woman, child, and 2177
animal in the town by name." [kunhardtB p243]

Infection – Exposures (to people)

⟨2⟩ When Lincoln left Springfield in 1861, he knew "every man, woman, child, and 2178
animal in the town by name." [kunhardtB p243]

⟨1⟩ "Knew every man, woman & child for miles around." – James Short [wilson 2179
p91]

⟨2⟩_c Lincoln did not shy away from the sick: 2180

⟨1⟩ 1820s: "Abe used to visit the sick boys & girls of his acquaintance" – Elizabeth 2181
Crawford [wilson p126]

Infection – Exposures (to people) (continued)

⟨H⟩ As a boy, consoles a friend, Hugh Brace, who has a deformed arm, and says   2182
a lot about physical aberrations. [paulmier pp13-18] *May all be fiction.*

⟨1⟩ 1831: On a return trip from New Orleans by boat, "his Comrades took sick ...   2183
he was very modest and Kind to all the sick which made him very Popular" –
J. Rowan Herndon [wilson p6] then later says it was 1832 [wilson p34]

⟨1⟩ Lincoln removed a needle from the finger of a young woman he "seemed to   2184
go for." – Elizabeth Bell [wilson p605]

⟨1⟩ Visited Ann Rutledge during her final illness [wilson pp21,387]. She died of a   2185
disease "of the head or brain" [wilson p394] – "brain fever" [wilson pp402,409].

⟨1⟩ "atentive [sic] to the sick" – J. Rowan Herndon [wilson p92]   2186

⟨1⟩ Feb. 1861: A man named John Shanks "has unfortunate red nose to which L.   2187
calls attention at table. L. is worried over it." Acetic acid is obtained. During
the night, too much is applied to the nose, leaving it "bleached & shrivelled
like wash-womans finger." At breakfast "L. will not meal to begin [sic] till
Shanks comes in. When he does, all laugh. L. asks why his nose is like black-
slider. No answer." – John Shanks [wilson p702]

⟨2⟩ Dec. 1861: Met with General McClellan while McClellan had typhoid fever   2188
[rafuse] [leech p154]

⟨2⟩ March 1863±: Lincoln visited Congressman Owen Lovejoy, recuperating   2189
from smallpox [aa71 p384]

⟨1⟩ Feb. 1864: Lincoln visited Owen Lovejoy "repeatedly" during the latter's ill-   2190
ness [carpenter p17]

⟨1⟩ April 1865: "Among the *last* acts of his life was to visit the hospitals of City   2191
Point, and it is perhaps the most pleasing reminiscence of their hospital life,
that our soldiers can recall the circumstances of his late visit. [parag.] The
convalescents from the wards were ranged in files along the streets of the
camp, and he passed from man to man, saluting each one wih a friendly
hand-shaking, and giving to many, kindly words of cheer and sympathy. But
he did not forget those who, unable to leave their beds, could not enjoy the
pleasure of of receiving him publicly, and retiring from the crowd, he passed
through all the wards, stopping at bed after bed, till every man had touched
his hand, and the whole five thousand of the camp had been treated with his
friendly salutation." [anonA] (See ¶1297ff.)

■ ○○○ *Project:* Was there a smallpox epidemic while a Congressman?   2192

⟨1⟩ Feb. 1857: "The first part of the winter was quiet, owing to so much sickness   2193
among children with scarlet fever, in several families some two & three children
were swept away" – Mary [turner p48]

■ Pre-Presidential: 2194

⟨2⟩ Lincoln was exposed to gigantic crowds of people. He gave speeches to   2195
crowds of 6 thousand, 20 thousand, 6-10 thousand, and 10-15 thousand [gary
pp81,80,101,114].

⟨2⟩ Sept. 18, 1858: Estimated 20,000 people attended debate with Douglas in   2196
Charleston, IL [arnold p147]

⟨1⟩ Oct. 1858: Spoke "to an audience of not less than two thousand people" –   2197
James Grimes [wilson pp377-378]

⟨2⟩ About 50-60 children attended a birthday party for Willie [randallC p88]   2198

⟨1⟩ August 8, 1860: "Lincoln made his appearance on the ground, Fair Grounds   2199
in a Carriage –. That the People Surrounded the carriage – sunk it in the
mud – stuck tight – broke in the top of the Carriage – Came near smothering

Infection – Exposures (to people) (continued)

Lincoln" – George Brinkerhoff [wilson p437] (Rest of the story tells of Lincoln's extraction from the carriage and transfer to a horse.)

⟨1⟩ Summer 1860: "... we have had immense crowds of strangers visiting us" – Mary [turner p66] · 2200

⟨1⟩ April 1859: "There is a good deal of scarlet fever around us." – Mary [turner p55] · 2201

⟨2⟩ Summer 1861: Epidemics of measles, mumps, and smallpox in Washington. By 1863, virtually no part of the city was smallpox-free [hopkinsB pp276-277]. · 2202

- Smallpox periodically swept through Washington. In 1861 a visitor to the White House tried to infect Lincoln (see Special Topic §4). In November 1863 Lincoln did develop smallpox (this is Special Topic §5). · 2203

- In the White House: · 2204
    ⟨2⟩ All rooms were open to the public except, on the first floor, the family dining rooms, and about half the rooms on the second floor. [donaldH p23] · 2205
    ⟨1⟩ "The ante-rooms were crowded all the time from morning till night, with men, women and children all anxious to see Mr Lincoln. ... That crowd swayed, and jostled against each other every day." – Robert Wilson [wilson p208] · 2206
    ⟨1⟩ After the Civil War began: "Those were exciting days when, for hours and hours, the anterooms and halls upstairs were so full that they would hold no more, and when this broad staircase itself was also packed and jammed, stair by stair, from top to bottom, so that you could hardly squeeze your way up or down. It was all cut short by one of Lincoln's decrees. ... The anxious throng of office-seekers long since dwindled from a river into a brook of manageable size." – [stoddardA p5] · 2207
    ⟨2⟩ "Any day's run in the White House was crowded, tiring, and strenuous." [randallB p5] · 2208
    ⟨2⟩ Lincoln had to wade through the crowd to get from his living space to his office. Finally, in winter 1864-1865: "By cutting doors and constructing partitions, a private passageway was made on the second floor of the mansion, so that the President could pass from his bedroom to his office without meeting the crowds of strangers in the hall." [leech p442] · 2209
    ⟨2⟩ Jan. 20, 1865: White House reception draws about 8000 people. Lincoln shakes hands. [harris p57] · 2210
    ⟨1⟩ March 4, 1865: Lincoln shakes 5000 hands [french p466]. See ¶1221. · 2211

⟨1⟩ Nov. 19, 1863, Gettysburg, PA: As soon as Lincoln got atop the horse he would ride to the dedication ceremony, "he was besieged by a crowd eager to shake hands with him ... the marshals had some difficulty in inducing the people to desist and allow him to sit in peace upon his horse" [nicolayG]. · 2212
    ▣ A photograph ([ostendorf #81]) shows a dense crowd around Lincoln at the dedication ceremony. · 2213

⟨1/q⟩ April 1865: Lincoln comes ashore in Richmond and is soon surrounded by a "very oppressive" crowd. Admiral Porter orders his men to fix bayonets and surround the President, later recalling "I thought we all stood a chance of being crushed to death." [browneF p692] · 2214

⟨2⟩ April 8, 1865: Visits 5000 wounded/ill troops in a hospital in City Point, VA [pfanz pp84-88]. (See ¶1297.) · 2215

- Tomcatting: · 2216

Infection – Exposures (to people) (continued)

⟨1⟩ "I think he had no desire for strange woman I never heard him speak of any *particular Woman* with disrespect though he had Many opportunities for doing so" – Abner Ellis [wilson p171] 2217

⟨1⟩ According to Geo. W. Glasscock (a man Lincoln later pardoned), "Mr L in his younger days was a Man of good habits ... had no desire for strange Woman" – Abner Ellis [wilson p162] (∈ ¶1346) 2218

⟨1⟩ 1830s: "I never knew him to ... fool nor seduce Women" – Henry McHenry [wilson p15] 2219

⟨1⟩ In the Black Hawk War: "Lincoln and myself were in Iles – Spy Battallion – Got to Galena – went to the hoar houses – Gen Henry went – his magnetism drew all the women to himself – All went purely for fun – devilment – nothing Else" – John T. Stuart [wilson p481] (Elijah Iles commaded the Spy Company [wilson p520]) 2220

⟨1/q⟩ 1835: "Up to the time of Anne [sic] Rutledge's death Lincoln was a pure perfectly chaste man. Afterwards in his misery – he fell into the habits of his neighborhood." – Herndon to Caroline Dall [tripp p230] citing journal entry for 29 October 1866 in the Dall papers at Bryn Mawr College 2221

⟨1⟩ After interviewing Joshua Speed in 1889, Herndon writes: "Mr. Speed told me this story of Lincoln. Speed about 1839-'40 was keeping a pretty woman in this City and Lincoln desirous to have a *little* said to Speed – 'Speed, do you know where I can get *some*; and in reply Speed said – 'Yes, I do, & if you will wait a moment, or so I'll send you to the place with a note. [Lincoln went.] ... Lincoln and the girl stript off and went to bed. Before any thing was done, [price was discussed – Lincoln was two dollars short.] Well said the girl – 'I'll trust you, Mr. Lincoln, for $2.. Lincoln thought a moment or so and said – 'I do not wish to go on credit. ... I cannot afford to Cheat you.' Lincoln after some words of encouragement from the girl got up out of bed, – buttoned up his pants [and left]." Several days later the girl told the story to Speed. Herndon: "Speed told me the story and I have no doubt of its truthfulness." [wilson p719] (See Special Topic §2 for discussion.) 2222

⟨1⟩ 1861: "Pretty woman there that took Abes Eyes – I assure you" – John Hanks [wilson p458] 2223

⟨1/q⟩ As President: Lincoln tells James A. Briggs of a woman who pled her case: "By degrees she came closer and closer to me as I sat in my chair, until really her face was so near my own that I thought she wanted me to kiss her; when my indignation came to my relief, and drawing myself back and straightening myself up, I gave her the proper sort of a look and said: 'Mrs. —, you are very pretty, and it's very tempting, BUT I WON'T.' " [tripp p229] citing the card catalog of the Illinois State Historical Library, and J Ill St His Soc 1939; 32: 399 (which mis-dates it). 2224

■ Co-sleeping, with or without more intimate physical contact, affords opportunities for infection. 2225

⟨1⟩ 1831 and/or 1832: "slept together in the same cott & when one turned over the other had to do likewise." – William Greene [wilson pp17-18] (See ¶2273.) 2226

⟨1⟩ New Salem: Lincoln shared a bed in a boardinghouse with Daniel Burner. Other boarders sometimes slept in the same bedroom. [templeB] 2227

⟨1/q⟩ New Salem: "Him and I slept in the same bed while he boarded with my uncle James Rutledge." – McGrady Rutledge [walsh p96] 2228

⟨1⟩ 1837: Lincoln walked into a store, looking for a lodging. He encountered 2229

Infection – Exposures (to people) (continued)

Joshua Speed, who replied "I have a very large room, and a very large double-bed in it; which you are welcome to share with me if you choose." [wilson p590]

⟨2⟩ Springfield: William Herndon and Charles R. Hurst also slept in the room with Speed and Lincoln. They were then clerks in Speed's store. [randallC p101] 2230

⟨2⟩ Judge David Davis "shared more beds with Lincoln and tried more cases in which he was involved than any other judge" [kunhardtA p77]. 2231

⟨1⟩ Herndon and Lincoln slept in the same bed at least once on the circuit. [hertz p96] 2232

⟨1⟩ "Lincoln didnt care what he ate – who who he ate with or where he slept or who he slept with." – Henry C. Whitney [wilson p648] 2233

⟨2⟩ 1858, campaigning against Douglas: Reporter Andrew Shuman "accompanied Mr. Lincoln through nearly all of the campaign, travelling with him by night sometimes occupying the same room, and when in crowded quarters, the same bed." [browneF p293] *See §1c for priceless details.* 2234

⟨2⟩ As President: Invites the captain of Company K to share his bed while Mary away [leech p374]. This was Capt. Charles Derickson [tripp pp16-17]. 2235

⟨1/q⟩ 1863: Asked about testimony of Charles Maltby, Lincoln said: "I know Maltby, for I slept with him six months, and he used to be an honest man." – James W. Simonton [tripp p128] citing [brooksO p253n4] 2236

⟨2/c⟩ In Lincoln's era, "Bed-sharing ... was about as common as , and indeed was very similar to, the way people today share apartments." [shenk p35] 2237

Joints

Many descriptions of Lincoln use the word "loose." Today, that word usually modifies "jointed," but in Lincoln's case I think it had more to do with his muscles. For a tabulation of this word's occurrence, see ¶3012. 2239

⟨s⟩ Some believe Lincoln's feats of strength would be impossible were his joints lax. [lattimerNY] 2240

⟨-⟩ *This argument is suspect. Joint laxity need not come into play when the muscles acting on it are balanced. That is, joints typically have opposing muscles. As long as they oppose each other with forces of approximately equal magnitude, the net stress on the joint is small, and so even a lax joint will not dislocate. Thus, a combination of strength and finesse is compatible with loose-jointedness and no history of joint dislocation.* 2241

⟨s⟩ Some believe lax joints are incompatible with wrestling prowess because "the opponent could take each finger of the man with Marfan syndrome and bend it backward. In fact, he could bend back the entire wrist and arm and thus escape from any 'hold' at all." [lattimerNY] *Difficult to accept. Do not wrestlers resist movement with their muscles more than they resist by an inability for a bone to move in a joint?* 2242

⟨1⟩ In wrestling against the 15-year-old Lincoln, Dennis Hanks says "he could bring me down by throwin' his leg over my shoulder. I always was a little runt of a feller." [wilsonR p29] *Hanks would then have been 25.* 2243

⟨1/q⟩ "He was full of pranks that showed his agility. I have seen him place a cup of water between his heels, and then folding his arms bend his tall form backward until he could grip the edge of the cup between his teeth and then straighten himself into an upright position without spilling the water. He was fond of backing up against the wall and stretching out his arms to their fullest extent, and I never saw a man 2244

Joints (continued)

with so great a stretch. He did a great many little things like these that pleased and amused people." – Daniel Green Burner, who shared a room with Lincoln in New Salem for four years [templeB] (Agrees with [sandburgP v1p471]) *This difficult-to-believe feat is discussed in* The Physical Lincoln. *Contortionist videos show that such a maneuver is possible.*

⟨1⟩ Mar. 1865: "he sat in a camp-chair with his long legs doubled up in grotesque attitudes ... he looked the picture of comfort and good-nature." [porterH] (For date, see ¶1272.)   2245

Legs

- Length (youth):   2246
  - ⟨1/q⟩ As a toddler (presumably): "I recollect how Tom joked about Abe's long legs when he was toddlin' round the cabin." – Dennis Hanks [wilsonR p21] (Part of ¶474)   2247
  - ⟨1/q⟩ When a stranger came down the road near the house, "Then Abe'd come lopin' out on his long legs, throw one over the top rail an' begin firin' questions. [To stop him,] Tom'd have to bang him on the side o' the head with his hat." – Dennis Hanks [wilsonR p27]   2248
  - ⟨2⟩ About age 17: "His feet and hands were large, arms and legs long and in striking contrast with his slender trunk and small head." [herndon p35] (∈ ¶492) *Herndon did not know Lincoln at age 17.*   2249
  - ⟨2⟩ In his "younger days:" was called "Long Shanks" [sandburgP v1p306]   2250
- Length (adult):   2251
  - ⟨1⟩ 1834: "his legs were long, feet large" – Robert Wilson [wilson pp201-202] (Part of ¶99)   2252
  - ⟨1⟩ "His legs & arms were abnormally – unnaturally long, & hence in undue proportions to the balance of his body. It was only when he stood up that he loomed above other men." [herndonC] (∈ ¶2) (Cognate in: [herndon p472].)   2253
  - ⟨1⟩ "limbs large and bony" – William Herndon [hertz p195] (∈ ¶87)   2254
  - ⟨2⟩ In Springfield, Lincoln's church pew was so shallow "it seemed impossible that he ever sat there and managed to stow away his grasshopper legs." [kunhardtB p270]   2255
  - ⟨1/q⟩ 1850s(?): "He was so long-legged that when he crossed one over the other, both feet seemed to rest on the floor." – Charles W. Nickum [ostendorfA p147] *Does this make sense?*   2256
  - ⟨1/q⟩ Autumn 1854: "a human being rising slowly, and unfolding his long arms and his long legs, exactly like the blades of a jack-knife.... his trousers did not reach to his socks." – J.B. Merwin [hobson p63] (∈ ¶142)   2257
  - ⟨1⟩ " long-limbed" – Leonard Swett [riceA p464]   2258
  - ⟨1⟩ "long limbs, large hands and feet" [arnold p441] (∈ ¶167)   2259
  - ⟨1/q⟩ "legs of more than proportionate length" – John Nicolay [meserve p5] (∈ ¶177)   2260
  - ⟨H⟩ In Indiana: Rejected by Susie Enlow because "my feet and hands were too big, and my legs and arms too long." [paulmier p26]   2261
  - ⟨1⟩ 1862: "long bony arms and legs, which, somehow, seem always to be in the way" [dicey v1pp220-221] (∈ ¶179)   2262
  - ⟨1⟩ As President: "long legs ending with feet such as I never saw before" [salmsalm p144] (∈ ¶190)   2263
  - ⟨1⟩ Mar. 26, 1865: rides a horse "with very long stirrup leathers, lengthened to their extreme to suit his extraordinarily long limbs." [barnesA]   2264

Legs (continued)

⟨1⟩ 1865: "long legs" [crookA p9] [crookK]   2265

⟨s⟩ Lincoln's legs were reminiscent of a great spider, e.g. a "daddy long legs."   2266
[sandburgP v2p303] cited by [schwartzA] *This cannot be taken too seriously; Sand-*
burg waxed eloquent (and loosely) in his Lincoln biography's first two vol-
umes.

⟨2⟩ Black hair on his legs [kunhardtA p321]   2268

⟨2⟩ "genu recurvatum is suggested in Herndon's description" [gordon] citing ?¶2   2269

🔘 Photographs showing the angle of his legs when seated. [ostendorf #49-53, 58-61, 66-67,   2270
70-74, 76, 100, 101]

⟨2⟩ "Seated, his knees poked up like prongs" [kunhardtA p280]   2271

⟨1/q⟩ "Such long legs! ... They stick up in the air, as he sits in an ordinary chair." –   2272
Benjamin Seaver [ostendorfA p191]

⟨1⟩ Spring 1831; "his thigs [sic] were as perfect as a human being Could be" – William   2273
Greene [wilson p17] Part of ¶394. (See ¶2226.)

⟨1⟩ 1830s: "Mr Lincoln would wait till all who were disposed to try their muscles had   2274
made their best jumps, then come forward with a heavy weight in each hand with
his long muscular legs raise himself from the ground and light far beyond the
most successful champion" – Dr. Jason Duncan [wilson p541] See ¶2850 for more on
jumping.

⟨1/q⟩ 1840: In a speech Lincoln says: I was a poor boy and "had only one pair of   2275
breeches and they were of buckskin now if you know the nature of buckskin when
wet and dried by the sun they would shrink and mine kept shrinking ... and whilst
I was growing taller they were becoming shorter: and so much tighter, that they
left a blue streak around my leg which you can see to this day." [wilson p447]

⟨1⟩ Agrees with: [herndon p157] who says 1839   2276

⟨1⟩ "Shin bones Sharp – blue & narrow" – Nathaniel Grigsby [wilson p118]   2277

⟨1/q⟩ Late 1850s: "Lincoln's favorite position when unraveling some knotty law point   2278
was to stretch both of his legs at full length upon a chair in front of him." – John
Littlefield [angle pp184-185]

⟨1⟩ As President: "... as he sat comfortably in his arm-chair, in his favorite position,   2279
with his legs crossed." [brooksC p298]

⟨1⟩ "His message to the last session of Congress was first written upon [a] white paste-   2280
board ... its stiffness enabling him to lay it on his knee, as he sat easily in his arm-
chair, writing..." [brooksR]. *Did his knees reach so high that it was convenient to*
write at that level?

Liver

■ Numerous references to "yellow," "sallow," and "saffron" skin, starting in youth.   2281
(See ¶3376ff.)

⟨1/q⟩ Nov. 1863: Was thought to be jaundiced during his bout of smallpox. See §5.70. –   2282
[barbeeP - box1 folder 51] transcript of Philadelphia Sunday *Dispatch* of Dec. 6, 1863

Lungs

⟨S⟩ It is worth remembering that people in the 19th century would have had very great exposures to burning wood – see ¶4307   2283

    ⟨2⟩ Springfield home was heated by wood fires [randallC p77]   2284

⟨1⟩ In Indiana: In and around a smoke-house, at least occasionally. [hobson p24] (∈ ¶2438)   2285

⟨2⟩ August 1864: Leaking overhead gaslight in the White House threatened Lincoln with asphyxiation. [beschlossB p97]   2286

Medications & Chemicals

■ Some ⟨Infection -- Exposures⟩ situations could also have exposed him to injurious substances.   2287

⟨1⟩ Summer 1835: Took "heroic doses of Peruvian bark, boneset tea, jalap and calomel" for a major febrile illness (probably malaria) [rankinA p74]. "Peruvian bark" is explained in ¶2005. See also ¶2008ff, ¶2695ff (which discusses potential toxicities), and Special Topic §1.   2288

■ 1860-1861: Lincoln took "blue mass" pills, which contained inorganic mercury (¶612) and possibly colocynth [turnerL]. There are no records of blue mass purchases from the Corneau & Diller drug store [hickey], but drug store owner Samuel Melvin sent Lincoln 5 boxes of pills in April 1861 [hirschhornC], a time when Lincoln is known to have been taking blue mass. Whether Lincoln took these pills during other years is unknown.   2289

    ⟨-⟩ For claims about mercury and Lincoln's mental status, see ¶2419ff. For constipation, see ¶612ff.   2290

    ⟨1⟩ "Samuel H. Melvin is listed in the Springfield city directories from 1860/61 through 1875. He is listed as owner of a drug store from 1860 to 1870. In 1869/70, the drug store appears as Melvin & Glidden. Apparently Melvin sold his interest to Glidden in 1870 as the drug store appears as Glidden's after that date." – Reference report from Illinois State Historical Library, Jan. 29, 1947, in Box 1, folder 1 of [shutesP]   2291

    ⟨2⟩$_c$ Lincoln may also have been taking calomel pills in 1853 [turnerL].   2292

■ In Springfield: [hickey] lists the Lincoln household's purchases of gastrointestinal remedies from the Corneau & Diller drug store from 1849 to 1860, including: 2293

    ⟨1⟩ calomel (Hg_2Cl_2) – 4 occasions   2294
    ⟨1⟩ Carminatives – 8 occasions (inlcuding 4 in one month in 1852)   2295
    ⟨1⟩ Castor oil – 9 occasions   2296
    ⟨1⟩ ipecac – 3 occasions (including 2 in one week in 1857)   2297
    ⟨1⟩ a bottle of "Dead Shot," used against bedbugs [shutes p57]   2298
    ⟨1⟩ Other: "emetic" (1), "cholera mix" (1), glycerine (1), magnesia (1)   2299
    ⟨2⟩ (See ¶627.)   2300
    ⟨S⟩ Commentary on a few purchases is in [shutes pp56-58].   2301

■ One purchase of Jayne's Carminative (named after a local physician – ¶3180) is recorded in [hickey]. It is described as an an anti-flatulence remedy [shutes p45].   2302

■ Lincoln purchased (¶2293) and took (¶2750) medicinal brandy.   2303

⟨1⟩ "Mr. Lincoln's law office smelled of tar in the summer because outside the window was a roof with pebbles on tar and the sun melted it." – Mary Brown [kunhardtC]   2304

Medications & Chemicals (continued)

⟨2⟩ It was on the second floor, overlooking a flat warehouse roof. "In the summer   2305
the tar softened and gave off a pungent, resinous odor which wafted through
the office on hot, breezy days." [kunhardtA p77]

⟨2⟩ August 1864: Leaking overhead gaslight in the White House threatened Lincoln   2306
with asphyxiation. [beschlossB p97]

Mental Status

Originally I hoped to avoid examining Lincoln's mental state (hence the title of the   2307
book), but once the hypothesis arose that Lincoln's facial expression was heavily influenced by physical factors ("pseudo-depression" – see ¶3028ff), ignoring the non-
physical Lincoln became impossible. This crumbled separation should have been anticipated earlier, as it is entirely typical of medicine: inevitably, exploring any physiological sub-system in detail will show it is related to numerous other sub-systems in
previously unsuspected ways.

Lincoln's mood has generated much discussion. I have not attempted to be compre-   2308
hensive. For extended treatments, see [burl pp92-122] [clark] [kempfB] [shenk] [shutesE]. The
historical evolution of this literature is helpfully reviewed by [shenk pp221-243]. This entire
body of literature should be re-evaluated in light of the pseudo-depression hypothesis.

Some have called Lincoln a "hypochondriac" [shutes p87]. This was incorrect, in the way   2309
the word is used today (imagined illness). Lincoln used the word "hypo" in two letters,
but in his time it was a word with multiple meanings. See ¶2741 and ¶2467. Lincoln-
the-hypochondriac would not have been so careless about his risk of assassination or
walking through the enemy capital less than 24 hours after it had been captured. When
Lincoln had smallpox, a staffer noted "He has not been alarmed about himself at any
moment" [stoddardA p109] (is part of §5d).

Based on an enormous clinical experience, Dr. Victor McKusick has stated "There is no   2310
characteristic personality of Marfan patients" [shenk p22].

The most revealing observation about Lincoln: "He was never quite as sad as he   2311
looked, and amid his heaviest responsibilities he generally decorated the situation with
a story, an allegory, or a joke... And on occasion he was not without real vigor." [croffut].
(But Croffut did see him look "very dejected" – ¶196.) *This is evidence that it was his
facial muscle tone that made him look sad, not his internal status.*

⟨1⟩ "Lincoln had poor judgments of the fitness and appropriateness of things. He   2312
would wade into a ballroom and speak aloud to some friend: 'How clean these
women look!' " – William Herndon [hertz pp76, 417]

⟨S⟩ "It is impossible for us to realize the spell he exercised by sheer personal presence,   2313
for cold print cannot recreate the magic with which he imbued his utterances...."
– Albert Beveridge [burl p9]

⟨1⟩ "The meanest man in the bar would always pay great deference & respect to   2314
Lincoln" – David Davis [wilson p351]

■ A little help from his friends: 2315
⟨S⟩ A theory in evolutionary psychology holds that depression can benefit its   2316
victims by attracting sympathetic acts of kinds from others [aa7 p1612] [shenk
pp37-38].

⟨1⟩ "He was a sad-looking man; his melancholy dripped from him as he walked.   2317
His apparent gloom impressed his friends, and created sympathy for him –

Mental Status (continued)

one means of his great success. ... The reader can hardly realize the extent of this peculiar tendency to gloom." [herndon p473]

⟨1⟩ "Men at once, at first blush, everywhere saw that Lincoln was a sad, gloomy man, a man of sorrow. I have often and often heard men say: 'That man is a man of sorrow, and I really feel for him, I sympathize with him.' This sadness on the part of Mr. Lincoln and sympathy on the part of the observer were a heart's magnetic tie between the two. This result gave Lincoln a power over men, rather it was self-inspired. All men and women always and everywhere treated him under all conditions with great and profound respect, and a close observer of human nature could see, detect that much of that deep respect issued from the heart." – William Herndon [hertz p122]   2318

⟨2⟩ In New Salem: After the Lincoln-Berry store failed, Lincoln had serious financial problems. Seeing him despondent, "friends engineered his appointment as town postmaster" [shenk p18] (Also: [wilson p540]). "Later, he was made deputy surveyor, too" [shenk p18].   2319

⟨2⟩ In New Salem: Creditors seized Lincoln's horse and surveying equipment. "James Short saw Lincoln moping about." Short bought the items at auction (for about $2500 in 2005 dollars) and returned them to Lincoln [shenk p18] (Also: [wilson p74])   2320

⟨2⟩ "When Lincoln was in distress, he could count on receiving aid as surely as he gave it to stray animals." [shenk p29]   2321

⟨1⟩ As a state legislator, personal feelings of other legislators toward Lincoln helped him pass at least one bill [nicolayO pp30-31]   2322

⟨2⟩ "Lincoln's friends didn't merely help him. According to Herndon, they 'vied with each other for the pleasure or honor of assisting him.' " [shenk p30] citing [hertz p123]   2323

⟨1⟩ Hearing Lincoln complain of poverty and loneliness, William Butler paid some of Lincoln's debts and had Lincoln come live with him and his wife. [nicolayO pp22-23]   2324

⟨2⟩ "In all the accounts of Lincoln's gloomy spells, there exists not a single instance in which one of his friends or colleagues asked him what he was *thinking* about." [shenk p111] *This is highly revealing. It means that all indicators of Lincoln's emotional state must derive from his facial expression, tears, or other objective signs.*   2325

⟨2⟩c "The most marked and prominent feature in Lincoln's organization was his predisposition to melancholy or at least the appearance thereof as indicated by his facial expression when sitting alone and thus shut off from conversation with other people. It was a characteristic peculiar as it was pronounced. Almost every man in Illinois I met ... reminded me of it ... My inquiry on this subject among Lincoln's close friends convinced me that men who never saw him could scarcely realize this tendency to melancholy, not only as reflected in his facial expression, but as it affected his spirits and well being." – Jesse Weik [shenk p109]   2326

- William Herndon: 2327
  ⟨-⟩ *Herndon fancied himself endowed with great psychological insights (¶12). His hard observations are more trustworthy than his soft conclusions.*   2328
  ⟨1⟩ "Mr. Lincoln is a sad, sad, melancholy man. This is so organically, or functionally, caused by conditions, etc. It is partly organic and partly caused by conditions [sic]. In the first place his grandmother was a halfway prostitute." [hertz pp51-52] *This is classic Herndon: presenting an observation, then launching into speculation about its cause.*   2329

Mental Status (continued)

⟨1⟩ "was a sad, gloomy, and melancholic man and wore the signs of these in ev-   2330
ery line of his face, on every organ and every feature of it; they were chiseled
deep therein, and now the question is: What were the causes of these? The
causes were, *first*, possibly heredity, and *secondly*, his physical *organization*."
[hertz p121]

⟨1⟩ "Lincoln kept aloof from men generally, few knew him; he would be cheerful   2331
and chatty, somewhat social and communicative, tell his stories, his jokes,
laugh and smile, and yet you could see, if you had a keen sense ... that Lincoln's soul was not present, that it was in another sphere; he was an abstracted and an absent-minded man; he was with you and he was not with
you; he was familiar and yet he kept you at a distance." [hertz p169] *Herndon, of course, believed he had a "keen sense." For abstractedness, see
¶2365]ff.*

⟨1⟩ "'Did his mind with his philosophy make him such – gloomy, etc. – or did his   2332
physical organism alone make him so?' It was his physical side that did it."
[hertz p167]

■ Lability: 2333

⟨-⟩ For changes in his face accompanying emotion, see ¶1798ff.   2334

⟨1⟩ "He was odd, but when that gray eye and that face and those features were   2335
lit up by the inward soul in fires of emotion, then it was that all those apparently ugly features sprang into organs of beauty or disappeared in the sea of
inspiration that often flooded his face. Sometimes it appeared as if Lincoln's
soul was fresh from its Creator." [herndon p475]

⟨1⟩ "lived continuously in three worlds, states, or conditions of his existence.   2336
First, he lived in the purely reflective and thoughtful; *secondly*, in the sad,
thoughtless, and gloomy; and, *thirdly*, he lived in the happy world of his
own levities. He was sometimes in the one state and then in another, and
at times the transition was slow and gradual and at times quick, quick as a
flash." – William Herndon [hertz pp123-124]

⟨1⟩ Herndon sometimes left the office when Lincoln was glum. Returning an   2337
hour later, Lincoln could "walk up and down the room, laughing the while,
and now the dark clouds would pass" [hertz pp133-134]

⟨1⟩ "Mr. L had a *double consciousness*, a double life. The two states, never in the   2338
normal man, co-exist in equal and vigorous activities though they succeed
each other quickly. ... This is the sole reason why L. so quickly passed from
one state of consciousness to another and a different state. In one moment
he was in a state of abstraction and then quickly in another state when he
was social, talkative, and a communicative fellow." Herndon would watch
the sitting, thinking Lincoln. "He would to the observer's surprise without
warning burst out in a loud laugh or quickly spring up and run downstairs
as if his house were on fire, saying nothing. Sometimes it took a strong effort on his part to awake, arouse himself from one condition on purpose or
with intent to live in another state of consciousness. ... The sharp points of
one state of consciousness touched the other state, and it was easy for him
to pass from one state to another and a different state. Such was the man
always." – William Herndon, 1891 [hertz p263]

⟨1⟩ More of William Herndon on abstractedness: [hertz p77] and ¶2365ff.   2339

⟨1⟩ "he was sad and cheerful by turns" – William Herndon [hertz p187]   2340

⟨1⟩ 1834: "when at ease had nothing in his appearance that was marked or Strik-   2341
ing, but when enlivened ... his countenance would brighten up the expres-

Mental Status (continued)

sion woul[d] light up not in a flash. but rapidly the muscles of his face would begin to contract. ... terminating in an unrestrained Laugh in which every one present willing or unwilling were compelled to take part." – Robert Wilson [wilson p202] (∈ ¶101)

⟨1⟩ March 1837: Arrives in Springfield, carrying all he owns in two saddlebags. 2342
Asks storekeeper Joshua Speed the price of wood to make a bedstead. Lincoln says he cannot afford it. Speed: "The tone of his voice was so melancholy that I felt for him. I looked up at him, and I thought then as I think now, that I never saw so gloomy, and melancholy a face." Speed offers to share his own room, rent-free. Lincoln takes his bags upstairs, sets them down, returns downstairs, and "with a face beaming with pleasure and smiles exclaimed 'Well, Speed I'm moved.'" [wilson p590]

⟨1⟩/q In Springfield, Lincoln telling stories in the center of a knot of people: "His 2343
eyes would sparkle with fun, and when he reached the [punch line] nobody's enjoyment was greater than his. An hour later he would might be seen in the same place or in some law office nearby, but, alas, how different! His chair, no longer in the center of the room, would be leaning back against the wall; his feet drawn up and resting on the front rounds so that his knees and chair were about on level; his hat tipped slightly forward to as if to shield his face; his eyes no longer sparkling with fun or merriment, but sad and downcast and his hands clasped around his knees. There, drawn up within himself as it were, he would sit, the very picture of dejection and gloom. Thus absorbed I have seen him sit for hours at a time defying the interruption of even his closest friends. No one ever thought of breaking the spell by speech; for by his moody silence and abstraction he had thrown about him a barrier so dense and impenetrable that no one dared to break through. It was a strange picture and one I have never forgotten." – Jonathan Birch [wilson pp727-728]

⟨1⟩ June 21, 1856: "He was grave, gloomy, thoughtful and abstracted." A "day 2344
or two later," Lincoln collects his earnings, packs his bag, and heads home. "I do not remember to have seen him happier." – Henry Whitney [angle p220] (Related: [wilson p734].)

⟨1⟩/q 1859: Watching lawyer Lincoln sitting in a courtroom: "his melancholy ex- 2345
pression had so impressed me that I should not have felt more solemn if I had been at a funeral." Lincoln then stood, addressed the court, and began telling a funny story. A "faint smile spread over his features." Lincoln sat down, and "It was but a few minutes until that old, sorrowful look came over him." – John Widmer [shenk p155]

⟨1⟩/q Feb. 11, 1860: "passing easily from grave to gay, and from gay to grave" – 2346
Chester County (Pennsylvania) *Times* [shenk p167]

⟨1⟩ May 19, 1860: A delegation is notifying Lincoln he is the Republican nominee 2347
for President. "He stood erect, in a stiff and unnatural position, with downcast eyes. [Delegation speaks its brief message.] Lincoln's reply was equally brief. With the utterance of the last syllable his manner instantly changed. A smile, like the sun shining through the rift of a passing cloud sweeping over the landscape, illuminated his face, lighting up every homely feature, as he grasped the hand" of a delegate. [coffinA pp172-173]

⟨1⟩ May 19, 1860, being notified of his nomination: "his face downcast and ab- 2348
solutely void of expression [until notification speech complete, then:] The bowed head rose as by an electric movement, the broad mouth, which had been so firmly drawn together, opened with a genial smile, and the eyes, that

Mental Status (continued)

had been shaded, beamed with intelligence." – William Kelley [riceA p258] (∈ ¶158)

⟨1⟩ "His Way of Laughing two was rearly funney and Such awakard Jestures be- 2349
longed to No other Man they actracted Universal attention from the old
Sedate down to the School Boy then in a few Minnets he was as Calm &
thoughtful as a Judge on the Bench" – Abner Ellis [wilson p161]

⟨2⟩ When telling a joke, Lincoln would laugh without restraint. "This picture of 2350
a mirthful, storytelling Lincoln played a role in making his melancholy so
shocking. No one could truly appreciate the gloom, said lawyer Orlando B.
Ficklin, without seeing the awful contrast between his face in pleasure and
in agony. Using shorthand, people often said that Lincoln had two distinct
moods. But those who knew him well saw, as Ficklin did, that he 'was naturally despondent and sad.' " [shenk p117]

⟨1/q⟩ 1845-1847: Lincoln often slipped away from conversations and fell into a 2351
"blue spell." Lincoln "wore a sad, or more correctly a far-away expression,
that made one long to wake him up, as it were, and bring him back to his
accustomed geniality and winning smile. ... It took me no great time to learn
that a very slight thing would break up his brooding." – Gibson Harris [shenk
p108]

⟨1⟩ "He was grave and gay alternately ... appeared to be either extremely mirthful 2352
or extremely sad although if he had griefs he never spoke of them in general
conversation" – Joseph Gillespie [wilson pp507-508]

⟨1/q⟩ Lincoln in animated conversation: "his expressive face beaming forth its joy, 2353
now seeming almost to laugh outright in its grimaces of fun, and now as
solemn and sorrowful as a tomb." – Amanda Hanks (daughter of Dennis)
[randallC p118]

⟨1/q⟩ As President-elect: "in good spirits" yet "There was a sort of sadness in his 2354
face... But he kept it under." – Samuel Weed [shenk p170] citing [NYTimes Feb. 14,
1932]

⟨1⟩ As President-elect, "laughter lighted up his otherwise melancholy counte- 2355
nance with thorough merriment." [villardM v1p143] (∈ ¶2409)

⟨H⟩ Mar. 7, 1861: The controversial "Diary of a Public Man" describes Lincoln 2356
laughing "but the gloomy, careworn look settled back very soon on the President's face" [angle p341].

⟨1⟩ Summer 1863: Fifteen minutes after being "a complete picture of dejection... 2357
the President seemed more cheerful. The dejected look was gone, and the
countenance was lighted up with new resolution and hope. The change was
so marked that I could not but wonder at it." [keckleyB pp118-119] (∈ ¶2533)

⟨1⟩ Sept. 7, 1863: "While I was speaking the expression of Mr. Lincoln's face had 2358
changed many times. He had never taken his eye from me." [harveyC] (∈ §6.6)

⟨1⟩ Sept. 9, 1863, after four days of meetings that saw Lincoln angry, sad, uproar- 2359
ious: "His face then beamed with such kind benevolence and was lighted by
such a pleasant smile that I looked at him, [and called him lovely]. He colored a little and laughed most heartily. ... his character had assumed so
many different phases, his very looks had changed so frequently and so entirely, that it almost seemed to me I had been conversing with half a dozen
different men." [harveyC] (∈ §6.11)

⟨1⟩ As President: "His countenance ... while in repose sometimes seemed sad; 2360
but it lighted up easily." [sumnerA pp132-133] (∈ ¶185)

⟨1⟩ Mar.-Apr. 1865: "After a moment's inspection, Mr. Lincoln left with you a sort 2361

Mental Status (continued)

of impression of vague and deep sadness. It is not too much to say that it was rare to converse with him a while without feeling something poignant. Every time I have endeavored to describe this impression, words, nay, the very ideas, have failed me.... He willingly laughed either at what was being said to him, or at what he said himself. But all of a sudden he would retire within himself; then he would close his eyes, and all his features would at once bespeak a kind of sadness as indescribable as it was deep. After a while, as though it were by an effort of his will, he would shake off this mysterious weight under which he seemed bowed; his generous and open disposition would again reappear. In one evening I happened to count over twenty of these alternations and contrasts." [chambrunA] (Cognate in [chambrunB p100].) (See ¶2383 for an example of this at Lincoln's inauguration.) *Chambrun says he cannot determine the cause of the sadness.*

⟨1⟩ April 3, 1865: Sees half-starved rebel prisoners. All happiness leaves his face. [crookA p49] (∈ ¶2556)   2362

⟨1⟩ April 14, 1865, late afternoon: "...was more depressed than I had ever seen him and his step unusually slow. ...earlier in the afternoon he had been extremely cheerful, even buoyant.... The depression I noticed may have been due to one of the sudden changes of mood to which I have been told the President was subject. I had heard of the transitions from almost wild spirits to abject melancholy which marked him. I had never seen anything of the sort, and had concluded that all this must have belonged to his earlier days. In the time when I knew him, his mood, when there was no outside sorrow to disturb him, was one of settled calm. I wondered at him that day and felt uneasy. [Lincoln goes to the War Dept., depressed [crookA p76].] He came out of the Secretary's office in a short time. Then I saw that every trace of the depression, or perhaps I should say intense seriousness, which had surprised me before had vanished." [crookA pp65-67]   2363

⟨2⟩ "According to those who witnessed his spells firsthand, the photographs do represent them, but not fully. Because LIncoln had to hold his expression for several minutes for the camera's long exposure, his countenance in the images did reflect his gloom. But his contemporaries said that no one could truly appreciate the gloom without seeing the awful contrast between his face when at ease and when in agony. 'The pictures we see of him only half represent him,' said the lawyer Orlando B. Ficklin. Observing him in the motion of storytelling, and then falling back into misery, made the latter state all the more dramatic." [shenk p155] *It is impossible to know what mental process occupied Lincoln's mind as he sat for photographs. An exposure time of "several minutes" is probably incorrect.*   2364

■ Abstracted: 2365

⟨$\frac{1}{q}$⟩ "I've seen him when he was a little feller, settin' on a stool, starin' at a visitor. All of a sudden he'd bust out laughin' fit to kill. If he told us what he was laughin' at, half the time we couldn't see no joke." – Dennis Hanks [wilsonR p21]   2366

⟨$\frac{1}{q}$⟩ In Indiana: "I noticed Lincoln out by an old stump, working very industriously at something. On going nearer, I saw that he was figuring or writing on a clapboard, which he had shaved smooth, and was paying no attention to what was going on around him. ... Many times have I seen him studying at odd moments, with a book or something to write on, when others were having a good time. That was what made him so great." – J.W. Lamar [hobson p23]   2367

Mental Status (continued)

⟨1⟩ "was social in spots, at courts on the circuit ... was not a warm-hearted man ... he was abstracted and absent-minded. When in one of his moods he was abstracted and absent-minded and would not notice a friend on the street, though spoken to pleasantly." Sometimes Lincoln did this to Herndon: "I know the man so well that I paid no attention to it, rather I have felt for him, sympathized with the suffering, sorrowful, sad man." – William Herndon [hertz p171]   2368

⟨1⟩ "His habits, like himself, were odd and wholly irregular. He would move around in a vague, abstracted way, as if unconscious of his own or anyone else's existence. ... But, however peculiar and secretive he may have seemed, he was anything but cold." [herndon p411] (∈ ¶1125)   2369

⟨1⟩ "Mr Lincoln was a man of thought. I have met him in the streets of this city possibly a thousand times and said to him: 'Good morning, Mr. Lincoln,' and he would spraddle, walk along as if I were not in existence, so abstracted was he." – WIlliam Herndon [hertz p95] *Earlier, this tendency may have been mistaken for "going crazy" – see ¶398.*   2370

⟨1⟩ Herndon tells an anecdote of being ignored, then concludes: "Sometimes this abstraction would be the result of intense gloom or of thought on an important law or other question." [hertz p99]   2371

⟨1⟩ "Of a Sunday, Lincoln might be seen ... hauling his babies in a little wagon up and down the pavement north and south on Eighth Street. Sometimes Lincoln would become so abstracted that the young one would fall out and squall, Lincoln moving on the while. Someone would call Lincoln's attention to what was going on; he would turn back, pick up the child..." – William Herndon [hertz pp104-105] ([randallC p80] says Lincoln would read from a book while pulling the wagon.)   2372

⟨1⟩ "he was embodied reflection itself; he was not only reflective, but abstracted." – William Herndon [hertz p120]   2373

⟨1⟩ "he could sit and think without rest or food longer than any man I ever saw." – William Herndon [hertz p196]   2374

⟨1⟩ "he was an abstracted and an absent-minded man" – William Herndon [hertz p169] (∈ ¶2331)   2375

⟨1⟩ Lincoln would not react to the havoc Willie and Tad created in the office "so abstracted was he and so blinded to his children's faults." – Herndon [hertz pp176-177]   2376

⟨1⟩ Sitting at the office table, after writing a few words, "and then become abstracted and wholly absorbed on some question; he would often put his left elbow on the table in his abstracted moods, resting his chin in the palm of his left hand. I have often watched Mr. Lincoln in this state while he was lost in the world of his thoughts, gazing in the distance. ... Occasionally I did ask him a question in his moods but he would not answer, probably for thirty minutes. In the meantime, I would quite forget that I had asked a question. To my surprise, say in thirty minutes, he would answer my question freely and accurately." Lincoln would look "sad and grim" when sitting abstracted. – William Herndon [hertz p214]   2377

⟨1/q⟩ In Springfield: "Thus absorbed I have seen him sit for hours at a time defying the interruption of even his closest friends. No one ever thought of breaking the spell by speech; for by his moody silence and abstraction he had thrown about him a barrier so dense and impenetrable that no one dared to break through." – Jonathan Birch [wilson p728] (∈ ¶2343)   2378

Mental Status (continued)

⟨1⟩ 1854: "One evening Bob and I were playing checkers. Mr. Lincoln was look-   2379
ing thoughtfully into the fire and apparently did not hear what Mary was
saying. Finally a silence. Mary put down her piece of embroidery and said,
'Your silence is remarkably soothing, Mr. Lincoln, but we are not quite ready
for sleep just yet.' As Mr. Lincoln did not seem to hear, Mary got up and
took his hand, 'I fear my husband has become stone deaf since he left home
at noon,' she said. 'I believe I have been both deaf and dumb for the last
half hour,' replied Mr. Lincoln, 'but now you shall not complain'; and he
launched into an anecdote of one of his clients which broke up the game
of checkers and left us all speechless with laughter." [helmB p110]

⟨1⟩ "When Lincoln was sitting at his office table writing and had paused, seem-   2380
ing to be meditating of what he should write, he usually placed his left elbow
on the table, ... with his thumb partly supporting the chin that rested in his
large hand. I have seen him, in the privacy of the office, maintain this position as immovable as a statue for more than half an hour, though generally
less time, if not writing, but while he was listening to someone addressing
him on a subject he was deeply interested in." [rankinA pp374-375]

⟨1⟩ As President: "Beneath this [sunny temper], however, ran an under-current   2381
of sadness; he was occasionally subject to hours of deep silence and introspection that approached a condition of trance." – John Nicolay[browneF p736]
(∈ ¶204)

⟨1⟩ As President: "I saw him every day, as he went in or came out of his office   2382
room, and I now and then had talks with him, but he was generally the most
absorbed and unconversational of men." [stoddardD p286]

⟨1⟩ Mar. 4, 1865 inauguration: "Hardly had he seated himself, when I saw him   2383
close his eyes and abstract himself completely, as though absorbed in deep
meditation. Far from seeking the glances of those who sought his own, he
seemed suddenly to become sad." [chambrunA] (See ¶2361.)

⟨2⟩ "his extraordinary moods of abstraction in which he was blind and deaf to   2384
all around him" [randallC p67]

⟨2⟩ "Matters concerning clothes did not register with this absent-minded man."   2385
_c [randallC p134]

⟨-⟩ *Anecdotes about Lincoln's inattention to his clothing suggests an "absent-*   2386
minded professor," e.g. [randallC p79[two]], [volk] *(¶516).*

⟨2⟩ Children romping noisily around the house would not disturb Lincoln's   2387
reading [randallC p94].

⟨2⟩ "He could sit lost in thought while his boys were shouting and turning the   2388
room upside down all around him." [randallC p107]

⟨1⟩ Confidence and mental stamina: 2389

  ⟨1⟩ "had unbounded and unlimited confidence in his own mental powers, he   2390
was himself and wholly self-reliant, asking no man anything..." – William
Herndon [hertz p85]

  ⟨1⟩ "he was self-reliant, self-helpful, self-trustful, never once doubting his own   2391
ability or power to do anything anyone else could do. Mr. Lincoln thought,
at least he so acted, that there were no limitations to the endurance of his
mental and vital forces." Herndon thinks such over-taxing and mental and
physical consequences. [hertz p120]

  ⟨1⟩ "He thought, at least he so acted, that there were no limitations to the force   2392
and endurance of his mental and vital powers." Would decompensate after
long study periods without food or drink. – William Herndon [hertz p124]

Mental Status (continued)

⟨1⟩ "Lincoln thought that he could do anything that other men could or would try to do; he had unbounded confidence in himself." – William Herndon [hertz p126] 2393

⟨1⟩ Tried to square the circle [hertz p126] [sandburgP p476] 2394

⟨1⟩ "he was intensely thoughtful, persistent, fearless, and tireless in thinking." – William Herndon [hertz p99] 2395

⟨1⟩ "he could sit and think without rest or food longer than any man I ever saw." – William Herndon [hertz p196] 2396

⟨1⟩ "One of Lincoln's striking characteristics was his simplicity, and nowhere was this trait more strikingly exhibited than in his willingness to receive instruction from anybody and everybody." – John Littlefield *I wonder if this was not, in fact, supreme self-confidence. (See ¶3833.)* 2397

⟨2⟩ Members of the Lincoln family, including cousins of Abraham, spoke of the "Lincoln blues" as a familial personality trait. [evans p329] 2398

⟨1⟩ "was cool and calm under the most trying circumstances" – William Herndon [hertz p82] *It is difficult to tell if Herndon observed this in Springfield or is talking about Lincoln's Presidency.* 2399

⟨1⟩ Mary would show off the children when "any big man or woman visited her house. ... she would become enthusiastic and eloquent over the children, much to the annoyance of the visitor and the mortification of Lincoln." – William Herndon [hertz p128] 2400

- Humor: 2401
  ⟨2⟩ Lincoln was the funniest President in American history [dole]. 2402
  ⟨1⟩ "He could make a cat laugh" [carrA p107] 2403
  ⟨2⟩ "was the sort of man who could tell jokes in a charnel house." [neelyL] 2404
  ⟨1⟩ "His conversation consists of vulgar anecdotes at which he himself laughs uproariously." – the Ambassador from Holland [donaldA p280] 2405
  ⟨1⟩ "If it were not for these stories – jokes – jests I should die; they give vent – are the vents of my mood & gloom." – Lincoln to Herndon [burl p106] 2406
  ⟨1⟩ 1850: Upon hearing a good joke from a companion in a stage coach: "Lincoln really laughed himself tired, kicked out, in fact, the bottom of the stage, tore out the crown of his hat by running his hand through it, etc., etc." – William Herndon [hertz p128] 2407
  ⟨1⟩ Late 1850s: "I have heard him relate the same story three times within as many hours to persons who came in at different periods, and every time he laughed as heartily and enjoyed it as it were a new story. ... I had to laugh because I thought it funny that Mr. Lincoln enjoyed a story so repeatedly told." – John Littlefield [angle p185] 2408
  ⟨1⟩ As President-elect: "The most remarkable and attractive feature of those daily 'levees,' however, was his constant indulgence of his story-telling propensity. ... His supply was apparently inexhaustible... None of his hearers enjoyed the wit and wit was an unfailing ingredient of his stories half as much as he did himself. It was a joy indeed to see the effect upon him. A high-pitched laughter lighted up his otherwise melancholy countenance with thorough merriment. His body shook all over with gleeful emotion, and when he felt particularly good over his performance, he followed his habit of drawing his knees, with his arms around them, up to his very face, as I had seen him do in 1858." [villardM v1p143] (Similar quote from Villard in [shenk p170].) 2409

Mental Status (continued)

⟨$\frac{1}{q}$⟩ Sept. 22, 1862: None of his Cabinet members laugh when Lincoln reads a funny story. "Gentlemen, why don't you laugh? With the fearful strain that is upon me night and day, if I did not laugh, I should die, and you need this medicine as much as I do!" [shutes pp102-103]   2410

⟨1⟩ Sept. 6, 1863: After telling a story to a petitioner, "You should have seen Mr. Lincoln laugh – he laughed all over, and fully enjoyed the point if no one else did." [harveyC] (∈ §6.4)   2411

⟨1⟩ Sept. 9, 1863, after a compliment: "He colored a little and laughed most heartily." [harveyC] (∈ §6.11)   2412

⟨$\frac{1}{q}$⟩ 1864: A comedian performs at the White House. The "voice and ringing laugh of the President" could be heard outside the Red Room. – Francis Carpenter [randallC p306]   2413

⟨$\frac{1}{q}$⟩ Enjoyed satirical column in the newspapers (e.g. Petroleum Nasby), sometimes reading them to visitor. "He offended many of the great men of the Republican party this way." – David Locke [shenk p181]   2414

⟨$\frac{1}{q}$⟩ "The theatre had great attraction for him, but it was comedy, not tragedy, he wanted to hear. He had great enjoyment of the plays that made him laugh, no matter how absurd or grotesque." – Hugh McCulloch [luthin p635]   2415

⟨1⟩ Re: his jokes: "He insisted sometimes that he had no invention, but only a memory." [sumnerA p134]   2416

⟨-⟩ More of Lincoln enjoying himself: ¶2527. His laughter: ¶3745 and ¶3751. ○○○ *Project:* My impression is that Lincoln as President was laughing more than he was crying. It would be interesting to see a quantitative comparison of incidents of each type. (Of course, he was working more than anything else.)   2417

⟨1⟩ A friend of Lincoln's, John T. Stuart, suggested a treatment for constipation: "I used to advise him to take blue-mass pills, and he did take them before he went to Washington, and for five months while he was President, but when I came to Congress he told me he had ceased using them because they made him cross." [herndon p473] See ¶612   2418

■ [hirschhornC] makes several claims related to mercury intoxication: 2419

  ⟨S⟩ Claim: "Lincoln's personality, at least, from the late 1830s, was one of rapidly shifting moods" (cites [wilsonB] and quotes several witnesses who testify to Lincoln's lability from the 1830s to 1860, e.g. ¶2490). Also claims the lability changed in the 1850s. *Lincoln's face was labile in the sense of being enormously expressive. See ¶2333ff.*   2420

  ⟨S⟩ Claim: Lincoln took mercury-containing "blue mass" pills because of his mood. *There is no direct evidence that Lincoln took blue mass pills for anything other than constipation [donaldA p164]. As shown in ¶612ff, all mentions of blue mass pills by Lincoln's contemporaries are connected with constipation. A second-hand report states John Stuart believed Lincoln's melancholy was caused by constipation, but available evidence is silent on whether Stuart urged Lincoln to take blue mass for constipation only, melancholy only, or for both. In that era, blue mass pills were taken for many possible reasons, mood disorder and constipation being just two of them.*   2421

  ⟨S⟩ Claim: Lincoln had "neurobehavioral consequences of mercury intoxication." *In 1861 Lincoln concluded that blue mass pills made him "cross." For that reason – at least – he stopped taking them.*   2422

Mental Status (continued)

⟨S⟩ Claim: Lincoln's labile mood was a neurobehavioral consequence of mer- 2423
cury intoxication. *This seems unlikely. Lincoln took blue mass pills for an unknown duration before becoming President and stopped five months into his term. Because crossness is the kind of adverse effect normally noticed after a few months of using a medicine – not years or decades – it is not likely he took blue mass pills for years or decades before becoming President. Thus any mood lability outside of 1860-1861 is difficult to ascribe to blue mass pills. Note that Lincoln had other exposure to inorganic mercury – e.g. ¶2294 discusses calomel – but the exposure quantity is wholly unknown.*

⟨–⟩ For constipation, see ¶612ff. Also see ¶2289ff. 2424

⟨$\frac{1}{q}$⟩ Weather effects: 2425
  ⟨$\frac{1}{q}$⟩ Bad weather was "verry [sic] severe on defective nerves" (his own nerves) – 2426
  Lincoln [donaldA p89]
  ⟨$\frac{1}{q}$⟩ After Ann Rutledge died, Lincoln said "I can never be reconciled to hear the 2427
  snow – rains & storms ... beat on her grave." [burl p96]
  ⟨1⟩ After Ann Rutledge died, "Lincoln bore up under it very well until some days 2428
  afterward a heavy rain fell, which unnerved him" – John Hill [wilson p23]
  ⟨2⟩ Yet, as President, Lincoln sometimes wandered "alone and unrecognized 2429
  through the streets of Washington, something he liked to do especially during storms." [kunhardtA p322]

⟨S⟩ John Nicolay wrote that Lincoln's melancholy spells ended after he married [evans 2430
p328]. This is widely disputed [evans pp329-331].

⟨$\frac{1}{q}$⟩ Youth: 2431
  ⟨$\frac{1}{q}$⟩ "I've seen him when he was a little feller, settin' on a stool, starin' at a visitor. 2432
  All of a sudden he'd bust out laughin' fit to kill. If he told us what he was laughin' at, half the time we couldn't see no joke." – Dennis Hanks [wilsonR p21]
  ⟨$\frac{1}{q}$⟩ "He was a 'bashful, somewhat dull, but peaceable boy.' " (speaker not 2433
  named) [kunhardtA p36]
  ⟨1⟩ Upon hearing a man had kiiled his wife, young Lincoln "was very sad," ac- 2434
  cording to Mentor Graham [hertz p132]
  ⟨$\frac{1}{q}$⟩ "he never got over the mizable way his mother died." – Dennis Hanks [wilsonR] 2435
  (∈ ¶4798)
  ⟨1⟩ 1820s: "While Abe was in Indiana he was or seemed to be always cheerful 2436
  and happy. I never discovered any Sadness or Melancholy in his appearance. ... In my first acquaintance with him in the year 1819 I discovered in him wit and humor ... This lively and jesting disposition seemed to be natural with him and continually growing on him." – David Turnham [wilson p518]
  ⟨2⟩ As a boy in Indiana, Lincoln would "get fits of blues, then he wouldn't study 2437
  for two or three days at a time" – James Grigsby [burl p93]

⟨$\frac{1}{q}$⟩ Jan. 20, 1828: "A great grief which affected Abe through life was caused by the 2438
death of his only sister, Sally. They were close companions and were a great deal alike in temperament. About a year after her marriage to one of the Grigsbys she died. This was a hard blow to Abe who always thought her death was due to neglect. Abe was in a little smoke-house when the news came to him that she had died. He came to the door and sat down burying his face in his hands. The tears trickled through his large fingers, and sobs shook his frame. From then on he was

Mental Status (continued)

alone in the world, you might say." – Captain J.W. Lamar [hobson p24] See [Sarah] [Death].

⟨2⟩ "Lincoln was not depressed in his late teens and early twenties." [shenk p16] *Seems* 2439
  c *to overlook ¶2438.*

⟨1⟩ 1830s: "When by himself, he told me that he was so overcome with mental depres- 2440
sion, that he never dare carry a knife in his pocket, And as long as I was intimately
acquainted with him, previous to his commencement of the practice of the law,
he never carried a pocket knife." – Robert Wilson [wilson p205]
  ⟨2⟩ Lincoln did carry a pen-knife, at least some times, e.g., using it to treat the 2441
      "stone bruise" of a friend's son [burl p59]

⟨1⟩ 1830s: "I think, that I never saw Mr Lincoln angry or desponding; but always 2442
cheerful, and his spirit and temper such as would engender the like cheerfulness
in all surrounding minds" – George Harrison [wilson p330] *But see ¶2708 for talk*
of suicide in 1835.

⟨1⟩ 1830s: "1st Lincoln was witty – humorous at 1832 & so down: the People would 2443
flock to hear him – loving jokes – humor &--. This quality of his nature declined.
When he first came among us his wit & humor boiled over. 2d My opinion is that
Mr Lincoln's sadness – melancholy – despair, grew on him – He had 2 Sentiments
– one to Stick his head in a hollow log, & see no one; & the other was to climb up –
to win the [tithes?] of his ambition 3d My own opinion is that Mr Lincoln's fancy
– Emotion, & Imagination dwindled – ie – that is to Say his reason & his Logic –
swallowed up all his being – ie became dominant 4th Mr Lincoln grew more.
more abstracted – Contemplative – &c. as he grew older." – James Matheny, 1866
[wilson pp431-432]
  ⟨2⟩ "Lincoln was *not* melancholy: that he was light-hearted & jovial always." – 2444
      James Matheny, 1887, as told by Henry Whitney [wilson p616]. Whitney, "sur-
      prised exceedingly" by this assessment, disagrees with it.

⟨1⟩ 1830s: New Salem, Lincoln the storekeeper: "Almost always Abe would be seated 2445
on a box in the front of the store, dejected and abstracted almost beyond belief.
The boy [Shastid's father] would sometimes have to go to him and shake him.
After he had waited on his customers, Abe would take his seat again." [shastid]

⟨2⟩ Spring 1833: marked depression [shutes p12] citing Dr. Duncan (¶3168) 2446
  ⟨1⟩ 1834-1835: "at this time he was greatly embarrassed in financial matters at 2447
      times seemed rather dispondent [sic]" – Dr. Jason Duncan [wilson p540] *Dun-*
      can dates this to the time Lincoln started reading law books: late 1834, at
      the earliest [donaldA p53].
  ⟨2⟩ Jan. 1833: Business is "slipping" at the store Lincoln owns with a partner. 2448
      Shortly afterwards it "winks out," leaving the partners with notes coming
      due on their purchase of the store [donaldA pp49-50, 52]. In late 1834, a court
      judgment is filed against Lincoln and his partner; the partner dies soon after,
      and Lincoln assumes the full debt; in March 1835, his goods are taken from
      him and sold at auction; a friend buys them and returns them to Lincoln
      [donaldA pp54-55]. It takes years to pay off the debt.
  ⟨1⟩ Lincoln's friends get him jobs (postmaster and surveyor) that "procured 2449
   q bread, and kept body and soul together." [shenk p18] citing [baslerA]

■ Summer 1835: depression-like episode after the death of Ann Rutledge, while ill 2450
with ?malaria. See ¶2695 for psychological aspects and ¶2008 for infectious aspects.

Mental Status (continued)

- Dec. 1836: Writes to Mary Owens of feeling "unwell" and having "spirits so low." 2451
  (See ¶2739.)

⟨1⟩ 1837: "The tone of his voice was so melancholy that I felt for him. I looked up at 2452
him, and I thought then as I think now, that I never saw so gloomy, and melancholy a face." – Joshua Speed's first meeting with Lincoln [wilson p590] (∈ ¶2342)

⟨1⟩ Jan. 20, 1840: "You know that I am never sanguine." [baslerA v1p185] *This remark* 2453
relates to an election prediction, so it is difficult to know if it applies only to
Lincoln-in-politics, or to Lincoln-in-general.

⟨2⟩ "He did forego in his later life the ugly tendency to belittle and wound others, but 2454
 c   he never lost his capacity for anger." [burl p xiv]

- Temper, pre-Presidential: 2455
  ⟨1⟩ "Abe never gave me a cross word or look and never refused in fact, or Even 2456
  in appearance, to do any thing I requested him" – Sarah Bush Lincoln [wilson
  p107]
  ⟨1⟩ "He would swear under strong provocation, but this was not often." – Daniel 2457
  Burner, who lived with Lincoln in the 1830s [templeB]
  ⟨2⟩ Late 1830s: "with his high temper still not under control, he was capable of 2458
  flaring up in debate" [donaldA p83]
  ⟨1⟩ 1830s: "I never in my life saw him out of humor. He never got angry." – James 2459
  Short [wilson p91]
  ⟨1⟩ "Mr Lincoln's temper both as a lawyer & politician was admirable But when 2460
  thoroughly roused & provoked he was capable of terrible passion & invec-
  tive" – Samuel Parks [wilson p239]
  ⟨1⟩ "he was good-natured generally, but it was terrible to see him mad" – William 2461
  Herndon [hertz p187]

⟨2⟩ Lincoln was an extraordinarily patient man as President, but Burlingame's chap- 2462
 c   ter on Lincoln's anger and cruelty [burl pp 147-235] makes it abundantly clear that
     Lincoln could (and did) become angry on occasion. There is an example in [NY-
     Times - Aug. 22, 1869].
  ⟨1⟩ "Does the good-natured, soft-hearted, easy-going ... tenant of the White 2463
   q   House ever really lose his temper? The country generally does not believe
       that he ever does or can, but the right answer to the question is that under
       exceedingly trying circumstances he *generally* succeeds in keeping down the
       storm..." –W.O. Stoddard [burl p208]

- Jan. 1841: Lincoln and Mary break up (see ¶2746ff and Special Topic §3): 2464
  ⟨1⟩ "With this exception he was always a man of very uniform character and 2465
  temper." – Orville Browning [nicolayO p2] (See ¶2720 and ¶2585.)
  ⟨2⟩ Dr. Anson Henry (¶3180) helped Lincoln recover from this episode. [shutes 2466
  p26-29] [shenk pp57-59]

- 1841±: The letter to Dr. Drake (see §2c): 2467
  ⟨2⟩ About the time Lincoln broke his engagement with Mary Todd he wrote a 2468
  letter to Dr. Daniel F. Drake, dean of the medical department at the College
  of Cincinnati. He described his symptoms and asked for a treatment recommendation. Drake replied that an in-person evaluation would first be necessary. There is no record of further communication, between them [shutes pp
  25-26], but it is likely that Lincoln did visit Drake [shenk p60n]. (Lincoln's friend,
  Anson Henry, had been a student of Dr. Drake (¶3184).)
  ⟨H⟩ William Herndon relates this letter to Lincoln having syphilis. See ¶2016 2469

Mental Status (continued)

⟨S⟩ Shutes believes the letter was a manifestation of hypochondriasis. [shutes pp25-28] 2470

⟨1⟩ 1842 (?): "during 1842 he [James Matheny] though [sic] that L would Commit Suicide" [wilson p251] *Matheny, recalling in 1866, probably meant 1841. See ¶2762.* 2471

⟨2⟩_c "The acute fits of his young manhood gave way to less histrionic, but more pervasive, spells of deep gloom." [shenk p23] 2472

⟨S⟩ Donald believes Lincoln did not fully grieve over his mother's death until 1844 [donaldA p116]. 2473

  ⟨S⟩ [burl p xvii] believes Lincoln never recovered from his mother's death. 2474

⟨1⟩ "Miss Todd didn't know her man. Lincoln was somewhat cold and yet exacting – blew up quickly" – Henry Whitney [wilson p623] 2475

⟨1⟩ "*he* was never himself – when I was not perfectly well" – Mary [turner p523] 2476

⟨1⟩_q 1837-1856: Had "a settled form of melancholy, sometimes very marked, and sometimes very mild, but always sufficient to tinge his countenance with with a shade of sadness, unless a smile should dispel it, which frequently happened, as he enjoyed humor and often indulged in it." – James Lemen Jr. [tarbellB pp226-227] 2477

  ⟨S⟩ Of Lemen's reminiscences about Lincoln, [tarbellB p227] adds: "I see no reason to doubt their genuineness [but] several serious historical students have challenged its genuineness." She believes Lemen exaggerated his intimacy with Lincoln. 2478

  ⟨S⟩ "However deep in melancholy Lincoln may often have sunk in 1837, it did not interfere with either his political or his professional activities. And this is true of all those periods of gloom through which he went at different times and which have been interpreted by his biographers as periods of practical insanity. A man who goes on with his work regularly and intelligently through a time of moral and mental abasement is not a carzy man. And Lincoln always did this. At the time of Ann Rutledge's death... it was only when he was absolutely prostrated by 'chills and fever' that he gave up. As soon as that illness had abated he went about his business." [tarbellB pp227-228] 2479

⟨1⟩_q 1847, as a freshman Congressman: Lincoln confessed to being approximately as nervous delivering speeches in the House of Representatives as he was speaking in court. [donaldA p121] citing [baslerA v1p430] 2480

⟨2⟩ January 31, 1850: "I have never been so happy in my life." – said by Lincoln the day before his son Edward died [kunhardtB p12] (¶3922). Eerily, see ¶2559. 2481

  ⟨1⟩ After Edward's death, Lincoln forces himself to eat [kunhardtC]. See ¶4381. 2482

  ⟨2⟩ "in William Herndon's voluminous oral histories, in which [Ann] Rutledge's death is mentioned scores of times, Eddie's death comes up not once. ... it does suggest that he [Lincoln] said or did little that registered with his contemporaries." [shenk p107] *Or: Herndon would have seen Lincoln daily after Eddie became ill, and so may not have felt the need to ask others about surrounding events or even write down what his informants said on the matter.* 2483

⟨S⟩ Jan. 1851: Lincoln's father dies. "To some extent, Lincoln's muted reaction can be accounted for by cultural norms." [shenk p107] 2484

⟨1⟩ 1850s: "Lincoln had no spontaneity – nor Emotional Nature – no Strong Emotional feelings for any person – Mankind or thing" – David Davis [wilson p348] 2485

Mental Status (continued)

⟨1⟩ "He was tender hearted without much shew of sensibility" – Joseph Gillespie [wilson p507]   2486

⟨1⟩ 1850s: Telling of his childhood, while riding on the circuit: "It was told with mirth and glee, and illustrated by pointed anecdote, often interrupted by his jocund laugh which echoed over the praries." – Leonard Swett [riceA p468]   2487

⟨2⟩ "At times he would talk to himself." – manuscript page in [randallP box 15] citing [whitney p68]. *This may be allusion to ¶3450.*   2488

⟨$\frac{1}{q}$⟩ Late 1850s: "He had three different moods: first, a *business* mood, when he gave strict and close attention to business, and banished all idea of hilarity, i.e., in counselling or in trying cases, there was no trace of the joker; second, his *melancholy* moods, when his whole nature was immersed in Cimmerian darkness; third, his *don't-care-whether-school-keeps-or-not* mood; when no irresponsible 'small boy' could be so apparently careless, or reckless of consequences." – Henry Whitney [angle pp166-167]   2489

⟨$\frac{1}{q}$⟩ Late 1850s: "In his melancholy moods, the exuberant fountains of his pleasantry and mimicry were completely sealed and frozen up, but when the black fit passed by, he could range from grave to gay, from lively to severe, with the greatest facility" [hirschhornC] citing [whitney p135 in a different edition].   2490

⟨$\frac{1}{q}$⟩ Oct. 4, 1854, preparing to speak: "It was a marked face, but so overspread with sadness that I thought that Shakespeare's melancholy Jacques had been translated from the forest of Arden to the capital of Illinois." – Horace White [shenk p132]   2491

- Jan. 1855, Loses election for U.S. Senate: 2492
  ⟨$\frac{1}{q}$⟩ "I never saw him so dejected." – Joseph Gillespie [shenk pp141-142]   2493
  ⟨$\frac{1}{1}$⟩ "I regret my defeat moderately, but I am not nervous about it." – Lincoln [shenk p142]   2494

⟨2⟩ 1855+: "Many of the most dramatic reports of Lincoln's gloomy spells came from men who only met him after 1854 – including, for example, Jonathan Birch (¶2343), Lawrence Weldon, Joseph Wilson Fifer, and Henry C. Whitney." [shenk p280n]   2495

⟨1⟩ 1855+: "With all the jollity of his every-day life, in all but the surface indications of his character, he was sad and serious." – Lawrence Weldon [riceB p139]   2496

⟨2⟩ 1856: Henry Whitney never saw Lincoln look so sad as when he (Lincoln) helped free his step-brother's son from jail. [randallC p116]   2497

⟨1⟩ 1857: Lincoln was in the audience at a public reading. "In the midst of one stanza, in which no effort is made to say anything particularly amusing, and during the reading of which the audience manifested the most respectful silence and attention, someone in the rear seats burst out into a loud, coarse laugh – a sudden and explosive guffaw. It startled the speaker and audience, and kindled a storm of unsuppressed laughter and applause. Everyone looked back to ascertain the cause of the demonstration, and was greatly surprised to find that it was Mr. Lincoln. He blushed and squirmed with the awkward diffidence of a schoolboy. What prompted him to laugh no one was able to explain. He was doubtless wrapped up in a brown study, and, recalling some amusing episode, indulged in laughter without realizing his surroundings. The experience mortified him greatly." [herndon p479]   2498

  ⟨1⟩ "He was a sad man – an abstracted man – have gone over to his house house many times – talked with my sister – Lincoln would lean back – his head   2499

Mental Status (continued)

against the top of a rocking Chair – sit abstracted that way for moments – 20 – 30 minutes – and all at once burst out with a joke – though his thoughts were not on a joke" – Frances Todd Wallace [wilson p486]

⟨2⟩ 1857: While arguing the case for acquitting Duff Armstrong of murder, "Real tears trickled down his homely face. 'But they were genuine' " [angle p178] reprinting Albert Woldman   2500

⟨1/q⟩ Nov. 1858, after losing election vs. Stephen Douglas for U.S. Senate: "I never saw any man so radically and thoroughly depressed, so completely steeped in the bitter waters of hopeless despair." – Henry Whitney [shenk p157]   2501

⟨1/q⟩ Jan. 6, 1859: "I shall never forget the day ... I went to your office and found Lincoln there alone. He appeared to be somewhat dejected – in fact I never saw a man so depressed. I tried to rally his drooping spirits ... but with ill success. He was simply steeped in gloom. For a time he was silent; finally he ... slid back into his chair again, blurting out as he sank down: 'Well, whatever happens I expect everyone to desert me now, but Billy Herndon.' " – Henry Whitney writing to William Herndon [hertz p10]   2502

⟨1/q⟩ 1859: "the thing that impressed me most of all in regard to Abraham Lincoln was the extreme sadness of his eyes. Lincoln had the saddest eyes of any human being that I had ever seen." – John Widmer [shenk p155] (∈ ¶150)   2503

- 1860, on the day Lincoln was nominated for President: 2504
    ⟨1⟩ "Lincoln played ball with me on that day ... L was nervous, fidgety – intensely excited Lincoln told stories – one of which was Washingtons picture in a necessary – privy in England – make an Englishman S–h–t." – Christopher Brown [wilson p438]   2505
    ⟨1⟩ "Lincoln went home from the Journal Office directly after his nomination for Presdt: he was agitated – turned pale – trembled." – James Gourley [wilson p453]   2506
    ⟨2⟩ As Lincoln was given the official notification that he was the Replication Presidential nominee: "Mr. Lincoln seemed to be calm, but a close observer could detect in his countenance the indications of deep emotion." – [lamonL p452] (reprinted [angle p277])   2507
    ⟨-⟩ More on that day: ¶1362   2508

⟨1/q⟩ Feb. 2, 1861: Ralph Waldo Emerson visits Lincoln and finds him to be a "frank, sincere, ... with a sort of boyish cheefulness." [kunhardtA p174]   2509

⟨1/q⟩ Feb. 24, 1861: During a photo session in Mathew Brady's studio, Lincoln "seemed absolutely indifferent to all that was going on about him, and he gave the impression that he was a man who was overwhelmed with anxiety and care." – George H. Story [kunhardtA pp24-25] (date is from [ostendorf #52])   2510

⟨2⟩ Mar. 4, 1861: Lincoln explodes in anger at son Robert, who mislaid the satchel containing the text of the inaugural address Lincoln was to deliver. [kunhardtA p26]   2511

⟨1⟩ Oct. 21, 1861: Lincoln goes into a room to talk with General McClellan. "Five minutes passed, and then Mr. Lincoln, unattended, with bowed head, and tears rolling down his furrowed cheeks, his face pale and wan, his heart heaving with emotion, passed through the room. He almost fell as he stepped into the street, and we sprang from our seats to render assistance, but he did not fall. With both hands pressed upon his heart he walked down the street, not returning the salute of the sentinel pacing his beat before the door." Lincoln had been told that his close friend, Edward Baker, had been killed in combat. [coffinA pp176-177]   2512

Mental Status (continued)

⟨1⟩ "Once he said that the keenest blow of all the war was ... the death of his beloved Baker." [brooksR]　2513

⟨1⟩ "I doubt if any other of the many tragic events of President Lincoln's life ever stunned him so much..." [coffinA p178]　2514

■ Feb. 1862: Lincoln's son Willie sickens and dies on the 20th.　2515

　⟨1/q⟩ Lincoln spends long hours with the ill Willie. "The President is nearly worn out, with grief and watching." – Attorney General Bates [kunhardtA p174]　2516

　⟨1⟩ It "wellnigh broke the President's heart, and certainly an affliction more crushing never fell to the lot of man. ... Strong as he was in the matter of self-control, he gave way to an overmastering grief, which became at length a serious menace to his health. ... A deep and settled despondency took possession of Mr. Lincoln; and when it is remembered that his calamity – for such it surely was – befell him at a critical period of the war, just when the resources of his mighty intellect were in most demand, it will be understood how his affliction became a matter of the gravest concern to the whole country." [lamonR p161]　2517

　⟨2⟩ In fact, Lincoln went only four days without writing official documents. [neelyL]　2518

　⟨2⟩ A week after Willie's death, Lincoln "shut himself up in his room" [kunhardtB p137]. (See ¶653.)　2519

　⟨1/q⟩ At some point Lincoln said: "I catch myself every day involuntarily talking with him as if he were with me." [kunhardtA p302]　2520

⟨1/q⟩ July-Sept. 1862: "The Prest. was in deep distress ... he seemed wrung by bitterest anguish – said he felt almost ready to hang himself." – Edward Bates [baslerA v5p486]　2521

⟨2⟩ Dec. 1862, after the battle of Fredericksburg: Lincoln particularly distressed. "He walked the floor of his office, moaning in anguish. ... Visitors to the White House often found Lincoln hopeless and distressed. He was awake at all hours of the night." A reported thought his eyes looked "sunken" and "deathly." [shenk pp186-187]　2522

⟨1/q⟩ Dec. 17, 1862: "I saw in a moment that he was in distress – that more than usual trouble was pressing upon him." – Orville Browning [shenk p187]-sal Browning 12/17/1862 text　2523

⟨1/q⟩ "You know I am not a man of very hopeful temperament." – Lincoln in 1862 [burl p106]　2524

　⟨1/q⟩ "You flaxen men with broad faces are born with cheer, and don't know a cloud from a star. I am of another temperament." – Lincoln [shenk p113]　2525

⟨2⟩ "Lincoln had always been one to upset hard and fast rules – he hated any procedure that could not be altered on the spur of the moment" [kunhardtB p231]　2526

■ Fun with guns (as President):　2527

　⟨1/q⟩ Test-fires a new weapon (early mitrailleuse) "and sent forth peals of Homeric laughter as the balls, which had not the power to penetrate the target set up at a little distance, came bounding back among the shins of the bystanders." – John Hay [angle pp435-436]　2528

　⟨1⟩ A man writes that he has invented a gun for cross-eyed shooters. "Mr. Lincoln laughed well over the cross-eyed letter." [stoddardD p246]　2529

　⟨1⟩ Lincoln is illegally firing a gun within the city limits of Washington. An angry police corporal commands him to stop, without at first recognizing who it is. The corporal beats a quick retreat. Lincoln laughed. [stoddardD p250]　2530

　⟨-⟩ See also ¶3839 and, for pre-Presidential, ¶2083.　2531

Mental Status (continued)

⟨$\frac{1}{q}$⟩ Feb. 6, 1863: "I observe that the President never tells a joke now." – diary entry of then-Captain John Dahlgren [kunhardtA p204]   2532

⟨1⟩ Summer 1863: "His step was slow and heavy, and his face sad. Like a tired child he threw himself upon a sofa, and shaded his eyes with his hands. He was a complete picture of dejection." After 15 minutes "on glancing at the sofa the President seemed more cheerful. The dejected look was gone, and the countenance was lighted up with new resolution and hope. The change was so marked that I could not but wonder at it." [keckleyB pp118-119] *Keckley thought Bible-reading effected the change.*   2533

⟨1⟩ Sept. 7, 1863: "The President bowed his head, and with a look of sadness I can never forget, said 'I never shall be glad any more.' All severity had passed from his face. He seemed looking backward and heartward, and for a moment he seemed to forget he was not alone; a more than mortal anguish rested on his face." [harveyC] (∈ §6.8)   2534

⟨1⟩ Nov. 18, 1863, on the train to Gettysburg: Lincoln borrows a newspaper. "He read for a little while and then began to laugh at some wild guesses of the paper about pending movements. He laughed very heartily and it was pleasant to see his sad face lighted up. He was looking very badly at that particular time, being sallow, sunken-eyed, thin, care-worn and very quiet. After a while he returned the paper and began to talk..." With other men on the train, "They told stories for an hour or so, Mr. Lincoln talking his turn and enjoying it very much." Excusing himself, Lincoln said "Gentlemen, this is all very pleasant, but ... I must give [tomorrow's speech] some thought." [cochrane]   2535

⟨1⟩ Dec. 15, 1863 (probably), watching Falstaff's antics in *Henry IV* at Ford's Theatre: "I watched his gloomy face in vain for any sign of a smile... At last the truth slowly dawned upon me that Mr. Lincoln was not there for the purpose of being amused. He had not come to laugh and therefore did not do so. His intention was rather a deep study of human nature as rendered by the great poet... I cannot find one other who was, in my opinion, so keenly capable of meeting another human being as a book to be opened and read on the spot, nearly through." [stoddardD p306]   2536

⟨2⟩ Feb.10, 1864: After the White House stables burn and two ponies die, Lincoln weeps [kunhardtB p297]. See ¶1100.   2537

⟨$\frac{1}{q}$⟩ Summer 1864: "A lady who saw Mr. Lincoln in the Summer of 1864 for the first time, and who had expected to see 'a very homely man,' says: 'I was totally unprepared for the impression instantly made upon me. So bowed and sorrow-laden was his whole person, expressing such weariness of mind and body, as he dropped himself heavily from step to step down to the ground. But his face! – oh, the pathos of it! – haggard, drawn into fixed lines of unutterable sadness, with a look of loneliness, as of a soul whose depth of sorrow and bitterness no human sympathy could ever reach. I was so penetrated with the anguish and settled grief in every feature, that I gazed at him through tears, and felt I had stepped upon the threshhold of a sanctuary too sacred for human feet. The impression I carried away was that I had seen, not so much the President of the United States, as *the saddest man in the world.*'" [browneF p670]   2538

⟨1⟩ Feb. 7, 1865: Lincoln, "when I entered the [Cabinet] room, was reading with much enjoyment certain portions of Petroleum V. Nasby to Dennison and Speed. The book is a broad burlesque on modern Democratic party men." [welles v2p238]   2539

Mental Status (continued)

⟨1⟩ Feb. 22, 1865: "The President was cheerful and laughed heartily" over a war story [welles v2p245] — 2540

⟨1⟩ Feb. 23, 1865: "apparently more depressed than I have seen him since he became President." [browning pp7-8] *Lincoln and Browning were discussing an imminent hanging.* (∈ ¶1209) — 2541

⟨1⟩ March 5, 1865: "very gloomy and dejected" over some political appointments – Henry C. Whitney [wilson p649] — 2542

⟨1⟩ March 1865: "Under this frightful ordeal his demeanor and disposition changed – so gradually that it would be impossible to say when the change began; but he was in mind, body, and nerves a very different man at the second inauguration from the one who had taken the oath in 1861. He continued always the same kindly, genial, and cordial spirit he had been at first; but the boisterous laughter became less frequent year by year; the eye grew veiled by constant meditation on momentous subjects; the air of reserve and detachment from his surroundings increased. He aged with great rapidity." – John Hay [hayA] — 2543

⟨1⟩ Mar. 26, 1865: Mary explodes in anger at a military review. That night, at 11pm, Lincoln, in the company of Mary, "seemed weary and greatly distressed, with an expression of sadness that seemed the accentuation of the shadow of melancholy which at times so marked his features... [The episode] bears upon the cause of the vein of sadness which ran through the naturally cheerful disposition of" Lincoln [barnesA]. — 2544

  ⟨1⟩ "In these perhaps unnecessary allusions to Mrs. Lincoln, there can be found the cause of the sadness and melancholy which were at times so apparent in Mr. Lincoln's expression." [barnesB] *Interesting that Barnes says "expression," not "conduct."* — 2545

⟨1⟩ Mar. 27, 1865, at Grant's headquarters: "He seemed in very good spirits." Listens to Admiral Porter's sea stories, "his face expressing in every feature the keenest enjoyment, he would stretch himself out, and look at the listeners in turn as though for sympathy and appreciation. General Grant did not have much, if any, humor..." [barnesB] — 2546

  ⟨1⟩ Mar. 1865: Grant tells a story. "Lincoln was as good at listening as he was at story-telling; and as [the story unfolded] he became so convulsed with laughter that his sides fairly shook." [porterH] — 2547

⟨1⟩ Late March 1865: "The President was evidently nervous; the enormous expense of the war seemed to weigh upon him like an incubus; he could not keep away from General Grant's tent, and was constantly inquiring when he was going to move.. ... he had a load to bear that few men could carry, yet he traveled on with it, foot-sore and weary, but without complaint; rather, on the contrary, cheering those would faint on the roadside." [porterD pp282-283] — 2548

⟨1⟩ Late March 1865: "I do think if I had given him two fence-rails to sleep on he would not have found fault. That was Abraham Lincoln in all things relating to his own comfort. He would never permit people to put themselves out for him under any circumstances." [porterD p285] — 2549

⟨1⟩ Late March 1865: "I never saw such a change in any one in my life as took place in Mr. Lincoln" when he was told Vice President Johnson and Preston King wished to see him. "The habitual benevolent expression had left his face; he was almost frantic." [porterD p287] — 2550

Mental Status (continued)

⟨1⟩ Mar. 30, 1865, Petersburg falls. "The President's heart was filled with joy, for he felt this was the 'beginning of the end.' " [porterH]   2551

    ⟨$\frac{1}{q}$⟩ When Petersburg fell: "I doubt whether Mr. Lincoln ever experienced a happier moment in his life" – Horace Porter [kunhardtA p268]   2552

⟨1⟩ "As March 31, 1865, drew near ... grew depressed," knowing Grant (and Robert) were soon to make an attack. "Anxiety became more intense" on April 1. "I have never seen such suffering in the face of any man was in his that night." Good progress makes Lincoln cheerful late on April 2. [crookA pp47-48]   2553

⟨1⟩ April 3, 1865: Hears Richmond has fallen: "Thank God that I have lived to see this! It seems to me that I have been dreaming a horrid dream for four years, and now the nightmare is gone." [porterD p294]   2554

    ⟨1⟩ April 3: "He was in high spirits, seemed not at all fatigued, and said that the end could not be far off." [barnesB]   2555

    ⟨1⟩ Says "Poor fellows!" when he sees half-starved rebel prisoners. "His face was pitying and sorrowful. All the happiness had gone." [crookA p49]   2556

⟨1⟩ Apr. 4, 1865: "never looked sadder in his life than when he walked through the streets of Richmond" [crookA p59]   2557

⟨1⟩ April 4, 1865: Lincoln happily receives his old friend Duff Green, but Green spews vitriol against Lincoln. "The smile left the President's lips ... and the softness of his eyes faded out. He was another man altogether. ... [Lincoln's] slouchy manner had disappeared, his mouth was compressed, his eyes were fixed, and even his stature appeared increased. ... his coarse hair stood on end, and his nostrils dilated like those of an excited race-horse. He stretched out his long right arm, and extended his lean forefinger until it almost touched Duff Green's face." (Lincoln then chews him out.) [porterD pp307-308]   2558

⟨2⟩ April 9, 1865: "I have never been so happy in my life." – said repeatedly by Lincoln after the surrender of Lee [kunhardtB p11]. Eerily, see ¶2481. *Lincoln lived less than a week after Lee's surrender – a clear example of the Agamemnon phenomenon* [aa91] *– feeling euphoric shortly before a health catastrophe.*   2559

⟨$\frac{1}{q}$⟩ April 10 (or so), 1865: "He had suddenly become, on the fall of Richmond and the surrender of the Confederate Army, April 9, at Appomattox, a different man. His whole appearance, poise, and bearing had marvelously changed. He was, in fact, transfigured. That indescribable sadness which had previously seemed to me an adamantine element of his very being had been suddenly changed for an equally indescribable expression of serene joy! – as if conscious that the great purpose of his life had been achieved. His countenance had become radiant, – emitting spiritual light something like a halo. Yet there was no manifestation of exaltation or ecstasy. He seemed the very personification of supreme satisfaction. His conversation was, of course, correspondingly exhilarating." – Senator James Harlan [helmB p253]   2560

    ⟨1⟩ "... didn't in late days dream of death – was cheery – funny – in high spirits" – Mary [wilson pp357,359]   2561

⟨1⟩ April 11-14, 1865: "No one was more joyous and happy than Mr. Lincoln. The dark clouds had disappeared" [arnold p428]   2562

⟨1⟩ April 13, 1865: "I noticed that he was in one of those moods when 'melancholy seemed to be dripping from him,' and his eye had that expression of profound weariness and sadness which I never saw in other human eye [sic]" [field p321]   2563

Mental Status (continued)

- April 14, 1865 (his last full day alive):   2564
  - ⟨$\frac{1}{q}$⟩ On that morning Lincoln's hair was combed, he (atypically) had breakfast   2565
    with the family, and according to Elizabeth Keckley, "his face was more
    cheerful than I had seen it for a long time." [keckleyB p138]
  - ⟨$\frac{1}{q}$⟩ Mary found him "cheerful ... even playful," looking forward to the future,   2566
    and quoted him saying: "between the war & the loss of our darling Willie –
    we have both, been very miserable." [turner p285] [donaldH p50]
  - ⟨$\frac{1}{q}$⟩ Mary to Abraham: "I have not seen you so happy since before Willie's death."   2567
    [helmB] *It is not apparent what the source of this quotation might have been.*
  - ⟨$\frac{1}{q}$⟩ In the Cabinet meeting: "I never saw Mr. Lincoln so cheerful and happy. The   2568
    burden which had been weighing upon him for four long years had been
    lifted. The weary look which his face had so long worn, and which could be
    observed by those who knew him well, even when he was telling stories, had
    disappeared. It was bright and cheerful." – Hugh McCulloch [luthin p622]
  - ⟨$\frac{1}{q}$⟩ Had a "shaved face, well brushed clothing and neatly combed hair and   2569
    whiskers" – Joshua Speed (presumably at Cabinet meeting) [luthin p622]
  - ⟨$\frac{1}{q}$⟩ Lincoln considered the war to have ended on this day. [randallC p342]   2570
- ⟨2⟩ April 14, 1865: While watching the play at Ford's Theatre "Mr. Lincoln seemed   2571
  weary and his face was serious. ... [He] frequently leaned forward and rested his
  chin in one hand." [kunhardtB pp28-29]
  - ⟨$\frac{1}{q}$⟩ "Many pleasant allusions were made to him in the play, to which the au-   2572
    dience gave deafening responses, while Mr. Lincoln laughed heartily and
    bowed frequently to the gratified people." – James Suydam Knox [luthin p635]
  - ⟨$\frac{1}{q}$⟩ "never applauded with his hands, but he laughed heartily on occasion, and   2573
    his face spoke plainly of his approval." – Helen Coleman [luthin p636]
- ⟨$\frac{1}{q}$⟩ "Doesn't it strike you as queer that I, who couldn't cut the head off of a chicken,   2574
  and who was sick at the sight of blood, should be cast into the middle of a great
  war, with blood flowing all about me?" [donaldA p514]. See ¶2083

- During the Civil War Lincoln lost a large number of people close to him: 2575
  - ⟨1⟩ His son, Willie   2576
  - ⟨2⟩ Elmer Ellsworth – Lincoln "loved him like a younger brother" [burl p80]   2577
  - ⟨2⟩ Ben Hardin Helm – "a surrogate son" [burl p104]. Also [randallC p294]   2578
  - ⟨2⟩ Edward D. Baker – Lincoln had named a son after him [burl p104]. This was the   2579
    "keenest blow of all the war" [brooksR]; see ¶2512.
  - ⟨2⟩ James S. Wadsworth [burl p104]   2580

- ⟨$\frac{2}{c}$⟩ "Perhaps the greatest strength of his character was his lack of egotism." [burl p xiii]   2581
  - ⟨-⟩ But there are several references to his ambition, e.g. [wilson p127], [burl pp245-257]   2582

- ⟨2⟩ "Lincoln often thought of committing suicide." – William Herndon [hertz p412] *I*   2583
  do not put much stock in this. The phrasing is suspiciously close to Men-
  tor Graham's comment, which probably referred to the Ann Rutledge episode
  ¶2708.

- Summary by friends: 2584
  - ⟨1⟩ "He had his moods like other men. ... He was sometimes mirthful and some-   2585
    times sad, but both moods passed away and left him always the same man.
    ... Nevertheless he always had these spells of melancholy. ... And many times
    even [in the White House], he used to talk to me about his domestic trou-
    bles." – Orville Browning [nicolayO pp2-3] (See ¶2720 and ¶2465.)

Mental Status (continued)

⟨1⟩ As President: "He had naturally a most cheerful and sunny temper, was highly social and sympathetic, loved pleasant conversation, wit, anecdote and laughter. Beneath this, however, ran an under-current of sadness; he was occasionally subject to hours of deep silence and introspection that approached a condition of trance." – John Nicolay[browneF p736] (∈ ¶204)   2586

⟨1⟩ "I remember his face. . . . And yet my memory of him is not of an unhappy man. I hear so much to-day about the President's melancholy. It is true no man could suffer more. But he was very easily amused. I have never seen a man who enjoyed more anything pleasant or funny that came his way. I think the balance between pain and pleasure was fairly struck..." [crookA p77-78]   2587

⟨1⟩ "He had been happy in life. He was not less happy in death." [sumnerA p131]   2588

⟨2⟩c Was "deeply mysterious to the people who knew him best." [shenk p216]   2589

⟨1⟩q "Those who have spoken most confidently of their knowledge of his personal qualities are, as a rule, those who saw least of them below the surface." – Alexander McClure [shenk p216]   2590

- Diagnoses: 2591

⟨S⟩ "Without question, he meets the U.S. surgeon general's definition of mental illness, since he experienced 'alterations in thinking, mood, or behavior' that were associated with 'distress and/or impaired functioning.' Yet Lincoln also meets the surgeon general's criteria for mental health: 'the successful performance of mental functions, resulting in productive activities, fulfilling relationships with other people, and the ability to adapt to change and to cope with adversity' " [shenk p25]. Still, [shenk pp21-23, 99] claims Lincoln had episodes of major depression in 1835 and 1841, and afterwards had a chronic mental affliction he (Shenk) cannot name.   2592

⟨S⟩ cyclic personality – Karl Menninger [evans p330]   2593

⟨S⟩ Three academic psychiatrists are highly confident Lincoln met standard criteria for "major depressive disorder, recurrent, with psychotic features" – DSM code 296.34 – and that the disorder was evident in office [davidsonJ]. *I have not seen evidence of psychotic features during Lincoln's presidency. Embarrassingly, the psychiatrists consulted only chapters in history books and in medical history books, eschewing primary sources and book-length biographies.*   2594

⟨S⟩ Based on [shenk], two physicians (probably psychiatrists) see "ample evidence [of] an enduring and at times near-fatal depression." [goldberg]   2595

⟨S⟩ [donaldA p164] acknowledges proposed physical causes for Lincoln's melancholy, but such explanations (as applied to the mid-1850s, at least) "missed the essential point that Lincoln was frustrated and unhappy with a political career that seemed to be going nowhere."   2596

⟨1⟩ "[James] Matheny said he wasnt melancholy at all" – Henry Whitney [wilson p626] (but: ¶2471)   2597

⟨S⟩ To explain Lincoln's rapid changes between pessimism and supreme confidence (¶2333ff), [shenk p37] offers: "Because he felt deeper and thought harder than others, Lincoln could be expected to alternate among states more quickly, returning, more often than not, to sadness, disquiet, perturbation, and gloom." *Implies all deep thinkers have labile moods. Seems highly questionable.*   2598

⟨1⟩q Herndon describes Lincoln as having 3 states: gloomy, "joky," and "kindly thoughtful." [shenk p216]   2599

Mental Status (continued)

⟨2⟩ "Ward Lamon, attributed his 'melancholy' to his lack of religious faith." [shutes p83] 2600

⟨s⟩ Lincoln's self-mastery over his emotions is an indication of his superiority as a man. [evans pp328-329] citing [nicolayS p69] 2601

⟨s⟩ [rubenzer] applied the NEO PI-R personality inventory to information from seven Lincoln historians, and found that Lincoln was "moderately Neurotic, Extraverted, Agreeable, and Conscientious." He also scored high on openness. 2602

■ Diagnoses, old or not to be taken seriously: 2603

⟨s⟩ "psychoneurotic temperament" [shutes p32&39] 2604

⟨s⟩ "Lincoln's athletic-asthenic physique, suggestive of a schizoid (dual) personality" [shutes p38]. 2605

⟨s⟩ Other: "psychotic," "schizoid-manic," "a mother fixation of unusual intensity" – cited by [burl p361] 2606

■ Etiological hypothesis: Pre-natal influence: 2607

⟨1⟩ "Nancy Hanks Lincoln – was in a constant trepidation and frequent affrights from reasons we have talked together about while she was pregnant & these affrights & trepidations made a maternal *ante natal* impression on our hero: that was the most of it. This melancholy was stamped on him while in the period of gestation: it was part of his nature and could not more be shaken off than he could part with his brains." – Henry Whitney [wilson p617] (See ¶612.) *Whitney labeled this passage "private" in an 1887 letter to William Herndon, and then crossed out the passage.* 2608

⟨1⟩ Whitney again alludes to his hypothesis of ante natal impressions in [wilson pp625-626]. 2609

■ Etiological hypotheses: Miscellaneous: 2610

⟨s⟩ Lincoln's eye deviation "would prove to be a definite factor in contributing to and precipitating minor attacks of depression" [shutes p67] 2611

⟨s⟩ [shastid], a self-described "oculist," is also convinced Lincoln's ocular misalignment caused Lincoln's "deep and protracted melancholy," which could have been treated with "a prism for hyperphoria." See ¶872. 2612

⟨s⟩ Of Lincoln's melancholy: "Stuart said it all arose from abnormal digestion – from the failure of his liver to work" – Henry Whitney [wilson p626] (See ¶612.) 2613

⟨s⟩ Others: malaria, bad teeth, bad feet – cited by [evans p329] 2614

⟨s⟩ "If Lincoln had given his wife syphilis and if he had, inadvertently, caused the death of his children, the fits of melancholy are now understandable – and unbearably tragic." [vidalA p667] 2615

⟨2⟩ Writing in 1922, psychologist G. Stanley Hall unequivocally links Lincoln's mental development to his physical state: "His height, long limbs, rough exterior, and frequent feeling of awkwardness must have very early made him realize that to succeed in life he must cultivate intrinsic mental and moral traits. ... Hence he compensated by trying to develop intellectual distinction." [burl pp256-257] 2616

Mental Status – Job Stress and

⟨2⟩ 1847 or 1848: Lincoln decided his wife and (then) two children were interfering with his work as a Congressman, so he had them go live with Mary's family in Kentucky. [kunhardtA p75] 2617

Mental Status – Job Stress and (continued)

⟨2⟩ᶜ "The campaign for president had been a time of great stress for Lincoln"   2618
[hirschhornC]. *Although sensible, this conclusion is based on a description of Lincoln's physical appearance (¶1120), i.e. it assumes no organic cause was affecting his appearance. This assumption cannot be accepted.*

⟨1⟩ Mar. 4, 1861: Later "He told me that the very first thing placed in his hands after   2619
his inauguration was a letter from Majr [sic] Anderson announcing the impossibility of defending or relieving [Fort] Sumter." [browning p476, July 3, 1861]

⟨1⟩ As President: "Mr. Lincoln spent most of his evenings in his office, though occa-   2620
sionally he remained in the drawing room after dinner, conversing with visitors
or listening to music... In his office he was not often suffered to be alone; he frequently passed the evening there with a few friends in frank and free conversation. If the company was all of one sort he was at his best; his wit and rich humor
had free play; he was once more the Lincoln of the Eighth Circuit, the cheeriest
of talkers, the riskiest of story tellers; but if a stranger came in, he put on in an
instant his whole armor of dignity and reserve." – John Hay [angle p437]

⟨1⟩ As President: "Anything that kept the people away from him he disapproved –   2621
although they nearly annoyed the life out of him by unreasonable complaints &
requests." – John Hay [wilson p331]

- March-April 1861: The crisis over Ft. Sumter, which led to the first shots of the   2622
  Civil War, extended over several weeks and caused Lincoln immense stress.
  - ⟨1⟩ "He told me that ... all the troubles and anxieties of his life had not equalled   2623
    those which intervened between this time [inauguration day] and the fall
    of Sumter." – Lincoln [browning p476, July 3, 1861] *If this was the worst that
    the White House dealt him, then how can psychosomatic illness explain
    the greater change in his appearance from 1864 to 1865, compared to the
    change from 1860 to 1861?*
  - ⟨H⟩ "... of all the trials I have had since I came here none begin to compare with   2625
    those I had between the inauguration and the fall of Fort Sumter. They were
    so great that could I have anticipated them, I would not have believed it pos-
    sible to survive..." – Lincoln [shutesE p135]. *Did Shutes invent this quotation?
    Browning's actual diary statement is above.*
  - ⟨H⟩ March 7, 1861: The controversial "Diary of a Public Man" describes a hag-   2626
    gard, worn look on Lincoln's face [angle p341].
  - ⟨1⟩q March 31, 1861 (Sunday): "On Friday he confessed to a friend of mine that   2627
    he was in 'the dumps' & yesterday Mrs Lincoln told Russell that her husband
    had keeled over with sick headache for the first time in years." – Sam Ward
    [shenk p285, citing S.L.M. Barlow papers in the Huntington Library] *"In years" implies that
    there had been previous episodes of keeling over.*
  - ⟨S⟩ "The pressure was so great that Mary Lincoln reported that he 'keeled over'   2628
    and had to be put to bed with one of his rare migraine headaches" [donaldA
    p289]. *Donald goes beyond the data. He assumes the episode was caused
    by pressure and that the headache was migrainous.*
  - ⟨2⟩ Great demands on Lincoln continued after the firing on Ft. Sumter (April   2629
    12, 1861), "but now that he could clearly see what had to be done, he bore
    up well under the strain" [donaldA p301]. A visitor found Lincoln looking "very
    fresh and vigorous ... thoroughly calm and collected" [donaldA p301].
  - ⟨1⟩ [grimsley] describes Lincoln starting work at 5 a.m. "often." She thought "his   2630
    keen sense of humor ... afforded a kind of 'safety valve' from" the pressures
    upon him. See ¶647

Mental Status – Job Stress and (continued)

⟨1⟩ 1861: "Shortly after Bull Run I spent a whole afternoon with him alone – he excluded every one & relaxed himself by telling me stories & giving me his whole theory of the rebellion & his plan for putting it down." – Henry C. Whitney [wilson p399] 2631

⟨1⟩ July 8, 1861: "President Lincoln, thus far, bears his load of responsibility wonderfully well. ... at times wears a wearied and harassed look..." [stoddardB p14] (∈ ¶1140) 2632

⟨1/q⟩ Aug. 1861: Lincoln was so badgered by office-seekers that he told Robert L. Wilson: "the only way he [Lincoln] could escape from them would be to take a rope and hang himself, on one of the trees on the lawn south of the President's house." [kunhardtA p154] 2633

⟨1/q⟩ Mar. 8, 1862: "He was as cheerful as he had been on the morning of the previous day." – L.E. Chittenden [angle p380] 2634

⟨1⟩ April 25, 1862: After a 90 minute visit with Orville Browning, that included poetry reading, Lincoln, with a headache (see ¶1145), "said a crowd was buzzing about the door like bees, ready to pounce upon him as soon as I should take my departure, and bring him back to a realization of the annoyances and harrassments [sic] of his position." [browning p543] 2635

⟨2⟩ Late June 1862: Union forces faring poorly in the Seven Days' Battles. Lincoln worried "incessantly" [donaldA p358]. See ¶655 and ¶1150. 2636

⟨1⟩ June 1862: Lincoln was once asked if he had ever despaired of the country. "When the Peninsular campaign terminated so suddenly at Harrison's Landing I was as nearly inconsolable as I could be and live." [ChicagoTribune - Dec. 3, 1865] 2637

⟨2⟩ Aug. 1862: During the Second Battle of Bull Run (August 28-30, 1862): "Exhausted from long hours spent in the telegraph office attempting to learn the news and trying to speed reinforcements to Pope's army, Lincoln fell into a deep depression." [donaldA p371] 2638

⟨1/q⟩ After the Union defeat at second Bull Run, and tormented by difficulties finding a competent general to command the Army, Lincoln told his cabinet "he felt almost ready to hang himself" [donaldA p372] 2639

⟨2⟩ The approaching 1862 mid-term elections stressed the President. "Ordinarily the master of his emotions, he let his self-control slip at times" [donaldA p382] 2640

⟨2⟩ Dec. 1862: "Visitors to the White House around this time often found Lincoln hopeless and distressed." [shenk p187] *There is no clear primary reference for this.* 2641

⟨2⟩ February 1863: Was "deeply despondent" [donaldA p426]. Admiral Dahlgren observed "the President never tells a joke now" [donaldA p426]. (∈ ¶2532) 2642

⟨2⟩ April-May 1863: "The weeks after the battle of Chancellorsville were among the most depressing of Lincoln's Presidency." [donaldA p437] 2643

⟨1⟩ "I shall never forget that picture of despair. ... I mechanically noticed that his face, usually sallow, was ashen in hue. The paper on the wall behind him was of the tint known as 'French gray' ... I vaguely took in the thought the thought that the complexion of the anguished President's visage was almost exactly like that of the wall. ... Never, as long as I knew him, did he seem to be so broken, so dispirited, and so ghostlike. Clasping his hands behind his back, he walked up and down the room, saying 'My God! My God! What will the country say! What will the country say!" – Noah Brooks [brooksC pp57-58] 2644

Mental Status – Job Stress and (continued)

⟨2⟩ After Chancellorsville: Secretary of War Stanton says Lincoln "was at the brink of suicide in the Potomac River." [shutesE p158]   2645

■ July 1863: After the battle of Gettysburg, General Meade did not pursue the rebel army: 2646

   ⟨$\frac{1}{q}$⟩ "On only one or two occasions have I ever seen the President so troubled, so dejected and discouraged." – Gideon Welles [angle p456]   2647

   ⟨2⟩ Robert "saw his father's head bowed in tears" [shutesE p160]   2648

   ⟨$\frac{1}{q}$⟩ Was "very unwell ... had scarcely tasted food during the day." [shutesE p160]   2649

⟨$\frac{1}{q}$⟩ July 4, 1863: After capture of Vicksburg "very happy in the prospect of a brilliant success" – John Hay [shenk p192] citing [hayD p61]   2650

⟨$\frac{1}{q}$⟩ August 1863: John Hay thought Lincoln "in fine whack. I have rarely seen him more serene & busy. He is managing this war, the draft, foreign relations, and planning a reconstruction of the Union, all at once." [burl p13] [kunhardtA p216]   2651

⟨$\frac{2}{c}$⟩ 1864: "From the dizzying heights of the year's early months, with Lincoln at the peak of his popularity, it was a long fall to where the President stood by summer. ... By August, Lincoln's re-election looked impossible." [kunhardtA p256]   2652

⟨1⟩ Feb. 1864: "This war is eating my life out." – Lincoln [carpenter p17]   2653

   ⟨$\frac{1}{q}$⟩ Lincoln also remarked (date not provided) that his life was being "eaten out from the inside." [kunhardtA p343]   2654

⟨1⟩ About 1864: "I have never known so great a change to take place in any man's appearance as in Mr. Lincoln's during the three years following the day when I first saw him – March 4, 1861. ... He had a very dejected appearance" [croffut] (∈ ¶196)   2655

⟨1⟩ Mar. 20, 1864 (per [miers]): Stoddard is in Lincoln's office on a sunny Sunday: "It is as good as medicine to find him so cheerful this morning. ... laughing silently ...[the conversation turns to the new Army commander, Grant] with such a look of almost relief upon his worn and wrinkled face. ... the long, quiet laugh which interrupts his humorous commentary convinces you that he is, indeed, feeling vastly relieved." [stoddardA pp125-126] (∈ ¶3001)   2656

⟨2⟩ May 1864: "During the first week of the battles of the Wilderness he scarcely slept at all. Passing through the main hall of the domestic apartment on one of these days, I met him, clad in a long morning wrapper, pacing back and forth ... his hands behind him, great black rings under his eyes, his head bent forward upon his breast" [carpenter p30]   2657

⟨1⟩ May-June 1864: Nearly constant fighting at Wilderness, Spotsylvania Court House, North Anna, Cold Harbor. "During those long days of terrible slaughter the face of the President was grave and anxious, and he looked like one who had lost the dearest member of his own family." [arnold pp374-375]   2658

⟨$\frac{2}{c}$⟩ July 1864: "One of the darkest seasons of Lincoln's presidency," owing to political and military difficulties. [kunhardtA p244]   2659

   ⟨$\frac{1}{q}$⟩ As rebel forces near Washington, Lincoln is "very much irritated" when evacuated from his summer residence, and is "greatly ... annoyed" to learn that a boat has been prepared to remove him from the city. – Noah Brooks [kunhardtA p245]   2660

⟨2⟩ July 12, 1864: Lincoln visits Ft. Stevens, where forces are engaged. "For the first time in his life Abraham Lincoln saw men in battle action go to their knees and   2661

Mental Status – Job Stress and (continued)

sprawl on he earth with cold lead in their vitals. ... While he stood watching this bloody drama, a bullet whizzed five feet from him, was deflected, and struck [a surgeon] in the ankle. While he yet stood there, within three feet of the President, an officer fell with a death wound. Those who were there that afternoon said he was cool and thoughtful, seemed unconscious of danger, and looked like a Commander in Chief." [angle pp469-470] excerpting Carl Sandburg

⟨2⟩ The surgeon was C.C.V.A. Crawford, of the 102nd Pennsylvania Volunteers; he lived [shutes p106]. 2662

⟨1/q⟩ "Amid the whizzing bullets" Lincoln held his place with "grave and passive countenance" – Nicolay and Hay [angle p470]. 2663

⟨2⟩ "The story goes" that a young Oliver Wendell Holmes (a future Supreme Court justice) scolded Lincoln to "Get down, you fool." [randallC p305] *I believe the exact quote was "you damn fool."* 2664

⟨2⟩ Lincoln may have visited the fort on another day, too. [randallC p305] 2665

⟨1⟩ Aug. 1864, after the Battle of Mobile Bay: "He was now buoyant with hope, and began to expect an early termination of the war." [arnold p383] 2666

⟨1⟩ Aug. 1864: The Governor of Wisconsin proposes "Why can't you seek seclusion, and play hermit for a fortnight? it [sic] would reinvigorate you." Lincoln replied "Aye, two or three weeks would do me good, but I cannot fly from my thoughts..." [carpenter p305] 2667

⟨1⟩ Jan. 17, 1865: At a Cabinet meeting "The President was happy." [welles v2p227] 2668

⟨1/q⟩ Jan. 31, 1865: When Congress passed the 13th Amendment (outlawing slavery), Lincoln was "filled ... with joy." That night he slept like never before, according to the daughter of his personal sevant. [kunhardtA p270] 2669

⟨2/c⟩ In his last two years Lincoln became more often "peevish," "petulant," and so forth because of "the protracted and irritable condition of his nervous system, resulting from excessive labor, mental suffering, and loss of sleep." [burl p205] citing [holland pp453,487] 2670

⟨1/q⟩ "Mr. Lincoln did not retain the external equanimity of his earlier days under the galling pressure of the burdens laid upon him in 1863." – W.O. Stoddard [burl pp205-206] 2671

⟨H⟩ An account of Lincoln noting "I become about as savage as a wild cat by Saturday night, drained dry of the 'milk of human kindness,' " is from an interview that is admittedly "overdrawn" [burl pp207,235] 2672

⟨1⟩ During Presidency: Friends "saw the wrinkles on his face and forehead deepen into furrows, the laugh of old days was less frequent, and it did not seem to come from the heart. Anxiety, responsibility, care, thought, disasters, defeats, the injustice of friends, wore upon his giant frame. ... During these four years he had no respite, no holidays." [arnold pp453-454]" (∈ ¶186) 2673

⟨1/q⟩ circa 1865: A visitor asks if shaking hands in a receiving line for two hours is harder than office duties. Lincoln replies: "Oh, no-no. Of course, this is tiresome physically; but I am pretty strong, and it rests me, after all, for nobody is cross or exacting, and no man asks me for what I can't give him." [harris p57] 2674

⟨1⟩ 1865: "Even when awakened suddenly from a deep sleep – ... the most searching test of one's temper that I know – he was never ruffled, but received the message and the messenger kindly. No employee of the White House ever saw the President moved beyond his usual controlled calm." [crookA p11] 2675

Mental Status – Job Stress and (continued)

⟨⅟q⟩ March 4, 1865: As Vice President Andrew Johnson delivered an "incoherent harangue" for an inauguration speech, Lincoln "bowed his head with a look of unutterable despondency" [burl p168] 2676

  ⟨2⟩ Recovering from typhoid fever, Johnson had taken three "stiff drinks" of whiskey beforehand to steady his nerves [leech p453]. Compounding this, even when sober he had an uncontrolled oratorical style when speaking extemporaneously that could "easily be mistaken for a drunkard" [kunhardtB p108]. 2677

⟨1⟩ March 15, 1865, at the theater: "I am hounded to death by office-seekers, who pursue me early and late, and it is simply to get two or three hours' relief that I am here." [wilsonR pp424-425] (∈ ¶1238) 2678

⟨2⟩ March 1865: "The war was being won, peace was in sight. ... He apparently relaxed and became domestic, confiding, and forthright, as he had been before the pressure of the presidency had made it well-nigh impossible for him to be Lincoln the husband." [evans p240] 2679

- April 1865: The end of the rebellion made Lincoln a happy man. (See ¶2551ff.) 2680

Mental Status – Women and

This collection was originally begun to show that, as an unattractive man with access to only a small gene pool, Lincoln may have been wounded by women more deeply than better looking men with more money. The theory is probably true, but it does not play a role in major themes of the physical Lincoln. 2681

⟨H⟩ In Indiana: Rejected by Susie Enlow because "my feet and hands were too big, and my legs and arms too long." [paulmier p26] 2682

- In recent years Lincoln students have debated his attitude toward women. [tripp], argues that Lincoln's inclinations were predominantly homosexual. Usefully, the book also includes essays by other scholars, some supporting and some countering Tripp's argument. [burl pp123-146] is a chapter on Lincoln's attitude towards women, by one of the scholars who disagrees with Tripp. The paragraph below, the second saddest herein, relates the effects of the physical Lincoln in youth upon the opposite sex. It is not hard to fathom how his mental state may have been influenced as a result. (See also ¶2616) 2683

  ⟨⅟q⟩ Girl #1 (knew him in Indiana): "I never found any fault with him excepting he was so tall and awkward. All the young girls my age made fun of Abe. They'd laugh at him right before his face, but Abe never 'peared to care. He was so good and he'd just laugh with them. Abe tried to go with some of them, but no sir-ee, they'd give him the mitten every time, just because he was so tall and gawky, and it was mighty awkward I can tell you trying to keep company with a fellow as tall as Abe was." [burl pp123-124] 2684

  ⟨2⟩ Girl #2: "his awkwardness and large feet" were unattractive [burl p124] 2685

  ⟨⅟q⟩ Girl #3: Lincoln "wus [sic] so quiet and awkward and so awful homely." The "girls did not much care" about him, and Lincoln "never made up to the girls." [burl p124] 2686

  ⟨⅟q⟩ Girl #4: Her friends "unmercifully" teased her because Lincoln, with his "coatsleeves and pantlegs always being too short," was courting her. [burl p124] 2687

⟨2⟩ It's been noted that all the women Lincoln loved were plump [donaldA p56] 2688

| Mental Status – Women and (continued) | Abraham |

⟨2⟩ "Frisky interest in his stepsister Matilda" [kunhardtA p38] *Maybe derives from* [hertz pp422-423]. 2689

⟨1⟩ "I never could get him in Company with women: he was not a timid man in this particular, but did not seek such company." – John Hanks [wilson p455] 2690

    ⟨1/q⟩ "He was very reserved toward the opposite sex." – Dr. Jason Duncan [walsh p101] 2691

⟨1/q⟩ "Lincoln ought never to have married anyone. He had no quality for a husband. He was abstracted, cool, never loved." – William Herndon [hertz p183] 2692

    ⟨1/q⟩ "so great & peculiar a man as Lincoln could not make any woman happy. I guess he was too much allied to his intellect to get down to the plane of the domestic relations." – Henry Whitney [burl p319] 2693

⟨1/q⟩ 1830s: "He frequently visited from 1833 to 1837 young ladies" – Caleb Carman [walsh p100] 2694

■ Summer 1835: Reaction to the death of Ann Rutledge on Aug. 25. For more than 100 years Lincoln students have argued whether Ann Rutledge was the great love of Lincoln's life (reviewed by [walsh]). This question is, fortunately, largely irrelevant to the physical Lincoln. After some introductory remarks, a summary of Lincoln's reaction to her death, chiefly from [wilson], is presented. 2695

    ⟨2⟩ The length of Rutledge's illness has been "variously estimated at a week or two to a month or more." [walsh p120] 2696

    ⟨-⟩ *Before and after Rutledge died, Lincoln was afflicted with a major febrile illness, probably malaria (¶2008ff and Special Topic §1). He took "heroic doses" of medicines for it, while spending significant time tending to the ill Rutledge. Lincoln's entire community was hard-hit by sickness that summer. He lost many friends and helped build many coffins.* [rankinA pp72-87] 2697

    ⟨1/q⟩ After Rutledge's death, "Lincoln bore up under it very well until some days afterward a heavy rain fell, which unerved [sic] him." – John Hill [walsh p64] 2699

    ⟨1⟩ "it was a great shock to him and I never seen a man mourn for a companion more than he did for her he made a remark one day when it was raining that he could not bare the idea of its raining on her Grave that was the time the community said he was crazy he was not crazy but he was very disponding a long time I Think that was in the year 34 or 35" – Elizabeth Abell [wilson p557] 2700

    ⟨1⟩ "The effect upon Mr Lincoln's mind was terrible; he became plunged in despair, and many of his friends feared that reason would desert her throne." – Robert Rutledge [wilson p383] 2701

    ⟨1⟩ "During her last illness he visited her sick chamber and on his return stopped at my house. It was very evident that he was much distressed. I was not surprised when it was rumored subsequently that his reason was in danger." – John Jones [wilson p387] 2702

    ⟨1⟩ Friends "were Compelled to keep watch and ward over Mr. Lincoln, he being from the sudden shock somewhat temporarily deranged. We watched during storms – fogs – damp gloomy weather Mr Lincoln for fear of an accident. He said 'I can never be reconcile to have the snow – rains & storms to beat on her grave.' " – William Greene [wilson p21] 2703

    ⟨1/q⟩ "Often heard Father tell of his having to lock Mr. Lincoln up in a room to prevent suicide after Ann Rutledge's death – Every effort was made to divert his mind – as a fact for a short time his mind wandered." – John Hill [walsh p168] 2704

191

Mental Status – Women and (continued)

⟨1⟩ "He may not have been for a time totally insane but he was so near that con- 2705
dition that everybody who saw and knew him at once set him down as insane." – William McNeely [walsh p104] *This is second-hand. See the reference
for a more extensive excerpt.*

⟨1/q⟩ "After Ann died I remember that it was common talk about how sad Lincoln 2706
was; and I remember how sad he looked. They told me that every time he
was in the neighborhood after she died, he would go alone to her grave &
sit there in silence for hours." – Jean Rutledge Berry [walsh p97] quoting from
diary of R.D. Miller as printed by Ida Tarbell

⟨1⟩ "with the death of one whom he dearly & sincerely loved, a momentary – 2707
only partial & momentary derangement." – Mentor Graham [wilson p11]

⟨1⟩ "Lincoln told Me that he felt like Committing Suicide often, but I told him 2708
God higher purpose [sic]" – Mentor Graham [wilson p243] *Probably, but not
certainly, refers to after Rutledge's death.*

⟨1⟩ "As to the condition of Lincoln's Mind after the death of Miss R. after that 2709
Event he seemed quite *changed*, he seemed *Retired*, & loved *Solitude*, he
seemed wraped [sic] in *profound thought, indifferent*, to transpiring Events,
had but Little to say, but would take his gun and wander off in the woods
by him self, away from the association of even those he most esteemed, this
gloom seemed to deepen for some time, so as to give anxiety to his friends
in regard to his Mind, But various opinions obtained as to the Cause of his
change, some thought it was an increased application to his *Law studies*,
Others that it was deep anguish of Soul (as he was all soul) over the Loss
of Miss R, My opinion is, & was, that it was from the Latter cause" – Henry
McHenry [wilson pp155-156] *The emphases are McHenry's. The mention of
Lincoln carrying a gun reduces the believability of this remembrance, as
Lincoln himself stated that he did not hunt (¶2083).*

⟨1⟩ After her death, "I thought he had lost some of his former vivacity" – John 2710
McNamar [wilson p253]

⟨1⟩ "Abe – Is it true – Said Cogdale, that you ran a little wild about the matter: 2712
[paragraph] I did really – I run off the track: it was my first. I loved the woman
dearly..." – Isaac Cogdal, recalling 1860 (or later) conversation with Lincoln
[wilson p440]

⟨1⟩ "you ask about the Crazy spell. It is my opinion that if Mr. Lincoln was craz 2713
[sic] it only technically so – and not radically & substantially so. We used to
say – you were Crazy about Ann Rutledge. He was then reading Blackstone
[a law book] – read hard – day & night – terribly hard – did love Ann Rutledge
for he told me so – was terribly melancholy – moody" – Isaac Cogdal [wilson
p441]

⟨1⟩ "as to Mr Lincolns Crazy Spell I do not recollect." – George Spears [wilson p410] 2714
⟨1⟩ "With regard to the crazy Spell of Mr Lincoln, I had never heard of it Before." 2715
– John McNamar. James Short told McNamar that Lincoln's spell related to
Mary Todd, later. [wilson p493] *McNamar did not hear about many things; he
was not in Illinois when Rutledge died.*

⟨1⟩ "know nothing of his crazy spell – do know of the one in Springfield in 1841 2716
– or 2" – John Stuart [wilson p519]

⟨2⟩ "A week after the burial of Ann Rutledge, Bill Green found him rambling 2717
in the woods along the Sangamon River, mumbling sentences Bill couldn't
make out. They watched him and tried to keep him safe among friends at
New Salem. And he rambled darkly and idly past their circle to the burying

Mental Status – Women and (continued)	Abraham

ground seven miles away, where he lay with an arm across the one grave" [sandburgP v1pp189-190]. Per [burk p49], this account is "more of poetry rather than sober historical writing."

⟨1⟩ Other accounts of his reaction: [wilson pp25 (see ¶95), 73, 80, 325, 397].　　2718

⟨1⟩ "It was said that after the death of Miss Rutledge & because of it, Lincoln was　2719 locked up by his friends – Saml Hill and others, to prevent derangement or suicide – so hard did he take her death." – Hardin Bale [wilson p13] (Hill was in love with Rutledge, too [wilson p397], but she had rejected him before accepting the suit of McNamar.)

⟨1⟩ Except for the 1841 episode with Mary (¶2746), "There was never any other　2720 occasion to my knowledge, in the whole course of his life which gave the least indication of any aberration of mind." – Orville Browning [nicolayO p3] (See ¶2465 and ¶2585.)

⟨1⟩ At Bowling Green's house, "kept him a week or two & succeeded in cheer-　2721 ing him Lincoln up though he was quite molencoly [sic] for months" – Mrs. Bowling Green [wilson p236]

⟨1⟩ "young Lincoln was heartbroken and prostrate. The histories have not ex-　2722 aggerated his pitiful grief. For many days he was not able to attend to busi-ness. ... His friends did everything that kindness could suggest, but in vain, to soothe his sorrow." [rossH pp100-101] *Ross talks about Lincoln crying "One stormy winter's night," but Rutledge died in August.*

⟨1⟩ Dec. 1866 letter to Herndon: "The point in the lecture that lacks, chiefly, is　2723 that, – at the death of Miss Rutledge, – when, apparently, Mr. Lincoln's mind gives away. You do not claim for Lincoln 'insanity' in your statement of the facts, yet in attendant circumstances you insinuate it, and in the words you put into Mr. Lincoln's mouth there is positive insanity. The phrase, 'insanity of Lincoln,' is a shock to all who did not know of the facts. [paragraph] I learn through my mother – who, personally, was acquainted with Miss Rutledge, – that Mr. Lincoln's grief, not 'insanity,' was well known. This charge is some-thing so entirely new – you being the first to publish the story, and for so long his law partner, – the world is asking you stern questions, and it will consider that you have overdrawn the picture from the fact of his sudden recovery." – Henry Rankin, 1866 [rankinA pp92-93]

⟨2⟩ Of the 24 people who provided Herndon with information about Rutledge's　2724 death, 17 of them "said, at least, that Lincoln had grieved to an unusual de-gree after Rutledge's death, and many considered that he had had a brush with insanity." [shenk p222] citing work of [wilsonH]

⟨2⟩ Was back on his surveying job by Sept. 24 at the latest. [donaldA p57]　　2726

■ Summer 1835: Speculations regarding Ann Rutledge (non-Herndon):　　2727

⟨2⟩c A book dedicated to the Ann Rutledge incident says that the depth and dura-　2728 tion of Lincoln's "depression" after her death is a "still-vexed" question [walsh p121].

⟨S⟩ "At the time of Ann Rutledge's death... it was only when he was absolutely　2729 prostrated by 'chills and fever' that he gave up. As soon as that illness had abated he went about his business." [tarbellB pp227-228](∈ ¶2479)

⟨S⟩ Could biological (physical) factors have influenced Lincoln's reaction? Hard　2732 data are scarce, but there is much room for speculation. (1) At a very general level, fever and mood are linked, as Osler half-jokingly suggests: "Notice the post-febrile frown. Toxins act on the frowning center" [aa15 p126]. (2) Severe

Mental Status – Women and (continued)

forms of malaria will involve the brain. (3) Lincoln's "heroic doses" of Peruvian bark, boneset tea, jalap and calomel [rankinA p74] are intriguing: (a) Peruvian bark contains quinine (¶2005). Even at low doses quinine can cause a hypersensitivity reaction. Higher doses may cause "cinchonism," a syndrome that, in its mildest form, includes tinnitus, headache, nausea, and disturbed vision. If usual dosing continues, or if there has been a large single dose, the nervous system may become involved with symptoms such as "apprehension, excitement, confusion, delirium" [aa99]. (b) Toxic doses of calomel (contains Hg_2Cl_2) can produce depression and many other symptoms [aa119]. If Lincoln were taking other mercury-containing medications at the same time (¶612ff), the likelihood of toxic effects would be increased. (c) "Boneset tea" is the benign-sounding name for an emetic [aa37 pp66-67] that includes hepatotoxic pyrrolizidine alkaloids from the plant *Symphytum officinale*. (d) Jalap, little discussed in today's medical literature, was a "well-known" purgative in 1870, whose action was generally increased by adding calomel [chambers v5pp673-674].

- Summer 1835: Herndon's views of Ann Rutledge incident (incomplete):   2733
  - ⟨1⟩ "You ask me if Mr. Lincoln was ever crazy in Mendard County – was insane   2734 in 1835; and in answer to which I say – he was, as the people in that region understood craziness or insanity, and I *fear* much worse than I painted it." (written Nov. 1866) [hertz p36]
  - ⟨1⟩ "Mr. Lincoln's mind was shocked, shattered, by Miss Ann Rutledge's death."   2736 [hertz p42]
  - ⟨1/ⓠ⟩ While recuperating at Bowling Green's house, his friends entertained him   2737 in many ways. "He evidently enjoyed all, as man scarcely ever enjoyed two weeks before, nor since." – Herndon [walsh p18]
  - ⟨1⟩ Herndon refers to the Rutledge incident in [hertz pp52, 64, 66, 154].   2738

- ⟨1⟩ Dec. 13, 1836, writing to girlfriend Mary Owens from Vandalia, IL: "I have been   2739 ill ever since my arrival here, or I should have written sooner. ... You recollect I mentioned in the outset of this letter that I had been unwell. That is the fact, though I believe I am about well now; but that, with other things I can not account for, have conspired and have gotten my spirits so low, that I feel that I would rather be any place in the world than here. I really can not endure the though of staying here ten weeks. Write back as soon as you get this, and if possible say something that will please me, for really I have not [been] pleased since I left you. This letter is so dry and [stupid] that I am ashamed to send it, but with my pres[ent feel]ings I can not do any better." [baslerA v1pp55-56] *Lincoln arrived in Vandalia no later than Dec. 5.*
  - ⟨S⟩ Shutes states that Lincoln had been physically unwell [shutes pp21-22]. *This is*   2740 *not clear from the letter itself.*

- ⟨1⟩ May 7, 1837: Writing to girlfriend Mary Owens, this time from Springfield, Lincoln   2741 complains of loneliness. "I have been spoken to by but one woman since I've been here, and should not have been by her, if she could have avoided it." In the next sentence he says he has not yet been to church, and probably will not go, "because I am conscious I should not know how to behave myself." The next paragraph reminds Owens of the poverty she must endure if she "cast[s] her lot" with him. Lincoln concludes by asking her to (a) write him a long letter and (b) stop her sister from discussing the possibility of him "selling out and moving. That gives me the hypo whenever I think of it." [baslerA v1pp79-80]

Mental Status – Women and (continued)

⟨2⟩ This is the first time Lincoln used the word "hypo" in a letter [shutesE p52]. 2742

⟨2⟩ For people of Lincoln's time, *hypo* meant "a morbid depression of spirits" [aa86]. For example, Melville's *Moby-Dick* (1851) uses *hypo* in its famous opening paragraph to mean "a state of depression somewhat more chronic and morbid than our 'blues'" [aa76 p12n]. Although *hypo* was short for *hypochondria*, modern readers should not confuse it with *hypochondriasis*, which is the erroneous belief of being afflicted by disease [shutesE p52]. 2743

⟨1/q⟩ After ending his courtship of Mary Owens, Lincoln wrote: "Others have been made fools of by the girls; but this can never be with truth said of me." [kunhardtA p55] 2744

⟨1⟩ "I knew Mr L well – he was a cold Man – had no affection – was not Social – was abstracted – thoughtful. ... Could not hold a lengthy Conversation with a lady – was not sufficiently Educated & intelligent in the female line to do so" – Elizabeth Todd Edwards [wilson p443] 2745

- January 1841: In low spirits after a rift with Mary Todd: 2746
  ⟨-⟩ See [randallC pp30-56] [shenk pp43-65] [wilsonH pp233ff] and Special Topic §3 for detailed treatments. 2747
  ⟨2⟩ In the first week of January Lincoln was still able to conduct business, but then took to bed for about a week, seeing less than a handful of people. By the end of January he was back at work, but listlessly and sporadically. [donaldA pp 87-88] 2748
  ⟨2⟩ "the proven fact that Lincoln attended the legislature on January 2 ... and that he made at least a brief appearance there every day except one (January 4) until January 13. He was then confined to the house for a week with a physical illness..." [randallC pp45-46] "what sounds very much like a severe case of the 'flu'" [randallC p48]. *There is too little information to support a specific diagnosis.* 2749
  ⟨1⟩ After the rift, "strong Brandy was administered freely for about one Week" – Abner Ellis [wilson p238] 2750
  ⟨1/q⟩ Jan. 12-19 ("the missing days"): Lincoln spent "several hours each day" with Drs Anson Henry and Elias Merryman – H.W. Thornton [wilsonH p235] 2751
  ⟨2⟩ Although stories later emerged about friends keeping all sharp objects away from him, the depth of his depression is uncertain [donaldA p87]. Orville Browning, for example said Lincoln was "incoherent and distraught," but this "was only an intensification of his constitutional melancholy" [shutes pp24-25]. H.W. Thornton said "His most intimate friends had no fear of him injuring himself" [wilsonH p35]. 2752
  ⟨1⟩ Jan. 27, 1841: "The Doctors say he came within an inch of being a perfect lunatic for life. He was perfectly crazy for some time, not able to attend to his business at all." – Jane Bell [wilsonH p237] 2753
  ⟨1⟩ "He was so much affected as to talk incoherently, and to be delirious to the extent of not knowing what he was doing. In the course of a few days it all passed off, leaving no trace whatever. I think it was only an intensification of his constitutional melancholy..." – Orville Browning [nicolayO p2] 2754
  ⟨1/q⟩ Jan. 16: "We have been very much distressed, on Mr. Lincoln's account; hearing that he had two Cat fits and a Duck fit since we left." [wilsonH p236] [burl p99] *An on-line thesaurus equates both "cat fit" and "duck fit" with "upset."* 2755
  ⟨2⟩ There were apparently physical consequences, too. See ¶1114 for weight loss note. 2756

Mental Status – Women and (continued)

⟨2⟩ "The period following the broken engagement was perhaps the lowest point in Abraham Lincoln's life." [turner p28] 2758

⟨-⟩ Lincoln wrote a mysterious letter to Dr. Daniel Drake about this time. (See ¶2467.) 2759

- January 1841: Herndon's view of mental break: 2760
  ⟨1⟩ "Did you know that Mr. Lincoln was *'as crazy as a loon' in this city in 1841;* that he did not sit, did not attend to the Legislature, but in part, if any (special session of 1841); that he was then deranged? Did you know that he was forcibly arrested by his special friends here at that time; that they had to remove all razors, knives, pistols, etc. from his room and presence, that he might not commit suicide?" Herndon then speculates on the cause of this spell. [hertz p37] 2761

⟨1⟩ At some point after the break-up, Mary tells Lincoln "he was in honor bound to marry her. ... Lincoln was crazy for a week or so – not knowing what to do" – James Matheny [wilson p251] 2762

  ⟨1⟩ "During 1842 he [Matheny] though [sic] that L would Commit Suicide" [wilson p251] *No cause for Lincoln's desperation is given. This statement appears in Herndon's 1866 interview of Matheny, two paragraphs after the statement about a Mary-crazed Lincoln (¶2762); so this almost certainly relates to 1841, not 1842. Unjustifiably, I believe,* [shenk pp95-96] *paints Matheny's remark as a concern that Lincoln was generally suicidal.* 2763

⟨2⟩ June 19, 1841: Writes a "cheerful" letter to Joshua Speed, relating "a delightful 'who-dunit,' skillfully told." [randallC p51] 2764

⟨2⟩ Third quarter, 1841: Visits Joshua Speed in Kentucky. 2765
  ⟨1/q⟩ Sept. 27, 1841, back in Illinois: Lincoln writes a thank-you note to Speed's sister, reminder her that he had to lock her in a room "to prevent your committing an assault and battery upon me." [randallC pp52-53] 2766

⟨2⟩ 1842: Lincoln and Mary keep secret their plans to marry until the morning of the wedding. [turner pp29-30] 2767

⟨1⟩ 1842, his wedding day: Lincoln "looked and acted as if he was going to the Slaughter" – James Matheny (the best man) [wilson p251] 2768

⟨S⟩ John Nicolay wrote that Lincoln's melancholy spells ended after he married [evans p328]. This is widely disputed [evans pp329-331]. 2769

⟨S⟩ Lincoln's relationship with Mary during their marriage was not always smooth. For examples, see ¶3433, ¶3589, ¶3593, ¶3595, ¶4372, ¶4373, ¶4382, ¶4393, ¶4399. Herndon said: "his domestic life was a hell, a burning, scorching hell" [hertz p204]. A fair or balanced account of their relationship is beyond the scope of this book. 2770
  ⟨2⟩ Circa 1862: "President and Mrs. Lincoln began to drift apart." [donaldH p93] 2771
  ⟨2⟩ Other communication difficulties mentioned Sept. 1862 [turner pp133-134] 2772
  ⟨2⟩ "In the last year of their life together, there appears to have been a lack of communication and considerable tension between the President and his wife." [turner p183] 2773
  ⟨-⟩ For sleeping apart, see ¶3438ff. 2774

Mouth

"The degree of fullness of the lips reflects the amount of prognathism of the upper and lower jaws." [aa89 p32] · 2775

⟨$\frac{1}{q}$⟩ Size: · 2776

   ⟨$\frac{1}{q}$⟩ About 1835: "big ears and mouth" – Nancy Rutledge Prewitt [walsh p42] (∈ ¶102) · 2777

   ⟨$\frac{1}{q}$⟩ "large mouth" – John Nicolay [meserve p5] (∈ ¶177) · 2778

   ⟨$\frac{1}{q}$⟩ "His mouth was large" [arnold p441] (∈ ¶167) · 2779

   ⟨1⟩ "capacious mouth" [piatt p347] · 2780

   ⟨1⟩ March 1861: "the mouth is absolutely prodigious" – William Russell [russell pp37-38] (∈ ¶161) · 2781

   ⟨1⟩ "his big mouth" [salmsalm p144] (∈ ¶190) · 2782

   ⟨$\frac{1}{q}$⟩ "small lascivious mouth" – Elliott Herndon [herndon p470n] (∈ ¶1604) · 2783

   ⟨$\frac{1}{q}$⟩ Mid 1863: "large and expressive mouth." – Silas Burt [wilsonR p332] (∈ ¶1621) · 2784

- Lips: · 2785

   ⟨2⟩ As a youth: Josiah (Old Blue Nose) "Crawford was the only one among his neighbors, so far as I know, that ever remarked Lincoln's habit of sticking out his left lower lip when his mind was concentrating in reading or thinking. This habit, fallen into in his youth, resulted in that protuberance of the lower lip which is a distinguishing feature of his face. Crawford used to banter the boy on his 'stuck out lip.' In 1844, after fourteen year's absence from southwestern Indiana, Lincoln came back in the Harrison campaign to speak at Rockport, his old county seat, and Josiah Crawford went down to hear him. In those days an Indiana audience measured the importance of a speaker by the numbers of books and pamphlets he brought with him. Lincoln came without a printed page, and it bothered Mr. Crawford. 'Where's your books, Abe?' he asked. 'I haven't any. Sticking out my lip is all I need.' The old man told this tale with glee to his death. It was their own little joke!" [tarbellB pp140-141] *Harrison ran in 1840, not 1844.* · 2786

   ⟨$\frac{1}{q}$⟩ "thin upper and somewhat thick under lip" – John Nicolay [meserve p5] (∈ ¶177) · 2787

   ⟨$\frac{1}{q}$⟩ June 21, 1860: "The lips were full of character" – newspaper reporter [linclore-HDE] (∈ ¶159) · 2788

   ⟨1⟩ March 1861: "the lips, straggling and extending almost from one line of black beard to the other, are only kept in order by two deep furrows from the nostril to the chin" – William Russell [russell pp37-38] (∈ ¶161) · 2789

   ⟨1⟩ 1862: "a close-set, thin-lipped, stern mouth" [dicey v1pp220-221] (∈ ¶179) · 2790

   ⟨1⟩ April 1865: "his lips at the same time thick and delicate" [chambrunA] (∈ ¶200) · 2791

   ⟨$\frac{1}{q}$⟩ "There is a peculiar curve of the lower lip" – Herndon [ostendorfA p46] (∈ ¶1606) · 2792

   ⟨1⟩ "His lower lip was thick – material and hanging undercurved, while his chin reached for the lip up curved." [herndonC] (∈ ¶3) *Cognate in* [herndon p472]: *"...his lower lip was thick, hanging, and undercurved, while his chin reached for the lip upcurved"* · 2793

   ⟨2⟩ Examining lips in the 1865 head cast (¶1914): "The lower is distinctly fuller than the upper, being about twice as thick, with a slight downward curve, or eversion. Its fullness is emphasized by the long thin upper lip" [shapiro]. *This description is interpreted as "distinctive"* [shutesE p206] *or as being "a perfect cupid's bow"* [shutesE p208]. · 2794

   ⟨2⟩ At some times "his thick lower lip hung down" [kunhardtA p9] (Part of ¶176) · 2795

Mouth (continued)

⟨²c⟩ "The left half of the upper lip is somewhat thicker than the right and less   2796
expressive, that is, less involitionally and volitionally active. The right half of
the lower lip protrudes markedly and is pulled toward the right by the mouth
and cheek muscles. " [kempfB p9]

⟨²c⟩ In photographs and life-masks "the right half of the lower lip always pro-   2797
truded more than the left half. ... Although a laugher, he tended to keep his
mouth closed firmly [in photographs], with more protrusion of the right side
of the lower lip than the left." [kempfB p17].

⟨○⟩ [ostendorfA p163] and [hamilton p163] note that an "odd lump" is present on the   2798
far right of Lincoln's lower lip in [ostendorf #85]. *It is present in many other
photographs.*

⟨¹q⟩ After seeing scenes of slavery: "I bite my lip and keep quiet." – Lincoln [baslerA   2799
v2p321] [randallC p147]

⟨²⟩ "The large, thick, and protruding under lip injures the general harmony and   2800
delicacy of the face in the estimation of some keen observers ... Were it not
for the high, firm chin, powerful jaw, and decided upper lip, all forming a
well-proportioned combination, and thus reducing the lower lip to a less
obtrusive effect, this member of the face would indeed seem unpleasantly
large. Still, it is to be remembered that the right kind of a thick lower lip is a
physiognomical mark of sensitiveness and tenderness of nature." – Truman
Bartlett [schurz pp24-25]

⟨○⟩ The lower lip looks especially large in [ostendorf #96].   2801

⟨²⟩ On the 1860 and 1865 head casts: "They show ... the same prominent right   2802
lower lip." [stewart]

⟨²c⟩ [fishman] ascribes asymmetries in the lips, nose, and ears of the 1865 cast of   2803
Lincoln's head (¶1914) to "extraneous" or "technical" factors associated with
the casting. *This seems unlikely, as the same asymmetries are present in
the 1860 cast (¶1905).*

⟨S⟩ "probably had a highly arched palate" [gordon] *Support for this statement is un-   2805
clear. Extrapolating?*

⟨¹q⟩ 1860: "His features are not handsome, but extremely mobile; his mouth particu-   2806
larly so. He has the faculty of contorting that feature to provoke uproarious merriment. Good humor gleams in his eye and lurks in the corner of his mouth." – "a
biographer" [meserve p4]

- Jaw: 2807

   ⟨1⟩ "his jaws were long and upcurved ... his chin was sharp and upcurved" [hern-   2808
don p472]

   ⟨¹q⟩ "strongly developed jawbones; chin slightly upturned" – John Nicolay [meserve   2809
p5] (∈ ¶177)

   ⟨1⟩ As President: "... my horrible lantern jaws" – Lincoln [healy pp69-70] (∈ ¶1722)   2810

   ⟨2⟩ "prognathism [is] suggested by Herndon's description" [gordon] citing ¶3   2811

   ⟨2̂⟩ "massive jaw" [kunhardtA p9] (Part of ¶176)   2812

   ⟨¹q⟩ "large, square jaws" – Elliott Herndon [herndon p470n] (∈ ¶1604)   2813

   ⟨²c⟩ [shapiro] refers to the "enormous width" of the jaw (the bigonial width). (See   2815
¶1652.) He also believes this is the basis for Herndon's impression of mas-
sivity and strength in the jaw.

   ⟨²c⟩ "The chin was not especially deep from the mouth down." [shapiro]   2816

- Dentistry and teeth: 2817

Mouth (continued)

⟨1⟩ Sept. 27, 1841: After seeing a dentist, probably in Louisville, KY, Lincoln wrote Joshua Speed's sister: "Do you remember my going to the city while I was in Kentucky, to have a tooth extracted, and making a failure of it? Well, that same old tooth got to paining me so much, that about a week since I had it torn out, bringing with it a bit of the jawbone; the consequence of which is that my mouth is now so sore that I can neither talk, nor eat. I am litterally 'subsisting on savoury remembrances' – that is, being unable to eat, I am living upon the remembrance of the delicious dishes of peaches and cream we used to have at your house." [baslerA v1pp261-262]   2818

⟨1⟩ "When I came to Washington in the fall of 1873 ... Dr. J.L. Wolf was one of the older dentists then in practice here. [I] heard Dr. Wolf tell of extracting a tooth for President Lincoln. [On] a number of occasions I heard him tell the story. ... One day the President came into his office and asked Dr. Wolf to extract a tooth. As Dr. Wolf started to do so the President asked him to wait a minute. He took from his pocket a small bottle of chloroform and took a few inhalations from it. He then told Dr. Wolf to remove the tooth, which he did. *So far as I know* that was the only visit the President made to Dr. Wolf's office. ... Dr. Wolf was a fine man and would not fake a story." – Dr. H.M. Schooley (dentist), July 1932 [shutesP] ([shutes pp88-89] also tells the story.) *Poor Lincoln must have been disappointed in the effect of the chloroform. If he was able to converse after taking the inhalations, he would have had little, if any, anesthetic effect from the gas.*   2820

⟨1⟩ 1862: "Mr Lincoln one evening at the White House was Suffering with pain caused by the extraction of a 'raging tooth' ... Mr Lincoln hearing our voices came in & Sat down ... and notwithstanding the pain that afflicted him chatted humorously" – John Littlefield [wilson pp514-515]   2821

⟨1⟩ 1862: "two rows of large white teeth" [dicey v1pp220-221] (∈ ¶179)   2822

⟨1⟩q "white teeth" – Ralph W. Emerson [shutesE p197]   2823

⟨1⟩ Sept. 7, 1863, perturbed: "Now every muscle in his face seemed to contract, and then suddenly expand. As he opened his mouth you could almost hear them snap as he said, '[whatever],' and closed his mouth as though he never expected to open it again, sort of slammed it to. [Then,] With the same snapping of muscle he again [replied]." [harveyC] (∈ §6.6)   2825

Muscle / Athletics

Interesting questions about Lincoln's strength can be asked. The first concerns his strength. Lincoln was reputed to have great muscular strength. He denied this, however, and ascribed his wrestling prowess to his long limbs. Even in his prime, he was said to *not* be muscular.   2826

The second question concerns his habit of "lounging" (¶2967) and his swinging-arm gait (¶1070). These suggest muscular hypotonia. As discussed in *The Physical Lincoln*, hypotonia has significant ramifications in understanding Lincoln's mental state and the symmetry of his face.   2827

In Marfan syndrome "Muscular underdevelopment and hypotonia is a frequent but by no means invariable feature" [mckusickA p52]. "Pronounced sparsity of subcutaneous fat is a striking feature of most cases" of Marfan syndrome [mckusickA p52], which could confuse visual assessment of muscle mass.   2828

- Also see: Gait, Handwriting   2829

Muscle / Athletics (continued)

- Axe use: 2830
    - ⟨$\frac{1}{q}$⟩ "though very young ... had an ax put into his hands at once; and from that   2832
      till within his twentythird year he was almost constantly handling that most
      useful instrument – less, of course in plowing and harvesting seasons." –
      Lincoln, writing in the third person [baslerA v4p63] *Lincoln implies this started
      upon moving to Indiana – age 7.*
    - ⟨1⟩ "When he was eighteen years old he could take an ax at the end of the handle   2833
      and hold it out on a straight horizontal line, easy and steady." [sandburgA p47]
    - ⟨1⟩ "Abe could sink an axe deeper in wood than any man I Ever Saw. ... he was a   2834
      strong man – physically powerful: he could strike with a mall a heavier blow
      than any man: he was long, tall and strong" – William Wood [wilson p124]
    - ⟨1⟩ "he was a good chopper." The type of axe used in Lincoln's youth (at least)   2835
      was "n use was a great clumsy tool ... weighing about Six pounds, the handle
      being round and Strait, which made it very difficult to hold when chopping
      requiring a gripe as Strong as was necessary to wield a Blacksmiths Sledge
      Hammer." – Robert Wilson [wilson p202] (Expanded in ¶99)
    - ⟨1⟩ In Springfield: "he sawed his own wood generally when at home" – James   2836
      Gourley [wilson p453]
    - ⟨1⟩ In Springfield: "I heard an axe ... Saw Mr Lincoln in his Shirt Sleeves Cutting   2837
      wood" – John B. Weber [wilson p389] (Part of ¶3435)
    - ⟨$\frac{1}{q}$⟩ April 1865: Reputed to give a remarkable wood-chopping demonstration at   2838
      City Point, VA – see ¶1297.
- ⟨$\frac{1}{q}$⟩ "In rasslin, running, an' hoss-back ridin' and log rollin', and railsplittin', he could   2839
  beat everybody." – Dennis Hanks [lattimerNY]
- ⟨1⟩ "He was a strong, athletic boy" – Leonard Swett, who did not witness this [riceA   2840
  p459]
- ⟨1⟩ "Lincoln was a powerful man in 1830 – Could Carry what 3. ordinary men would   2841
  grunt & sweat at – Saw him Carry a chicken house made of poles pinned together
  & Covered that weighed at least 600 if not much more." – Joseph Richardson [wilson
  p120]
- Feats of strength (1) - the barrel: 2842
    - ⟨1⟩ "Physically, Mr. Lincoln was the strongest man I ever knew. That is saying a   2843
      good deal. Let me tell you what I saw him do. He took a full barrel of whisky
      [sic], containing forty-four gallons, gripping each end with one hand, raised
      it deliberately to his face and drank from the bunghole. In doing this he won
      a $10 hat from Bill Green. In the grocery I have often seen him pick up a
      barrel of whisky, place it on the counter, and then lower it on the other side."
      – Daniel Burner, who lived with Lincoln in the 1830s [templeB]
    - ⟨1⟩ "The Whiskey Barrell story so help me god is true..." – William Greene [wilson   2844
      p33]
    - ⟨1⟩ "Trials of strength were very common among the pioneers. Lifting weights,   2845
      as heavy timbers piled one upon another was a favorite pastime, and no
      workman in the neighborhood could at all cope with Mr Lincoln in this di-
      rection. I have seen him frequently take a barrel of whiskey by the chimes
      and lift it up to his face as if to drink out of the bung-hole." – Robert Rut-
      ledge [wilson p387]
    - ⟨1⟩ "I am inclined to believe that ... Herndon, drew largely on his imagination   2846
      when he told these stories." [rossH pp100, 125-126]

Muscle / Athletics (continued)

⟨2⟩ Circa 1831: Lincoln thought "the best use he could put his life to was to become a blacksmith" [kunhardtB p290].   2847

⟨1/q⟩ Perhaps 1832: While speaking to a crowd, Lincoln saw someone attack a friend. He left the speaking platform, grabbed the ruffian, "threw him some ten feet," then resumed his speech [angle p50] (reprinting Nicolay & Hay)   2848

⟨1/q⟩ 1858: "The strongest man I ever looked at" – Mayor Henry Sanderson of Galesburg, who saw Lincoln bathing [meserve p2]   2849

- Jumping: 2850
    ⟨1⟩ 1830s: "Mr Lincoln would wait till all who were disposed to try their muscles had made their best jumps, then come forward with a heavy weight in each hand with his long muscular legs raise himself from the ground and light far beyond the most successful champion" – Dr. Jason Duncan [wilson p541]   2851
    ⟨1⟩ "was seldom ever Beat Jumping" – William Miller [wilson p363]   2852
    ⟨-⟩ More leaping: ¶1096, ¶1100   2853

⟨1⟩ "During Lincoln's youth he had everywhere been distinguished as the crowning athlete of the neighborhood in which he lived." – Leonard Swett, who did not witness this [riceA p463]   2854

⟨1⟩ "Very few men in the army could succesfully compete with Mr Lincoln, either in wrestling or swimming; he well understood both arts." – George Harrison [wilson p554] *As a youth, however, could not swim. See ¶3561.*   2855

- Feats of strength (2) - 1000 pounds of stones: 2856
    ⟨1⟩ "I saw him Lift Betwen 1000 and 1300 lbs of Rock waid in a Boxx"– J. Rowan Herndon [wilson p7]   2857
    ⟨1⟩ About 1835: "he made a box in the mill – put stones in it and raised one thousand, by throwing straps across his shoulders – he getting on some logs. I saw the box – rocks & straps & it is said by good men & true that he lifted the thousand pouns." – Harding Bale [wilson p13] *Bale was apparently not, therefore, an eye-witness.*   2858
    ⟨1⟩ "He lifted 1000 pounds of shot by main strength." – James Short [wilson p73]   2859
    ⟨1⟩ "He was a great fellow to try projects – invented a wheel – fixd a box – strapt himself and weighed a thousand or more pounds" –Hardin Bale [wilson p528]   2860
    ⟨1⟩ [rossH pp125-126] says Herndon invented this story.   2861

- Wrestling: 2862
    ⟨1⟩ "he Became very Poupelar whilst in the army he Could throw Down any man that took hold of him he Could out jump the Best of them he Could out Box the Best of them" – J. Rowan Herndon [wilson pp6-7]   2863
    ⟨1⟩ "He was a great wrestler – wrestled in the black Hawk war: his mode – method – or way – his Specialty was side holds: he threw down all men." – James Gourley [wilson p451]   2864
    ⟨1⟩ "I remember one time wrestling with him, two best in three, and ditched him. He was not satisfied, and we tried it in a foot-race for a five-dollar bill. I won the money, and 'tis spent long ago." – William Wilson, 1882 recollection [wilson p707] *Is probably referring to era of Black Hawk War. This letter exists in copy only.*   2865
    ⟨1⟩ "Saw Lincoln Catch a man by the Nape of the neck and a– of the breeches and toss him 10 or 12 feet, Easily" – James Herndon [wilson p460]   2866
    ⟨1⟩ Lincoln dislocated William Bolen's shoulder – Samuel Kercheval [wilson p645]   2867

Muscle / Athletics (continued)

⟨1⟩ "One man in the army alone could throw him and that man's name was   2868
Thompson" – William Greene [wilson p19]; also [wilson p12]

⟨1⟩ "Very few men in the army could succesfully compete with Mr Lincoln... in   2869
wrestling" – George Harrison [wilson p554] (∈ ¶2855)

⟨1⟩ "was fond of wrestling, in which he excelled" – James Short [wilson p91]   2870

⟨2⟩ Accounts of Lincoln's famous wrestling match against local champion Jack   2871
_c_ Armstrong vary [donaldA p40]. There is at least one account where Armstrong
"grabbed Lincoln by the thigh and threw him in a second," after which Lincoln got up "pretty mad" [burl p159].

⟨1/q⟩ Lincoln was a reluctant wrestler – he did not like all the "wooling and   2872
pulling" involved [donaldA p40].

⟨2⟩ 1858: Lincoln remarks that he has never been "dusted" (laid on his back in a   2873
wrestle) and would like to have "tussled" with George Washington [kunhardtB
p291]

⟨1/q⟩ "All I had to do was extend one hand to a man's shoulder, and with weight of   2874
body and strength of arms give him a trip that generally sent him sprawling
on the ground, which would so astonish him as to give him a quietus." –
Lincoln, overheard by Thomas D. Jones in 1860 [meserve p5]

⟨2⟩ [lattimerNY] thinks Lincoln's height was a disadvantage in wrestling. *"Wrest-*   2875
ing" in the 19th century was probably a different sport than in the 20th
century.

■ Other sports: 2876

⟨1⟩ Circa 1833: "His playful hours for these years was pitching quoits – jumping   2877
– hopping – Swimming – Shooting" – Mentor Graham [wilson p10]

⟨1⟩ Early to mid-1830s: "would play at varis [sic] games – jumping – running –   2878
hopping" – Hardin Bale [wilson p13]

⟨1⟩ Late 1830s: "We played the old fashioned town ball – jumped – ran – fought   2879
& danced. Lincoln played town ball – he hopped well – in 3 hops he would
go 40.2 on a dead level." – James Gourley [wilson p451]

⟨1⟩ "Lincoln was a good player – could catch a ball: he would Strip and go at it –   2880
do it well" – James Gourley [wilson p451]

⟨1⟩ "In 1844 I used to play ball with Abe Lincoln ... the game was Called fives   2881
– Striking a ball with our hands against a wall that Served as alley. In 1860
Lincoln & myself played ball – this game" – James Gourley [wilson p453] *This*
has been interpreted as being handball [randallC p86].

⟨1⟩ "Lincoln played ball pretty much all the dy [sic] before his nomination –   2882
played at what is called fives – Knocking a ball up against a wall that served
as an alley – He loved this game – his only physical game – that I Knew of
– Lincoln said – This game makes my shoulders feel well." – Charles Zane
[wilson p492]

⟨1⟩ Lincoln's physical Exercise running – jumping – pitching quoits – hopping   2884
swimming – shooting" – William Greene [wilson p21]

⟨1⟩ "Mr L. was very fond of out door recreation & sports, and excelled in them."   2885
– James Short [wilson p73]

⟨1⟩ "he was fond of Exercise such as Jumping Rasling Paying Ball and all Kinds   2886
of funn" – J. Rowan Herndon [wilson p92]

⟨1⟩ Illinois: "he used to run footraces & jump with the boys and also play ball" –   2887
Abner Ellis [wilson p170]

⟨1⟩ 1840s or 1850s: "he used to Saw wood for exercise –: he really loved to do it"   2888
– Frances Todd Wallace [wilson p485]

Muscle / Athletics (continued)

⟨1⟩ 1848±: "Congressman Lincoln was very fond of bowling. ... He was a very   2889
awkward bowler, but played the game with great zest and spirit, solely for
exercise and amusement." – Samuel Busey [busey p27] (Busey was a physician:
¶3202)

⟨1⟩ "Mr. Lincoln's remarkable strength resulted not so much from muscular power   2890
as from the toughness of his sinews. He could not only lift from the ground enormous weight, but could throw a cannon-ball or a maul farther than anyone else in
New Salem. I heard him explain once how he was enabled to thus to excel others.
He did not attribute it to a greater proportion of physical strength, but contended
that because of the unusual length of his arms the ball or projectile had a greater
swing and therefore acquired more force and momentum than in the hands of an
average man." [herndon p70]

⟨1⟩ 1840: "the Cannon ball thrown by Lincoln went Some four or Six feet further   2891
than any one Could throw it." – Andrew Kirk [wilson p603]

⟨1⟩ "a great big, angular, strong man" – William Herndon [hertz p195] (∈ ¶87)   2892

⟨2⟩ "No little of Lincoln's influence with the men of New Salem can be attributed to his   2893
extraordinary feats of strength. By an arrangement of ropes and straps, harnessed
about his hips, he was enabled one day at the mill to astonish a crowd of village of
celebrities by lifting a box of stones weighing near a thousand pounds. There is no
fiction, either, as suggested by some of his biographers, in the story that he lifted a
barrel of whisky from the ground and drank from the bung; but in performing this
almost incredible feat he did not stand erect and elevate the barrel, but squatted
down and lifted it to his knees, rolling it over until his mouth came opposite the
bung." [herndon pp102-103]

⟨2⟩ Mentions immense physical strength [donaldA pp40-41&46].   2894

⟨1⟩ "Physically, he was a very powerful man, lifting with ease four hundred, and in   2895
one case six hundred pounds." [herndon p471]

⟨1⟩ "capable of immense physical & mental labor ... He was verry [sic] powerful   2896
physically" – Joseph Gillespie [wilson p186]

⟨1⟩ "not *muscular*, weighed from 160 to 180 pounds." – Herndon [hertz p186] (∈ ¶327)   2897

⟨1⟩ "He died at the age fifty-six years a sinewy tough iron-framed man; he had no   2898
extra flesh on him, but was all nerve and sinew; he was not what is generally
termed a muscular man, but a sinewy one and a very strong and glorious
one." – William Herndon [hertz p440]

⟨1⟩ "was not what is called muscular, but was sinewy, wiry" – Herndon [hertz p196]   2899
(∈ ¶88)

⟨$\frac{1}{q}$⟩ Lincoln described himself as having "strong muscles" [donaldA p575]. See ¶1297   2900

⟨S⟩ McKusick notes that Lincoln's "legendary strength ... does not exclude Marfan   2901
syndrome by any means." [mckusickB]

⟨2⟩ As President: "His upper body still showed the remarkable muscle formation that   2902
Leonard Volk had commented on in 1860," when sculptor Volk had seen Lincoln
shirtless. [kunhardtA p321] *I have not seen a primary source for this statement.*

⟨1⟩ "He was very athletic ... and of great physical strength. There was no grace in his   2903
movements, but an expression of awkwardness, combined with force and vigor."
[arnold p441] (∈ ¶167)

⟨1⟩ "enormous muscular strength" [crookA p74]   2904

203

Muscle / Athletics (continued)

⟨1⟩ "Abraham Lincoln was an unusually tall man, although he did not seem slender. He appeared to be as lean and his muscles as hard as a prize-fighter. He was obviously a very strong, powerful man, physically capable of immense endurance." – Senator James Harlan (date of recollection unknown) [helmB p166] Part of ¶173   2905

⟨2⟩ "long stringy musculature and scant subcutaneous fat" [gordon]   2906

- Awkward: (for ungainly, see ¶103)   2907
  - ⟨1⟩ About age 10: "long tall dangling award drowl looking boy" [sic] – ¶481 [wilson p120]   2908
  - ⟨$\frac{1}{q}$⟩ Girl #1: Before 1830: "he was so tall and awkward. All the young girls my age made fun of Abe." – ¶2684 [burl pp123-124]   2909
  - ⟨2⟩ Girl #2: "his awkwardness and large feet" ¶2685 [burl p124]   2910
  - ⟨$\frac{1}{q}$⟩ Girl #3: "so quiet and awkward and so awful homely" – ¶2686 [burl p124]   2911
  - ⟨$\frac{1}{q}$⟩ In Indiana: "Dressed in the frontiersman's coonskin cap, deerskin shirt, and home-made trousers, he was indelibly impressed upon my memory as being one of the gawkiest and most awkward figures I ever saw." – J.W. Lamar [hobson p22]   2912
  - ⟨1⟩ 1830±: "a long awkward gawky looking boy." – Jesse Dubois [nicolayO p30]   2913
  - ⟨2⟩ About 1831: "awkward step" – ¶95 [wilson p24]   2914
  - ⟨1⟩ 1832 or 1833: "would enforce his ideas with awkward gestures" – ¶1122 [wilson p384]   2915
  - ⟨$\frac{1}{q}$⟩ 1847: "Tall, angular, and awkward" – Elihu Washburne [hunt p228]   2916
  - ⟨$\frac{1}{q}$⟩ "His Way of Laughing two was rearly funney and Such awakard Jestures belonged to No other Man" – ¶3118 [wilson p161]   2917
  - ⟨1⟩ "awkward" – Herndon [hertz p125]   2918
  - ⟨1⟩ 1848: "his manifest awkwardness" – ¶138 [wilson p699]   2919
  - ⟨1⟩ 1849: "He was a very awkward bowler" – ¶2889 [angle pp144-145]   2920
  - ⟨1⟩ 1857: "blushed and squirmed with the awkward diffidence of a schoolboy" – ¶2498 [herndon p479]   2921
  - ⟨1⟩ 1858: "singularly awkward, almost absurd ... movements of his body" – ¶145 [kunhardtA p108]   2922
  - ⟨$\frac{1}{q}$⟩ 1858: "His gesture was awkward." – ¶3719 [kunhardtA p110]   2923
  - ⟨2⟩ 1858: "moved his arms and hands awkwardly" – ¶91 [donaldA p215]   2924
  - ⟨1⟩ Feb. 27, 1860: "so angular and awkward that I had, for an instant, a feeling of pity" – eyewitness [brooksA p186] (∈ ¶156)   2925
  - ⟨1⟩ 1860: "Every movement was awkward in the extreme." [piatt p345] (∈ ¶152)   2926
  - ⟨1⟩ Probably about 1860: "his awkward manner" – ¶3720 [angle p177]   2927
  - ⟨$\frac{1}{q}$⟩ June 21, 1860: "After you have been five minutes in his company you cease to think that he is either homely or awkward." – Utica newspaper reporter [lincloreHDE] (∈ ¶159)   2928
  - ⟨1⟩ Pre-1861: "At first he was very awkward ... apparent diffidence and sensitiveness ... added to his awkwardness" – ¶90 [herndon p331]   2929
  - ⟨1⟩ 1860s: "I have heard it said that he was ungainly, that his step was awkward. He never impressed me as being awkward. ... when you were near him you never thought whether he was awkward or graceful; you thought of nothing except, What a kindly character this man has!" [dana p173] (∈ ¶183)   2930
  - ⟨1⟩ March 1861: "the awkward bonhommie of his face" – William Russell [russell pp37-38] ¶161   2931
  - ⟨$\frac{1}{q}$⟩ 1862: "There is no describing his awkwardness, nor the uncouthness of his movements." [hawthorne p309] (∈ ¶178)   2932

Muscle / Athletics (continued)

⟨1⟩ Sept. 8, 1863: "was very tall and moved with a shuffling awkward motion." [harveyC] (∈ §6.9) 2933

⟨1⟩ 1864: "For such an awkward fellow, I am pretty surefooted. It used to take a pretty dextrous man to throw me." – Lincoln [hayD p244] (∈ ¶1097) 2934

⟨1⟩ "his gait was not altogether awkward" [lamonL p470] (Part of ¶1081) 2935

⟨1⟩ "he was homely, awkward, diffident" [arnold p46] 2936

⟨2⟩ "When people talked about Lincoln, it was nearly always about one or more of these five things: (1) how long, tall, quick, strong, or awkward in looks he was..." – ¶1106 [sandburgP v1p200] 2937

■ Of Lincoln's nude remains, on autopsy table, a few hours post-mortem: 2938

⟨1⟩ "A smooth clear skin fitting cleanly over well-rounded muscles, sinewy and strong – the physique of an athlete in training. Easily understood now is that physical prowess of former years, when none might stand up in a wrestling bout before the rail-splitter of Illinois, and in later days the untiring endurance, physical and mental both." – Edward Curtis, MD, recalling in 1908 [curtis] *The skin description sounds unlikely – see ¶3416.* 2939

⟨1/q⟩ "I was simply astonished at the showing of the nude remains, where well rounded muscles built upon strong bones told the powerful athlete. Now did I understand the deeds of prowess recorded of the President's early days." – Edward Curtis, MD, one week post-autopsy [lattimerNY] and [lattimerBk p38] citing [curtis]. *Unfortunately, [curtis] does not contain this text. His better documented quotations are in ¶2939 and ¶3416.* 2940

⟨2⟩c "Judged by modern standards of athletes, Abraham Lincoln would certainly qualify as a topflight all-American in several fields of sports and with proper training as a young man would have returned from the Olympics with several gold medals." [montgomeryJ] *As the basis of this hyperbolic statement, Dr. Montgomery cites ¶2940.* 2941

⟨1⟩ "I knew [Chauncey] Depew knew Lincoln. ... I remember him repeating one observation over and over: He said he never could figure out why Mr. Lincoln had the reputation of being awkward and ungainly. He said he always had marveled at the grace and ease, the *economy*, of his movements. He said that big man just got himself out of chairs all in one piece, with a single motion, while smaller men were struggling and squirming. He said that he walked with dignity and sureness, handled objects with delicacy, used his hands gracefully and without wasting energy. He talked especially about Lincoln's beautiful hands. ... Lincoln's every movement, according to Depew, was made with the greatest control and economy – and, therefore, grace." – Marie de Montalvo, 1948 letter to J.G. Randall [randallP box 15] 2942

⟨1⟩ "Lincoln had the grace of pose and action." – William Herndon [hertz p194] 2943

⟨2⟩ Oct. 1849: Enthusiastically pitched wood aboard a steamboat racing another [randallC p123] 2944

⟨1⟩ May 19, 1860: Meeting a formal delegation: "He bowed, but it was not gracefully done. There was evident constraint and embarrassment." [coffinA p172] 2945

⟨1⟩ 1862: "an air of strength, physical as well as moral" [dicey v1pp220-221] (∈ ¶179) 2946

⟨1⟩ Sept. 1863: "His face was peculiar; bone, nerve, vein, and muscle were all so plainly seen" [harveyC] (∈ §6.2) *Suggests thin, translucent skin.* 2947

⟨1⟩ Sept. 7, 1863: almost snapping use of mouth muscles [harveyC]. See §6.6. 2948

⟨1⟩ April 1865: "his arms were strong and ... his gestures were vigorous and supple, re-   2949
vealing great physical strength and an extraordinary energy for resisting privation
and fatigue" [chambrunA] (∈ ¶200)

Muscle Energy

"Muscle energy" is an invented term. I am using it to record observations about Lin-   2950
coln's muscle use. Muscle energy differs from muscle strength because it relates to the
expenditure of energy during sub-maximal muscular effort. Thus, muscular energy
encompasses both muscle tone (i.e., the standard medical concept known as "neuromuscular tonus") and manifestations of muscular energy conservation. Examples of
the latter include the posture Lincoln assumed while sitting or reading, the apparently
unrestrained way his arms swung when he walked, etc.

- See also Muscle / Athletics , Nervous System , Energy .   2951

- Youth: 2952
  - ⟨2⟩ Around his 16th year he was growing so fast that "he was tired all the time,   2953
  and he showed a notable lack of enthusiasm for physical labor." Dennis
  Hanks describe him as "lazy" and a neighbor remembered "he was no hand
  to pitch in at work like killing snakes" [donaldA p33]. (∈ ¶1109)
  - ⟨1⟩ "Lincoln was lazy – a very lazy man – He was always reading – scribbling –   2954
  writing – Ciphering" – Dennis Hanks [wilson p104]
  - ⟨1⟩ "he was no hand to pitch in at work like killing Snakes but he would take hold   2955
  of his work as camely and pleasant as his maner was other ways" – Elizabeth
  Crawford [wilson p335]
  - ⟨1⟩ "he didn't like physical labor" – Lincoln's step-mother [wilson p106]   2956
  - ⟨1⟩ About 1829: "Abe was awfully lazy: he worked for me – was always reading &   2957
  thinking – used to get mad at him – He worked for me in 1829 pulling fodder
  – I Say Abe was awful lazy: he would laugh & talk and crack jokes & tell stories
  all the time, didn't love work but did dearly love his pay ... Lincoln said to me
  one day that his father taught him to work but never learned him to love it."
  – John Romines [wilson p118]

- ⟨S⟩ "The neuromuscular tonus of his body was more relaxed than in the average man.   2958
That was shown in the slow, drawling, staccato monotone of his speech..." [kempfB
p6]

- ⟨1⟩ "His organization – rather his structure and functions – worked slowly. His blood   2959
had to run a long distance from his heart to the extremities of his frame, and his
nerve force had to travel through dry ground a long distance before his muscles
were obedient to his will. ... The whole man, body and mind, worked slowly, as
if needing oiling. ... His mind was like his body, and worked slowly but strongly."
[herndon p471]

- ⟨$\frac{1}{q}$⟩ Nov. 1860: "slouchy ... round shouldered, leans forward" – Thomas Webster [ran-   2960
dallC p163] (∈ ¶160)

- ⟨1⟩ April 12, 1861: "He was bent until he almost appeared to stoop" [stoddardD p221] (∈   2961
¶1139)

- ⟨1⟩ Mid 1863: "The drooping eyelids, looking almost swollen ... the deep marks about   2962
the large and expressive mouth; the flaccid muscles of the jaws, were all so majestically pitiful." – Silas Burt [wilsonR p332] (∈ ¶1621)

Muscle Energy (continued)

⟨1⟩ Early 1864: "He looked wearied, and when he sat down in a chair, looked as   2963
though every limb wanted to drop off his body." – Henry Beecher [riceA pp249-250]
(∈ ¶195)

◻ July 11, 1864: [ostendorf #127] is a rare unposed photograph of Lincoln (if it is Lin-   2964
coln). It shows him propping himself against the railing of a Coast Guard cutter.
[ostendorfA p370]

⟨1⟩ As President: Chauncey Depew "always had marveled at the grace and ease, the   2965
economy, of his movements. He said that big man just got himself out of chairs all
in one piece, with a single motion, while smaller men were struggling and squirming. He said that he walked with dignity and sureness, ... used his hands gracefully
and without wasting energy. ... Lincoln's every movement, according to Depew,
was made with the greatest control and economy – and, therefore, grace." [randallP
box 15] (∈ ¶2942)

⟨1/q⟩ April 14, 1865: "never applauded with his hands, but he laughed heartily on occa-   2966
sion, and his face spoke plainly of his approval." – Helen Coleman [luthin p636]

■ "Lounging:"   2967

  ⟨2⟩c "Lincoln did not complain of physical fatigue, but he would move to a lounge   2968
  as an habitual smoker reaches for a cigarette. When one was unavailable,
  he sought an approach to the horizontal position by placing his chair and
  shoulders against a wall and his feet on the highest rung or, preferably, on
  a table. Herndon said that his partner usually arrived at their office at nine
  o'clock, that the first thing he did was to lie down on the sofa, one leg on
  a chair, and read the newspapers. Throughout Lincoln literature, he can
  be found lying on the grass, on the floor, or on a sofa. An excerpt from
  the Boston *Daily Advertiser* (April 20, 1865) is a reflection of his lounging
  reputation: 'Our interview left no grotesque recollections of the President's
  lounging...' " [shutesE p105]. (Is quoting [hertz p176], too.)

  ⟨2⟩ "The habit of lounging [was] peculiarly pronounced in him" [shutesE p106].   2969
  ⟨c/q⟩ In youth: "Abe'd lay on his stummick by the fire, an' read out loud" – Dennis   2970
  Hanks [wilsonR p26]
  ⟨1/q⟩ "An' when he come to the house at night, he'd tilt a cheer back by the chim-   2971
  bley, put his feet on the rung, an' set on his back-bone an read." – Dennis
  Hanks [wilsonR p26]
  ⟨1⟩ In Indiana: "take down a book – Sit down on a chair – Cock his legs up as   2972
  high as his head and read" – John Hanks [wilson p455] (∈ ¶591)
  ⟨2⟩ In New Salem: "He was often seen seated against the trunk of a tree, or lying   2973
  on the grass under its shade, poring over his books, changing his position as
  the sun advanced, so as to keep in the shadow." [arnold p40]
  ⟨2⟩ "Stretched under an ancient shade tree wchich stood just outside the door of   2974
  his store, his long bare feet resting high on th ebark of the tree, Abe Lincoln
  read..." [angle p90, quoting Albert Woldman's 1936 book]
  ⟨1⟩ In New Salem: "He read aloud very often; and frequently assumed a lounging   2975
  position when reading." – James Short [wilson p90]
  ⟨1⟩ 1840s: "His favorite way of reading when at home was lying down on the   2976
  floor   I fancy I See him now lying full length in the *Hall of his old home*
  reading" – Harriet Chapman [wilson p407]
  ⟨1⟩ 1840s: "You wish to know if Mr Lincoln read news papers. *He did* yes and   2977
  often vary late at night. ... his usual way of reading was lying down in warm
  weather he Seemed to prefer the floor he would turn a Chair down on the

Muscle Energy (continued)

floor and put a pillow on it and lie thare for hours and read." – Harriet Chapman [wilson p512]

⟨1⟩ 1848±: "When about to tell an anecdote during a meal he would lay down his knife and fork, place his elbows upon the table, rest his face between his hands, and begin with the words 'that reminds me'..." – Samuel Busey (¶3202) [busey p25]   2978

⟨1/q⟩ In Springfield: "His chair ... would be leaning back against the wall; his feet drawn up and resting on the front rounds so that his knees and chair were about on level" – Jonathan Birch [wilson p727] (∈ ¶2343) *This picture is unclear to me.*   2980

⟨1⟩ In Springfield: "... lying on the lounge looking skyward" when there was trouble at home [herndon p348] (∈ ¶3433)   2981

⟨1⟩ In Springfield: "L's old office ... a small dirty bed – one buffalo robe – a chair and a bench – L would lounge in it all day reading – '*abstracting*' – 'glooming' && c" – James Matheny [wilson p251]   2982

⟨1⟩ In Springfield: "Lincoln would lean back – his head against the top of a rocking Chair – sit abstracted that way ... 20 – 30 minutes" – Frances Todd Wallace [wilson p486] (∈ ¶2499)   2983

⟨1⟩ In Springfield: Habitually would "come into the office, pick up book, newspaper, etc., and sprawl himself out on the sofa, chairs, etc., and read aloud.... Sometimes in reading he would have his body on the sofa, one foot on one chair and one foot on the table. He spilt himself out easily over one-quarter of the room. ... In reading at his private home he would turn his chair down, upside down, lean it down, turn it over, and rest his head on the back of the chair, it forming an inclined plane, his book and body on the carpet." – William Herndon, 1885 [hertz p95]   2984

⟨1⟩ "Lincoln would sometimes lie down in the office to rest on the sofa, his feet on two or three chairs or up against the wall. In this position he would reflect, decide... and then he would jump up, pick up his hat and run, the good Lord knows where. " – Herndon [hertz p178]   2985

⟨1⟩ William Herndon (¶2377) and Henry Rankin (¶2380) tell of Lincoln sitting for 30 minutes and more, silent, with his left arm and hand supporting his chin.   2986

⟨1⟩ On the circuit: "In the Evening Lincoln would strip off his coat and lay down on the bed – read – reflect and digest – After Supper he would Strip – go to bed – get a Candle – draw up a chair or table and read till late of night" – John Stuart [wilson p519]   2987

⟨1⟩ June 19, 1856: "Lincoln sat awkwardly in a chair tilted up after his fashion" – Henry Whitney [angle p218]   2988

⟨1⟩ 1858: "sat tilted back in one chair with his feet upon another in perfect ease." – David Locke [meserve p2] (∈ ¶991)   2989

⟨1⟩ Late 1850s: "Lincoln's favorite position when unraveling some knotty law point was to stretch both of his legs at full length upon a chair in front of him." – John Littlefield [angle pp184-185]   2990

⟨1⟩ 1860: "I was well tired out, and went home to rest, throwing myself down on a lounge in my chamber." – Lincoln [brooksR] (∈ ¶907)   2991

⟨1⟩ April 1860: "I found him in the United States District Court-room ... his feet on the edge of a table, one of his fingers thrust into his mouth, and his long, dark hair standing out at every imaginable angle, apparently uncombed for a week." [volk]   2992

Muscle Energy (continued)

⟨1⟩ As President: "... as he sat comfortably in his arm-chair, in his favorite position, with his legs crossed." [brooksC p298] 2993

⟨1⟩ As President: typically reclined on a horsehair sofa when visiting the telegraph office. [NYTimesTeleg] (∈ ¶2103) 2994

⟨1/q⟩ As President: "Even when he crosses his spiderlike legs or throws them over the arms of a chair he does it with a natural grace." – Daniel Voorhees [gordon] (∈ ¶184) 2995

⟨1⟩ Spring 1862: "He sat in his chair loungingly, giving no evidence of his unusual height. [Later,] Mr. Lincoln (who had been sunk down in his big chair up to this time) began to rise, and as I looked he went up and up and up" [bancroft] (∈ ¶182) 2996

⟨1⟩ 1862: "In lounged a tall, loose-jointed figure" [hawthorne p309] (∈ ¶178) 2997

⟨1/q⟩ April 1862: During a 2-hour conversation (¶720), "He sat before the open fire in the old Cabinet room, most of the time with his feet up on the high marble mantel." – A.K. McClure [angle p401] 2998

⟨1⟩ Summer 1863: "Like a tired child he threw himself upon a sofa, and shaded his eyes with his hands. He was a complete picture of dejection." [keckleyB pp118-119] (∈ ¶2533) 2999

⟨1⟩ Sept. 1863: "as he sat in a folded up sort of way in a deep arm chair, one would almost have thought him deformed. ... When I first saw him his head was bent forward, his chin resting on his breast, and in his hand a letter... He threw himself around in the chair, one leg over the arm, and again spoke..." [harveyC] (∈ §6.2, §6.3) 3000

⟨1⟩ Mar. 20, 1864 (per [miers]): W. O. Stoddard returns to White House after an illness.. The offices are empty; Lincoln's door is closed. He enters Lincoln's office. The President "is lying on the lounge, just as if he were resting." A conversation starts. "The President half lay down again ... but now he very nearly sits up, laughing silently." ... Grant seems to be doing a good job. 'If so, there is no wonder that he [Lincoln] can lie here upon his lounge, this sunny Sunday afternoon, with such a look of almost relief upon his worn and wrinkled face. ... Once more the half-reclining form comes up to a sitting posture... The President is sitting straight up, now..." [stoddardA pp125-126] 3001

⟨1⟩ Spring 1864, a Sunday in the White House: "... he was actually lying down upon the sofa... with his hands folded over his head and looking as if he did not care two cents for the past, present, or future. He half arose as I came in..." [stoddardD p318] (Same incident as ¶3001.) 3002

⟨1⟩ Summer 1864: "So bowed and sorrow-laden was his whole person, expressing such weariness of mind and body, as he dropped himself heavily from step to step down to the ground." – a lady [browneF p670] (∈ ¶2538) 3003

⟨1⟩ Oct.± 1864: "The President lay on a sofa, apparently very weary." [stoddardD p339] 3004

⟨2⟩ General William T. Sherman recalled that, at rest or listening, Lincoln sat with his arms hanging as if lifeless and his face dull; he would light up when he talked. [currentBk p248] 3005

⟨1⟩ As President: "I knew when he threw himself (as he did once when I was there) on a lounge, and rattled off story after story, that it was his method of relief" – Chauncey Depew [riceA p428] 3006

⟨1⟩ April 12 (11?), 1865: Mary enters a White House room without knocking, after Lincoln had made a speech. "There was Mr. Lincoln, stretched at full length, resting on a large sofa from his oratorical efforts.... he rose impulsively... I did 3007

Muscle Energy (continued)

not stay too long, in order to let him rest" [chambrunB p93]

⟨2⟩ Adulthood: "He often read in a reclining position on a couch or the floor" [kempfB p14]. *Kempf ascribes this to an effect of Lincoln's oculomotor problems – see* Eyes -- Motor . 3008

⟨2⟩ "Resting his chin on the palm of his left hand, he would sit for hours in silence" [donaldA p163]. 3009

⟨2⟩ Robert Lincoln thought that George P.A. Healy's portrait of Lincoln, "which showed him, nearly lifesize, seated with legs crossed, one finger along his cheek, the other hand clutching the chair arm," to be the best likeness of his father ever painted. [anonB] 3010

⟨S⟩ Lounging diagnosis: In 1926, Dr. E.E. Maxey suggested that Lincoln's lounging "was an instinctive search for a less tiring position for his eyes" [shutes p70]. (See ¶917.) *This seems unlikely, but is the only medical hypothesis I have seen.* 3011

■ "Loose:" 3012
  ⟨1/q⟩ Jan. 1, 1841: "slender, and loosely built" – Quincy *Whig* [shenk p263] (∈ ¶335) 3013
  ⟨1⟩ Pre-Presidency: "His structure – his build was loose and leathery. His body was shrunk and shrivelled" [herndonC] (∈ ¶1) (Cognate in: [herndon p471].) 3014
  ⟨1/q⟩ "a tall, homely, loose-jointed man" – recollection of an Illinois attorney [burl p76] 3015
  ⟨1/q⟩ 1860: "His loose, tall frame is loosely thrown together." – Gideon Welles [kunhardtB p65] (∈ ¶154) 3016
  ⟨1⟩ March 27, 1861: "a shambling, loose, irregular, almost unsteady gait" – William Howard Russell [russell pp37-38] (∈ ¶161) 3017
  ⟨1⟩ Spring 1862: "homely of face, large-boned, angular, and loosely put together" [bancroft] (∈ ¶182) 3018
  ⟨1⟩ 1862: "In lounged a tall, loose-jointed figure" [hawthorne pp309] (∈ ¶178) 3019
  ⟨1/q⟩ "enormously long loose arms" – Princess Salm-Salm [salmsalm] (∈ ¶190) 3020
  ⟨1⟩ Clothes "hung loosely on his giant frame." [herndon p332] (∈ ¶401) 3021
  ⟨2⟩ "What some observers took to be a loose, lank, awkward physical frame operated to hide from them the fact that Lincoln was all his life an athlete, sometimes slow to get going but when in stride having panther quality." – Carl Sandburg [meserve p4] 3022
  ⟨2/c⟩ "unnaturally long loose arms and legs" [gordon] (∈ ¶208) 3023

■ Gait: 3024
  ⟨1⟩ Sept. 4, 1861: "the peculiar swinging gait that characterizes the old 'Rail splitter.'" [french p373] 3025

■ Riding: 3026
  ⟨1⟩ Nov. 1863: He rode a horse to the ceremonies at Gettysburg Cemetery. "Before he reached the grounds he was bent forward, his arms swinging, his body limp, and his whole frame swaying from side to side. He had become so absorbed in thought that he took little heed of his surroundings, and was riding just as he did over the circuit in Illinois" [carrB p39]. *Perhaps he was not feeling well. See Special Topic §5.* 3027

■ Lincoln's face: 3028
  ⟨-⟩ *The Physical Lincoln concludes that Lincoln had "pseudo-depression." That is, hyptonia of the facial muscles caused his face to sag, mimicking sadness, when he was not necessarily sad.* 3029
  ⟨2/c⟩ "subnormal neuromuscular tonus of the left side" [kempfB p4] 3030

Muscle Energy (continued)

⟨$\frac{1}{q}$⟩ When Lincoln became abstracted, his facial expression was described by friends as "ugly and stupid looking," "dull," "sad and abstract," "detached," and "withdrawn." [kempfB p12] 3031

⟨2⟩ "Upon being stimulated in a way that aroused emotivating interest, his facial expression was observed to change quickly from dull indifference to animated interest, with a tendency to smile and laugh." [kempfB p12] 3032

⟨2⟩ "Strangers who estimated the man by his dull, perplexed face and sad, tired eyes were always astonished by the quick change of his expression to alertness when he became interested in their conversation and wanted to make some contribution to it." [kempfB p16] 3033

⟨$\frac{1}{q}$⟩ cheeks were 'leathery and flabby, falling in loose folds at places, looking sorrowful and sad" – William Herndon [herndonC] (∈ ¶3) 3034

⟨1⟩ 1863: "The drooping eyelids, looking almost swollen; the dark bags beneath the eyes; the deep marks about the large and expressive mouth; the flaccid muscles of the jaws, were all so majestically pitiful..." – Col. Silas Burt [wilsonR p332] 3035

⟨1⟩ "His very prominent features in repose seemed dull and expressionless. ..." – undated clipping from Terre Haute newspaper [wilson p641] (∈ ¶139) 3036

⟨2⟩ Apparently could whistle: [sandburgC v2p302] – see ¶3114. 3037

⟨$\frac{1}{q}$⟩ Springfield years: "Always his thoughtful face was bent forward, as if thinking out some deep problem." – Philip Ayres, recalling his mother's recollections [ayres] 3038

Neck

⟨$\frac{1}{q}$⟩ "a thin but sinewy neck, rather long" – John Nicolay [meserve p5] (∈ ¶177) 3039

• Larynx: 3040

⟨2⟩ 1857: "his large Adam's apple" – Albert Woldman [angle p177] *This may reflect a thin neck rather than an enlarged larynx or thyroid.* 3041

⟨2⟩$_c$ "his larynx was large" [kempfB p9] 3042

⟨$\frac{1}{q}$⟩ Oct. 13, 1858: "His neck ... long and sinewy..." – Carl Schurz [angle p243] (∈ ¶149) 3043

⟨$\frac{1}{q}$⟩ Feb. 1860: Photographer Mathew Brady later recalled "When I [first] got him before the camera I asked him if I might arrange his collar. 'Ah,' said Mr. Lincoln, 'I see you want to shorten my neck.'" [ostendorfA pp13, 36]. 3044

⟨2⟩ 1860: New York Republicans advise Lincoln to grow a beard and "wear standing collars" to improve his appearance [kunhardtA p13]. See ¶1421. 3045

⟨1⟩ Feb. 27, 1860: "long and lean head-stalk" – eyewitness [brooksA p186] (∈ ¶156) 3046

⟨$\frac{1}{q}$⟩ March 1861: "a sinewy muscular yellow neck" – William Russell [russell pp37-38] (∈ ¶161) 3047

⟨1⟩ 1862: "a long scraggy neck" [dicey v1pp220-221] (∈ ¶179) 3048

⟨2⟩ 1865: neck was "leathery and wrinkled" [kunhardtB p49] 3049

▣ Neck wrinkles are appreciated in stereo view [zeller] and monocular view of [ostendorf #88, 89]. 3050

⟨1⟩ April 14, 1865: "he slowly walked with bowed head and drooping shoulders" [lealeA p3] (∈ ¶207) 3051

⟨2⟩ As President: "his long throat" [NYTimes - Aug. 22, 1869] 3052

⟨2⟩ "Mrs. Lincoln was always so solicitous about his going out without a muffler or something about his throat" [shutes p74]. (See ¶2064.) 3053

Nervous System

Older writings in the Lincoln literature attach superior intelligence to persons with the   3054
Marfan syndrome, e.g., [kempfB p2], [schwartzA]. I have seen no hard data on this topic. (See
¶2310 for personality and Marfan syndrome.) MEN2B is a different story, however. *The
Physical Lincoln* presents some biologically-based speculations that link the disease to
mental function.

More importantly, the lesson of Lincoln is one of hard work, humility, and diligent self-   3055
improvement. These resources are available to everyone.

Nevertheless, it is interesting to catalog the intellectually-related advantages Lincoln   3056
may have had, whatever their source (nature and/or nurture). One was his good memory, present even in childhood and apparently a family trait (¶5185). His great talent
for story-telling, also present in his father (¶5174), was another. Less evident in the historical record, but perhaps most important, was his curiosity (see Appendix, ¶3768ff).
From this alone, anything is possible.

Lincoln was photographed swaying as he stood without support (¶3144). This is akin   3057
to, but not actually, a Romberg sign of posterior column dysfunction. His eyes were
almost closed in these pictures, making the finding even more Romberg-like. The finding raises intriguing diagnostic possibilities: (1) Perhaps Lincoln was deficient in vita-
min B_{12} as a result of his weight loss (¶438). Are cold extremities part of this syndrome
(¶1210)? They might have been numb and been able to steam without being painful.
(2) Is the swaying related to the de Musset sign of aortic regurgitation (¶1975ff)? (3) Is
swaying a sign of muscular weakness or hypotonia or fatigue? (4) Is swaying a sign of
Lincoln's practice of standing with his feet even (¶966), producing an unsteady base?
The Physical Lincoln discounts most of these possibilities.

- See also: Handwriting and Gait   3058

⟨1/q⟩ "Will was the true picture of Mr. Lincoln, in every way, even to carrying his head   3059
slightly inclined toward his left shoulder." – Springfield neighbor [burl p66] citing
[NYHerald - May 26, 1861] *Given Lincoln's left hyperphoria, one would expect tilt
toward the right shoulder. See ¶1827.*

⟨S⟩ Charles Zane, who practiced law in Springfield and who became William Hern-   3060
don's law partner after Lincoln assumed the Presidency, provides a detailed analysis of Lincoln's memory, intellect, and psychology in [wilson pp487-490].
  ⟨1⟩ "I should say he had greater natural mental cabilre [sic] than any man I ever   3061
  knew" – Joseph Gillespie [wilson p507]

- Memory (also see Reading & Learning):   3062
  ⟨1⟩ "... he must understand Every thing – even to the smallest thing – Minutely &   3063
  Exactly –: he would then repeat it over to himself again & again – sometimes
  in one form and then in another & when it was fixed in his mind to suit him
  he became Easy and never lost that fact or his understanding of it" – Sarah
  Bush Lincoln [wilson p107]
  ⟨1⟩ "He would hear sermons preached – come home – take the children out – get   3064
  on a stump or log and almost repeat it word for word" – Sarah Bush Lincoln
  [wilson p107]
  ⟨1/q⟩ "Abe had a powerful good memory. He'd go to church an' come home an'   3065
  say over the sermon as good as the preacher. He'd often do it for Aunt Sairy,
  when she couldn't go, an' she said it was jist as good as goin' herself. He'd say

Nervous System (continued)

over everything from beloved brethern to amen..." – Dennis Hanks [wilsonR p28]

⟨1⟩ "Abe could Easily learn & long remember and when he did learn anything   3066
he learned it well and thoroughly. What he thus learned he stowed away in his memory which was Extremely good – What he learned and Stowed away was well defined in his own mind – repeated over & over again & again till it was so defined and fixed firmly & permanently in his Memory" – Sarah Bush Lincoln [wilson p108]

⟨1⟩ "He would repeat the sermon over again to the children. The sight of such a   3067
thing amused all and did Especially tickle the Children." – Sarah Bush Lincoln [wilson p108]

⟨1⟩ In Indiana: "He had a great memory, and for hours he would tell me what he   3068
had read." – Henry Brooner [hobson p19]

⟨1⟩ March 1831: Guided a flatboat from Illinois to New Orleans. Having "a good   3069
pair of eyes and a good memory," he saw navigational hazards (e.g. "snags, sandbars, overhanging trees") and remembered them. This secured him a job as a steamboat pilot the next year. [rossH p110]

⟨1⟩ 1830s: "... seemed hardly ever to forget anything he had read." – Daniel   3070
Burner [templeB]

⟨1⟩ "No one had a more retentive memory. If he read or heard a good thing it   3071
never escaped him." [herndon p39]

⟨1⟩ "I first became acquainted with 'Abe' Lincoln when he was about 14 years of   3072
age ... He read the life of Washington – Histories – some poetry, – all he could get & learned most of it by heart quickly & well & always remembering it." – John Hanks [wilson p43]

⟨1⟩ "Abe could when 15 years of age or in the year 1824, could hear a Sermon –   3073
Speech or remark and repeat it accurately ... Could do the Same in what he heard and read." – Dennis Hanks [wilson p104]

⟨1⟩ "his memmory [sic] was remarkably tenacious. hardly ever forgetting any   3074
thing which he read possessing any interest in his mind" – Dr. Jason Duncan [wilson pp540-541]

⟨1⟩ "His memory was a great Store house" – Robert Wilson [wilson p204]   3075

⟨1⟩ "He remembered everything he read, and could afterwards without appar-   3076
ent difficulty relate it." [herndon pp93-94]

⟨1⟩ "I once remarked to him that his mind was a wonder to me – That impres-   3077
sions were easily made upon it and never effaced – 'No said he you are mistaken – I am slow to learn and slow to forget that which I have learned – My mind is like a piece of steel, very hard to scratch any thing on it and almost impossible after you get there to rub it out' – I give this as his own illustration of the character of his mind – it is as good as any I have seen" – Joshua Speed [wilson p499] [herndon p420] [kunhardtB p298]

⟨1⟩ "Mr. Lincoln had an astonishing memory I never found it at fault He could   3078
recall every incident of his life particularly if any thing amusing was connected with it" – Joseph Gillespie [wilson p187]

⟨1⟩ "He never forgot any thing espically [sic] any personal kindness" – Joshua   3079
Speed [wilson p158]

⟨1⟩ "He never forgot anything" – Matilda Johnston Moore [wilson p110]   3080

⟨1⟩ "he was much Devoted to Reading and had the Best memory of any man i   3081
Ever Knew he Never forgot any thing he Read Nor any friends" – J. Rowan Herndon [wilson p7]

Nervous System (continued)

⟨1⟩ "he allways Remembered what he Red" – J. Rowan Herndon [wilson p92]   3082

⟨1⟩ As President, "he seemed to know more about the general topography of the County than any person he ever say discribed ery house and farm hill Creek and family that lived here when he was a boy." – Charles Friend, speaking of Larue County [wilson p676]   3083

⟨1⟩ "Abraham Lincoln wrote to me that his first recollections were of Knob Creek residence" – Samuel Haycraft [wilson p67]   3084

⟨1⟩ "He read very thoroughly, and had a most wonderful memory. Would distinctly remember almost everything he read." – James Short [wilson p90]   3085

⟨1⟩ "Never forgetting what he read" – David Turnham [wilson p121]   3086

⟨1⟩ 1827: After hearing a sermon, "Abe Said he could repeat it and we boys got him at it ... He did preach almost the identical Sermon. It was done with wonderful accuracy." – David Turnham [wilson p123]   3087

⟨1⟩ 1830s: "He was a good reader rather than a 'much reader' as the Indian would Say: what he read he read thoroughly & well & never forgot it." – Caleb Carman [wilson p374]   3088

⟨1/q⟩ "full of wit, facts, dates ... if I beat him my victory will be hard won" – Stephen A. Douglas [kunhardtA p108]   3089

⟨1/q⟩ Lincoln could repeat "almost word for word anything he had read" – General Viele [kunhardtB p298]   3090

⟨1⟩ "He helped his memory by the conscious and strict observance of the truth. He may not have remembered so much as many others; but within the limits which for good reasons undoubtedly he set to his recolection [sic] he was very exact and reliable." – Charles Zane [wilson p488] *Zane provides a detailed analysis of Lincoln's memory, intellect, and psychology. See* [wilson pp487-490].   3091

⟨1⟩ "All of them [Lincoln and his parents] had good memories" – Dennis Hanks [wilson p598]   3092

⟨2⟩ "He continually astounded people with his memory of names, dates, and facts, and with his ability to quote long passages of poetry after a single reading." [kunhardtA p328]   3093

⟨2⟩ "his remarkable memory for long passages" of Shakespeare [randallC p28]   3095

⟨1⟩ Re: his jokes: "He insisted sometimes that he had no invention, but only a memory." [sumnerA p134]   3096

⟨1⟩ "His memory was strong, ready, and tenacious." Example: He was introduced to a Swede and a Norwegian at the White House. "Immediately he repeated, to their delight, a poem of some eight or ten verses descriptive of Scandinavian scenery, and an old Norse legend. He said he had read the poem in a newspaper some years before, and liked it, but it had passed out of his memory until their visit had recalled it." [arnold p443]   3097

⟨1⟩ "He's got a mighty fine memory, but an awful poor forgetery." – a soldier [porterH]   3098

⟨2⟩ "Lincoln's memory was extraordinarily retentive, and without conscious effort he stored in his mind every whimsical or ludicrous narrative which was read or heard. ... After rehearsing a portion of [a] letter to his guests at the Soldiers' Home one evening, a sedate New England gentleman expressed surprise that he could find time for memorizing such things. 'Oh,' said Lincoln, 'I don't. If I like a thing, it just sticks after once reading it or hearing it.'" [browneF p645]   3099

■ Memory – for people: 3100

Nervous System (continued)

⟨2⟩ "Lincoln never forgot anybody." [tarbellB p185]　　3101

⟨1⟩ 1860-1861: "we had spoken over old times – persons – Circumstances – in　3102
which he showed wonderful memory" – Isaac Cogdal [wilson p440] *Lincoln
and Cogdal had known each other since 1831.* [walsh p83] *thinks Lincoln
prepared for this meeting.*

⟨1⟩ In 1860 greets a man: "You and I are no strangers; we dined together at Gov-　3103
ernor Lincoln's [of Massachusetts] in 1848." – Henry Gardner [wilson p699]

⟨1⟩ Two men, Nelson and Hammond, met Lincoln in spring 1849. A comet was　3104
then in the sky. Nelson told Lincoln that he thought the world "would follow
the darned thing off." Nelson and Lincoln became acquainted over the years.
In 1861, while looking for Lincoln in a crowded hotel dining room, "a long
arm and reached to my shoulder and a shrill voice exclaimed 'Hello, Nelson!
do you think, after all the world is going to follow the darned thing off?' It
was Mr. Lincoln." – undated article in Terre Haute newspaper [wilson pp641-
642] [angle pp160-161]

■ Poor memory:　　3105
　⟨1⟩_q 1860: Does not remember shaking hands with Henry Whitney an hour be-　3106
　fore. [hirschhornC]
　⟨2⟩ Complaining he'd not previously heard about a planned military operation,　3107
　talks "of going back to Illinois if his memory has become as treacherous as
　that." [burl p181]

⟨1⟩ Age 9: Horse-kick to head causes unconsciousness [herndon pp51-52]. (See ¶3568.)　3108

⟨1⟩ "Mr Lincoln had the appearance of being a slow thinker　My impression was　3109
that he was not so slow as he was careful　He never liked to put forth a propo-
sition without revolving it over in his own mind but when he was compelled to
act promptly as in debate he was quick enough" – Joseph Gillespie [wilson p186]

■ Mimicry:　　3110
　⟨2⟩_c "He was especially good at cruel mimicry of accents, mannerisms, gestures,　3111
　and physical defects. [burl p149]
　⟨1⟩_q "unequaled power of mimicry" – Herndon [burl p149]　　3112
　⟨1⟩ "He was a good Mimic in Words & Jestures do you remember his Personating　3113
　J.B. Thomas how he Made Thomas Cry" – Abner Ellis [wilson p161]
　⟨2⟩ "He could imitate a stutterer he knew who had a trick of whistling between　3114
　stuttered syllables." [sandburgC v2p302]
　⟨2⟩_c "talented as a mimic" [currentEB]　　3115

⟨2⟩ Apparently could whistle: [sandburgC v2p302] – see ¶3114.　　3116

⟨1⟩ "He often said that he could think better after Breakfast – and better walking, than　3117
sitting, lying, or standing" – Joshua Speed [wilson p499] [herndon p420]

⟨1⟩ "His Way of Laughing two was rearly funney and Such awakard Jestures belonged　3118
to No other Man they actracted Universal attention from the old Sedate down to
the School Boy then in a few Minnets he was as Calm & thoughtful as a Judge on
the Bench" – Abner Ellis [wilson p161]

⟨M⟩ "Mr Lincoln appreciated the beautiful he had emotions of beauty. His taste was　3119
not cultivated in many directions viz. his power of judging the beauty or deformity
of objects." – Charles Zane [wilson p489]
　⟨1⟩ "Mr nor Mrs Lincoln loved the beautiful" – Frances Todd Wallace [wilson p486]　3120
　(See ¶2052)

Nervous System (continued)

- Mathematics – ability and interests (see ¶4971). 3121
  - ⟨1⟩ In youth: "When the wood was got in and Cut up then Lincoln & father would 3122
    sit up till midnight or later calculating the figures &c." – Elizabeth Herndon
    Bell [wilson p606]
  - ⟨1⟩ 1836: "was a tolerably good mathematician, as he was surveyor of Sangamon 3123
    County." – William Herndon [hertz p85]
  - ⟨-⟩ See ¶3824ff for Euclid and for squaring the circle! 3124

- ⟨$\frac{1}{q}$⟩ "His quickness of perception often astonishes me. Long before the statement of 3125
  a complicated question is finished his mind will seem to comprehend the whole
  subject better than the person who is stating it." – Ulysses Grant [porterH]

- ⟨1⟩ "His organization – rather his structure and functions – worked slowly. His blood 3126
  had to run a long distance from his heart to the extremities of his frame, and his
  nerve force had to travel through dry ground a long distance before his muscles
  were obedient to his will. ... The whole man, body and mind, worked slowly, as
  if needing oiling. ... His mind was like his body, and worked slowly but strongly."
  [herndon p471]

- ⟨1⟩ Seasickness? Mar. 23-24, 1865: Upset stomach after nautical trip. Unclear if it 3127
  was seasickness. See ¶1261 and ¶658ff. (Other, erroneous, dates sometimes reported.)

- Syncope (fainting): 3128
  - ⟨1⟩ Age 9: Horse-kick to head causes unconsciousness [herndon pp51-52]. (See 3129
    ¶3568.)
  - ⟨1⟩ July 27, 1848: "I never fainted from the loss of blood." – Lincoln [baslerA v1p511] 3130
    A facetious reference to battles with mosquitoes during his militia service.
  - ⟨2⟩ March 30, 1861: Recently "had keeled over with sick headache for the first 3131
    time in years." [shenk p285]. (∈ ¶2627) *Phrasing suggests previous episodes.*
    Called a migraine headache by [donaldA p289], *but see ¶2628 for caveats.*
  - ⟨2⟩ Feb. 6, 1865: Faints after standing up quickly and angrily. He is then put to 3132
    bed. [shutes pp108-109]. See ¶1203.

- ⟨S⟩ Absent more definitive sources, it is reasonable to conclude that Lincoln was 3133
  right-handed. If he was worried about his signature on the Emancipation Proclamation after shaking thousands of hands earlier that day, then it follows that he
  signed his name using the same hand with which he shook hands, i.e. the right.
  See ¶1557

- ⟨1⟩ Was an enthusiastic chess player, with Judge Samuel Treat. "When the opportu- 3134
  nity offered indulged in the game." [wilson p725]
  - ⟨2⟩ "was very fond of a game of chess" [ChicagoTribune - Aug. 6, 1871] 3136

- Music (for singing, see ¶3700): 3137
  - ⟨2⟩ "... he was so tone-deaf that he could barely distinguish 'Dixie' from 'The 3138
    Star-Spangled Banner.' " [kunhardtB p302] *This is an exaggeration. Near the*
    end of his life Lincoln frequently made comments about "Dixie" and there
    is an account of him especially enjoying that tune in the 1850s [wilson p648].
  - ⟨2⟩$_c$ "Lincoln had no musical ability, but had an ear for rhythm." [angle p60] 3139
    (reprinting [bartonB]) *Barton may, like other observers, have been referring*
    to Lincoln's keen sense for the rhythm of words.
  - ⟨1⟩ "loved military music" [brooksC p51] 3140

Nervous System (continued)

⟨$\frac{1}{q}$⟩ "His musical tastes, says Mr. Brooks, 'were simple and uncultivated, his 3141
choice being old airs, songs, and ballads, among which the plaintive Scotch
songs were best liked.' " – Noah Brooks [browneF p644]

⟨1⟩ April 1865: "the 'Marseillaise' ... he had a great liking for that tune" [chambrunA] 3142

⟨1⟩ Of music: "he had an especial liking, though he was not versed in the science 3143
and preferred simple ballads to more elaborate compositions." – John Hay
[angle p437]

[□] October 1862: In two posed photographs [ostendorf #63,64], a standing "Lincoln is 3144
slightly blurred from swaying" [kunhardtA p311]. Figure 5 discusses one of the photographs at length.

⟨1⟩ The day before these pictures were taken, Lincoln wrote his wife: "Gen. Mc- 3145
Clellan and myself are to be photographed to-morrow A.M. by Mr. Gardner
if we can be still long enough. I feel Gen. M. should have no problem on his
end but I may sway in the breeze a bit." [ostendorfA p326]

⟨-⟩ *In at least some studio photographs, a hidden iron support helped Lincoln* 3146
steady his head during the camera exposures [meserve p4]. *See* [ostendorf #75]
for a visible example [ostendorfA p140].

⟨-⟩ *See also the cardiovascular considerations discussed in* ¶*1975ff.* 3147

⟨2⟩ April 14, 1865: Lincoln could shiver. See ¶697 3148

⟨$\frac{1}{q}$⟩ Post-mortem brain weight was unremarkable. (See ¶3303.) 3149

Physicians

This section lists people who were, or who may have been, Lincoln's physicians. The 3150
hope is that documents from these individuals will some day turn up and shed light
on Lincoln's health. (The hope is likely to be in vain, rather like hoping the medical
records department will turn up a patient chart previously declared "missing.")

Physicians who left memoirs include Jayne (¶3187), Busey (¶3202), Browne (¶3194), 3151
Graham (¶5187), and assassination & autopsy physicians.

⟨2⟩ [markens] attempts a complete listing of physicians with whom Lincoln had signifi- 3152
cant interactions, providing brief information for each.

⟨2⟩ Shutes names several physicians near the Lincoln's Kentucky home before and 3153
after Lincoln's birth [shutes p2]. One can read subtleties into Shutes' descriptions of
their comings and goings. The list below ignores the subtleties:

⟨2⟩ Dr. Ebenezer B. Goodletter, 1807-? 3154

⟨2⟩ Dr. Thomas Essex, from England, 1809-1811 (moved on) 3155

⟨2⟩ Dr. William Sulcer, of Holland, 1809-1811 (moved on) 3156

⟨2⟩ Dr. Daniel B. Potter, 1811-1814 (died). "Dr. Potter of Elizabethtown attended 3157
the Lincoln family in Kentucky" [shutesP: Letter from William E. Barton, Mar. 29, 1928].
Also see ¶5188

■ In Indiana: 3158

⟨2⟩ There was no physician within 30 miles of Gentryville [shutes p5]. *This is hard* 3159
to square with later references to specific physicians – see below.

⟨2⟩ However, Josiah Crawford was a "yarb and root" doctor who could apply 3160
plasters, pull teeth, give hot foot-baths, apply incantations, dispense blue-
mass pills – and let blood. Lincoln occasionally split rails for him, and nicknamed him "Old Blue-Nose Crawford." [shutes pp5-6] *"Blue-nose" implies*
some degree of color vision! See ¶*844.*

Physicians (continued)

⟨-⟩ The account of Lincoln's sister's death mentions two physicians, Fred Lively and William Davis, who perhaps lived closer than 30 miles. See below and ¶5019-¶5021.   3161

⟨1⟩ Dr. Fred Lively, who was born "back of Hawesville Ky." and is [perhaps] buried near Grandview, IN, was "a drunk – too drunk - to care for Sarah Lincoln Grigsby & her baby – both of whom died." [shutesP: Feb. 20, 1933 letter from Charles T. Baker] (Baker was editor of a Grandview newspaper, *The Monitor*.)   3162

⟨1⟩ The letter from Charles Baker in [shutesP] also mentions "Dr. 'Bill' Davis, of Warrick Co., and Dr. Anderson, of New Boston" and further says "both have been called to the Lincoln home at one time or another."   3163

⟨2⟩ When Lincoln was a militia captain in the Black Hawk War, his regimental surgeon was Dr. Jacob M. Early. [shutes p11]   3164

⟨S⟩ Shutes speculates that Early would also have tended to Lincoln during the latter's second tour with the militia. [shutes p11].   3165

⟨2⟩ Early was from Springfield. He "commanded the third Black Hawk War unit in which Lincoln served." [wilson p372n] Also: [wilson p520]   3166

⟨2⟩ Dr. Early was a Democratic leader and, therefore, political opponent of Lincoln in 1836. Lincoln's reply to him in a public address "completely crushed" Early with "wit, anecdote and ridicule," to a degree that was remembered even decades later. [burl p150]   3167

- Dr. Jason Duncan of New Salem, IL: 3168
  ⟨2⟩ Was "the only doctor of medicine who left any memoirs of the young Lincoln." Duncan also helped Lincoln become village postmaster in 1833. [shutes p12] *Other physicians left memoirs (¶3151).*   3169

  ⟨1⟩ Duncan "knew Lincoln well ... D & Lincoln were great friends" – Johnson Greene [wilson p365]   3170

  ⟨1⟩ Duncan's long letter to William Herndon is: [wilson pp539-542]   3171
  ⟨1⟩ Duncan is also mentioned in [wilson pp367,370,380]   3172

- Other physicians (and healers) of Lincoln's acquaintance during his New Salem, IL days: 3173
  ⟨2⟩ Dr. Nelson, Dr. Abbott, Dr. John Marsh [shutes pp9-11]; Dr. Francis Regnier, Dr. Bennett (first name Newton or Richard E.), Dr. David Meeker [shutes pp15-16]   3174

  ⟨2⟩ Dr. Bennett Abell [shutes p21] wife's sister was Mary Owen, whom Lincoln courted [donaldA pp67-68].   3175

  ⟨2⟩ Lincoln made calls with Dr. John Allen in summer 1835 [shutes p17] (see ¶2008). He was a Dartmouth graduate [donaldA p41]. Shutes ascribes great influence on Lincoln from Allen [shutes p20]. Allen arrived in New Salem on Aug. 28, 1831 [angle p61, reprinting bartonB]. "There Dr. Allen was doubtless his attending physician and he is an interesting character and not difficult to learn about. His daughter is still living or was a few years ago. I have interviewed her" [shutesP: Letter from William E. Barton, Mar. 29, 1928]. William Herndon called Allen (if it is the same one) "a great blow" and more [hertz p140]. Allen is extensively described in [rankinA pp73-82].   3176

  ⟨2⟩ Dr. Charles Chandler was instrumental in Lincoln's rise. It was through a contact of his that Lincoln was invited to deliver the career-igniting "Cooper Union" speech [shutes pp13-15].   3177

  ⟨1⟩ Two sons of Matthew Rogers were reading medicine "under the tutoring of Dr. Gershom Jayne." [rankinA p67]   3178

218

Physicians (continued)

⟨2⟩ James Pantier, a "yarb doctor" (see ¶3158), did not accept fees for his ser-   3179
vices! [shutes p10]

■ Physicians (and healers) of Lincoln's acquaintance during his Springfield, IL days: 3180
  ⟨2⟩ 1835 (two years before Lincoln moved there): Springfield had 12 practicing   3181
  physicians [shutesE p45].
  ⟨2⟩ "The family physician in Springfield, at least during the early years, was Dr.   3182
  H. E. Henry, as you will learn in 'Women Lincoln Loved.'" [shutesP: Letter from
  William E. Barton, Mar. 29, 1928] [bartonW]
  ⟨2⟩ Dr. Elias H. Merryman was Lincoln's second in a duel [shutes p23&31] and prob-   3183
  ably helped steer Lincoln into it [donaldA pp91-92]. He is said to have removed
  a lump from Lincoln's cheek (¶1850). He helped Lincoln during the 1841 rift
  with Mary [wilsonH p35] (¶2746). Has been spelled "Merriman" [pearson]. See
  also ¶3183.
  ⟨2⟩ Dr. Anson Henry was a staunch friend. Helped Lincoln recover after break-   3184
  ing up with Mary Todd (see ¶2746). Henry had been a student of Dr. Drake in
  Cincinnati (see ¶2467). Lincoln appointed Henry surveyor-general of Washington Territory [shutes pp46-49]. Henry consoled the surviving Lincolns after
  the assassination: he was also with Robert at the White House memorial service and accompanied the family to Chicago [shutesP: typewritten 5-page essay on
  Dr. Anson Henry in box 1, folder 1]. The Lincoln Presidential Library in Springfield
  holds the Henry papers [shenk p293].
  ⟨1⟩ Lincoln asked Dr. Daniel Drake for medical advice in a letter (see ¶2016 and   3185
  ¶2467). Joshua Speed notes: "Chs D. Drake of St Louis may have his Fathers
  papers" [wilson p431]
  ⟨2⟩ Mary's uncle was Dr. John Todd [evans p327] [baker p75]   3186
  ⟨2⟩ The Jaynes: As President, Lincoln appointed Dr. William Jayne to be territo-   3187
  rial governor of Montana, Idaho, and the Dakotas. His father, Dr. Gershom
  Jayne, was also a physician in Springfield, and was the force behind Jayne's
  Carminative, a flatulence remedy (see ¶2302) [shutes pp44-45]. William Jayne
  left reminiscences [jayne].
  ⟨2⟩ Many others, listed in [shutes pp49-53]   3188
  ⟨2⟩ R.W. Diller was the Springfield druggist. Diller stated that Dr. Wallace was   3189
  the Lincoln family physician and that Dr. Meredith S. Helm (trained in ob-
  stetrics) was called at times. [shutes p53].
  ⟨1⟩ Dr. B.B Lloyd – a dentist [wilson p425]   3190
  ⟨2⟩ His dentist, about the time of Robert's birth (1843) was Dr. French. [kunhardtA   3191
  p90]
  ⟨1⟩ Dr. Richard F. Barrett [wilson p8]   3192
  ⟨2⟩ Dr. John Henry Shearer lived across the street (Eighth Street). Mary corre-   3193
  sponded with his wife. [turner p54]. The Shearers traveled with the Lincolns for
  part of the 1861 train ride to Washington [turner p81n].
  ⟨2⟩ As a child, Robert H. Browne knew Lincoln in Springfield. He later became a   3194
  physician. Late in life he wrote a "very poorly organized" biography [linclore-
  HZA] [browneR].

■ Dr. William Wallace was married to Mary's sister Frances [shutes pp44-45], and was   3195
the Lincoln family physician in Springfield. The Lincoln's named their third son
after him.
  ⟨2⟩ Immediately after marrying, the Lincoln's moved into Wallace's old room at   3196
  the Globe Tavern. [randallC p69]
  ⟨-⟩ He attended Mary during at least one delivery – see ¶4648.   3197

Physicians (continued)

⟨-⟩ He is said to have operated on Robert's eye(s) (¶4929) and Tad's lip (¶5466).   3198

⟨2⟩ 1850s(?): Mary "was fearful about his health, which her brother-in-law, Dr.   3200
Wallace (¶3195) warned her to watch." [helmB p115]

⟨2⟩ Wallace was in charge of Lincoln's health during the 1861 trip from Spring-   3201
field to Washington [shutes p76].

- 1848±: Dr. Samuel C. Busey, "a young physician," lived in the same boarding   3202
house as Lincoln during Lincoln's term in Congress. His description of Lincoln
is thin on medical observations. [busey].

- The Lincoln family physician in the White House was Dr. Robert King Stone (1822-   3203
1872). A brief biography is in [shutes pp142-143].

⟨2⟩ Stone was Professor of Medicine at Georgetown University [pearson] who con-   3204
centrated on private practice after "a disabling carriage accident" about 1860
[crellin].

⟨2⟩ Received M.D. degree in 1845 from the University of Pennsylvania [rossC] and   3205
had special training in eye diseases [crellin].

⟨2⟩ Stone either did [crellin] or did not [pearson] keep good records of his patients.   3206
His case books are at Duke University [crellin].

⟨2⟩ Although "politically unsympathetic" to Lincoln, Stone "became a more or   3207
less frequent caller on the President and his family" [shutes p79]. Stone's only
known statement about Lincoln is: "It is the province of a physician to probe
deeply the interior lives of men; and I affirm that Mr. Lincoln is the purest
hearted man with whom I ever came in contact" [carpenter p81].

⟨2⟩ Stone was a Virginian. "He was the cousin of Robert E. Lee, and his wife   3209
was the daughter of Thomas Ritchie, long the renowned editor of the *Richmond Enquirer*." – from a 23-page manuscript titled "John F. Parker: Much
Maligned Virginian" in [barbeeP - box 2 folder 133] *Parker was the guard who
accompanied Lincoln to Ford's Theatre.*

- Dr. Stone's medical skills seem to admit of several lapses: 3210
⟨2⟩ Stone (incorrectly) prognoses that Willie will recover from his Feb. 1862 ill-   3211
ness.

⟨2⟩ Lincoln has smallpox and Stone sees him, but the diagnosis is made by an-   3212
other physician, Dr. Van Bibber (See ¶3215.)

⟨2⟩ Stone may also have mis-diagnosed Tad's November 1863 illness if, like Lin-   3213
coln, Tad had smallpox.

⟨2⟩ Stone gives brandy to the comatose, dying President, who "almost strangled"   3214
on it [kunhardtA p357]. ¶558

⟨2⟩ A Dr. Van Bibber, of Baltimore, made the diagnosis of varioloid in President Lin-   3215
coln (see Special Topic §5). In terms of comportment, Van Bibber was "of the
old school" [finney p259]. His office moved to 47 Franklin Street in Baltimore in
Dec. 1863 [Baltimore Sun, Dec. 10, 1863].

- Physicians Lincoln knew in Washington: 3216
⟨1⟩ Dr. Henry W. Bellows of "The Sanitary Commission" – see ¶654   3217
⟨1⟩ Dr. William A. Hammond was surgeon general of the Army. He was court-   3218
martialled, dismissed from the Army, but, according to [shutesP], "finally ex-
onerated."

⟨1⟩ 1865: "the White House physician," Surgeon General Joseph K. Barnes, "was   3220
often" there [crookA p29] *Is calling him "White House physician" an error?*

⟨2⟩ Wrote orders to physicians during the war; some are listed in [shutes pp104-105].   3221

Physicians (continued)

⟨2⟩ Physicians at Lincoln's death-bed: Charles Augustus Leale, Charles Sabin Taft, John Frederick May [kunhardtB p182], Robert King Stone (¶3203), Joseph K. Barnes (surgeon general of the Army), Charles H. Crane (assistant Army surgeon general), Neal Hall, C.H. Lieberman, Beecher Todd (a cousin of Mary's), a Dr. Ford, C.D. Gatch, E.W. Abbott [shutes p114].   3222

    ⟨2⟩ A different list: Leale, Taft, Charles A. Gatch, Africanus F.A. King in the Theater. Additional physicians in Peterson House: Barnes, Stone, Abbott, Crane, Curtis, Ford, Hall, Notson, Lieberman, May, Todd, Woodward. [kunhardtA pp356-358]   3223

    ⟨2⟩ The physicians who cared for Lincoln after his shooting marched as a unit in his Washington, DC funeral procession [kunhardtB p131] and had a place of honor at his Capitol funeral service [kunhardtB p132].   3224

    ⟨-⟩ Unflattering disclosures about Dr. Taft are in [markens] and Special Topic §7.   3225

    ⟨1⟩ Leale's obituary [NYTimes - June 14, 1932] says he was a student of Austin Flint. Leale was the last surviving witness of Lincoln's death [barbeeP - box 2 folder 137].   3226

■ Physician records of Lincoln's last hours alive: (See ¶3270 for autopsy records.)   3227

    ⟨2⟩ Leale made notes "within days" of Lincoln's death [good p59]. *Where are they now?*   3228

    ⟨1⟩_q Leale wrote letters in May 1865 (to a friend) [lattimerBk p41, excerpt] and in 1867 (to Benjamin Butler) [good pp59-62, excerpt].   3229

    ⟨1⟩ Leale: A copy of his report to the Surgeon General, "undated, but evidently written a day or two after the assassination" is in [barbeeP].   3230

    ⟨1⟩ Leale: News coverage: [WashingtonStar - April 17, 1865] [NYTribune - April 17, 1865] [NYHerald - April 18, 1865] (from [barbeeP])   3231

    ⟨1⟩ Leale: "Vivid description" in New York *World*, July 3, 1881 (in [barbeeP])   3232

    ⟨1⟩ Leale: In 1909 gave an address to the Loyal Legion and wrote a long account that appeared as a book [lealeA] and as an article in *Harper's Weekly* of Feb. 7, 1909. Account is reprinted in [lattimerBk pp28-32].   3233

    ⟨1⟩ Taft wrote an article for an April 22, 1865 medical journal [taft], reprinted in §7i.   3234

    ⟨1⟩ Taft's notes about Lincoln's death-night once belonged to collector Abraham Simon Wolf [anonB].   3235

    ⟨2⟩ Taft's 9 1/2-page letter about Lincoln's death-night and autopsy, written under the order of Edwin Stanton, came to light in 1995 and was auctioned [anonC]. *I do not know if this is the same as the "notes" described in 1937, above.*   3236

    ⟨2⟩ Taft wrote an article in *The Century* magazine in February 1893, according to [good p62].   3237

    ⟨1⟩ Stone gave brief testimony about the death-night and the autopsy at the trial of the conspirators. [pitman pp81-82] largely reprinted in [purtle].   3238

■ For physicians at the autopsy, see ¶3270.   3239

Post-Mortem

This section continues where `Death Watch` ended. Because DNA recovered from tissue samples of the long-dead can be analyzed and, in some cases, make a diagnosis, Lincoln's tissue samples are an item of interest. This is especially true in Lincoln's case, since he is buried under tons of concrete and cannot be exhumed. (In 1876 grave-robbers had his coffin halfway out of his tomb when they were apprehended [kunhardtA p398].) For the next 25 years Lincoln's body was in various secret locations. Finally, in   3240

Post-Mortem (continued)

1901, he was buried in an iron cage atop a four-foot thick slab of concrete. Then another four feet of concrete was poured over the coffin. Thus, he is now "in a place only a bomb could reach." [kunhardtA pp398-399]

⟨$\frac{1}{q}$⟩ Soon after death Lincoln's face assumed a look of "unspeakable peace" [kunhardtA p359] 3241

  ⟨1⟩ See Maunsell Field's account of Lincoln's death [NYTimes - April 17, 1865], reprinted in §7e. 3242

  ⟨-⟩ See also: ¶1797 and ¶3307. 3245

- Lincoln scholars have no doubt expended much effort on establishing the provenance of every artifact said to contain Lincoln tissue, and I can of course do no better than them. The list below may, however, give the reader some idea of the range of artifacts that may be considered, should medical interrogation of Lincoln's tissue ever be attempted. 3246

  ⟨2⟩ Lincoln bled on (at least) the collar of his overcoat [kunhardtB p1]. *Probably not Rathbone's blood...* 3247

  ⟨2⟩ Dr. Leale saved his blood-stained cuffs [shutes p117] 3248

  ⟨2⟩ Lincoln's head wound bloodily soaked two pillows on his death-bed. One pillow was thrown out the window of the house [kunhardtB pp82,97]. The other appears in a photograph [kunhardtB p82]. A piece of a blood-stained pillow case was (is?) in the collection of the College of Physicians in Philadelphia [purtle]. 3249

  ⟨1⟩ A resident of the Peterson house mailed "a piece of cloth which was placed between the President's head and the pillow, and is saturated with blood" to a Reverend Russell of Zion Church in New York City. [NYTimes - April 21, 1865] 3250

  ⟨2⟩ Whenever Mary entered the death-chamber to see her husband, towels were placed over the bloody pillows. The Lincoln National Life Foundation owns swatches of the towels. [kunhardtB pp 104, 311] 3251

  ⟨2⟩ At autopsy, Dr. C.H. Lieberman snipped lockets of hair from Lincoln's head surrounding the fatal wound [purtle]. Portions were presented to the surgeons present, and to Mrs. Lincoln. Two of these were later donated to the Army Medical Museum [purtle]. 3252

  ⟨$\frac{1}{q}$⟩ March 1905: John Hay presented Theodore Roosevelt with a ring containing hair from Lincoln's head, writing "Dr. Taft cut it off the night of the assassination, and I got it from his son." [beschlossB p154] 3253

  ⟨1⟩ The collection of Louise Taper included samples of Lincoln's hair, samples of Willie's hair, and blood stained white gloves that Lincoln carried to Ford's Theatre [ferguson p126]. 3254

  ⟨2⟩ Willie Clark claimed to have samples of Lincoln's hair and brain. The brain has vanished. [ferguson pp128, 135] 3255

  ⟨1⟩ The quantity of saved Lincoln hair is so large ("fistfuls" held by the Chicago Historical Society alone) as to be impossible. [ferguson pp126-127] 3256

  ⟨2⟩ Less than two hours after Lincoln's death, relic hunters descended on the house where he died. Many blood-stained items were taken away. [kunhardtB p97] 3257

  ⟨2⟩ Lincoln's blood stained Laura Keene's dress. She was the star actress in the play Lincoln watched that night and came to his box soon after the shooting, supposedly to render assistance [helmB pp258-259] [kunhardtB pp44-45]. Keene preserved the dress for many years, but it was ultimately lost, except for five swatches stained with Lincoln's blood [swansonB]. 3258

Post-Mortem (continued)

⟨1⟩ Ford's Theatre displays clothes Lincoln wore the night of his death. There are blood stains on his frockcoat, overcoat, and pants (knees). [ruane]   3259

⟨2⟩ "The bloodstained cuffs of the undershirt Dr. Curtis was wearing at the time of the autopsy, and a splinter of skull bone from the fatal wound area" were donated to the Army Medical Museum in 1947 by Dr. Curtis' son [purtle].   3260

⟨2⟩ The lethal bullet was transferred to the Army Medical Museum in 1956 [purtle].   3261

⟨H⟩ At the Harlan-Lincoln House in Mt. Pleasant, IA: "a collar fragment believed to be worn when President Lincoln was assassinated" (Internet)   3262

⟨2⟩ As of the 1990s, the National Museum of Health and Medicine owned: the surgical probe inserted in Lincoln's skull to locate the pistol ball, the ball itself, two locks of hair from Lincoln's head (about 180 strands), about 10 grams of skull tissue in 7 fragments, and Dr. Curtis' cuffs. The National Army Museum was the former owner. [reilly] *I believe the ball is normally displayed at Ford's Theatre.*   3263

⟨1⟩ Non-assassination-related: After taking the oath of office for his second term, Lincoln kissed the Bible on a spot later marked by Chief Justice Chase. The Bible was presented to Mary. [brooksC pp240-241]   3264

⟨2⟩ Besides President and Mrs. Lincoln, two other people were in box #7 at Ford's Theatre that night: Major Henry Rathbone and his fiancee, Clara Harris (daughter of a New York Senator) [kunhardtB p26]. Rathbone lunged at the assassin, who then tried to stab him in the chest. Rathbone parried, and received a two-inch-deep cut just above the elbow. This wound dripped and, later, spurted, blood [kunhardtB pp39,41,48]. Rathbone later became unconscious from loss of blood [kunhardtB p48].   3265

⟨2⟩ After Lincoln was carried from the box, it was "one pool of blood" [kunhardtB p98]. *Thus, any blood sample from the box would most likely include some of Rathbone's blood.*   3266

⟨2⟩ Rathbone had red-hair [kunhardtB p48] *Thus, interrogation of melanin genes could determine if a blood sample was Rathbone-free.*   3267

⟨1/q⟩ Lincoln's remains were taken to the White House. "I saw them taken from the box in which they were enclosed, all limp and warm, and laid upon the floor, and then stretched upon the cooling board." – Benjamin French [kunhardtA p362]   3268

⟨1/q⟩ "The corpse was laid out in the room on the North side of the second story, opposite Mrs. Lincoln's room. His eyes were both very much protruded – the right one most – and very black and puffy underneath. No other disfiguration. The skull was opened under the supervision of Surgeon General Barnes and Dr Stone, and the ball removed. It was a Derringer ball, much flattened on both sides. It entered at the base of the brain an inch and a half or two inches back of the left ear, ranging upward and transversely in the direction of the right eye, lodged in the brain about two thirds of the way from where it entered to the front. He never had a moment's consciousness after he was shot." – Orville Browning (diary entry) [kunhardtA p363]   3269

- Physicians at the autopsy: 3270

  ⟨2⟩ Edward Curtis [curtis] and Joseph Janvier Woodward performed the procedure. Both were pathologists at the Army Medical Museum and held the rank of Assistant Surgeon [kunhardtB p93].   3271

  ⟨2⟩ Also present: Joseph K. Barnes (Army Surgeon General) (¶3222), Robert Stone (¶3203), Charles Taft (¶3222), [Charles] Crane (Assistant Army Surgeon General) (¶3222), and a Dr. Notson (Assistant Surgeon) [kunhardtB p93].   3272

Post-Mortem (continued)

⟨1⟩ Autopsy performed by: "Surgeon General Barnes, Dr. Stone ...; Drs. Crane,   3273
Curtis, Woodward, Toft [sic] and other eminent men" [NYTimes - April 17, 1865].

⟨2⟩ "Dr. Leale declined an invitation to be present" [shutes p116].   3274

■ Physician records of the autopsy (see ¶3227 for records of dying):   3275

⟨2⟩ Curtis wrote a letter to his mother soon after the autopsy (excerpt in [kunhardtA   3276
p363] [kunhardtB pp93, 95] ¶3291 and mis-cited in [lattimerNY]).

⟨2⟩ "Dr. Curtis wrote an account of the autopsy which was published in the New   3277
York Sun for Sunday, April 12, 1903" [purtle].

⟨1⟩ Curtis wrote an address in 1908 [curtis].   3278

⟨1/q⟩ Woodward wrote the official military report. [lattimerBk pp34-35] (See ¶3293.)   3279

⟨1⟩ Taft wrote a report for a medical journal [taft], reprinted in §7i. See ¶3270 for   3280
more Taft.

⟨1⟩ Stone hand-wrote a $2\,^1/_2$-page report (with diagram) that was lost until 1965   3281
[lattimerAu].

⟨2⟩ Stone "read a paper before the Medical Society of the District of Columbia,   3282
describing the death and autopsy findings" on May 3, 1865 [shutes p142]

⟨1⟩ Stone gave brief testimony about the death-night and the autopsy at the trial   3283
of the conspirators. [pitman pp81-82] largely reprinted in [purtle].

⟨-⟩ For physician descriptions of Lincoln on the autopsy table, see ¶2938ff.   3284

■ Autopsy 1 - preparatory: 3285

⟨2⟩ Was conducted in the room at the front right-hand corner of the second floor   3286
of the White House. [kunhardtB p92]

⟨2⟩ Began at 11 am (less than four hours after Lincoln died), by sawing Lincoln's   3287
skull "straight around on a line above his ears so that the top could be lifted
off." [kunhardtB p93]

⟨2⟩ Southern sources bitterly maintained that "the blood drained out of Lincoln   3288
at autopsy was 'sacredly preserved' and already worshiped as a sacred relic."
[kunhardtA p223]

⟨-⟩ Physicians at the autopsy are listed in ¶3270ff.   3289

■ Autopsy 2 - procedure described by Dr. Edward Curtis in a letter: 3290

⟨1/q⟩ "A week ago today Dr. [J. Janvier] Woodward and myself were ordered by the   3291
surgeon general to make a post-mortem examination, in his presence, on
the body of the President. Accordingly, at 11 o'clock we assembled at the
White House in the room where the body lay. ... It contained but little fur-
niture: a large, heavily curtained bed, a sofa or two, bureau, wardrobe, and
chairs composed all there was. Seated around the room were several general
officers and some civilians, silent or conversing in whispers, and to one side,
stretched upon a rough framework of boards and covered only with sheets
and towels, lay – cold and immovable – what but a few hours before was the
soul of a great nation. ... The Surgeon General was walking up and down the
room when I arrived and detailed me the history of the case. He said that the
President showed most wonderful tenacity of life, and, had not his wound
been necessarily mortal, might have survived an injury to which most men
would succumb. Dr. Woodward and I proceeded to open the head and remove the brain down to the track of the ball. The latter had entered a little to
the left of the median line at the back of the head, had passed almost directly
forwards through the center of the brain and lodged. Not finding it readily,
we proceeded to remove the entire brain, when, as I was lifting the latter

Post-Mortem (continued)

from the cavity of the skull, suddenly the bullet dropped out through my fingers and fell, breaking the solemn silence of the room with its clatter, into an empty basin that was standing beneath. There it lay upon the white china, a little black mass no bigger than the end of my finger – dull, motionless and harmless, yet the cause of such mighty changes in the world's history as we may perhaps never realize." [kunhardtA p363] [kunhardtB pp93, 95]

⟨1⟩ Autopsy 3 - reports: 3292

  ⟨1/q⟩ Drs Woodward and Curtis performed the autopsy. Woodward's official report   3293
is reprinted in §7f.

  ⟨1⟩ The New York *Times* published a summary [NYTimes - April 17, 1865]. It is   3294
reprinted in §7g.

  ⟨1⟩ "... at the back of the head, low down and a little to the left, a small round   3295
blackened wound, such as is made by a pistol-shot at close range. There is
no counter-opening, so the missile has lodged and must now be found." –
Edward Curtis, MD [curtis]

  ⟨1⟩ The only non-traumatic skull finding at autopsy was "orbital plates very   3296
thin" [lattimerAu].

■ Contemporary academic discussions: 3297

  ⟨S⟩ [shutesP] mentions: July 22, 1865 *Lancet*: How where [sic] the fractures of the   3298
orbital plates of the frontal bone of the Late President Lincoln produced? –
W.F. Teevan

  ⟨S⟩ [shutesP] mentions: June 17, 1865 *Lancet*: Note on some of the injuries sus-   3299
tained by the late President of the U.S. – T. Longmore

⟨2⟩ Undertaker Dr. Charles D. Brown (of Brown and Alexander) and his assistant   3300
drained Lincoln's blood through "the" jugular vein. Through a cut on the inside
of the thigh (presumably to access the femoral artery) they embalmed the body.
"The face was shaved except for a small tuft left at the chin. The eyes were closed,
the eyebrows arched, the mouth set in the slightest of smiles." The black stain in
Lincoln's face had spread down his cheeks. Edwin Stanton decided the undertakers should not remove it: "No, this is part of the history of the event." [kunhardtB
p95]

  ⟨2⟩ The papers of the man who embalmed Lincoln were in the collection of   3301
Louise Taper. [ferguson p125]

  ⟨2⟩ Henry P. Cattell prepared the body. He drained the blood via a jugular vein   3302
and performed arterial embalming via a femoral artery. No cavity treatment
was given. [ferguson p221] quoting a brochure from the Museum of Funeral
Customs in Springfield, IL.

⟨1/q⟩ As the undertakers worked, Curtis suggested that Lincoln's brain be weighed: "...   3303
silently, in one corner of the room, I prepared the brain for weighing. ... The
weighing of the brain ... gave approximate results only, since there had been some
loss of brain substance, in consequence of the wound, during the hours of life after the shooting. But the figures, as they were, seemed to show that the brain
weight was not above the ordinary for a man of Lincoln's size." [kunhardtB p95]

⟨2⟩ The coffin was 6 feet 6 inches long [kunhardtB p120].   3305

■ Most Lincoln post-mortem services and ceremonies were open-casket.   3306

  ⟨2⟩ At the White House service: Lincoln's dark complexion was now "unpleas-   3307
antly lighter, a grayish putty color." He still had the faintly happy expression
of ¶3241 (and see ¶3300 and ¶1797). [kunhardtB p124]

Post-Mortem (continued)

⟨2⟩ Lincoln's face had to be re-chalked in Harrisburg "to hide the growing discoloration" of the face [kunhardtB p144]. 3308

⟨2⟩ Also in Harrisburg "the body literally had to be dusted," as the face, hair, and beard seemed to "attract particles out of the air" [kunhardtB p144] 3309

⟨2⟩ April 24, 1865 (±), in New York "the blackness had really started to distress viewers. Lincoln looked shriveled, his coffin many sizes too big for him. To many, his cheeks seemed hollow and pitted. ... After New York, with constant care and powdering from the undertaker, Lincoln's appearance had seemed to improve." [kunhardtB p237, 240] (Date is from [kunhardtB p166].) 3310

⟨2⟩ "By the time Lincoln's body reached Chicago, blackness had spread over the entire face, but constant powderings kept it presentable." [kunhardtA p383] 3311

⟨2⟩ By the time Lincoln reached Springfield, the undertaker (Dr. Charles D. Brown), "in great distress, said he had no idea how to remedy the totally black condition of Lincoln's face." A "very thick" layer of rouge chalk and amber was able to "completely hide" the blackness. [kunhardtB p256] 3313

⟨2⟩ At Lincoln's final burial in 1901 a hole was cut in his coffin just over his face. After escape of a pungent odor, 17 citizens of Springfield peered in to confirm Lincoln was in the coffin. "There was the face, still white from the chalk applied by the undertaker on the funeral trip west back in 1865. There were the nose and chin, as prominent as in life. There were the little black bow tie in place, and the suit of black cloth Lincoln had worn at his second inauguration, now whitened with mildew. There was the head, fallen to one side on the sunken pillow." [kunhardtA p399] 3314

Reading & Learning

⟨1⟩ Studied books. His knowledge surprised neighbors when "not mor'n seven." [browneR v1p83] (∈ ¶1762) 3315

⟨1/q⟩ "the things I want to know is in books. My best friend is the man who who'll git me one." – Lincoln, per Dennis Hanks [wilsonR p25] 3316

⟨2⟩ Could not write at the time his family left Kentucky (in 1816) [donaldA p23]. 3317

⟨2⟩ Oct. 1818: When mother died, wrote David Elkin, asking him to preach at her funeral [hobson p20]. 3318

⟨2⟩ His lifetime formal schooling totaled less than a year – [baslerA v4p63] (also outlines schools attended) 3319

⟨1/q⟩ "It pestered Tom a heap to have Abe writin' all over everything, but Abe was jist wropped up in it. ... When Tom got mad at his markin' the house up, Abe tuk' to markin trees Tom wanted to cut down." – Dennis Hanks [wilsonR p24] 3320

⟨1/q⟩ "bashful – Somewhat dull ... not a brilliant boy – but *worked* his way by toil: to learn was hard for him, but he walked Slowly, but Surely." – John Hanks [wilson p454] 3321

⟨2⟩ [donaldA p29] has "worked slowly" instead of "walked slowly." Both [wilson p454] and [kunhardtA p36] (see ¶1030) say "walked." 3322

- Lincoln's learning style: 3323

⟨1/q⟩ "He must understand every thing – even to the smallest thing – minutely and exactly. ... He would then repeat it over to himself again and again – some times in one form and some times in an other and when it was fixed in his mind to suit him he ... never lost that fact or his understanding of it." – Lincoln's step-mother [donaldA p29] and [wilson p107] 3324

226

Reading & Learning (continued)

⟨1/q⟩ Lincoln recalled that even as a child he would get "irritated" when he could not understand what others were saying, and would be unable to sleep until he had "bounded" the idea completely and could "put it in a language plain enough ... for any boy I knew to comprehend. This was kind of a passion with me, and it has stuck with me." [kunhardtA p37]   3325

⟨2⟩ During his brief formal schooling, Lincoln was "a good reader, an excellent speller, a good penman, and was able to compose well" [angle p25] (reprinting [bartonB])   3326

⟨1⟩ "Lincoln had a strong mind. I was older than we was by 6 years and further advanced – but he soon outstript me" – David Turnham [wilson p121]   3327

  ⟨1⟩ "What Lincoln read he read and re-read – read & Studied thoroughly –. He was generally at the head of all his classes whilst at school – in fact was nearly always so" – David Turnham [wilson p121]   3328

⟨1⟩ Age 15+: "The Schools we went to taught Spelling – reading – writing and Ciphering to single rule of 3 – no further —. Lincoln got ahead of his masters – Could do him no further good: he went to school no more." – Anna Gentry [wilson p131]   3329

  ⟨1⟩ "he aways was at the head of his cllass" [sic] – Nathaniel Grigsby [wilson p94]   3330

⟨1⟩ 1832-1833: Lincoln "*Devoured* all the Law Books he could get hold of" – William Greene [wilson p12]   3331

⟨1⟩ February 1833: "he Commenced to study the English grammar with me" – Mentor Graham [wilson p10]   3332

  ⟨1⟩ "all the instruction he ever had in Grammar he rec'd from me" – Lynn Greene [wilson p80]   3333

⟨1/q⟩ 1835+: County surveyor wants Lincoln as his deputy. Lincoln protests ignorance. Surveyor: "'they tell me you can learn anything." – per Allen Brooner [hobson p35]   3334

  ⟨2⟩ It took Lincoln six weeks, "working all day and far into the night," and with the assistance of a friend (Mentor Graham [wilson p10]) to "master" a book on surveying. [shutes pp12-13]   3335

    ⟨1⟩ Other references to learning surveying: [wilson pp10,14,18] [baslerA v4p66]   3336

⟨1⟩ In New Salem: "He read aloud very often; and frequently assumed a lounging position when reading." – James Short [wilson p90]   3337

⟨2⟩ "Lincoln was admitted to the bar in 1836. The kind of examination that was given in those days by a friendly elder lawyer needed just seven words – 'In what direction does the Mississippi flow?'" [kunhardtB p270] *This is unrelated to medicine, but the anecdote was too good to pass up.* :-)   3338

  ⟨2⟩ [angle pp93-94] says the only requirement to practice was an attestation of "good moral character" from some court   3339

⟨1⟩ Herndon wrote: "Lincoln never read any other way but aloud" Lincoln's explanation: "When I read aloud two senses catch the idea: first, I see what I read; second I hear it, and therefore I can remember it better." [herndon p268]   3340

⟨1⟩ "I doubt if he ever read a single elementary law book through in his life. In fact, I may truthfully say, I never knew him to read through a law book of any kind." [herndon p271]   3341

  ⟨1⟩ "The truth about Mr. Lincoln is that he read less and thought more than any man in his sphere in America." [herndon p477]   3342

⟨1/q⟩ Due to "an untoward domestic situation," Lincoln was "a constant attendant" at the state library, where he read widely – J.G. McCoy (a Springfield friend) [burl p325]   3343

Reading & Learning (continued)

⟨2⟩ [burl p325] presents opinions of Benjamin Thomas and Henry Whitney, saying Lincoln learned much by endeavoring to live with his wife.   3344

⟨$\frac{1}{q}$⟩ Lincoln was not rigid about spelling [burl p161]   3345

    ⟨1⟩ As President: "He said that with him punctuation was a matter of feeling, not of education. But his punctuation, it may be added, was always good." [brooksC p299]   3346

⟨1⟩ "Abe allways was trubled Bout words what they Ment" – Dennis Hanks [wilson p147]   3347

⟨$\frac{1}{q}$⟩ 1861: After watching Willie solve a problem, Lincoln said: "I know every step of the process by which that boy arrived at his satisfactory solution of the question before him, as it is just by such slow methods I attain results." [grimsley]. (See ¶5763.) *The problem was an inter-personal one, not a mathematical or peda-gogical one.*   3348

Reproductive

One textbook mentions neurogenic impotence in men who have MEN2B [aa153 p933], but does not quantify prevalence or age at onset.   3349

⟨1⟩ "I have heard him say over & over again about sexual contact: 'It is the harp of a thousand strings.' Oliver Davis thought his mind run on sexual [matters?]" – Henry Whitney [wilson p617]. *This part of Whitney's letter to Herndon has been struck out, but is still readable.*   3350

- Herdon comments on Lincoln's "passions" (see Special Topic §2 for details):   3351
  - ⟨1⟩ 1835-36: "a devlish passion" [hertz p259]   3352
  - ⟨1⟩ "Lincoln was a man of terribly strong passions" [hertz pp259-260]   3353
  - ⟨1⟩ "goaty" [kunhardtB p291] (∈ ¶89)   3354
  - ⟨1⟩ "I have seen women make advances and I have seen Lincoln reject or refuse them. Lincoln had terribly strong passions for woman, could scarcely keep his hands off them" [hertz p247]   3355
  - ⟨2⟩ "a strong, if not terrible passion for women. He could hardly keep his hands off a woman, and yet, much to his credit, he lived a pure and virtuous life." [weik p81]   3356

Skin

Comments about Lincoln's facial skin tone are in Head & Face. Comments about skin in general are here.   3357

⟨1⟩ "Lincoln was a vegetable – His skin performed what other organs did for the [sic] He was sluggish – apathetic –" – John T. Stuart [wilson p482] *This difficult-to-interpret sentence probably refers to Stuart's theories about Lincoln's consti-pation – see ¶612*   3358

- How much sun exposure did his face get?   3359
  - ⟨1⟩ In Indiana: "wore Coon skin Caps – Sometimes for Skin & possum Skin Caps" – David Turnham [wilson p121]   3360
  - ⟨1⟩ In Indiana: "coonskin cap" – J.W. Lamar [hobson p22] (∈ ¶2912)   3361
  - ⟨$\frac{1}{q}$⟩ Spring 1831: wore a "Common Chip hat" – William Greene [wilson p17]   3362
  - ⟨1⟩ About 1831: wore a "Plug hat" [wilson p593]   3363
  - ⟨2⟩ About 1831: "a sealskin cap" – from *Menard Axis*, 1862 [wilson p24] (Part of ¶95)   3364

Skin (continued)

⟨1⟩ "While in the army he Kept a handkerchif [sic] tied round him very near all the time for wrestling purposes" – William Miller [wilson p363] *To prevent hair-pulling?* 3365

⟨1⟩ "I heard him make his first speech after returning from the Black Hawk War ... 'My personal appearance is rather shabby & dark. I am almost as red as those men I have been chasing through the praries & forests' " – Henry McHenry [wilson p15] 3366

⟨1⟩ 1830s: "he Wore a Calico Shert Such as he had in the black Hawk War he wore coarse Brogans Tan Couler Blue Yarn Socks & straw Hat – old style and without a band" – Abner Ellis [wilson p170] plus [wilson pp170, 171, 210] 3367

⟨1⟩ In New Salem, habitually read under a tree: "changing his position as the sun advanced, so as to keep in the shadow." [arnold p40] 3368

⟨1⟩ Summer 1833: Buys a new wardrobe that includes a "buckeye hat" [rossH p109] 3369

⟨1⟩ 1858: Makes a speech. Wears a silk hat. [rossH p119-120] 3370

⟨1⟩ 1858: "he usually wore in his great canvass with Douglas a linen coat, generally without any vest, a hat much the worse for wear, and carried with him a faded cotton umbrella which became almost as famous as in the canvass as Lincoln himself." – Jonathan Birch [wilson p728] 3371

⟨1⟩ Oct. 1858, at last Lincoln-Douglas debate: "sunburned" – Gustave Koerner [angle p247] 3372

⟨2⟩ June 1864: "Tired and sunburned" after visiting the troops at City Point, Virginia (near Petersburg) for two days [donaldA p516] 3373

⟨1⟩ April 1865: "his complexion sunburned, like that of a man who has spent his youth in the open air, exposed to all inclemencies of the weather and to all hardships of manual labor" [chambrunA] (∈ ¶200) 3374

▢ Referring to a photograph: "The 1860. one that was from the 'Century' magazine picture was taken: you will observe that the wrinkles are considerably smoothed out of it, but I think they are the best that are available." – Henry Whitney [wilson p621] *He seems to be suggesting something was done to minimize the appearance of the wrinkles.* 3375

■ Texture / complexion / color – per William Herndon: 3376

⟨1⟩ "his dark, yellow face, wrinkled and dry." [herndon p331] Part of ¶90 3377

⟨1⟩ "his cheeks were leathery and saffron-colored' " – William Herndon [kunhardtB p291] (∈ ¶89) 3378

⟨1⟩ " His structure – his build was loose and leathery. His body was shrunk and shrivelled – having dark skin – dark hair – looking woe struck." [herndonC] (∈ ¶1) (Cognate in: [herndon p471].) *Does "leathery" apply to the skin?* 3379

⟨1⟩ "His face was long – sallow – cadaverous – shrunk – shrivelled – wrinkled, and dry, having here and there a hair on the surface. His cheeks were leathery and flabby, falling in loose folds at places, looking sorrowful and sad." [herndonC] (∈ ¶3) (Cognate in: [herndon p472].) 3380

■ Texture / complexion / color – per others: 3381

⟨1⟩ Age 15+: "long – thin – leggy – gawky boy dried up & Shriveled" – Anna Gentry [wilson p131] (∈ ¶486) 3382

⟨1q⟩ 1820s: "His skin was shriveled and yellow" – Kate Roby, a school friend. [herndon p35] *There is no mention of a Kate Roby in* [wilson]. *From* [wilson pp131-132], *she is clearly the same person as Anna Caroline Gentry, above and in ¶486.* [herndon p35] *seems not to have recognized this. The date is from* [wilson p131]. *Gentry's maiden name was Roby* [wilson p132]. *Anna was two* 3383

Skin (continued)

years older than Lincoln [wilson p749]. *It is possible that Weik embellished the Anna Gentry remark and substituted the name Kate (as a nickname?).*

⟨2⟩ "of a leathery complexion" at about age 17 [warrenY p154] 3384

⟨1/q⟩ Textural features of Lincoln's skin are noticeable in the casts made of his hands (¶1524) and head (¶1941) – sculptor Avarel Fairbanks [purtle]. 3385

⟨1⟩ In late teens: "dark Skinned" – Joseph Richardson [wilson p119] 3386

⟨1⟩ "Abraham L__ he was rether dark complextion ... Abraham he was tall like his mother and dark skin" – John Hanks [wilson p615] *Filed here because, although the wording is ambiguous, the skin description appears to be about Abraham and not his mother.* 3387

⟨1/q⟩ Aug. 1858: He "was as swarthy as an Indian" – Martin Rindlaub [ostendorfA p19] (∈ ¶148) 3388

⟨1⟩ Oct. 13, 1858: "swarthy face" – Carl Schurz [angle p243] (∈ ¶149) 3389

⟨1/q⟩ 1859: "he had a very pale, long face" – John Widmer [shenk p155] (∈ ¶150) 3390

⟨1/q⟩ Dec. 1859: "dark complexion" – part of Lincoln's self-description [donaldA p237] (∈ ¶151) 3391

⟨1⟩ April 1860: "bronzed cheeks" [volk] 3392

⟨1⟩ 1860s: "His complexion was dark and quite sallow." [dana p173] (∈ ¶183) 3393

⟨1⟩ March 1861: "a sinewy muscular yellow neck" – William Russell [russell pp37-38] (∈ ¶161) 3394

⟨1⟩ July 8, 1861: "a little thinner and paler than on the day of his inauguration" [stoddardB p14] (∈ ¶1140) 3395

⟨1⟩ 1862: "His complexion is dark and sallow" [hawthorne p310] (∈ ¶178) 3398

⟨1⟩ Nov. 18, 1863: "He was looking very badly... sallow" [cochrane] (∈ ¶2535) 3399

⟨1/q⟩ Nov. 1863: Was thought to be jaundiced during his bout of smallpox. See §5.70. – [barbeeP - box1 folder 51] transcript of Philadelphia Sunday *Dispatch* of Dec. 6, 1863 3400

⟨1/q⟩ 1864: "His complexion was inclined to sallowness, though I judged this to be the result, in part, of his anxious life in Washington." [carpenter p218] 3401

⟨1⟩ About 1864: "he became constantly more lean and sallow" [croffut] (∈ ¶196) 3402

⟨1/q⟩ "dark complexion" – John Nicolay [browneF p736] [meserve p5] (∈ ¶177, ¶204) 3403

⟨1⟩ Sept. 1863: "His face was peculiar; bone, nerve, vein, and muscle were all so plainly seen" [harveyC] (∈ §6.2) *Suggests thin, translucent skin.* 3404

- Fingerprints: 3405
  ⟨2⟩ The Illinois Historical Society owns a Lincoln fingerprint. When Lincoln autographed a piece of scrap paper for John Hay's undersecretary, Gustave Matile, the pen left a drop of ink on the paper, where Lincoln then happened to put his finger. Matile left a note saying "The finger marks are also his." [matile] 3406

  ☐ A fingerprint is visible on the note Lincoln wrote Nov. 27, 1863, while ill with smallpox (¶1585). This is not provably Lincoln's print, but given the nature of smallpox, it is likely he was febrile and sweating, which renders him the most likely person to have left the print. 3407

- Perspiration: 3408
  ⟨-⟩ See also Endocrine. 3409
  ⟨1⟩ 1830s: "shirt wet with sweat" while doing manual labor – Erastus Wright [walsh p81] 3410
  ⟨1⟩ ca. 1837-1841: On a warm August day, carries red handkerchief to wipe sweat while walking. [rossH pp113-115] 3411

Skin (continued)

⟨2⟩ Oct. 13, 1858: Undergoes a "run sweat" [shutes pp60-61], unless the story was 3412 apocryphal [turnerL]. (See ¶708.)

⟨1⟩ 1860: On a "blazing hot" day, was wearing "a linen duster, the back of which 3413
_q had been marked by repeated perspirations and looked somewhat like a rough map of the two hemispheres." – Carl Schurz [angle pp290-291]

⟨2⟩ April 4, 1865: Walking through Richmond on a hot day, sweats profusely. 3414 [donaldA p576] (See ¶1285ff.)

▢ Stereo-photograph in [zeller] shows prominent wrinkling of the skin on his left 3415 hand's finger II and, to a lesser degree, finger III in [ostendorf #69].

⟨1⟩ On autopsy table, a few hours post-mortem: "A smooth clear skin fitting clearly 3416 over well-rounded muscles" – Edward Curtis, MD [curtis] (Part of ¶2939.) *This appears to be the only description of Lincoln's non-sun-exposed skin. Observers (and photographs) universally describe Lincoln's sun-exposed skin as precisely the opposite of "smooth" or "clear."*

Sleep & Circadian Rhythms

Sleep apnea is common in persons with Marfan syndrome, and common in persons 3417 with myopathy. Lincoln certainly had psychological reasons to have insomnia. For snoring, see ¶3515.

⟨1⟩ Lincoln recalled that even as a child he would get "irritated" when he could not 3418
_q understand what others were saying, and would be unable to sleep until he had "bounded" the idea completely and could "put it in a language plain enough ... for any boy I knew to comprehend." [kunhardtA p37] (Part of ¶3325)

⟨1⟩ 1818 and after, in the log cabin: "Abe slept up stairs – went up on pins stuck in the 3419 logs ... He read diligently – studied in the day time – didnt after night much – went to bed Early – got up Early & then read – Eat his breakfast – go to work in the field with the men" – Sarah Bush Lincoln [wilson p106]

⟨1⟩ "He rose Early – went to bed Early, not reading much after night." – Sarah Bush 3421 Lincoln [wilson p108]

⟨1⟩ 1820s: "He usually read till near midnight reading – rose early" [sic] – Green Taylor 3422 [wilson p130]

⟨1⟩ In youth: "When the wood was got in and Cut up then Lincoln & father would 3423 sit up till midnight or later calculating the figures &c." – Elizabeth Herndon Bell [wilson p606]

⟨1⟩ After hearing more about a defendant who pleaded insanity and whom Lincoln 3424 had vigorously prosecuted, Lincoln admitted to Joseph E. McDonald that "his [own] sleep had been disturbed by the fear that he had been too bitter and un-relenting in his prosecution of him. 'I acted,' he said, 'on the theory that he was "possuming" insanity, and now I fear I have been too severe and that the poor fel-low may be insane after all. If he cannot realize the wrong of his crime, then I was wrong in aiding to punish him.' " [herndon p278]

⟨1⟩ "Lincoln would go and tell his jokes ... People in town would gather around him – 3425 He would keep them there till midnight or longer telling stories ... I would get tired – want to go home" –Dennis Hanks [wilson p105] *This seems to be about Abraham, but the text could also be construed to refer to Thomas.*

Sleep & Circadian Rhythms (continued)

⟨1⟩ In New Salem: "Used to sit up late of nights reading, & and would recommence in the morning when he got up. He was not an unusually early riser – at least it was not considered early for country habits, though for the City it would be very early. ... Didnt sleep very much as he always sat up late." – James Short [wilson p90] 3426

⟨1⟩ Early 1830s: "I also remember that he used to sleep in the store on the Counter when they had two Much Company at the Tavern." – Abner Ellis [wilson p170] 3427

- 1830s: 3428
  - ⟨1⟩ "I Know he sat up late and at night and studied hard – rose tolerably Early." – Caleb Carman [wilson p374] 3429
  - ⟨1⟩ Upon beginning to study law: "read & study at late hours after the business of the day was disposed of" – Robert Rutledge [wilson p426] 3430

⟨1⟩ "he Set up Late & Rose Early ... he scearsly ever went to Bed Befor 12 and was up By Day Light and often set up Later" – J. Rowan Herndon [wilson p92] 3431

- William Herndon observations: 3432
  - ⟨1⟩ "I could always realize when he was in distress, without being told. He was not exactly an early riser, that is, he never usually appeared at the office till about nine o'clock in the morning. I usually preceded him an hour. Sometimes, however, he would come down as early as seven o'clock – in fact on one occasion i remember he came down before daylight. If, on arriving at the office, I found him in, I knew instantly that a breeze had sprung up over the domestic sea, and that the waters were troubled. He would either be lying on the lounge looking skyward or doubled up in a chair.... He would not look up on my entering, and only answered my 'Good morning' with a grunt. ... [the] melancholy and distress was so plain, and his silence so significant, that I would grow restless myself." [herndon p348] 3433
  - ⟨$\frac{1}{q}$⟩ "Lincoln was a good sleeper scarcely ever getting out of bed before 7-8 unless *Mrs.* Lincoln chunked beat him out" [sic] [randallC p111] *Unclear if "good sleeper' is an observation or a deduction.* 3434

⟨1⟩ 1840s or 1850s: "One night he Came home late at night. I heard an axe: it rang out at Lincoln's – got up – Saw Mr Lincoln in his Shirt Sleeves Cutting wood – I suppose to cook his supper – it was between 12 & 1 o'cl. This I remember well – used to tell it on the stump and in Conversation – told him so ... Mr L did not say aye or nay – yet he took it as intended – Complimentary." – John B. Weber [wilson p389] 3435

⟨1⟩ June 1848: "I was so tired and sleepy, having ridden all night" [donaldH p70] 3436

⟨1⟩ Spring 1849: Soundly asleep around daybreak in a stage coach that arrives in Terre Haute. Appears to wake up quickly. See ¶139. 3437

- Sleeping arrangements: 3438
  - ⟨2⟩ By the mid-1850s Abraham and Mary Lincoln had separate, but connecting, bedrooms. This was fashionable for well-to-do couples. [donaldA p198] 3439
  - ⟨S⟩ [donaldA p198] speculates this might have also improved Mary's quality of sleep, and notes that such an arrangement does not imply an end to intimacy between Abraham and Mary. 3440
  - ⟨2⟩ The house was enlarged in 1856 to provide separate bedrooms [burl p322] 3441
  - ⟨2⟩ Separate, adjoining bedrooms in the White House [donaldH p25], but this may not have started immediately (see ¶3499). 3442

Sleep & Circadian Rhythms (continued)

⟨2⟩ "After the death of Willie [Feb. 1862], Tad was so lonely and so subject to nightmares that he was regularly allowed to sleep in his father's bed." [donaldH p43] — 3443

⟨2⟩ According to Herndon, Lincoln often left for work at 7 or 8 a.m. and would not return until midnight or later [burl p321] — 3444

⟨2⟩ Lincoln placed a six-and-a-half-foot couch in his law office so he could sleep there "on nights of domestic discord" – according to the inheritor of the couch, 1934 [burl p272] — 3445

    ⟨1⟩ There was "a small dirty bed" in Lincoln's "old office up stairs above the Court Room" – James Matheny [wilson p251] — 3446

- As a lawyer in the 1840s and 1850s, Lincoln "rode the circuit" several months of each year. That is, he and other attorneys would travel from town to town, to argue cases before a judge making the same travels. — 3447
  - ⟨2⟩ On the circuit: "The lawyers generally slept two to a bed" [gary p7]. — 3448
  - ⟨2⟩ Often slept "two in a bed and eight in a room" [randallC pp70-71] — 3449
  - ⟨1⟩_q Latter 1850s, on the circuit: Henry Clay Whitney and Lincoln were sharing a bed in Danville, Illinois when "I was awakened early – before daylight – by my companion [Lincoln] sitting up in bed, his figure dimly visible by the ghostly firelight, and talking the wildest and most incoherent nonsense all to himself. A stranger to Lincoln would have supposed he had suddenly gone insane. Of course, I knew Lincoln and his idiosyncrasies, and felt no alarm, so listened and laughed. After he had gone on in this way for, say, five minutes, while I was awake, and I know not how long *before* I was awake, he sprang out of bed, hurriedly washed, and jumped into his clothes, put some wood on the fire, and then sat in front of it, moodily, dejectedly, in a most somber and gloomy spell, till the breakfast bell rang, when he started, as if from sleep, and went with us to breakfast. Neither Davis nor I spoke to him; we knew his trait; it was not remarkable for Lincoln."– Henry Whitney, reprinted in [angle p169-170] — 3450
    - ⟨2⟩ Whitney apparently thought this was a nightmare [donaldA pp163-164]. *The phenomenon is a parasomnia, and may or may not be a nightmare.* — 3451
    - ⟨S⟩ [hirschhornC] dates this episode to either May 1857 or May 1859. — 3452

- More from Henry C. Whitney, a lawyer who traveled the circuit with Lincoln in the latter 1850s: — 3453
  - ⟨1⟩ "we slept together on the circuit" – Henry C. Whitney [wilson p617] — 3454
  - ⟨1⟩ "During the sitting of the 1st Phila. Convention in '56, Lincoln was attending a special term of Court in our County –. Davis, L., and my self roomed together" – Henry C. Whitney [wilson p406] (There is some doubt about the first sentence [wilson p406n].) — 3455
  - ⟨1⟩ In Danville, Illinois: Judge Davis slept in "a three-quarter bed, and Lincoln and I in the other one, jointly.' – Henry C. Whitney [wilson p647] — 3456
  - ⟨1⟩ "Lincoln didnt care what he ate – who who he ate with or where he slept or who he slept with." – Henry C. Whitney [wilson p648] — 3457

- Other observations of Lincoln's sleep habits from the circuit: — 3458
  - ⟨1⟩ "In travelling on the circuit he was in the habit owing to his regular hours of rising earlier than his brothers of the bar, on such occasions he was wont to sit by the fire having uncovered the coals, and muse ponder and soliloquize wisper no doubt by strange psychological influence" – Lawrence Weldon, who saw such an incident in 1861 [wilson p88] — 3459

233

Sleep & Circadian Rhythms (continued)

⟨¼⟩ "would frequently lapse into reverie and remain lost in thought long after the rest of us had retired for the night." – Lawrence Weldon [hirschhornC]   3460

⟨1⟩ "read till late of night" – John T. Stuart [wilson p519]   3461

⟨2⟩ "Frequently ... the lawyers had to rise before dawn and drive all day and into the night to reach the next court on time." – [angle pp163-164] reprinting Benjamin Thomas (not [thomas])   3462

⟨1⟩ Herndon tells of Lincoln studying Euclid by candlelight until midnight or 1 a.m. [hertz p96]. In general, however, evenings on the circuit were generally devoted to joke- and story-telling, "till one or two o'clock in the night, and thus night after night till the court adjourned for that term" [hertz p101].   3463

⟨1⟩ 1858, while traveling on a train: "Presently he arose, spread the cloak over the seat, lay down, somehow folded himself up till his long legs and arms were no longer in view, the drew the cloak about him and went to sleep." – Jonathan Birch [wilson p728]   3464

⟨¼⟩ 1858: After retiring at 8 pm to "load up with all the sleep I can get," almost loses his cool trying to sleep in a bedbug-infested room. Ends up sleeping very well – on the floor. [browneF pp294-296] See §1c.   3465

⟨1⟩ 1860, in the sculpture studio of Leonard Volk: Lincoln "gave me on this day a long sitting of more than four hours, and when it was concluded, went to our family apartment ... to look at a collection of photographs which I had made in 1855-6-7, in Rome and Florence. While sitting in the rocking-chair, he took my little son on his lap and spoke kindly to him, asking his name, age, etc. I held the photographs up and explained them to him, but I noticed a growing weariness, and his eyelids closed occasionally as if he were sleepy, or were thinking of something besides Grecian and Roman statuary and architecture. Finally he said: 'These things must be very interesting to you, Mr. Volk, but the truth is I don't know much of history, and all I do know of it I have learned from law-books.'" [volk]   3466

- Other pre-presidential schedules: 3467
  ⟨1⟩ "You wish to know if Mr Lincoln read news papers. He did yes and often vary late at night. he was not a vary early riser." – Harriet Chapman [wilson p512]   3468
  ⟨1⟩ "Lincoln came to his office about 9 or 10 o'clock A.M. – sometimes sooner" – Newton Bateman [wilson p436]   3469
  ⟨1⟩ One night "L Came off the Circuit – went to P.O after Eating his Supper – read the letters – Cracked jokes &c – till about 11oc (Night time.)" Rather than disturb his family at home, he spent that night at the home of A.Y. Ellis – P.P. Enos [wilson p449]   3470
  ⟨1⟩ "In all his habits of eating, sleeping – reading Conversation & study – he was If I may so express it regularly irregular – That is he had no stated time for eating, no fixed time for going to bed or getting up" – Joshua Speed [wilson p498] [herndon p420]   3471

⟨2⟩ Nov. 1860, Election night: Lincoln went home to sleep at 1:30 a.m. [kunhardtA p130]   3472

⟨1⟩ Jan. 1861: "I can't sleep nights" – Lincoln, discussing the effect of the secession crisis [whitney p492]   3473

- Feb. 1861: Lincoln travels by rail from Springfield to Washington, under constant heavy guard.   3474
  ⟨1⟩ Allan Pinkerton recalled that, nearing Washington, "Mr. Lincoln was cool, calm, and self possessed – firm and determined in his bearing. He evinced   3475

234

Sleep & Circadian Rhythms (continued)

no sign of fear or distrust, and throughout the entire night was quite self possessed" [wilson p323].

⟨1⟩ In fact, during this leg of the trip, Lincoln "made several witty remarks show-   3476
ing that he was as full of fun as ever" [wilson p286].

⟨1⟩ In New York he "looked very pale, and fatigued" [wilson p278]   3477

⟨1⟩ In Philadelphia "he was rather exhausted from the fatigues of travel and re-   3478
ceptions" [wilson p320]

⟨1⟩ Between Philadelphia and Havre de Grace, Maryland, Lincoln does not sleep   3479
[wilson p323]

⟨1⟩ Leaving Baltimore at 4:15 am, Lincoln may or may not have been awake –   3480
Allan Pinkerton's description is unclear [wilson p286]

⟨2⟩ On the train from Baltimore to Washington "Lincoln was pushed up into a   3481
sleeping berth far too short for him, so that his huge legs had to be doubled
up" [kunhardtA p19].

■ Presidential schedule (see ¶3505 for 1865):   3482

⟨1⟩ "he worked by no rule – Saw people at all hours ... He was irregular in his   3483
habits of eating and Sleeping. I remember asking him on one occasion,
when he slept – his answer was – 'just when every body else is tired out.'"
– Joshua Speed [wilson p255]

⟨1⟩ 1861: "was often summoned as early as five o'clock in the morning to the   3485
Cabinet Room" [grimsley] (∈ ¶647) *Was this peculiar to the Ft. Sumter crisis
(¶2622)?*

⟨1⟩ Feb. 1863: "My dear sir never aspire to the Presidential chair I have neither   3486
rest by day nor sleep by night." – Lincoln, related by Charles Hart [wilson p222]

⟨1⟩ "The labor caused by the breaking out of the war ... imposed on him more   3487
work than one man could do. He adopted no hours for business, but did
business at all hours, rising early in the morning, and retiring late at night,
making appointments at very early, and very late hours. He never had any
time for rest and recuperation." – Robert Wilson [wilson p207]

⟨1⟩ "Mr Lincoln would let in People indiscriminately – Member of Congress   3488
Could get to see him most any time – when possible. House opened from
7 o'cl am & 11 o'cl P.M." – Ward Hill Lamon [wilson p466]

⟨1⟩ "The President usually came to us morning, noon and night for his news." –   3489
David Homer Bates, of the War Dept. telegraph office [NYTimesTeleg]

⟨$\frac{1}{q}$⟩ "I consider myself fortunate if at eleven o'clock, I ... find myself in my ... room   3490
and ... my tired and weary Husband is there ... to receive me – to chat over
the occurrences of the day." – Mary [kunhardtA p284]

⟨$\frac{1}{q}$⟩ "Lincoln went to bed ordinarily from ten to eleven o'clock, unless he hap-   3491
pened to be kept up by important news, in which case he would frequently
remain at the War Department until 1 or 2. He rose early. When he lived in
the country at Soldiers' Home he would be up and dressed, eat his breakfast
(which was extremely frugal, an egg, a piece of toast, Coffee, & c), and ride
into Washington, all before 8 o'clock. In the winter at the White House he
was not quite so early. He did not sleep well but spent a good while in bed.
Tad usually slept with him." – John Hay, 1866 [wilson p331] [herndon p415] *This
would today be labeled "poor sleep efficiency."*

⟨$\frac{1}{q}$⟩ "The President rose early, his sleep was light and capricious" – John Hay [angle   3492
p435] *This seems to be habitual.*

⟨2⟩ "sometimes ... had trouble sleeping, especially in winter, and lay in bed well   3494
past dawn, wrapped in his long yellow nightshirt, lost in thought." [kunhardtA

Sleep & Circadian Rhythms (continued)

p321] *One senses this is extrapolated from Hay's account, above.* [kunhardtA p322] *parrots another portion of Hay's account.*

⟨2⟩ "The President was an early riser. In the morning he would devote two or three hours to correspondence, with a glance at the newspapers. He would have breakfast about nine, then walk over to the war department building." [randallB p5] based on *Cincinnati Daily Gazette*, 12 Dec. 1863, p. 1, col. 4.   3495

⟨$\frac{1}{q}$⟩ Sept. 11, 1861: When the wife of a reprimanded general demanded at midnight to have an audience with Lincoln, he replied "Now, at once." [kunhardtA p159]   3497

  ⟨2⟩ When awakened to receive a caller in the middle of the night, Lincoln would say "You did just right to wake me." [kunhardtB p231]   3498

⟨$\frac{1}{q}$⟩ Dec. 12, 1861: "Mrs. Lincoln has for three nights slept in a separate apartment." – Lincoln [burl p284]. See ¶3438 for sleeping arrangements.   3499

⟨2⟩ 1862: When Willie and Tad were ill with "bilious fever," Lincoln sat up with them "night after night." He "was able to transact little business, and he seemed to stumble through his duties." [donaldA p336]   3500

⟨$\frac{1}{q}$⟩ April 1862, during Shiloh battle: "I called on Lincoln at eleven o'clock at night and sat with him alone until after one o'clock in the morning. He was, as usual, worn out with the day's exacting duties." – A.K. McClure [angle p401]   3501

⟨2⟩ Dec. 1862±: "He was awake at all hours of the night." [shenk p187] *Has no clear primary source.*   3502

⟨1⟩ Sept. 7, 1863: "I asked if he slept well, and he said he was never a good sleeper, and, of course, slept less now than ever before." [harveyC] (∈ §6.8)   3503

⟨1⟩ July 1864 (probably): "I enjoy my rations, and sleep the sleep of the innocent." – Lincoln [riceB p350]   3504

■ Presidential schedule 1865, per William Crook (see ¶3482 for other dates and sources):   3505

  ⟨1⟩ Jan. 9, a little after 11pm: Lincoln walks to War Department [crookA p7-10]. "For the next three weeks, while I was on duty the first half of the night, I went to the War Department with Mr. Lincoln every evening" [crookA p10]. Starting Feb. 1, Crook's shift began at midnight. "Often I had to wait for the President to return from the War Department; even when he came back comparatively early it was midnight before he got to bed" [crookA p11].   3506

  ⟨1⟩ "He was not interrupted after he retired unless there were important telegrams. Even when awakened suddenly from a deep sleep – which is the most searching test of one's temper that I know – he was never ruffled, but received the message and the messenger kindly." [crookA p11]   3507

  ⟨1⟩ Feb. 1-14 (presumably): "Usually the household, with the exception of Mr. Lincoln, was asleep when I began my watch." [crookA p12] [crookK]   3508

  ⟨1⟩ "He was an early riser; when I came on duty, at eight in the morning, he was often dressed and reading in the library." [crookA p14] [crookK]   3509

  ⟨1⟩ "Mr. and Mrs. Lincoln breakfasted at nine" [crookA p15].   3510

  ⟨1⟩ "...from half-past nine, when he came into his office, until midnight, when he went to bed, his work went on, almost without cessation." [crookA p15] [crookK]   3511

  ⟨1⟩ Mar. 23, on a ship, sailing to City Point: "It was nearly midnight when he went to bed" [crookA p39]. "Toward morning" Lincoln is awake to check on Tad [crookA p40]. On Mar. 24, ashore, "Everybody was up until late," in good spirits [crookA p41].   3512

Sleep & Circadian Rhythms (continued)

⟨1⟩ April 4: Checks on Tad during the night. [crookA p57]   3513

⟨2⟩ Jan. 31, 1865: Lincoln "slept like never before" the night after Congressed passed   3514
the 13th Amendment [kunhardtA p270]. See ¶2669.

⟨1⟩ Feb. 1865: "When in my patrol I came near to the door of the President's room I   3515
could hear his deep breathing. Sometimes, after a day of unusual anxiety, I have
heard him moan in his sleep. ... I would stand there and listen..." [crookA p13] [crookK]
This is as close as I've seen to hard evidence that Lincoln snored. It can be
considered only suggestive, not definitive.

    ⟨2⟩ Various Presidents, including Lincoln, "are proven or believed on a thick web   3516
of circumstance" to have been snorers [dugan]. *No further information is*
provided.

⟨1⟩ March 3, 1865 (the night before his second inauguration): Stays up with the Cab-   3517
inet at the Capitol until at least midnight [welles v2p251]

⟨2⟩ March 17, 1865: Day ends 'beyond midnight" [shutesE p177]. Apparently has a sound   3518
sleep [shutesE p177].

⟨1⟩ Late March 1865: Asked how he slept his first night aboard USS *Malvern*: "I slept   3519
well." (Then mentions bed was too short for him.) [porterD p285]

⟨2⟩ April 1, 1865: Staying aboard the *River Queen*, "walks deck most of night" [miers   3520
v3p324] citing [crookB]

⟨1⟩ April 1865: "I retired very late. I had been up waiting for important dispatches   3521
from the front. I could not have been long in bed when I fell into a slumber, for I
was weary. I soon began to dream." He dreamed of being killed (¶3547). "I slept
no more that night." – Lincoln [lamonR pp116-117] *Unlikely Lincoln would have said*
"soon began," since sleepers are insensible to time.

⟨2⟩ April 14, 1865: Woke up about 7 a.m. [shenk p209]   3522

- The demands of the Presidency interfered with Lincoln's sleep.   3523
  - ⟨2⟩ March-April 1861: The crisis over Ft. Sumter, which would ultimately be the   3524
    site of the Civil War's first battle, brewed over several weeks. On a day he
    received news forcing his hand, Lincoln slept "not at all" that night [donaldA
    p288]. (See ¶2622.)
  - ⟨2⟩ July 21, 1861, the night of the Battle of (First) Bull Run: Lincoln did not go to   3525
    bed. He stretched out on a couch in the Cabinet room of the White House
    [donaldA p307].
  - ⟨2⟩ Late June 1862: Lincoln was worrying "incessantly" and, according to Mary,   3526
    got very little sleep at night. [donaldA p358]
  - ⟨2⟩ May 1864: "During the first week of the battles of the Wilderness he scarcely   3527
    slept at all." [carpenter p30] (∈ ¶2657)

- Secondary summaries: 3528
  - ⟨2⟩ Lincoln was not a good sleeper [neelyL]   3529
  - ⟨2⟩ [donaldA p198] implies Lincoln had insomnia.   3530
  - ⟨2⟩ [donaldH p42] describes Lincoln's nights as "generally sleepless"   3531
  - ⟨2⟩ "Frequently at night he cold not sleep, and rose to wander from room to   3532
    room." – Helen Nicolay [angle p368]

Sleep – Dreams

Dreaming occurs predominantly in REM (rapid eye movement) sleep, although not exclusively. Thus, reports of dreaming affect the odds that a person is having REM sleep. REM sleep may be absent in certain disease states, e.g., sleep apnea. A temporary increase in REM sleep, known as "REM rebound" can occur after deprivation of REM sleep is cured, and is often accompanied by vivid dreams. The science of sleep is not sufficiently advanced to allow useful conclusions about Lincoln's sleep architecture, based on his available dream information. 3533

- Attitudes: 3534
  - ⟨2⟩ Lincoln had "a well-known propensity to dream and talk about his dreaming" [currentBk p70] 3535
  - ⟨1/q⟩ 1865: "It seems strange to me how much there is in the Bible about dreams. ... Nowadays dreams are regarded as very foolish, and are seldom told, except by old women and by young men and maidens in love...." – Lincoln [kunhardtA p334] 3536
  - ⟨1⟩ "There was more or less superstition in his nature, and, although he may not have believed implicitly in the signs of his many dreams, he was constantly endeavoring to unravel them." [herndon p352] 3537
  - ⟨1⟩ April 1865: Lincoln took his assassination dream seriously [lamonR p116] (See ¶3521 and ¶3547.) 3538

- Family dreams: 3539
  - ⟨1⟩ April 1848: a "foolish dream about dear Bobby" [kunhardtA p75] [angle p147] 3540
  - ⟨1⟩ Dreams about Willie after Willie's death [wilson p679] [brooksB] 3541
  - ⟨1/q⟩ June 1863: "an ugly dream" about the pistol recently given to Tad. Lincoln wires Mary, asking her to take the pistol from Tad. [donaldA p446] [kunhardtA p212]. 3542

⟨1⟩ Latter 1850s: Henry C. Whitney, sharing a bed with Lincoln, saw him sitting up and talking while apparently asleep [angle pp169-170]. (Fully quoted in ¶3450) 3543

⟨1⟩ April 1865: While on a trip, Lincoln dreamed the White House was on fire [wilson pp358,359]. 3544
- ⟨2⟩ He told this to Mary, who sent two enquiring telegrams to the White House [donaldA p572]. 3545
- ⟨1⟩ Mary suggests Lincoln sent her back to Washington because of the dream [wilson pp358,359]. *Other reasons sent her back (¶4694).* 3546

⟨1⟩ April 1865: It is reported [lamonR p116], "though not so well documented," that Lincoln dreamed of his assassination not long before it happened. The "pat, made-up quality" of this report also undermines its legitimacy [currentBk p70]. Lincoln said he actually dreamed it "was not me, but some other fellow, that was killed" [lamonR p118]. (See ¶3521.). 3547

⟨1⟩ April 13-14, 1865, in his last sleep: Lincoln dreamed he was on the sea, in a vessel of unknown type, "moving with great rapidity towards an indefinite shore." [welles v2p282] 3548
- ⟨1⟩ This was a recurring dream that previously "preceded nearly every great and important event of the War" [welles v2p282]. "He had this dream preceding Sumter, Bull Run, Antietam, Gettysburg, Stone River, Vicksburg, Wilmington, etc." [welles v2pp282-283] 3549
- ⟨2⟩ Lincoln also had the dream the night before Eddie's death [kunhardtC] 3550
- ⟨-⟩ *The relationship among recurrent dreams, anxiety, and stress is still being worked out* [aa60 p757] 3551

Speech

- See also ⌐Voice⌐   3552

⟨1⟩ "He was a good debater. ... He was a natural talker." – Daniel Burner, who lived   3553
with Lincoln in the 1830s [templeB]

⟨2⟩ As a lawyer, Lincoln would plead "his own cases in the slow drawl he had become   3554
famous for" [kunhardtA p80].

⟨1⟩ Herndon wanted Lincoln to talk faster in the courtroom ("Speak with more vim   3555
and arouse the jury – talk faster and keep them awake"). Lincoln responded with
a story comparing a short-bladed knife and a long-bladed knife. "Just so with the
long, labored movements of my mind. I may not emit ideas as rapidly as others, because I am compelled by nature to speak slowly, but when I do throw off a
thought it seems to me, though it comes with some effort, it has force enough to
cut its own way and travel a greater distance." [herndon p273]

⟨2⟩ As President-Elect: "Visitors to his office often felt stunned by the sheer volume   3556
of his words. He showered upon them opinions, ideas, and anecdotes concerning
almost every subject in the world." [donaldA p259]

⟨2⟩ "some listeners detected a strong Kentucky accent" [donaldA p464]   3557

⟨1⟩ "The Inlow family were slow spoken rather drawling in their manner of conver-   3558
sation. Lincoln had the voice of the Inlows." – Michael Cassidy [wilson p615] *Some
cite a member of the Enloe family as Lincoln's father. See ¶44.*

⟨1⟩ "Lincoln's tones were high-pitched and often disagreeable. He spoke distinctly,   3559
however, and very regularly – almost staccato." – Thomas Shastid, recalling his
father's description [shastid]

Trauma

- For head trauma, see ¶1871ff. For hand trauma, see ¶1489ff.   3560

⟨$\frac{1}{q}$⟩ In youth, month of June: "We concluded to cross the creek to hunt for some par-   3561
tridges ... The creek was swollen by a recent rain, and, in crossing on the narrow
footlog, Abe fell in. Neither of us could swim. I got a long pole and held it out
to Abe, who grabbed it. Then I pulled him ashore. He was almost dead and I
was badly scared. I rolled and pounded him in good earnest. Then I got him by
the arms and shook him, the water meanwhile pouring out of his mouth. By this
means I succeeded in bringing him to, and he was soon all right." – Austin Golla-
her [tarbellE p44] *Lincoln apparently learned to swim later. See ¶2855.*
     ⟨H⟩ Another time with Gollaher, Lincoln narrowly escaped the fall of a large rock.   3562
      [paulmier p19]

- Corporal punishment: 3563
     ⟨2⟩ "The worst trouble with Abe was when people was talking – if they said   3564
      something that wasn't right, Abe would up and tell them so. Uncle Tom had
      a hard time to break him of this." – a third-hand recollection [burl p38].
     ⟨$\frac{1}{q}$⟩ [burl p38] relates examples of Thomas striking Abraham in the face or giving   3565
      Abe "a little drilling"
     ⟨1⟩ "Abe was one of those forward Boys I have seen his father Nock him Down   3566
      of the fence when a Stranger would Call for Information to neighbor house
      Abe always would have the first word" – Dennis Hanks [wilson p176]

- Age 9: Was kicked in the forehead by a horse. He was unconscious overnight. (See   3568
§1a.)
     ⟨1⟩ Herndon describes the episode in [herndon pp51-52] and [hertz pp72-73]. (See §1a.)   3569

Trauma (continued)

⟨2⟩ Secondary accounts: [donaldA p26] [shutes p6]. 3570

⟨1⟩ "In his tenth year he was kicked by a horse, and apparently killed for a time." 3571
– Lincoln, writing in the third person [baslerA v4p63]

⟨1⟩ "About 1826 & 7 ... It must have been about this time that Abe got kicked by 3572
a horse in the mill and who did not Speak for several hours and when he did
speak – he ended the sentence which he Commenced to the horse as I am
well informed & blieve [sic]." – Dennis Hanks [wilson p42] *Age estimate differs*
sharply from Lincoln's.

⟨1⟩ "Saw old Man Gordons Mill – rather the near ruins of it. This is the Mill where 3573
Abe got Kicked by a horse" – William Herndon, Sept. 1865 [wilson p118]

⟨S⟩ "... Lincoln's brain had been injured in childhood, leaving residual impair- 3574
ments of certain highly necessary nervous functions that had been coun-
terbalanced by developing special volitional compensations, repeated constantly to maintain normal mental integrity." [kempfB v1p xvi].

⟨2⟩ "There is an unusual depression in the Volk mask with a palpable edge near 3575
the midline above the left eye. I have examined the Mills mask and found a
similar depression in its forehead. ... The sharp depression in the forehead
above the left eye with a definitely palpable edge, in the life masks, shows
where his skull had been fractured," which led to differing neuromuscular
tones on each side of the face. [kempfB pp8-9, 9-10] *The masks are discussed in*
Head -- Casts *and* ¶*1942ff.*

⟨S⟩ The kick "evidently fractured the skull at the point of impact and must have 3576
violently snapped the head and neck backward. The size and depth of the
depression is evidence of its severity." Speculates that a subdural hematoma
and other hemorrhages occurred, with involvement of the frontal lobe and
consequent change in personality. [kempfB p11]

⟨S⟩ "A blow from an unshod hoof would be unlikely to produce a localized, de- 3577
pressed skull fracture and no such scarred depression can be found on careful examination of the original Volk lifemask in the Smithsonian Institution
or on any of the many Lincoln photographs." [shutesE p195]

⟨S⟩ "Since the facial muscles on both sides have bilateral cortical innervation," 3578
compensation would largely have occurred, "within a few months." [kempfB
p11]

⟨S⟩ "... the only disorder worthy of relating was the *petit-mal*-like call to the 3579
horse. ... It was a concussion with recovery and no psychosomatic sequels.
If the injury was more violent than here suspected, the so-called laws of
chance again were kind to Lincoln." [shutesE p196] *Given that MEN2B in-*
volves neuronal growth, we could reasonably wonder if it is associated with
better neuronal survival after injury. Perhaps it was the laws of biology
rather than the laws of chance which allowed Lincoln to escape serious
injury here.

⟨S⟩ *Rapid backward displacement of the head can cause the anterior cord syn-* 3580
drome, affecting the spinal cord. One sign of such an injury is pronounced
swinging of the arms during walking – which Lincoln had (¶*1070*).

⟨2⟩ Cold injury of feet while crossing the frozen Sangamon River in winter 1830-1831. 3581
See ¶930

⟨2⟩ 1828: Traveled to New Orleans with Allen Gentry where "one night they were at- 3582
tacked by seven negroes with intent to kill and rob them. They were hurt some
in the melee, but succeeded in driving the negroes from the boat, and then 'cut
cable' 'weighed anchor' and left." – Lincoln [baslerA v4p63]

Trauma (continued)

⟨2⟩ The attackers had hickory clubs and attacked while Lincoln and Gentry were asleep [angle p32] (reprinting [beveridge])   3583

⟨1⟩ "Abe fought the Negroes" – Anna Gentry [wilson p131]   3584

⟨1⟩ "at the Gentry landing – Give about 2 m. Lincoln was attacked by the Negroes   3585
– no doubt of this – Abe told me so – Saw the scar myself." – John Romines [wilson p118]

⟨2⟩ Ward Lamon mentions a scar resulting from this incident (¶1876) [shutesE   3586
p197]

⟨1⟩ Lincoln emerged from a hatchway, and an attacker "struck him a blow with   3587
a heavy stick, but the point of the stick reached over his head, and struck the floor beyond, at the same time, thus lightening the blow on his head, but making a scar which he wore always, and which he showed me at the time of telling this story." – Leonard Swett [riceA pp461-462]

⟨1⟩ Although the reference is unclear, it appears that several men in Lincoln's com-   3588
pany during the Blackhawk War were injured by a stampede of horses ¶2145. Lincoln is not mentioned to have sustained injury.

⟨1⟩ Mary struck Abraham "on [the] head with a piece of wood while reading paper in   3589
South Parlor – cut his nose – lawyers saw his face in Court next day but asked no questions" – Margaret Ryan, lived with Lincolns until February 1860 [wilson p597]

⟨1/q⟩ Agrees with: [burl p273] who somehow quotes more detail   3591

⟨2⟩ Maybe agrees with: [baker p134], who also says Mary threw books at him   3592

⟨1⟩ In Springfield: "Ms L. had some aristocratic company from Ky and met L & D. as   3593
they came in the door. Upon opening the paper of meat she became enraged at the Kind L had bought. She abused L. outrageously and finally was so mad she struck him in the face. Rubbing the blood off his face" Lincoln and "D." left. – Jesse Dubois ("D.") [wilson p692]

⟨2⟩ Other domestic violence: 3595

⟨1/q⟩ 1850s: Mary "was seen frequently to drive him from the house with a broom-   3596
stick" – daughter of a Lincoln neighbor [burl p277]

⟨2⟩ A neighbor saw Mary, with a knife in her hand, chase Lincoln down the street   3597
in 1856 or 1857 – recalled by Stephen Whitehurst in 1867 [currentBk p49]

⟨2⟩ She threw hot coffee in his face [burl p277]   3598

⟨1/q⟩ She threw potatoes at him (poorly) [burl p277]   3599

⟨1/q⟩ November 1863: During an argument she "made a mad dash at his cravat,   3600
and captured a part of his whiskers" [burl p287]

⟨1⟩ 1865(?): "Mrs. Lincoln struck Mr Lincoln in the face on a boat going to or   3601
at Richmond – Struck him hard – damned him – cursed him" – Ward Hill Lamon, second-hand from a White House employee [wilson p467]

⟨2⟩ Sept. 13±, 1862: Sprains wrist checking his runaway horse during morning ride   3602
from Soldiers' Home to White House. [thelincolnlog - 13 Sept. 13. 1862] citing [Washington-Star - Sept. 13, 1862]

⟨2⟩ Lincoln often went out unguarded [donaldA p548]. In August 1864 a shot was fired   3603
at him while riding in Washington, leaving a bullet hole in the crown of his hat [donaldA pp549-550].

⟨1⟩ [bancroft] shows, however, that a close watch was kept on all who visited Lin-   3604
coln.

Travel & Dwellings

A travel history is useful in determining possible infectious exposures. See also 3605
Infection -- Exposures . More usefully, many events in Lincoln histories have the
place specified, but not the date. A travel history can, therefore, help supply the date.
[gary] records Lincoln's travels in detail. The items below are odds and ends culled from
other readings.

- Kentucky home #1:   3606
  ⟨2⟩ Born "at Buffalo, Hardin (now La Rue) County, Ky." [lea p86]   3607
  ⟨1⟩ "on the road from Bardstown Ky. to nashville Tenn. at a point three, or three   3608
      and a half miles South or South-West of Atherton's ferry on the Rolling Fork."
      – Lincoln [baslerA v4p62]
  ⟨2⟩ Lincoln lived there the first two years of his life [angle p7]   3609
  ⟨2⟩ Synonyms: Sinking Spring farm [angle p7], Rock Spring Farm [tarbellE p232], Creal   3610
      Place [tarbellE p232], Big South Fork of Nolin Creek [tarbellE p42].
  ⟨2⟩ It was 3 miles from Hodgensville and 14 miles from Elizabethtown [tarbellE   3611
      p43].
  ⟨1/q⟩ Jacob Brother [hobson pp13-14] recounts the fate of Lincoln's farm and log cabin.   3612

- Kentucky home #2:   3613
  ⟨2⟩ Ten miles north and east of Kentucky home #1 [angle p9]   3614
  ⟨2⟩ Synonyms: "Knob Creek farm" [angle p9]   3615
  ⟨2⟩ Knob Creek flows into Rolling Fork which flows into Salt River which flows   3616
      into the Ohio River [angle p9]
  ⟨2⟩ "The Knob Creek farm provided a reasonably sure living with a minimum of   3617
      physical exertion. ... [It] was on the main road from Louisville to Nashville.
      Travelers went by every day. ... The farm was subject to sudden rise of water."
      [angle pp14-15] (reprinting [bartonB])
  ⟨2⟩ A suit filed against Thomas Lincoln in 1816 sought to take his farm's title   3618
      from him. He decided to move to Indiana, where land was acquired directly
      from the U.S. government [angle p16].

- Indiana home: 3619
  ⟨2⟩ Synonyms: "Little Pigeon Creek homestead" [angle p18], "Spencer County" [an-   3620
      gle p30]
  ⟨2⟩ The site was 1.5 miles east of Gentryville [angle p18] and 15 miles north of the   3621
      Ohio River [hobson p17]. *I estimate the distance from Knob Creek to Little
      Pigeon Creek at about 65 miles, as the crow flies.*
  ⟨2⟩ For the first year, the Lincolns lived in a temporary shelter that was closed   3622
      on three sides and open on the fourth, while Thomas built a log cabin. The
      cabin had no door, windows, or floor for the first year or two the Lincolns
      lived in it. [angle p18]
  ⟨2⟩ Operated a ferry on the Ohio River for a time [angle p30]   3623
  ⟨2⟩ This was Perry County when the Lincolns settled. Became Spencer County   3624
      in 1818. [hobson p17]

- Macon County, Illinois home: 3625
  ⟨1⟩ "settled a new place on the North side of the Sangamon river, at the junction   3626
      of the timber-land and prairie, about ten miles Westerly from Decatur." –
      Lincoln [baslerA v4p64]
  ⟨1⟩ Coming to Illinois, "passed the first year in Macon County" – Lincoln [arnold   3627
      p15]

Travel & Dwellings (continued)

⟨1⟩ About March 1, 1831: Took a flatboat "from Beardstown, Illinois to New Or- 3628
leans." Returned by July 1831. – Lincoln [angle pp37, 38]

⟨1⟩ Returned from New Orleans by boat. Visited parents in Coles County. [rossH 3629
p111]

- During the Black Hawk War (1832): 3630
  ⟨2⟩ Mustered into state service on April 28 at Beardstown, IL; mustered into fed- 3631
  eral service on May 9 at Rock island, IL; re-enlisted on May 26 (Alexander
  White's company); re-enlisted on June 16 (Dr. Jacob Early's company ¶3164);
  mustered out on July 16 at Black River, Wisconsin [thomas p56]
  ⟨1⟩ "Lincoln never got out of Ills – never got into the Wisconsin line – was in no 3632
  battle – Demint scoured the N. western part of Ills. Lincoln was with him." –
  Royal Clary [wilson p372] It is doubtful, however, that Lincoln served with this
  man, Maj. John Dement [wilson p372]. See also ¶1032.
  ⟨2⟩ [lincloreFDH] lists 24 places Lincoln transited during his term of service. 3633
  ⟨1⟩ He walked "from Wisconsin back to New Salem" after his horse was stolen 3634
  near the end of his militia service [kunhardtA p44].
  ⟨2⟩ Lincoln arrived back in New Salem 10 days before the local elections [angle 3635
  p46] (reprinting Nicolay and Hay)

- New Salem: 3636
  ⟨2⟩ July 1831 to spring 1837 [angle p89] 3637
  ⟨1⟩ New Salem was "in Sangamon, now in Menard County" – Lincoln [angle p37], 3638
  14 miles from Springfield [arnold p40]
  ⟨2⟩ Appointed postmaster May 7, 1833 [angle p56] 3639
  ⟨2⟩ Fall 1835 ("almost certainly October"): Visited father and step-mother in 3640
  Coles County, IL, per Usher Linder [walsh p128]
  ⟨1⟩ New Salem "never had three hundred people living in it" – Lincoln [angle p93] 3641
  q

- 1834-1842: Lincoln is a member of the Illinois Legislature [angle p99]. The capital 3642
  until 1839 was in Vandalia [angle p67].

- Springfield: 3643
  ⟨2⟩ January 1840: "No street lights, no sidewalks, and the mud so thick it was 3644
  hard for the stage to pull through." – Mrs. Benjamin Edwards [randallC p1] ([ran-
  dallC p3] states there are many references to mud in letters of that time from
  Springfield.)
  ⟨2⟩ Hogs had free roam of the town [randallC p76]. (See ¶2045.) 3645

- Springfield residences, after marriage: 3646
  ⟨2⟩ 1842-1843: A hotel-boardinghouse called the Globe Tavern [turner p30]. 3647
  ⟨2⟩ winter 1843-1844: Rented three-room frame cottage at 214 South Fourth 3648
  Street [turner p31].
  ⟨2⟩ May 1844-1861: House on the corner of Eighth and Jackson [kunhardtA p70]. 3649

- April 12, 1837 to early 1841: Partnered with J.T. Stuart in the practice of law in 3650
  Springfield [angle pp94&98]
  ⟨2⟩ Began to ride the circuit [angle p96]. "Traveling was a real hardship" [angle p97]. 3651
  ⟨2⟩ Dec. 3, 1839: "Admitted to practice before the courts of the United States" 3652
  [angle p98]

- Spring 1841 to fall 1844: Partnered with Stephen T. Logan in the practice of law in 3653
  Springfield [angle p109]
  ⟨2⟩ Travelled the circuit six months out of the year [turner p31], usually three 3654
  months in the spring and three in the fall [randallC p70].

Travel & Dwellings (continued)

⟨2⟩ July-Aug. 1841: Visits Joshua Speed in Kentucky, near Louisville, for five weeks [shenk p63]. ([wilsonH pp249, 250] says end-summer to September.) — 3655

- Congress, 1847-1849: — 3656
  ⟨2⟩ Lincoln, Mary, Robert, and Eddie arrive in St. Louis about Oct. 28, 1847. Then to Lexington, KY to visit Mary's family for about three weeks. Arrived in Washington on Dec. 2. Congress started Dec. 6. [randallC pp92-94] *It is curious, but correct, that Lincoln was elected to Congress in 1846, but began serving at the end of 1847.* — 3657
  ⟨2⟩ In Washington, lived at the boarding house of Mrs. Sprigg, located on Capitol Hill where the Library of Congress is today. [angle p116 following, in photograph legend] — 3658
  ⟨2⟩ April 1848: Back in Lexington by this date [randallC p96] — 3659
  ⟨2⟩ June 1848: Attended Whig National Convention in Philadelphia [angle p153] (reprinting Benjamin Thomas (not [thomas])) — 3660
  ⟨2⟩ Fall 1848 trip: Washington, New England, Buffalo, Chicago (was there Oct. 6), Springfield (was there Oct. 10). Returned east in November 1848. [randallC pp112-113] — 3661
  ⟨2⟩ March 31, 1849: Returns to Springfield [randallC p113] — 3663
  ⟨1⟩ 1849: "On the adjournment of Congress, the 30th, he passed through some of the New England States, making some speeches for Taylor as I remember it." – William Herndon [hertz p207] — 3664

- The Circuit, II: — 3665
  ⟨2⟩ He began riding the circuit again in fall 1849, traveling the whole circuit. [angle pp163, 166] reprinting Benjamin Thomas (not [thomas]) — 3666
  ⟨1⟩ Was on the circuit six to eight months per year and would not come home in the middle [hertz p177, 178]. *I think there were two circuit seasons per year.* — 3667

- Other trips before Presidency: — 3668
  ⟨-⟩ Trips to New Orleans in 1828 (¶3582) and 1831 (¶3628) — 3669
  ⟨2⟩ Summer 1840: Made political speech in Rocheport, Missouri [turner p14] — 3670
  ⟨2⟩ Oct.-Nov. 1849: To Lexington, KY with Mary and sons, after death of Mary's father. [randallC p123] — 3671
  ⟨2⟩ Early spring 1850: To Lexington, KY with Mary and family after death of Mary's maternal grandmother. Lincoln returned to Springfield ahead of Mary.[randallC pp125, 130] — 3672
  ⟨-⟩ Jan. 1854(?): Terre Haute for "mad stone" treatment of Robert after a dog bite – see ¶4953. — 3673
  ⟨1⟩ Summer 1857: Pleasure trip with Mary (?and sons) to "Niagara, Canada, New York & other points of interest" – Mary [turner pp50, 45] — 3674
  ⟨2⟩ September 1857: In Chicago almost entire month [turner p51n] — 3675
  ⟨2⟩ In the 18 months after the 1858 Senate election, "Lincoln traveled frequently and extensively, often taking his wife with him" [turner p53] — 3676
  ⟨2⟩ February 1859: On legal business in Chicago [turner p53n] — 3677
  ⟨2⟩ June 1859: To Chicago with Willie [randallC pp156-157] — 3678
  ⟨2⟩ Summer 1859: Trip of 1100 miles with Mary (?and sons) to inspect property of Illinois Central Railroad [turner p58] — 3679
  ⟨2⟩ August 1859: Business trip to Iowa [turner p55n] — 3680
  ⟨1⟩ Sept. 1859: Speaking tour to Columbus, Cincinnati, and other parts of Ohio with Mary and one son. [turner p59] [randallC p157] — 3681
  ⟨1⟩ October 1859: Speaking in Wisconsin [turner p59] — 3682
  ⟨2⟩ Dec. 1859: Kansas [randallC p158] — 3683

Travel & Dwellings (continued)

Abraham

⟨2⟩ February 1860: New York City (for Cooper Union address) and Exeter, New   3684
Hampshire (to visit Robert) [turner p62]

- Washington: 3685
  - ⟨1/q⟩ 1861: "It was then an unattractive, straggling, sodden a town, wandering up   3686
    and down the left bank of the yellow Potomac, as the fancy can sketch. Penn-
    sylvania Avenue ... was the only paved street of the town. The other streets,
    which were long stretches of mud or deserts of dust and sand, with here and
    there clumps of poorly built residences with long gaps between them. ... Not
    a sewer blessed the town, nor off of Pennsylvania Avenue was there a paved
    gutter. Each house had an open drain from its rear, out across the sidewalk.
    As may be supposed, the Capital of the Republic had more malodors than
    the poet Coleridge ascribed to ancient Cologne. There was then the open
    canal, a branch of the Chesapeake and Ohio, from Rock Creek to Anacosta
    [sic], breeding malaria, tadpoles, and mosquitoes. The Tiber of the day, an-
    cient 'Goose Creek,' stagnated from the highlands through the Botanic Gar-
    dens, and Slash Run overflowed the northwest wastes of the swampy city
    plat." [angle p318] reprinting [riddle]
  - ⟨1⟩ 1861: "Along the north edge of the Mall slowly crept and soaked through the   3687
    city a fetid bayou called, by courtesy, 'The Canal,' floating dead cats and all
    kinds of putridity and reeking with pestilential odors. Cattle, swine, goats,
    sheep, and geese ran at large everywhere. There were only two short sew-
    ers in the entire city, and these were so choked as to back the contents into
    cellars and stores on Pennsylvania Avenue. Happy hogs wallowed in the gut-
    ters. ... On wet days Pennsylvania Avenue was a river of mud and filth in
    which carts and even light buggies were often mired." [croffut]
  - ⟨1/q⟩ 1861: "The population of the District was then about 75,000, of which the   3688
    city of Washington contained 61,000; 15,000 of these were colored, including
    a fraction over 3,000 slaves." [angle p319] reprinting [riddle]
  - ⟨2⟩ 1865: "Washington was sprawling, simple city of about seventy-five thou-   3689
    sand people. It was a city of little frame houses and raggedy, unpaved streets,
    in the midst of which [were] half a dozen great marble buildings." [kunhardtB
    p111]

- Travels while President: 3690
  - ⟨2⟩ Spring 1863: To Aquia Creek, VA aboard the "little steamer" *Carrie Martin*,   3691
    to visit Hooker's army with Mary and Tad. [randallC pp288-289]
  - ⟨2⟩ November 1863: Gettysburg, PA   3692
  - ⟨2⟩ March 22, 1864: Did **not** visit City Point, as [porterH] and [badeau p356] claim.   3693
  - ⟨2⟩ June 16-17, 1864: To Philadelphia, by train. Bried stops in Baltimore and   3694
    Wilmington, DE. [thelincolnlog]
  - ⟨2⟩ June 20-23, 1864: City Point, VA [donaldA pp515-516]   3695
  - ⟨2⟩ Feb. 3, 1865: Is in Hampton Roads, VA, meeting with rebel leaders. [shutesE   3696
    p172][browneF pp678-679]
  - ⟨2⟩ March 23 to April 9, 1865: City Point, VA and Richmond, VA [donaldA pp571, 580]   3697

Voice

"The voice in patients with Marfan syndrome sometimes is rather high pitched, with a   3698
timbre sufficiently characteristic that one author thought he could recognize affected
persons over the telephone" [mckusickA p106].

Voice (continued)

- See also [Speech] 3699

- Singing (for music, see ¶3137): 3700
  - ⟨2⟩ About age 15: "When father & Mother would go to Church ... Abe would take down the Bible, read a verse – give out a hymn – and we would sing – were good singers." – Matilda Johnston Hall Moore [wilson p109] 3701
  - ⟨1⟩ 1830s: "Lincoln couldn't sing any more than a crow." – Daniel Burner [templeB] 3702
  - ⟨1/q⟩ "he could not sing very well" – Sarah Rutledge Saunders [walsh p45] 3703
  - ⟨1⟩ "...devoid of any natural ability as a singer." [herndon p48] 3704
  - ⟨1/q⟩ "Could Lincoln sing? Can a pig whistle?" – William Herndon [walsh p43n] citing (incorrectly) [hertz p138] 3705
  - ⟨1⟩ "Songs he Sang was a great many" – Caleb Carman [wilson p429] 3706
  - ⟨1⟩ "He was always quoting Poetry – singing songs – 'Old Suekey blue Skin'" – Caleb Carman [wilson p374] 3707
  - ⟨1⟩ Played the "boy's harp" – "probably a jew's harp, or harmonica" [wilson p647(n)] 3708
  - ⟨1/q⟩ 1849: "I never sung in my life and never was able to" – Lincoln [kunhardtA p332]. In the same conversation, a friend says "Abe has a great reputation as a singer. It is quite a common thing ... to invite him to farm auctions and have him start off the sale of stock with a good song" [shenk p120]. 3709
  - ⟨1⟩ As President: Lincoln visited a camp of refugee slaves and asked them to sing. "President Lincoln took off his hat and sang too. ... he had a good voice. ... [On the last song] he joined in the chorus and sang as loud as anyone there. She said he certainly had a sweet voice, and it sounded so sad, when he tried to follow her with the first tune." [washington pp85-86] 3710

- Talented as a mimic – see ¶3110. 3711

- Lincoln the orator (also see ¶1122 and [Voice]): 3712
  - ⟨1⟩ "When he began speaking, his voice was shrill, piping, and unpleasant." [herndon p331] 3713
  - ⟨1⟩ "As he proceeded with his speech the exercise of his vocal organs altered somewhat the tone of his voice. It lost in a measure its former acute and shrilling pitch, and mellowed into a more harmonious and pleasant sound." [herndon p333] 3714
  - ⟨1⟩ 1847: "Mr. Lincoln slowly got up, and in his strange, half-erect attitude and clear, quiet accent began... Then rising to his full height, and looking upon the defendants with the compassion of a brother, his long right arm extended towards the opposing counsel..." – George Minier [wilson p708] 3715
  - ⟨1/q⟩ Autumn 1854: "pathetic voice" – J.B. Merwin [hobson p63] (∈ ¶142) 3716
  - ⟨1⟩ 1858: "He used singularly awkward, almost absurd, up-and-down and sidewise movements of his body to give emphasis to his arguments. His voice was naturally good, but he frequently raised it to an unnatural pitch." – Henry Villard [kunhardtA p108] (Part of ¶145) 3717
  - ⟨1/q⟩ Summer 1858: As an orator, in contrast to being in repost,"he was a man of magnificent presence and remarkably impressive manner." – Rev. George C. Noyes [browneF pp289-290] 3718
  - ⟨1/q⟩ Oct. 14, 1858: "His gesture was awkward. He swung his long arms sometimes in a very ungraceful manner. Now and then he would, to give particular emphasis to a point, bend his knees and body with a sudden downward jerk, and then shoot up again with a vehemence that raised him to his tip-toes and made him look much taller than he really was – a manner of enlivening a speech which at that time was, and perhaps still is, not uncommon in the 3719

Voice (continued)

West, but which he succeeded in avoiding at a later period." – Carl Schurz [angle p245] (is continuation of ¶3730))

⟨1/q⟩ Lincoln's effect on audience members: "Then vanished all consciousness of 3720 his uncouth appearance, his awkward manner, or even his high-keyed unpleasant voice, and it required extraordinary effort of the will to divert attention to the man, so concentrated was every mind upon what he was saying." – Judge Abram Bergen [angle p177] reprinting Albert Woldman

⟨1/q⟩ "He sometimes stopped for repairs before finishing a sentence, especially at 3721 the beginning of a speech." – Horace White [randallC p154]

⟨1⟩ "The Inlow family were slow spoken rather drawling in their manner of conver- 3722 sation. Lincoln had the voice of the Inlows." – Michael Cassidy [wilson p615] *Some cite a member of the Enloe family as Lincoln's father. See ¶44.*

⟨1⟩ 1848: "When he was announced [to speak], his tall, angular, bent form, and his 3723 manifest awkwardness and low tone of voice, promised nothing interesting. But he soon warmed to his work." – Henry Gardner [wilson p699]

⟨1⟩ "Lincoln's tones were high-pitched and often disagreeable. He spoke distinctly, 3724 however, and very regularly – almost staccato." – Thomas Shastid, recalling his father's description [shastid]

■ Voice descriptions: 3725

⟨1/q⟩ 1836: Lincoln's first campaign: "for the first time, developed by the excite- 3726 ment of the occasion, he spoke in that tenor intonation of voice that ultimately settled down into that clear, shrill monotone style of speaking that enabled his audience, however large, to hear distinctly the lowest sound of his voice." – Robert(?) Wilson [lamonL p188]

⟨1/q⟩ 1850s: "With a voice by no means pleasing, and, indeed, when excited, in 3727 its shrill tones sometimes almost disagreeable; without any of the personal graces of the orator..." – Thomas Drummond [angle p185]

⟨1/q⟩ 1850s: "kind [but] austere voice" – James Sebree [ChicagoTribune - Feb. 2, 1937] 3728

⟨1/q⟩ 1854: "thin, high-pitched falsetto" – Horace White [shenk p137] 3729

⟨1/q⟩ Oct. 14, 1858: "His voice was not musical, rather high-keyed, and apt to turn 3730 into a shrill treble in moments of excitement; but it was not positively disagreeable. It had an exceedingly penetrating far-reaching quality. The looks of the audience convinced me that every word he spoke was understood at the remotest edges of the vast assemblage." – Carl Schurz [angle p245] (continues in ¶3719)

⟨1/q⟩ Feb. 27, 1860, an indoor speech: "He began in a very low tone of voice – as if 3731 he were used to speaking out-doors and was afraid of speaking too loud." – eyewitness [brooksA p186] (∈ ¶156)

⟨1⟩ 1861, while looking for Lincoln in a crowded hotel dining room, "a long arm 3732 and reached to my shoulder and a shrill voice exclaimed 'Hello, Nelson! ...' It was Mr. Lincoln." – undated article in Terre Haute newspaper [wilson pp641-642] (Part of ¶3104)

⟨1⟩ 1862 or 1863: "... a low voice at my shoulder said to me..." [stoddardD p288] 3733

⟨1⟩ 1863: "those, clear, ringing, earnest tones, which once heard could never be 3734 forgotten" [carrA p252]. Also: "those high, clarion tones. ... His was a voice that, when he made an effort, could reach a great multitude, and he always tried to make everyone hear" [carrB p57].

⟨1⟩ Jan. 9, 1865: "his slow, soft voice" in speaking to his bodyguard [crookA p9] 3735 [crookK]

Voice (continued)

$\langle\frac{1}{q}\rangle$ March 4, 1865: "high pitched, but resonant" voice to deliver second inaugural address [shenk p173] — 3736

$\langle 1 \rangle$ March 4, 1865: "a clear but at times saddened voice" [arnold p403] — 3737

$\langle 1 \rangle$ April 4, 1865: "his voice was gentle and soft" [barnesB] ($\in$ ¶1286) — 3738

- Secondary descriptions: — 3739
  $\langle 2 \rangle$ "Lincoln spoke in a piercing tenor, which at times became shrill and sharp." [donaldA p214] — 3740

  $\langle\frac{1}{q}\rangle$ Springfield era: A worked-up Lincoln is described in the courtroom, probably second-hand: he "rose, turned, and ... cried in a shrill voice, overflowing with the hottest indignation: 'Gentlemen of the jury...' " [burl p156] — 3741

  $\langle 2 \rangle$ 1863: "high, penetrating voice" when delivering the Gettysburg address [donaldA p464] — 3742

  $\langle 2 \rangle$ 1865: Delivering his second inaugural address: "his clear, high-pitched voice that reached even the outer edges of the huge crowd" [donaldA p566] — 3743

$\langle 2 \rangle$ In at least one indoor speech (? Cooper Union), Lincoln had someone stand at the back of the auditorium with a cane and a hat, with instructions to put the hat on the cane and wave it if Lincoln's voice became difficult to hear [holzerB]. — 3744

- Audible laughter: — 3745
  $\langle\frac{1}{q}\rangle$ March 7, 1841, with Lincoln in a funk because of troubles with Mary: "No more will we the merry peal of laughter ascend *high in the air*" – James Conkling [randallC p48] — 3746

  $\langle 1 \rangle$ 1857: "... someone in the rear seats burst out into a loud, coarse laugh – a sudden and explosive guffaw" [herndon p479] ($\in$ ¶2498) — 3747

  $\langle 2 \rangle$ 1860: "at the punch line his high-pitched laughter rang through the capitol." [donaldA p259] *"Capitol" is the Illinois state capitol building.* — 3748

  $\langle 1 \rangle$ "fairly shrieked with laughter" [brooksC pp288-289] *It was rueful laughter.* — 3749

  $\langle 1 \rangle$ "an indescribable chuckle" [brooksC p300] — 3750

- Silent laughter: — 3751
  $\langle 1 \rangle$ Aug. 1863: "Lincoln was laughing silently when I began [reading] and loudly when I ended." [stoddardD p321] — 3752

  $\langle 1 \rangle$ Spring 1864: "at this point he again held in for another long, quiet fit of laughter." [stoddardD p319] — 3753

$\langle 1 \rangle$ In Illinois, prob. 1858: "To see Lincoln ... on an open prairie, the central figure of ten thousand people ... his voice clear and powerful, and of a key that could be distinctly heard by all the vast multitude..." [arnold pp90-91] *Quoted more extensively in The Physical Lincoln.* — 3755

$\langle\frac{1}{q}\rangle$ Feb. 11, 1861: Leaving Springfield, his voice "quivered with emotion so deep as to render him almost unable to utter a single word." – Henry Villard [shenk p171] — 3756

$\langle 2 \rangle$ Feb. 1861: As Lincoln slowly journeyed from Illinois to take office in Washington, he accepted innumerable requests to speak. "At times he lost his voice." [donaldA p275] (Agrees with [kunhardtA p6].) — 3757

$\langle\frac{1}{q}\rangle$ March 1861: An eyewitness recalled Lincoln delivering his first inaugural address in a voice "though not very strong or full-toned" that "rang out over the acres of people before him with surprising distinctness and was heard in the remotest part of his audience" [donaldA p283]. — 3758

  $\langle 1 \rangle$ "In the open air, and with a voice so clear and distinct that he could be heard by thrice ten thousand men, he read his inaugural address..." [arnold p190] — 3759

Voice (continued)

⟨1⟩ 1862: Robert Wilson was with Lincoln the night after the first Battle of Bull Run. Army regulations prohibited Lincoln from telling news of the battle to Wilson. Wilson tried a different approach: "I said to him then, I don't ask for the news, but you tell me the quality of the news, – is it good, or is it bad. Placing his mouth near my ear he said in a sharp shrill voice, 'damned bad.'" [wilson p207] 3760

⟨1⟩ Nov. 1863: Delivering the Gettysburg Address: "slow and very impressive and far-reaching utterance" [macveagh] 3761

⟨1⟩ March 1865: Delivering his second inaugural address: "Every word was clear and audible as the ringing and somewhat shrill tones of Lincoln's voice sounded over the vast concourse." [brooksC p239] 3762

⟨1/q⟩ "His voice had something peculiarly winning about it, some quality which I can't describe, but which seemed to thrill ever fiber of one's body." – a recollection 45 years after the fact [burl p9] 3763
  ⟨1/q⟩ Nicolay thought Lincoln had a "subtle and indefinable magnetism" [burl p12] 3764
  ⟨1/q⟩ Another observer thought Lincoln had "a deep, unfathomable sense of power" [burl p12] 3765

⟨S⟩ [kempfB pp11,12] believes the horse-kick to Lincoln's head (see ¶3568) was responsible for impairing the laryngeal muscles, resulting in Lincoln's "high pitched, rasping voice" and a compensatory "slow staccato monotone." 3766

Weight

See Build -- Adult . 3767

Appendix – Mental Explorations

This appendix explores a very few aspects of the mental Lincoln, chiefly (but not exclusively) his intellectual interests. This departure from our usual emphasis on his physical features supports a chapter in *The Physical Lincoln*. 3768

Astronomy & Physics 3769

⟨1⟩ About 1826: Anna Roby, sitting with Lincoln on the banks of the Ohio River one evening, remarks that the moon is going down. Lincoln responds by explaining the motion of the earth and moon, and how the moon "don't really go down." Roby responds "Abe – what a fool you are." – Anna Roby Gentry [wilson p132] 3770

⟨2⟩ Used an almanac of lunar phases to clear a client of murder (Duff Armstrong) [kunhardtB p294] 3771

⟨2⟩ Sept. 14, 1858, at Jonesboro, IL: With Horace White, looked at Donati's comet for an hour. [randallC p153] 3772
  ⟨1/q⟩ "Mr. Lincoln greatly admired this strange visitor, and he and I sat for an hour or more in front of the hotel looking at it." – Horace White [ChicagoTribune - Sept. 17, 1858] 3773

⟨1/q⟩ Sept. 1862: Chicago ministers suggest he free the slaves in the south. "Now, gentlemen, if I cannot enforce the Constitution down South, how am I to enforce a mere Presidential proclamation? Won't the world sneer at it as being as powerless as the Pope's bull against the comet?" [riceA p334] 3774

Appendix – Mental Explorations (continued)

⟨2⟩ Visits to the Naval Observatory (e.g. Aug. 22, 1863 [hayD]). Viewed the moon and Arcturus. [hermanJ]   3775

⟨1⟩ On one of these visits, "Lincoln had come unattended through the dark streets to inquire why the moon had appeared inverted in the telescope. Surveyors' instrument, which he had once used, show objects in their true position" [hallA p93].   3776

⟨1⟩ "He invited me one day at Washington to call upon him in the evening when he said he would go to the observatory and take a look at the moon through the large telescope   It proved to be cloudy and I did not go" – Joseph Gillespie [wilson p506]   3777

⟨1⟩ "I have heard him decant upon the problem whether a ball discharged from a gun in a horizontal position would be longer in reaching the ground than one dropped at the instant of discharge from the muzzle the gun [sic] and he said it always appeared to him that they would both reach the ground at the same time even before he read the philosophical explanation" – Joseph Gillespie [wilson pp505-506]   3778

⟨1⟩ 1836-1840: Sees the first house in the region with a lightning rod. No one can tell him how it works. "He rode into town, bought a book on the properties of lightning, and before morning knew all about it." – Joshua Speed [wilson p589] *But Lincoln also used the rod in a speech to evoke religious paranoia in his listeners* [wilson p589].   3779

⟨1⟩ May 1860: Had celestial globe in his office at home [coffinA]. (∈ ¶3905)   3780

Biology – Himself   3781

⟨1⟩ Would speculate on his interruption and resumption of speech after bring kicking in the head by a horse during childhood. See §1a.   3782

⟨1⟩ Checks whether circulatory pulsations in his leg blurred a photograph. (See ¶1975.)   3783

⟨1⟩ Investigates his double vision. (See ¶907.)   3784

⟨1⟩ As President: Is watching soldiers clearing a forest in Virginia, but mentally comparing the length of his arms to theirs. (See ¶247.) [rothschild p26]   3785

■ Testing his height against other tall men: see ¶443.   3786

Biology – Not Himself   3787

■ Evolution: 3788

⟨1⟩ "He was an evolutionist" – William Herndon 1882 [hertz p90]   3789

⟨1⟩ "grew into the belief of a universal law, evolution, and from this he has never deviated. Mr. Lincoln became a firm believer in evolution and of the law." – William Herndon [hertz p407] (Also repeats that Lincoln read parts of Darwin's book.)   3790

⟨1⟩ watching stallions with a mare: "Lincoln always attended" – John Hill [wilson p23]   3791

⟨1⟩ Sept. 18, 1858: "[The People] plainly see that Judge Douglas is playing cuttlefish, a small species of fish that has no mode of defending itself when pursued except by throwing out a black fluid, which makes the water so dark the enemy cannot see it and thus it escapes." – Lincoln [baslerA v3p185]   3792

Appendix – Mental Explorations (continued)

⟨1⟩ June 1862: Notices a large spiderweb in the War Department's Telegraph Office (where spent much time). Some 6 or 7 spiders appeared on it one day. "Lincoln was much interested in the performance and thereafter, while writing at the [nearby] desk, would often watch for the appearance of the visitors." [angle pp404-405] quoting Thomas Eckert — 3793

⟨1/q⟩ Observing there weren't enough offices to satisfy all the office seekers, Lincoln said, "There are too many pigs for the tits" [kunhardtA p278]. — 3794

⟨2⟩ April 1865: "On the way back from City Point by train, Lincoln noticed a terrapin sunning himself by the roadside. He asked to have the train stopped and the terrapin brought in, whereupon he and Tad had a happy time watching the creature's ungainly movements." [randallC pp337-338] — 3795

⟨1⟩ April 1865: Lincoln has his carriage stop near Petersburg, to examine "a very tall and beautiful tree." "He admired the strength of its trunk, the vigorous development of branches, reminding one of the tall trees of Western forests, compared it to the great oaks in the shadow if which he had spent his youth, and strove to make us understand the distinctive character of these different types. The observations thus set forth were evidently not those of an artist who seeks to idealize nature, but of a man who seeks to see it as it really is; in short, that dissertation about a tree did not reveal an effort of imagination, but a remarkable precision of mind." [chambrunA] — 3796

Biology – "Coarse"
3797

⟨1/q⟩ He told anatomically correct jokes, e.g. a fish that was not a fish [shenk p116] — 3798

⟨1⟩ In open court he mocked an opposing witness: "there is Busey – he pretends to be a great heart smasher – does wonderful things with the girls – but I'll venture that he never entered his flesh but once and that is when he fell down & stuck his finger in his – – –" [wilson p630] — 3799

⟨1⟩ Talks of grabbing a preacher by the "____" [wilson p483] — 3800

⟨1⟩ "Jim Matheny think that Lincoln's mind ran to filthy stories – that a story had no fun unless it was dirty and I must admit it looks very plausible. I can't think he gloated over filth, however. I think he was some like Linder in that he had great ideality and also a view of grossness which displaced the ideality." – Henry Whitney [wilson p617]. — 3801

⟨1⟩ Story about Lincoln's ascending tickling of girls [wilson p90]. — 3802

⟨2⟩ A probably apocryphal story of a bullet wound that would not have injured a woman [neelyL] — 3803

⟨1⟩ Keen sense of humor; stories of "grosser" nature [lamonL pp479-480] — 3804

⟨1⟩ 1859: "a farmer Said – Lincoln, why do you not write out your stories & put them in a book?' Lincoln, drew himself up – fixed his face, as if a thousand dead carcusses – and a million of privies were Shooting all their Stench into his nostrils, and Said 'Such a book would Stink like a thousand privies.'" – Henry E. Dummer [wilson p442] — 3805

General Inquiry
3806

⟨1⟩ "Lincoln had a remarkably inquiring mind and I have no doubt he roamed over the whole field of knowledge" – Joseph Gillespie [wilson p506] (∈ ¶3873) — 3807

Appendix – Mental Explorations (continued)

⟨1⟩ "Where did this vast body of water come from?" – Lincoln at Niagara. (a view   3808
into the way he evaluated the world) [wilson p569] *This seems to reveal something
about Lincoln's way of thinking.* [randallC p113]*'s suggestion that the comment
was a tease at Herndon is refuted by reading* [wilson p569].

History and Biography   3809

⟨1⟩ "L. had a contempt for all history and biography; he knew how it was written; he   3810
knew the motives and conscience of the writers of history and biography. Lincoln
wanted to know the whole truth and nothing less." – William Herndon [hertz p152]

⟨1⟩ "'Biographies as written are false and misleading. The author of the Life of his love   3811
paints him as a perfect man, magnifies his perfections and suppresses his imperfections, describes the success of his love in glowing terms, never once hinting at
his failures and his blunders...' This Mr. Lincoln said to me in substance just as I
have it." – William Herndon [hertz p175]

⟨1⟩ "Let us believe, as in the days of our youth, that Washington was spotless; it makes   3812
human nature better to believe that one human being was perfect: that human
perfection is possible." [angle p170, quoting Henry Whitney quoting Lincoln]

Invention and Technology   3813

⟨$\frac{1}{q}$⟩ Lincoln thought mankind's greatest invention was the written word, "enabling us   3814
to converse with the dead, the absent, and the yet unborn" [kunhardtB p298]. *Are not
genes the same?*

- His lecture on science and inventions: 3815
  ⟨2⟩ Twice delivered a lecture in Springfield. He foresaw harnessing the wind,   3816
  taming the tides, expanding the use of steam, and mastery of the sun's explosive heat and firepower [kunhardtA p328]
  ⟨1⟩ His lecture on science: "his purpose was to analyze inventions and discov-   3817
  eries – 'to get at the bottom of things' – and to show when, where, how, and
  why such things were invented or discovered; and, so far as possible, to find
  where the first mention is made of some of our common things. The Bible,
  he said, he found to be the richest store-house for such knowledge." [brooksR]
  ⟨2⟩ Gave the lecture in April 1858 to a full house in Bloomington. [randallC p151]   3818
  ⟨1⟩ Herndon says (somewhere) that the lecture was terrible and that Lincoln   3819
  could not have made a living as a lecturer.
  ⟨1⟩ Text of lecture is in [baslerA].   3820

⟨1⟩ About 1855: Herndon buys a small book called *The Annual of Science* and takes it   3821
back to the office. Lincoln begins looking at it and quickly understands "the purpose and object of the book[:] to record, teach, and fully explain the *failures* and
successes of experiments of all philosophies and scientists, everywhere, including
chemistry, mechanics, etc. He instantly rose up and said that he must buy the
whole set, started out, and got them. On returning to the office, he said: 'I have
wanted such a book for years, because I sometimes make experiments and have
thoughts about the physical world that I do not know to be true or false. I may,
by this book, correct my errors and save time and expense. I can see where scientists and philosophers have failed and avoid the rock on which they split or can
see the means of their success and take advantage of their brains, toil, and knowledge. Men are greedy to publish the successes of efforts, but meanly shy as to
publishing the failures of man. Many men are ruined by this one-sided practice

Appendix – Mental Explorations (continued)

of concealment of blunders and failures.' This he said substantially to me with much feeling, vim, and force." – William Herndon, 1885 [hertz p113]

⟨2⟩ Another invention: a new method of steering a wagon wherein the axle was rigid and the front wheels free-moving. [kunhardtB p292]　3822

⟨2⟩ 1860: Lincoln offers his basement as a darkroom, watching "with interest the development of the picture." [ostendorfA p60]　3823

Mathematics　3824

⟨1⟩ He had a "bias for mathematics and the physical sciences　I think he bestowed more attention to them than upon metaphysical speculations" – Joseph Gillespie [wilson p505]　3825

- Euclid:　3826
  - ⟨1⟩ "Lincoln from 1849 to 1855 became a hard student and read much, studied Euclid and some mathematical books." – William Herndon, 1887 [hertz p172]　3827
  - ⟨1⟩ After opposing President Polk on the Mexican War, "Mr. Lincoln knew that he was politically dead and so he went most heartily to knowledge; he took Euclid around with him on the circuit and of nights and odd times he would learn Euclid's problems. ... He would study till twelve or one o'clock in the night." Read by "tallow candlelight." – William Herndon, 1885 [hertz p96]　3828
  - ⟨1⟩ "I have seen him myself, upon the circuit, with 'a geometry,' or 'an astronomy,' or some book of that kind, working out propositions in moments of leisure." – Leonard Swett [riceA p467]　3829
  - ⟨1⟩ Herndon refutes the idea that Lincoln studied Euclid in the 1830s [hertz p403]　3830
  - ⟨1⟩q "read no histories, novels, biographies, etc., studied Euclid, the exact sciences" – David Davis [hertz p426]　3831

⟨1⟩ "He thought that he could completely demonstrate, square rather, the circle; he purchased tools, etc., with which to make the attempt, but failed. ... Lincoln thought that he could do anything that other men could or would try to do; he had unbounded confidence in himself." [hertz p126]　3832

⟨1⟩ "Lincoln was keenly sensitive to his failures, and it would not do to mention them in his presence." [hertz p126]　3833

⟨1⟩ "I never knew him to thoroughly understand any thing in law mathamatics ... anatomy" and many other fields – Elliott Herndon [wilson p460]　3834

Mechanics　3835

⟨1⟩q 1854: Lincoln and Herndon took the patent-dispute case of Alexander Edmonds, who had invented a mechanical baby-cradle rocker. "There was something about it that attracted the attention of Mr. Lincoln." Herndon remembered that "Mr. Lincoln, owing to his natural bent for the study of mechanical applications, soon became so enamoured of the case that he assumed entire charge of our end of it. The model of the machine ... eventually reached our office where Mr. Lincoln became deeply absorbed in it. He would dilate at great lengths on its merits for the benefit of our callers or anyone else who happened into the office and manifested the least interest in it." [angle p172] reprinting Jesse Weik　3836

⟨1⟩q "He had a good mechanical mind and knowledge" – David Davis [hertz p426]　3837

⟨1⟩ "He had a great deal of Mechanical genius, could understand readily the principles & mechanical action of machinery" – Grant Goodrich [wilson p510]　3838

- Weapons-testing (reviewed in [bruce]):　3839

Appendix – Mental Explorations (continued)

$\langle\frac{1}{q}\rangle$ In evaluating proposed weapons, "had a quick comprehension of mechani-   3840
cal principles, and often detected a flaw in an invention which the contriver
had overlooked." – John Hay [angle p435] (See ¶2528.)

$\langle\frac{1}{q}\rangle$ Test-fired early mitrailleuse (¶2528). Also "practised in the trenches his long-   3841
disused skill with the rifle. A few fortunate shots from his own gun..." – John
Hay [angle pp435-436]

$\langle 1 \rangle$ Was granted a patent by the U.S. Patent Office   3842

$\langle 1 \rangle$ About 1835: "invented a wheel – a water wheel – which ran under water: it   3843
promised at the time of some value. I do not know what became of it." – Hardin
Bale [wilson p13]

Medicine   3844

$\langle 1 \rangle$ 1827±: Applies first aid (?tourniquet) to his step-sister's severely bleeding thigh,   3845
lacerated when she fell on an axe. [hertz pp422-423]

$\langle 1 \rangle$ 1838: Speaking of some gamblers: "If they were annually swept, from the stage   3846
of existence, by the plague or small pox, honest men would, perhaps, be much
profited, by the operation" [baslerA v1p111].

- Lincoln often used medical facts and similes in his writings. [carman] provides sev-   3847
eral excerpts, the best being, from 1858: "As thin as the homeopathic soup that
was made by boiling the shadow of a pigeon that had starved to death." (Also in:
[shutes p94].) Also told medical jokes, e.g. a malingerer who's rump boils are cured
by hearing enemy troops [shutes pp103-104], and quinine tonic with whiskey [porterH].

$\langle 2 \rangle$ In Springfield: Lincoln spent hours in his local health-care facility – the Corneau   3848
and Diller drug store. [turnerL]

$\langle 2 \rangle$ "Once at a political rally Lincoln and Long John [Wentworth] had spent their time   3849
counting, not potential votes, but how many women in the audience were nursing
babies." [kunhardtB p237]

$\langle 2 \rangle$ 1840s: Soon after Robert's birth, Lincoln told his dentist, Dr. French, that he had   3850
feared the baby would have one long leg like his and "and one short one, like
Mary's." [kunhardtA p90]

$\langle 2 \rangle$ 1840s: Writes a poem about a friend, Matthew Gentry, who had gone "furously   3851
mad" when Lincoln was 16 [shenk p78]

$\langle 1 \rangle$ 1854: Of slavery: "Thus, the thing is hid away, in the constitution, just as an af-   3852
flicted man hides away a wen or a cancer, which he dares not cut out at once, lest
he bleed to death; with the promise, nevertheless, that the cutting may begin at
the end of a given time." – Lincoln [baslerA v2p275]

$\langle 1 \rangle$ 1850s: Clearly distinguishes between medical treatments based on superstition   3853
and those based on experimental data. [wilson p182] (See ¶4953.)

$\langle 2 \rangle$ 1857: While arguing the case of Duff Armstrong: "Lincoln had mastered some   3854
technical questions in anatomy and explained his theory that it was more likely
that [the murder victim] had died, not from any wound inflicted by Duff, but
rather from the blow of Norris' club or from repeated falls from his horse." [an-
gle pp177-178] reprinting Albert Woldman

$\langle 1 \rangle$ Feb. 1861: Lincoln "calls attention" to a man's red nose at dinner. The man applies   3855
acetic acid to the nose overnight, making it bleached and shriveled at breakfast.
All laugh at him. [wilson p702] (∈ ¶2187)

Appendix – Mental Explorations (continued)

⟨2⟩ Jan. 12, 1864: Assesses chances that he gave smallpox to another person (his sometime valet) [baslerC]. See §5g. 3856

⟨1⟩_q Described the 13th Amendment as the "King's cure for all the evils" of slavery, using a term from tuberculosis medicine. [kunhardtA p270] [carman] 3857

⟨1⟩ "His favorite illustration in the discussions in those days with his confidential friends was, that a faithful surgeon must always strive to save both life and limb, even though the limb was gangrened and diseased; but when that was impossible, then, at all hazards, he must save life and sacrifice limb." [riceA p333] 3858

⟨2⟩ Watched a soldier's arm being amputated: "He was greatly interested but evidently had little fondness for surgery." More than likely the operation would have been done without anesthesia. Lincoln overheard another surgeon congratulate the operating surgeon and then added, as a "solemn inquiry, 'But how about the soldier?' " [shutes p 96] 3859

⟨2⟩ There were two hospitals on the grounds of the White House. Lincoln "gave much thought to hospital construction" [shutes pp97-98] 3860

⟨2⟩ As President: Anesthesia had only been known since 1848, yet Lincoln tried it on himself in a dentist's chair [kunhardtB p292] [shutes p89]. 3861

⟨2⟩_c *His assessment of the madstone's therapeutic properties against rabies* [wilson p182] *is shockingly modern.* (See ¶4953.) 3862

⟨1⟩ Attended sanitary fairs and established a sanitary commission for "relief, health, and comfort" of soldiers. [arnold pp406ff] 3863
  ⟨1⟩ Attended the Great Sanitary Fair in 1864 [wilson p223] 3864

⟨1⟩_q "I am not yet ready to sell my bones to a physician" – Lincoln's reply when he was offered the chance to buy life insurance [shutes p107]. *Life insurance was then new. Remark seems more like a dig at the word "sell" than at physicians.* 3865

⟨1⟩_q "he had the *molera-corbus* [cholera-morbus] pretty bad" – Lincoln word-play in a long story [tripp p37] 3866

⟨2⟩ The Lincoln-Herndon law office library contained three medical books: Dean's *Medical Jurisprudence*, Taylor's *A Treatise on Poisons in Relation to Medical Jurisprudence*, and *A Synopsis of Practical Surgery* [shutes p62]. 3867

Practical 3868

⟨1⟩ "Mr. Lincoln was practical and thought things useless unless they they could [be] of utility, use, practice, etc., etc.; he would read awhile, read till he got tired, and then he must tell a story, crack a joke, make a jest to ease himself,; he hated study except for the practical to be applied right off as it were." – William Herndon [hertz p95] 3869

⟨1⟩ "was not a speculative-minded man; was, like Washington, severely practical ... was always directing the ideas and feelings of men to purely practical ends, to something that would end in good." – William Herndon [hertz pp82-83] 3870

⟨1⟩ "What he read, he read for a proximate, near end; he was not a general reader" – William Herndon [hertz p120] 3871
  ⟨1⟩_q "He made no attempt to keep pace with the ordinary literature of the day. Sometimes, he read a scientific work with keen appreciation, but he pursued no systematic course." – John Hay [angle p437] 3872

Appendix – Mental Explorations (continued)

⟨1⟩ "Lincoln had a remarkably inquiring mind and I have no doubt he roamed over the whole field of knowledge   There were departments however upon which he fixed his attention with special interest   Those which were of a practical character and having a solid and indisputable basis he made himself master of so far as time & opportunity would allow" – Joseph Gillespie [wilson p506]   3873

Psychology and Related   3874

⟨1⟩ Feb. 22, 1842: Of alcohol, in a temperance speech: "The victims to it were pitied, and compassionated, just as now are, the heirs of consumptions, and other hereditary diseases. Their failing was treated as a *misfortune*, and not as a *crime*, or even as a *disgrace*." – Lincoln [baslerA v1pp275-276]   3875

   ⟨2⟩_c "His practical advice on the psychotherapy of alcoholism and other psychopathological frustrations, as suggested in his lectures ... preceded by 100 years similar methods being applied today in the best psychiatric institutions." [kempfB pp xix-xx]   3876

⟨1⟩ "He used to say that the attempt to ascertain wherein wit consisted baffled him more than any other undertaking of the kind   That the first impression would be that the thing was of easy solution but the varieties of wit were so great that what would explain one case would be wholly inapplicable to another" – Joseph Gillespie [wilson p506]   3877

Readiness to Relieve Suffering   3878

⟨1⟩ "In this connection may be mentioned the extreme tenderness and sympathy of Mr. Lincoln for all forms of suffering." [arnold p409]   3879

⟨1⟩ 1822: Helps suffering student trying to spell a word out loud! [wilson p131]   3880

⟨2⟩ 1830: Rescues a dog from a frozen Illinois river in winter. [wilson p718] (See ¶2109.)   3881

⟨2⟩ 1832: While in the militia, prevents his fellow militiamen from killing an old Indian who wandered into camp, almost coming to blows with them [angle p44, quoting Benjamin Thomas].   3882

⟨1⟩ 1839: Lincoln is riding with a group of lawyers from one town to another. They were riding in pairs, Lincoln alongside John Hardin. At one point the group noticed Hardin was alone, and asked him what happened to Lincoln. "When I saw him last, he had caught two little birds in his hand, which the wind had blown from their nest, and he was hunting for the nest." Lincoln found the nest, replaced the birds, and later said, "I could not have slept tonight if I had not given those two little birds to their mother." [wilson p590] [arnold p55]   3883

⟨1⟩ Picks up a drunk [arnold p27].   3884

⟨1⟩ Rescues lamb stuck in water-hole [shutesE pp29-30]   3885

⟨2⟩ At peril to himself, rescues dog from frozen river as a youth or young man.   3886

⟨2⟩ The man who wanted to live in a world of cold reason [donaldA] cast aside his reason to take Robert to Terre Haute for the "madstone" folk-remedy to prevent rabies.   3887

⟨1⟩ 1865: "...we were on our way to the War Department, when we passed a ragged dirty man in army clothes lounging just outside the White House enclosure. He had evidently been waiting to see the President, for he jumped up and went toward him with his story. He had been wounded, was just out of the hospital – he looked forlorn enough. There was something he wanted the President to do; he had papers with him. Mr. Lincoln was in a hurry, but he put out his hands   3888

Appendix – Mental Explorations (continued)

for the papers. Then he sat down on the curbstone, the man beside him, and examined them. When he had satisfied himself about the matter, he smiled at the anxious fellow reassuringly and told him to come back the next day; then he would arrange the matter for him. A thing like that says more than any man could express." [crookA p78]

Secretiveness

3889

⟨$\frac{1}{q}$⟩ Was, in William Herndon's "oft-cited phrase," "the most secretive – reticent – shut-mouthed man that ever existed" [shenk p108, citing Herndon to JE Remsberg, 9/10/87, Published by HE Barker 1917, copy in Ill. St. Hist. Lib.]

3890

⟨1⟩ "He was a man of quite infinite silences and was thoroughly and deeply secretive, uncommunicative, and close-minded as to his plans, wishes, hopes, and fears. His ambition was never satisfied; in him it was a consuming fire which smothered his [undeciphered] feelings. ... He was skeptical, cautious, and terribly secretive, confiding his plans and purposes, ambitions and ends, to no man." – William Herndon [hertz p88]

3891

⟨1⟩ "In one of your letters you ask me this question in substance: 'Do you think Lincoln wished to be known, thoroughly known?' and to which I answer emphatically: 'No, he was a hidden man and wished to keep his own secrets.' " – William Herndon Aug. 22, 1887 [hertz p202]

3892

⟨1⟩ "was a secretive, silent, and a very reticent-minded man, trusting no man, nor woman, nor child with the inner secrets of his ambitious soul." – William Herndon [hertz p124]

3893

⟨1⟩ Refused to "tell all the secrets of his soul to any man" – William Herndon [hertz p159]

3894

⟨1⟩ "reticent, secretive, incommunicable, in some, many, lines of his character." – William Herndon [hertz p169]

3895

⟨1⟩ "This terribly reticent, secretive, shutmouth man never talked much about his history, plans, designs, purposes, intents ... Lincoln had profound policies and never revealed himself to any man or woman, and this his nature caused the devil domestically. Lincoln is unknown and possibly always will be." – William Herndon [hertz p204]

3896

⟨1⟩ "Mr. Lincoln never had a confidant, and therefore never unbosomed himself to others. He never spoke of his trials to me or, so far as I knew, to any of his friends." – William Herndon [randallC p110] *In context, "trials" seems to refer to domestic tribulations.*

3897

⟨1⟩ More of William Herndon on secretiveness: [hertz p77]

3898

⟨1⟩ "It is all new to me" – Joshua Speed's reaction to Herndon's 1866 lecture on Ann Rutledge [wilson p431] *So, apparently, Lincoln never told the story to Speed.*

3899

Teaching Himself – Day to Day

3900

⟨$\frac{1}{q}$⟩ On the circuit: "We frequently talked philosophy, politics, political economy, metaphysics and men; in short, our subjects of conversation ranged through the universe of thought and experience." – Henry Whitney [angle p168].

3901

⟨$\frac{1}{q}$⟩ On the circuit: "At another time the doctrine of metempsychosis was discussed by the whole crowd, i.e. the doctrine that when one man dies, a child is born which inherits the vital principle – the soul – of the departing one." – Henry Whitney [angle p169]

3902

Appendix – Mental Explorations (continued)

⟨1⟩ On the circuit: Lincoln quietly steals back to his room, having seen a show in town for the second night in a row. He "entertained us with a description of new sights – a magic lantern, electrical machine, etc. I told him I had seen all these sights at school. 'Yes,' he said, sadly, 'I now have an advantage over you in, for the first time in my life, seeing these things which are of course common to those, who had, what I did not, a chance at an education, when they were young.' " – Henry Whitney [angle p168]   3903

⟨1⟩ Herdon would have philosophical discussions with Lincoln in the office [hertz p116]   3904

⟨1⟩ May 1860: Lincoln's library in Springfield: "There were miscellaneous books on the shelves, two globes, celestial and terrestrial, in the corners of the room, a plain table with writing materials upon it." [coffinA p174]   3905

Teaching Himself – Learned Men   3906

⟨1⟩ January 15, 1865: Lincoln meets noted scientist Louis Agassiz and "shares insights into ancient science that even Agassiz hadn't considered." Lincoln admits that "many years ago he tried his hand at a lecture on inventions and discoveries but never finished;" Agassiz urges him to finish it. Lincoln surprises others by asking Agassiz not about glaciers and ice ages, but about academic techniques. Lincoln says: "Why, what we got from him isn't printed in books, the other things are." [brooksR]   3907

⟨2⟩ Lincoln and Joseph Henry [kunhardtA p326] "discussed everything from climatology ... to such questions as the use of balloons. ... The President had been the first to urge Dr. Henry to see the aeronaut, Thaddeus T. C. Lowe, and talk over his plan for the use of balloons in war [kunhardtB pp293-294]. (Goes on about other technologies, e.g. telegraph lines across Russia, gunpowder, ...)   3908

⟨2⟩ Jan. 2, 1865: Interviewed by *Scientific American* magazine [miers on that date] *I cannot find the interview in the magazine of 2, 9, or 14 Jan. 1865.*   3909

Unpretentious   3910

⟨$\frac{1}{q}$⟩ "Wealth is simply a superfluity of what we don't need." – Lincoln [riceA p452]   3911

⟨$\frac{1}{q}$⟩ "Simple in his habits, without pretensions of any kind, and distrustful of himself" – Thomas Drummond [angle p187]   3912

Lincoln, Edward

child #2

Edward

Chronology

▪ Lived March 10 1846 [baslerA v1p392] to Feb. 1, 1850 [templeC]   3913

Introduction & Sources

▪ Little is known of Edward. Unfortunately, the diary of Orville Browning starts a few months after Edward's death.   3914

Appearance

[◎] [ostendorfA pp364-365] states "A long lost daguerreotype of Edward Baker Lincoln ... has come to light. ... here first published through the courtesy of the owner, Keya Mazhari, of Keya Gallery, New York City." The daguerreotype's case bears an inscription identifying the youngster as Edward Lincoln, and was found in the collection of Herbert Wells Fay, who was an early custodian of the Lincoln tomb. *The image is apparently genuine. Medical factors add to the belief it is genuine.*   3915

Build

In Marfan syndrome, excess length may be demonstrable at birth and throughout childhood and adolescence [mckusickA p53].   3916

⟨1/q⟩ At age 7 months: "He is very much such a child as Bob was at his age – rather of a longer order. Bob is 'short and low,' and, I expect, always will be." – Lincoln (Oct. 22, 1846) [prattA] [kunhardtA p90] [burl [61]   3917

[◎] After Edward died, Mary gave his clothes to a neighbor, Mary Remann. Her son, Henry Remann, was photographed wearing them. [kunhardtA pp92-93] ○○○ *Project:* It would be interesting to know Henry's age in the photo. It might be possible to deduce the extent to which Edward was tall for his age, based on the fit of his clothes on a presumably normal Henry Remann.   3919

Death

⟨1⟩ "The day after Grandpa Remann's funeral on Dec. 11, 1849, little Eddie Lincoln took sick and he had all the symptoms Grandpa had. He died Feb. 1, at 6 in the morning." – Mary Edwards Brown, 1956, recalling a family story [kunhardtC].   3920

 ⟨2⟩ Remann died of "chronic consumption" [kunhardtC]   3921

⟨1⟩ "... we lost our little boy. He was sick fiftytwo days & died the morning of the first day of this month." – Lincoln [baslerA v2p78]   3922

 ⟨2⟩ [donaldA p153] says "fifty-two days of acute illness." *Justification is unclear, especially since census says "chronic" – see ¶3928.*   3923

 ⟨2⟩ Three days before Eddie's death, Lincoln did not mention illness when writing to Orville Browning [shutesM].   3924

Death (continued)

⟨2⟩ The day before Edward's death, Lincoln said "I have never been so happy in   3925
my life" [kunhardtB p12] (¶2481). *Assuming Lincoln would not say this if his*
son were at death's door, it suggests a misquote, or that Eddie's illness
worsened abruptly in less than 24 hours.

⟨2⟩ Lincoln had what was, or would become, a recurring dream the night before   3926
Eddie's death [kunhardtC]. (See ¶3548.)

⟨2⟩ The rate at which the Lincolns purchased items from the Corneau & Diller Drug   3927
Store [hickey] suggests that the parents were not idle during Eddie's illness. Between
Dec. 12 (presumably the first of the 52 days of illness) and Feb. 1, the Lincolns
made purchases on 24 different days, including Christmas. In only one other *year*
from 1849 to 1860 did they make purchases on 24 different days.

- Cause of death: 3928
  ⟨1⟩ The 1850 U.S. census for Sangamon County, Illinois, contains the following   3929
  record under "Persons who Died during the Year ending 1st June, 1850, in
  Springfield" [templeC]:

Name of the person who died	= Edward Lincoln
Age	= 4
Sex	= M
Place of birth	= Illinois
The month in which the person died	= Feb.
Disease or cause of death	= same [Consumption]
Number of days ill	= C.

  ⟨1⟩ The line above Edward's record lists "same" for cause of death; the line above   3930
  that lists "Consumption." [templeC] cites a reference as equating "C" with
  "chronic."

  ⟨2⟩ "pulmonary tuberculosis" [donaldA p153], "tuberculosis" [baker pp125&136]   3931

  ⟨2⟩ "The cause of death was either consumption, as the U.S. Census of 1850   3932
  ᶜ stated, or pulmonary tuberculosis, as researchers today believe." [kunhardtA
  p90] *Tuberculosis was one cause of "consumption."*

- "Fifteen days" account: 3933
  ⟨2⟩ Writing in 1933, [shutes p54] says 15 day illness, but no source given. *For ram-*   3934
  ifications, see ¶3938.

  ⟨2⟩ Writing in 1955, [shutesM] reports that Nicolay and Hay (? [nicolayB]) misread   3935
  Lincoln's letter, changing 52 days to 15 days.

- Other diagnostic considerations: 3936
  ⟨2⟩ Cholera had been in the area [durham].   3937
  ⟨S⟩ Without supporting arguments, two physicians in the 1930s cited diphtheria   3938
  as the cause of death [shutes p54] [evans pp139-140]. This diagnosis was made when
  it was thought Eddie had been ill for 15 days (see ¶3933). It has been coun-
  tered that Edward was ill for 52 days and that diphtheria's course is, classically, shorter [randallA p28] [durham] [baker p125] [templeC]. Even after the correction
  to 52 days, [shutesM] believed diphtheria was possibly the cause of death.

  ⟨2⟩ diphtheria [turner pp xvi, 40] [lincloreIGI]   3939

Eyes

▣ The daguerreotype of Eddie (¶3915) shows his left eye turned inwardly and the   3940
left eye socket seated higher than the right.

Feet

⟨1⟩ "Eddy's dear little feet" – Mary [randallC p97] *Probably not a true size indication.*   3941

General

⟨s⟩ Was likely breast fed, given that Mary breast fed a neighbor baby. (See ¶4647.)   3942

⟨1⟩ May 1848: "Our little Eddie has recovered from his spell of sickness" –Mary [angle p148]   3943

⟨1⟩ 1848: "After Congress adjourned in Sept. of that year Mr. L. accompanied by my two little boys and myself, visited B[oston] & remained there 3 weeks, detained by the illness of our youngest son, whom we lost a year afterwards." – Mary Lincoln, writing on Dec. 16, 1867 [turner p463]   3944

    ⟨-⟩ *Saying "the illness" instead of "an illness" lends an impression that the Boston illness and Edward's final illness were the same. This, however, may be reading too much into what could be simply an idiosyncrasy of expression. Nevertheless, others have drawn conclusions from the coupling of this illness with the final illness, as noted below.*   3945

    ⟨2⟩_c "There is some evidence that Eddie had been chronically ill all his life; certainly there was a long sickness in 1848." [baker p125] *Baker cites no evidence for chronicity beyond the 1848 illness. Also see ¶3955*   3946

    ⟨2⟩ Was "always a feeble child." [donaldA p153] *The source Donald cites for this statement (and another) does not state that Eddie was always a feeble child. I suspect Donald is echoing and extending Baker, whom he read* [donaldA p622n153].   3947

    ⟨2⟩_c [turner p453n] notes that, in another part of this letter, Mary has remembered Boston events incorrectly.   3948

Hair

⟨2⟩ "his hair fell over his brow in silken waves" [kunhardtB p134]   3949

Head & Face

⟨▢⟩ The daguerreotype of Eddie (¶3915) shows: (a) the right side of the head tilted downwards, (b) the left eye socket seated higher than the right, (c) the left ear sits higher than the right, and (d) unusual lips (see ⟨Mouth⟩).   3950

Heart & Circulation

⟨1⟩ The *Illinois Daily Journal* of Feb. 7, 1850 contained an unsigned 24-line poem mourning the death of a boy named Eddie. The poem included the lines: "And the crimson tinge from cheek and lip / With the heart's warm life has flown." [prattA]   3951

    ⟨-⟩ *This could be a reference to vasodilation or be poetic license.*   3952

    ⟨s⟩ The general consensus is that Mary wrote the poem, if for no other reason than Lincoln spelled his son's name "Eddy." [baker p126]   3953

Infection

⟨1⟩_q Herndon thought the Lincoln sons might have had congenital syphilis. See ¶2023. *Why would he think this? It suggests the boys had something "not right" that casual observation disclosed.*   3954

⟨2⟩ Fall 1847: Lincoln leaves Springfield to assume office as a Congressman in Washington: "he took with him his twenty-eight-year-old wife, their four-year-old-son   3955

Infection (continued)

Robert, and Eddie, their one-and-a-half-year-old son, who already showed signs of the tuberculosis that killed him in less than three years." [baker p136]

⟨-⟩ *It seems unlikely that Baker has hard evidence for this statement about* ⟨3956⟩ *Edward. More likely, she is extrapolating from her assertion that he was chronically ill (see ¶3944). The sentence about Edward is but one of several in a paragraph. The only source cited for the paragraph is an August 15, 1847 letter from David Davis that talks about Mary's social hopes in Washington. The full text of the letter is unavailable to me. However, because the paragraph excerpts this letter, and because other sources have not mentioned this letter in connection with Edward, I do not believe the un-excerpted portions discuss Edward.*

⟨2⟩ Lincoln's term in Congress began in March 1847. It was common for families ⟨3957⟩ to stay behind when the husband/father went to Congress. [rossA p136]

Infection – Exposures

⟨2⟩ May 1848: Brought home a stray kitten while visiting his mother's family in Lex- ⟨3958⟩ ington, KY. Mary's step-mother quickly ejected the animal. [burl p294] [angle p148]

Lungs

⟨1⟩ May 1848: He could scream "long and loud" [angle p148] (see ¶3965) *This says* ⟨3959⟩ *something about lung function.*

Mental Status

⟨1⟩ May 1848: Lincoln was in Congress while Mary and the children were in Kentucky. ⟨3960⟩ Mary closes a letter to Lincoln with: "Do not fear the children have forgotten you. I was only jesting. Even E's eyes brighten at the mention of your name." *what does "Even" say about Edward's usual attitude?*

Mouth

⌐○⌐ The daguerreotype of Eddie (¶3915) shows asymmetric lips and a thick lower lip. ⟨3961⟩ The copy available to me is too unfocused to show bumps in the lips.

Nervous System

⟨2⟩ "It is known he was of superior intelligence." [durham] ⟨3962⟩

⟨-⟩ *The basis for this statement is unknown. Durham may have read too much* ⟨3963⟩ *into a mother's effusive letter about her son.*

Travel & Dwellings

⟨2⟩ 1847-1849: To Washington, Lexington, New England, Niagara Falls, and Chicago ⟨3964⟩ with his mother, connected with Lincoln's term as a Congressman. [randallC pp92-96, 112-113]. (See ¶4709 and ¶4710.)

Voice

⟨1⟩ May 1848: His grandmother ejected his new pet kitten from the house, leaving ⟨3965⟩ "Ed screaming and protesting loudly against the proceeding. She [grandmother] never appeared to mind his screams, which were long and loud, I assure you." – Mary [angle p148]

Lincoln, Mary Todd

wife

Mary

Chronology

Mo.	Yr	Age	Home	Event	Ref.	3966
Dec.	1818	0	Lexington, KY	born	[evans p65]	
July	1825	6	"	Mother dies	[evans p65]	
fall	1826	7	"	Father remarries	[evans pp67&77]	
summer	1837	18	(Springfield, IL)	3 month visit with sister	[helmA] [randallC p23]	
	1839	20	Springfield, IL	lives with sister	[evans pp86&113]	
Nov.	1842	23	"	marries	[evans p79]	
Oct.	1847	28	(Lexington, KY)	3 week visit en route to DC	[turner p35]	
Nov.	1847	28	Washington, DC	Lincoln in Congress		
April±	1848	29	Lexington, KY	stays while Lincoln in Congress	¶4709	
fall	1848	29	(eastern USA)	travels	¶4710ff	
March	1849	30	Springfield	re-settles before Lincoln	[randallC p113]	
Feb.	1850	31	"	son Eddie dies		
summer	1851	32	(Lexington, KY)	visit	[helmB p102]	
Jan.	1861	42	(New York City)	shopping trip	[turner p69]	
Mar.	1861	42	Washington	First Lady		
May	1861	42	(Phila./Bost./NYC)	travel	[turner p87]	
Feb.	1862	43	Washington	son Willie dies		
April	1865	46	"	husband murdered		
May	1865	46	Chicago	lives there	[evans p193]	
Oct.	1868	49	Germany	"	[turner p489]	
Sep.	1870	51	England	"	[turner p573]	
April	1871	52	Sails for New York		[rossA p300]	
May	1871	52	Chicago	lives there		
July	1871	52	"	son Tad dies		
May	1875	56	Batavia, IL	institutionalized	[evans p224]	
Sep.	1875	56	Springfield	released from institution	[evans p225]	
Oct.	1876	57	Pau, France	lives there (with some travel)	[evans p227]	
Oct.	1880	61	Springfield	"	[evans p227]	
late	1881	62	New York City	winters there, into early 1882		
March	1882	63	Springfield	dies		

∎ Special Topic §9 lists additional travels and events, beginning in 1865. See also `Travel & Dwellings`. 3967

⟨1⟩ The 1850 U.S. census lists Mary's age as 28; she was 31. The 1860 census lists her age as 35; she was 41. Census-takers obtained ages by personal interview. [templeC] 3968

Chronology (continued)

See ¶5

⟨S⟩ [templeC] believes Mary lied about her age – apparently a Todd habit: see [helmB] note.   3969

⟨-⟩ Other instances of Mary altering her age: ¶3971, ¶4657   3970

- When did Mary first meet Lincoln?   3971

  ⟨2⟩ [randallC p23] says 1839, while [evans p338] says 1840.   3972

  ⟨1⟩ "He was 14 years and 10 months older than myself, & was from my eigh-   3973
  teenth year – Always – lover – husband – father & all all to me." – Mary Lincoln, 1869 [turner p534] *This would suggest they met in 1837, during Mary's
  visit to Springfield, but Mary's age-lowering propensities (¶3968) make
  this less than a straightforward conclusion. Lincoln was almost 10 years
  older than her.*

  ⟨1⟩ "soon after her arrival [in Springfield] in 1839" – Mary's nephew, Albert Ed-   3974
  wards, recalling in 1897 or later [stevens p113]

Introduction & Sources

Because Mary Todd Lincoln was not related by blood to Abraham Lincoln, she may   3975
seem biologically irrelevant to his medical history. This is false for two reasons.

First, she and Lincoln had contributed equally to their sons' genes. Thus, any use of   3976
the sons' conditions to illuminate Lincoln's conditions must be performed in light of
Mary's conditions. This is notably true in interpreting Tad's learning difficulties (see
Tad -Reading & Learning) and his inter-ocular spacing (¶5337).

Second, the medical history of a patient's spouse is pertinent because of potential di-   3977
rect influence on the patient, e.g. transmitting infection, involvement in domestic violence, affecting moods, etc.

That said, Mary presents her own diagnostic conundrum. Reduced to the starkest   3978
choices, either she was mentally healthy but with an extraordinarily unpleasant personality, or her behavior stemmed from a chronic neuropsychiatric disorder. Some
would strongly argue there is a third choice – that history's unflattering portrait of Mary
Lincoln is unfair and inaccurate. For this reason Mary is a highly controversial figure.
In keeping with the approach physicians take to the medical history, all *potentially* relevant data are herein recorded, and their interpretation deferred until an appropriate
time. Some preliminary comments about her mental problems begin in ¶4314.

As careful readers will immediately see, her history is not as well organized as the oth-   3979
ers in this book. In part, this is due to (a) the volume of the medical complaints she expressed during her life, (b) the variety of her medical complaints, which do not neatly
segregate into organ systems and organ functions, and (c) the simple fact that Mary's
ailments, although pertinent to diagnosing Lincoln, are not central to diagnosing him.

Readers with a deep interest in Mary's medical history should study Special Topic §9,   3980
which extracts – but does not organize – the medically-related comments from letters
she wrote during widowhood.

⟨2⟩ Over 600 of Mary's letters still exist [turner p xxi]. Mary and Robert "destroyed the   3981
letters she received with such efficiency that less than fifty addressed to her are
still in existence" [turner p xxiii]). The surviving correspondence between Mary and
her husband, whom she accused as "not *given* to letter writing," is sparse [burl

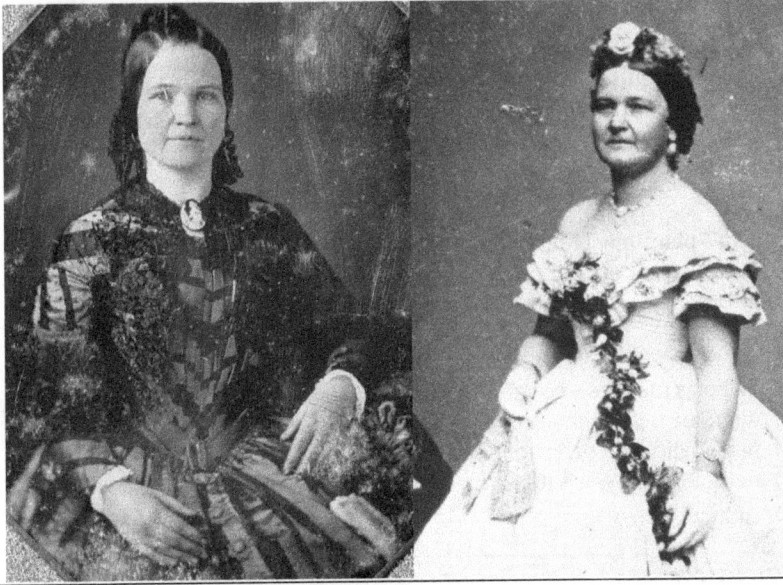

Figure 6. Mary Todd Lincoln. The Library of Congress attributes the left photograph to 1846 or 1847, and the right to 1860-1865. Figure 7 discusses her eyebrows and eye separation. Mary resembled her sister Ann in personality as well as facially (¶5880, ¶5893). Both photographs courtesy of the Library of Congress (LC-USZ6-2094, LC-USZ62-4681, respectively).

Mary

Introduction & Sources (continued)

p359]. All letters available as of 1972, along with their sources [turner pp xxii-xxiii], are included in [turner].

⟨1⟩ Twenty-five previously unknown letters, written by Mary in 1872-1878, were found in summer 2005 [emersonA]. They were published in a 2007 book [emersonB] I have not yet reviewed.   3982

⟨2⟩ The oldest letter in Mary's hand is from 1840. Only two others exist from before her marriage. The chief source of information about Mary's childhood is a letter written by Elizabeth Humphreys Norris 70 years after she shared a room with Mary in the 1820s [turner p5]. Excerpts from the letter appear in [turner pp5ff], [helmA], and [helmB]. According to [turner p7], information about Mary's teenage years comes from [helmB] and [townsend].   3983

⟨2⟩ Using information from William Herndon requires care. "She hates me," wrote Herndon in 1866 [hertz p40]. Mary's apologists think "Herndon hated Mrs. Lincoln" [randallC p363], but in my opinion Herndon's letters show great sympathy for Mary.   3984

⟨□⟩ [ostendorfM] reviews the photographs of Mary known through 1968. Figure 6 shows the oldest, made about 1846 [kunhardtA p66]. A daguerreotype, taken about 1839, was the basis for a portrait [helmB] [evans p275] [kunhardtA p62]. In her later years a photograph, at least partially fabricated, shows the spirit of her husband with his hands on her shoulder [kunhardtA p397].   3985

⟨2⟩c "There has never been a good clinical study of Mary Lincoln and the etiology of her illness. [evans] is disorganized and thin." [turner p xv]   3986

Family History

- Consanguinity: 3987
  ⟨2⟩ Mary's parents "were cousins" [turner p3] 3988
  ⟨2⟩ "Her father and mother ... were cousins." [randallC p16] 3989
  ⟨-⟩ *If true, this is fascinating. Mary and her sister Ann, the two most difficult* 3990
  personalities among the siblings, strongly resembled each other (¶5880).
  In fact, some photographs give them a syndromic appearance.

⟨2⟩_c Based on a painting of Mary's father, [randallC p73] sees a family resemblance. 3991

Diagnoses

- Diagnoses: 3992
  ⟨S⟩ diabetes mellitus – see ⟦Endocrine⟧ 3993
  ⟨S⟩ migraine headache – see ⟦Head & Face⟧ 3994
  ⟨S⟩ personality and behavior – see ¶4535ff 3995
  ⟨S⟩ neurological – see ¶4616 3996
  ⟨1⟩ cataracts – see ⟦Eyes⟧ 3997

Appearance

⟨1/q⟩ As a child: "She had clear, blue eyes, long lashes, light brown hair with a glint of 3998
bronze, and a lovely complexion. Her figure was beautiful, and no old master ever
modeled a more perfect arm and hand." [evans p276] quoting [helmB p52] quoting Mrs.
Norris. Also [angle pp122-123]

⟨1⟩ As a "young lady:" "Her features were not regularly beautiful, but she was cer- 3999
tainly very pretty, with her lovely complexion, soft brown hair, and clear blue eyes,
and intelligent bright face that, having once seen, you would not easily forget."
[helmA]

⟨2⟩ As a young woman: "... although not strictly beautiful, was more than pretty. She 4000
had a broad, white forehead, eyebrows sharply but delicately marked, a straight
nose, short upper lip, and an expressive mouth curling into an adorable, slow-
coming smile that brought dimples into her cheeks and glinted long-lashed, blue
eyes. ... Spirited carriage of her head. ... Plump round figure ... intelligent bright
face ... lovely complexion ... soft brown hair." [evans p276] quoting [helmB p52] and
perhaps Emilie Todd Helm

⟨1⟩ "I think that Miss Todd was a very shrewd girl, somewhat attractive." – William 4001
Herndon [hertz p137] (∈ ¶4368)

⟨1⟩ "Mrs Lincoln at the time of her marriage was a bright, lively, plump little woman – 4002
a good talker ... Fifteen & twenty years after marriage she became fleshy & stout in
personal appearance – The last year of her life she was in poor health & lost flesh
– when I last looked upon her upturned face when she was laid out in her coffin
I thought she looked (save the difference of years) much as she did when I knew
her so well in her girlhood days." – William Jayne [wilson pp624-625]

⟨○⟩ Figure 6 shows photographic portraits taken of Mary in the 1840s and the 1860s. 4003

⟨1/q⟩ According to Herndon (who did not like Mary), she was "the exact reverse" of Lin- 4004
coln in "figure and physical proportions, in education, bearing, temperament,
history – in everything." [burl p269] *They were similarly ambitious, however.*

266

Appearance (continued)

⟨1/q⟩ About 1856: "... soft brown hair ... clear blue eyes ... a plump, rounded figure and was rather short in stature" – H.B. Rankin [evans p277]   4005

⟨1⟩ Feb. 1861: "She is a plump, amiable, modest pleasant, round faced, agreeable woman with no silly airs."– George C. Shepard, 1861, typed transcript in [randallP box 15]. Original in Burton Historical Collection, Detroit Public Library   4006

Mary

⟨1/q⟩ 1861: "Fair, of about medium height" – her future daughter-in-law's father [evans p279] citing [helmB p167]   4007

⟨2⟩ "Miss Helm, writing of the same period, said she was still strikingly youthful and attractive in appearance. She was 'fair and forty,' but not fat, as she weighed only a hundred and thirty pounds. 'Her hair, a lovely chestnut, with glints of bronze, had as yet not a gray thread. Her beautiful shoulders and arms gleamed like pearls. She held her head high, slightly tilted back, possibly because she had so tall a husband to look up to. ... More than merely pretty, she was both brilliant and fascinating.' Miss Helm's is much the most flattering description of her aunt's appearance in 1861 to 1865 that has come from any source." [evans p279] citing [helmB p175]   4008

⟨1⟩ Jan. 1865: "We all thought Mrs. Lincoln looked handsome. To my mind she was a pretty woman, small and plump, with a round, baby face and bright black eyes." [crookA p6] [crookK]   4009

Arms

⟨2/c⟩ "Her arms were also good. The Springfield *Journal* said [metaphorically] that she was a woman of great strength. ... There are pictures of her, however, which show arms that might have had strong muscles." [evans pp283-284]   4010

   ⟨2⟩ "lovely arms" [kunhardtB p135]   4011

⟨2⟩ Age 40±: "'Her beautiful shoulders and arms gleamed like pearls'" [evans p279] citing [helmB p175] (∈ ¶4008)   4012

Build

⟨1/q⟩ Spring 1840: "my blooming partner" (later allusions make it clear she is gaining weight) – James Conkling [randallC p3]   4013

   ⟨1/q⟩ Another friend Dr. Elias Merryman (¶3183), jests about her weight in a poem [randallC p4].   4014

⟨1⟩ Dec. 1840: "I am still the same ruddy *pineknot*, only not quite as great an exuberance of flesh, as it was once my lot to contend with, although quite a sufficiency" [turner p22]   4015

⟨1⟩ As a "young lady:" "She had a plump, round figure, and was rather short in stature." [helmA]   4016

⟨1⟩ About 1842: "plump little woman" – William Jayne [wilson pp624-625] (∈ ¶4002)   4017

⟨1⟩ April 1848: Mary is free of [?spring] headaches for the first time in years, and Lincoln ponders her good health: "I am afraid you will get so well and fat and young as to be wanting to marry again." [angle p147] *Lincoln liked plump women ¶2688, so perhaps her weight was down at this time.*   4018

⟨1/q⟩ About 1856: "plump, rounded figure and was rather short in stature" – H.B. Rankin [evans p277] (∈ ¶4005)   4019

Build (continued)

⟨1⟩ About 1857-1862: "Fifteen & twenty years after marriage she became fleshy & stout in personal appearance" – William Jayne [wilson pp624-625] (∈ ¶4002)   4020

⟨2⟩ About 1858: "'fair and forty,' but not fat, as she weighed only a hundred and thirty pounds." [evans p279] (∈ ¶4008)   4021

⟨1⟩ May 1860: "a little short woman" – Lincoln [lamonL p452] (reprinted: [angle p278])   4022

⟨1/q⟩ 1861: "inclined to stoutness" [keckleyB pp82]   4023

⟨1/q⟩ August 1863: "fleshy" – a newspaper correspondent [randallC p292]   4024

■ Secondary descriptions: 4025
  ⟨2⟩ "short and plump" [randallA p6]   4026
  ⟨2⟩ "She had a rounded figure, buxom and ideally suited to the fashions of the day." [turner p7]   4027

⟨2c⟩ "In what was written of Miss Todd in her young womanhood, we find no reference to shortness or plumpness. ... The descriptions of her written after 1850 all include some reference to shortness and plumpness. This impression, which most people had of her, was partly due to contrast with her long, lean husband and partly to the styles. In 1860 dresses made the wearers appear latitudinous. But a part of Mrs. Lincoln's apparent dumpiness was due to the individual and not to the height of her husband nor to her clothes. She was stout, and her features carried a definite impression of fatness." [evans pp277-278]   4028

⟨2⟩ "No weight over a hundred and thirty [pounds] is recorded, but she must have weighed more than that part of the time. The impression she gave was that of an underheight, overweight woman – at least, after 1855 and until about 1876." [evans p284]   4029

⟨1⟩ Jan. 1865: "small and plump" [crookA p6] (∈ ¶4009)   4030

⟨2⟩ May 11, 1871: "is as stout as ever" [ChicagoTribune - May 16, 1871] (∈ ¶4169)   4031

⟨2⟩ Height: 4032
  ⟨2⟩ "I have found no very definite statement as to Mrs. Lincoln's height. We read that she was not short as compared with other women. She stood erect. Her posture was good." [evans p284]   4033
  ⟨2⟩ After quoting a doubtful story in which Lincoln, beside Mary, announces "Ladies and Gentlemen, here is the long and short of the Presidency," William Barton explains: "The long was six feet four. The short, five feet nothing." [evans p278] citing "Mr. and Mrs. Lincoln" by William E. Barton in *Woman's Home Companion*, February 1930. *It is unclear from Evans' excerpt if Barton is quoting an actual height for Mary or is using "nothing" to emphasize the difference in height.*   4034
  ⟨1/q⟩ Sept. 4, 1870: "about 5 feet 3 inches" – Benjamin Moran [randallC p379]:   4035
  ⟨2⟩ "a mere five feet four" [kunhardtA p96]   4036
  ⟨○⟩ [ostendorfA p96] juxtaposes "accurately scaled and matching portraits" of Lincoln and Mary to show how they looked side by side. "The contrast is obvious and amusing." *Scaling the pictures is problematic given the uncertainty in Mary's height. Furthermore, in the dress she is wearing it is impossible to accurately judge where her feet are.*   4037

⟨2⟩ "Some time after 1876 Mrs. Lincoln lost flesh. Her relatives in Springfield describe her as being thin as well as short. They give her weight in that period as a hundred and ten pounds or even less." [evans p279]   4038

Build (continued)

⟨2⟩ Evans refers to two descriptions from B.F. Stoneberger: (1) a frail, small woman who would go into a dry-goods store, purchase some dress-goods by the yard, throw her purchases across her arm, and go away [evans p230], and (2) small and thin, almost wizened [evans p279]. Stoneberger's father rented the Lincoln house; the family lived there for "several years" [evans p155].   4039

⬚ "... there is no photograph of Mrs. Lincoln taken after her weight had fallen to a hundred and ten pounds." [evans p283]   4040

Mary

⬚ The "last known" photograph of Mary, taken in the "late 1870's" [turner p165 opposite] shows a very round-faced Mary. The photograph was made by a "spirit photographer" [kunhardtA p397]. *Although clearly altered by the spirit photographer, it is unlikely he would have substantially changed Mary's appearance.*   4041

⟨2⟩ August 1878: Weighed 110 lb after a bout of boils the previous month [evans p227]. See ¶4176 and ¶4670.   4042

⟨1/q⟩ October 1879: "I enclose a card of my exact weight nearly a month ago – since then, as a matter of course many pounds of flesh have departed ... I am now, just the weight I was, when we went to Wash[ington] in 1861– Therefore I may conclude, my great bloat has left me & I have returned to my natural size." [turner p690]   4043

⟨1/q⟩ January 16, 1880: "I have now run down to 100- pounds, EXACTLY." [turner p693]   4044

⟨1/q⟩ When she returned from Europe in 1880 she was "little and thin, wrinkled and gray, and she looked like an old woman" [evans p279] – it is unclear whom he is quoting.   4045

⟨1⟩ "The last year of her life she was in poor health & lost flesh" – William Jayne [wilson pp624-625] (∈ ¶4002)   4046

Chest & Shoulders

■ Chest clothing: 4047
  ⟨1⟩ "She had a beautiful neck and arm, and low dresses were becoming to her." [keckleyB p101]   4048
  ⟨1⟩ Lincoln, at least once, admonished her about the low cut of a dress [keckleyB p101]   4049
  ⟨1/q⟩ "Her only ambition seems to be to exhibit her own milking apparatus to the public gaze" – an Orgeon Senator [burl p298]   4050

■ Secondary: 4051
  ⟨2⟩ "She had a rounded figure, buxom and ideally suited to the fashions of the day." [turner p7]   4052
  ⟨2⟩ "She had great pride in her elegant neck and bust" [burl p298]   4053
  ⟨2⟩ "exquisite bosom" [kunhardtB p135]   4054

Death & Final Illness

⟨2⟩ "She died at the age of sixty-four in her sister's home, where she had spent her last three months in seclusion, sleeping on one side of the bed only, reserving the other space for the President." [turner p xix] *She was 63.*   4055

⟨1⟩ Mary Edwards Brown, then 16, helped care for her great-aunt Mary in winter 1882. Over 70 years later she recalled: 4056

Death & Final Illness (continued)

⟨1⟩ "Every day she [Mary] got up and went through those trunks for hours.   4057
Grandmother said it was funny, if Aunt Mary was so sick, that she was able
to be up all day bending over her trunks." [kunhardtA pp396-397]

⟨1⟩ Mary had "terrible headaches" and was "puffed up," forcing her to remove   4058
her wedding ring. She thought she had a disease "where her blood was turning to water, and when too much water hit her heart she would die." [kunhardtA
p397] *Of note, Tad died with fluid in his chest.*

⟨1⟩ "She took a lot of bottles of 'restorative,' it was called, and it had paregoric   4059
in it, same as opium," but was non-prescription. – Mary Edwards Brown
[kunhardtA p397]

⟨1⟩ "Mrs. Abraham Lincoln breathed her last at the residence of the Hon. Ninian Ed-   4060
wards, her brother-in-law, this evening at 8:15 o'clock. Since Mrs. Lincoln's return
from New York City last March she has confined herself closely to her room, and
has received very little company excepting relatives and very intimate friends. It
has been her habit to take little or no exercise, though she was not confined to her
bed, and for several weeks of late she has been greatly troubled by boils, which
made their appearance on every part of her body, due to her peculiar disease and
sedentary habits. Mrs. Lincoln's health was considered as improved when she last
returned to this city, but has gradually failed of late, and a trip to the seashore had
been planned, in the hope of regaining some of her former vitality. The fulfillment
of this plan was prevented by a rapid wasting away of her vital energy, resulting in
death. Yesterday she was able to move about her room with assistance until afternoon, when her strength failed her completely, and it became apparent that she
was in a dangerous condition. Up to this time Mrs. Lincoln strenuously objected
to the attendance of a physician, but with her consent the family practitioner was
called, and remained in attendance until this morning. During part of Saturday
evening she was so far conscious as to recognize the fact that she was nearing her
end, and remarked that she was dying. Her mind was not then entirely clear, and
she expressed no care for the future, nor did she have any message to leave behind. Later she lost control of her vocal organs, and answered questions by the
opening and closing of her eyes, which was the only sign she was able to make.
About 1 o'clock this morning she passed into stupor, which lasted until her death.
Her end was peaceful and serene. No symptoms of pain marred her visage, nor
was she in a condition to suffer. At 8 o'clock this morning the attending physician
announced there was no hope, and her bedside was attended during the day by
loving relatives, who but awaited the end. Slowly and by degrees she passed away,
breath coming only at intervals, and the pulse stopped while one of the watchers
held a watch to note its beating." [ChicagoTribune - July 17, 1882, page 2 col. 4]

⟨-⟩ *The reference to skin lesions in the same sentence as "sedentary habits"*   4061
raises the possibility of decubitus ulcers. True boils remain more likely,
however.

⟨1/q⟩ "Within the past few days Mrs. Lincoln has been suffering from an attack of boils   4062
which caused her great pain and, no doubt, greatly increased her nervousness.
On Friday, last, she was up and walked across the room. Again, on Saturday, she
walked across the room with a little assistance; but grew worse later in the day
and about nine o'clock in the evening experienced a paralysis which seemed to
involve her whole system, so that she was unable to articulate, to move any part
of her body, or to take food. She soon afterward passed into a comatose state and
so continued, breathing stertorously up to 8.15 p.m., Sunday, when she died." –
Illinois State Journal, Monday, July 17, 1882 [evans pp343-344]

Death & Final Illness (continued)

⟨1/q⟩ The death certificate, prepared by Dr. T.W. Dresser, lists "paralysis" as cause of death [evans p344]   4063

⟨1⟩ "In the late years of her life certain mental peculiarities were developed which finally culminated in a slight apoplexy, producing paralysis, of which she died." – Dr. Dresser [wilson p671] (Also reprinted by [herndon p351])   4064

Mary

⟨2⟩ [evans p344] thinks Dresser was equating apoplexy and paralysis.   4065

⟨c⟩ *Dr. Dresser's statement clearly links a chronic process with her acute demise. He does not say what the chronic process was. In 1882 a list of specific disorders that produce chronic "mental peculiarities" and lead to a "slight apoplexy" plus paralysis would have been short. I can think only of epilepsy and syphilis. Vascular conditions such as atherosclerosis (stroke) would be on a modern list, but this was all but unknown in 1882. There is no record that Mary ever had a seizure, an event that is usually appreciated even by laypersons. One is, therefore, left with the possibilities that Dr. Dresser was (a) mistaken, (b) dissembling, (c) referring to a syndrome unknown to me, or (d) speaking, very subtly, of syphilis.*   4066

⟨S⟩ "There is considerable suspicion of diabetic coma, in some degree, during the last week of her life." [evans p344] See ¶4083   4067

⟨1⟩ "Her end was peaceful and serene, in marked contrast to her life" [ChicagoTribune - July 17, 1882]   4068

⟨2⟩ Autopsy: 4069
  ⟨2⟩ There was no autopsy [evans p344].   4070
  ⟨2⟩ The story that an autopsy showed "cerebral deterioration" seems to have occurred by mistake. [hirschhorn] writes: "despite diligent searches ... we have been unable to find any evidence for an autopsy."   4071
  ⟨1⟩ "Years ago a doctor friend in Chicago told me that an autopsy had been performed on Mrs. Lincoln (but only on the head, an odd procedure even then) and that the brain was found to have physically deteriorated, ruling out mere neurosis, the usual explanation for her behavior. I didn't write about this [in the novel *Lincoln*] and have never followed it up." [vidalA p692]   4072
  ⟨1⟩ "The autopsy on Mary Todd showed a physical deterioration of the brain consistent with paresis." [vidalA p667]   4073
  ⟨◎⟩ A lock of Mary's hair, snipped "right after she died," was in the collection of Dorothy Kunhardt [kunhardtA p xi].   4074

Diet & Digestion

⟨2⟩ March 1861: "Every member of the household became ill from eating too well of the unaccustomed Potomac shad." [shutes p77] (See ¶640.)   4075

⟨1/q⟩ August 1881: "her disease is of such a nature that requires her to consume a great deal of food" [hirschhorn] quoting [NYTimes - Aug. 4, 1881].   4076

⟨1⟩ 1882: She kept a commode beside her bed – Mary Edwards Brown [kunhardtC]   4077

Ears

⟨2⟩ Late 1880 or after: hearing problems [baker p365] (∈ ¶4181)   4078

Endocrine

⟨S⟩ "In her youth, Mrs. Lincoln was sometimes overactive. This might have been the   4079
result of hyperthyroidism. In her later life – before the loss of weight which occurred as her final years approached – she appeared short and fat. ... Some of
Mrs. Lincoln's pictures – those taken toward the evening of her life – are indicative
of myxoedema." [evans pp340-341] *In his next paragraph,* [evans p341] *may shrink
from this conclusion – the wording is ambiguous.*

- For a discussion on the "Queen Anne" eyebrow sign of hypothyroidism, see   4080
  ¶4114.

⟨2⟩ 1880 on: "She was likely to be dressed in black, and sometimes overdressed." [evans   4081
p229] See ¶4513
  ⟨-⟩ *The meaning of "overdressed" is not quite clear. One interpretation is*   4082
  that she wore more clothes than temperatures demanded – a possible sign
  of cold intolerance.

- Evidence suggesting Mary had diabetes mellitus (also see §2i):   4083
  ⟨$\frac{1}{q}$⟩ May 1875: "She had been very thirsty" recently – Dr. Willis Danforth [evans   4084
  p25] (See ¶4489.)
  ⟨2⟩ Circa 1876-1880: Drank Vichy water, which "enjoyed some reputation in   4085
  connection with this disorder" [evans p342]. (∈ ¶4302) *Recently discovered
  letters from Mary (¶3982) suggest that she may have taken the waters at
  Vichy for boils and/or pain – see ¶4671.*
  ⟨2⟩ Circa 1876-1880: "continual running waters, so disagreeable and inconve-   4086
  nient" [evans p342] (See ¶4302.)
  ⟨2⟩ Boils in July 1878 and early summer 1882 [evans pp227, 228, 342] (See ¶4670 and   4087
  ¶4672.)
  ⟨2⟩ August 1878: "Though hitherto a fat woman," she now weighed 110 pounds   4088
  [evans p342] (See ¶4176.)
  ⟨$\frac{1}{q}$⟩ August 1881: "her disease is of such a nature that requires her to consume a   4089
  great deal of food" [hirschhorn] (See ¶4076.)
  ⟨$\frac{1}{q}$⟩ January 1882: "chronic disease of the kidneys" [hirschhorn]. (See ¶4304.) (∈   4090
  ¶4183)
  ⟨$\frac{1}{q}$⟩ Fall 1881: she "underwent treatment for a disease of the eyes and for dia-   4091
  betes" [ChicagoTribune - July 17, 1882, p2, col4]
  ⟨S⟩ [evans p345] concludes that Mary "probably did have" diabetes, "perhaps after   4092
  1875."
  ⟨S⟩ [baker p365] says Mary "possibly" had diabetes while living with sister Elizabeth   4093
  after October 1880.
  ⟨S⟩ [hirschhorn] calls diabetes a "diagnosis we can be sure of."   4094
⟨S⟩ Diabetes onset: A photograph from the "late 1870's" shows a very round-faced   4096
Mary (see ¶4041), not compatible with a large weight loss.

Energy

⟨$\frac{1}{q}$⟩ As a youth she "was a bundle of nervous activity, wilful [sic] and original in plan-   4097
ning mischief, and so the inevitable clashes with her very conventional young
stepmother." [burl p293] citing [helmB p17]

⟨1⟩ May 1848: Commenting about her inability to remember the day of the week   4098
(¶4587) "I feel wearied and tired enough to know this is Saturday night, our babies
are asleep..." [angle p147]

⟨1⟩ March 1870: Would take Tad on a trip "if I were not so fatigued. ... The doctor has   4099
just left me and says he wonders to find me sitting up." [helmB pp281-282]

Energy (continued)

⟨1⟩ Jan. 26, 1871: "I scarcely imagined when I began this letter that my strength would hold out for more than three pages." – Mary [helmB p290] 4100

⟨1⟩ October 1874: "Nervous exhaustion .. confined to her room for the past five months" [NYTimes - Oct. 18, 1874] (Part of ¶4606.) 4101

Mary

Eyes

- For eyebrows, see [Hair]. 4102

- Eye color: 4103
  ⟨2⟩ In childhood: "clear blue eyes, long lashes" [evans p276] (Part of ¶3998.) 4104
  ⟨1⟩ As a "young lady:" "clear blue eyes" [helmA] (∈ ¶3999) 4105
  ⟨2⟩ 1840: "long-lashed, blue eyes" [evans p276] (Part of ¶4000.) 4106
  ⟨1⟩ About 1855: "eyes gray-blue" – Isaac Arnold [evans p277] 4107
  ⟨1⟩ About 1856: " clear blue eyes" – H.B. Rankin [evans p277] (Part of ¶4005.) 4108
  ⟨2⟩ Agrees with: blue eyes [randallA p6] 4109
  ⟨1⟩ Jan. 1865: "bright black eyes" [crookA p6] (∈ ¶4009) 4110

- Eye separation: 4111
  ⟨2⟩c "The space between Mrs. Lincoln's eyes and between her eyebrows was broad." [evans p280] 4112
  ⊙ Figure 7 shows wide spacing between Mary's eyes. 4113

- Eyebrows: 4114
  ⟨2⟩ "eyebrows sharply but delicately marked" [evans p276] (∈ ¶4000) 4115
  ⊙ Figure 7 shows that the lateral half of Mary's right eyebrow is thin, if not absent. 4116
  ⟨S⟩ Based on eyebrow appearance, [evans p280] suspects that Mary wore make-up 4117
  ⟨-⟩ *Bilateral absence of the lateral third of the eyebrows is the Queen Anne sign of hypothyroidism* [aa100 pp124-125]. *It also occurs in Hansen disease and syphilis* [aa111 pp573, 574] *(§2a).* 4118

⟨2⟩c "In photographs taken in later years there is not the same domination of the whole by the expression of the eyes. [Part of this appearance] results from the pose, and a larger part from the relative size of the aperture of the lids. ... Mrs. Lincoln's later pictures do not indicate that her eyes were prominent. They appear to be somewhat small and inconspicuous features in a broad, fat face. Whatever the cause may have been, the effect was that her face lost one of its best features – the expression of her youthful eyes – as she acquired age." [evans pp280-281] 4119

⟨1⟩ July 1865: "I have almost become blind, with weeping, and can scarcely, see sufficiently to trace these lines" [turner p257] 4120
  ⟨2⟩ In addition to the 1882 ocular problems (see ¶4129), "Mary Lincoln added another reason for her poor eyesight: She had been blinded by tears, the physical stigmata of her sorrows. And she had been, at least to the extent that her weeping had caused the surface of her corneas to become swollen and edemous [sic]. Like rubbing a blister, blinking hurt. So she closed her eyes and sat in the dark..." [baker p365] 4121
  ⟨-⟩ *[baker]'s text is extremely difficult to parse. The qualifier, "to the extent," robs all belief from the statements that weeping caused Mary corneal problems and that blinking hurt. Examination of the cited sources (Congressional Record, 47th Congress, First Session and* [NYTimes - July 27, 1881]*) may be illuminating. Baker also cites 1986 personal communication from Johns Hopkins ophthalmology giant Edward Maumenee, but this is likely* 4122

Eyes (continued)

to have been interpretive assistance, rather than access to primary sources. From what I can tell, [baker] *cites no evidence to place this event in 1882. I believe she has applied Mary's 1865 statement to a later year.*

⟨2⟩ [turner pp266-267] observes that despite her eye problems, "she was after 1865 a more compulsive newspaper reader" than previously, despite the "microscopic print" they used.   4123

⟨1⟩ February 1866: "My eyes pain me so much, I can scarcely see." [turner p409]. More clinical detail: "Owing to an intense headache, I was unable to read you kind note of yesterday until this morning, and I avail myself, of a moment's respite of sitting up, to reply to it." *This was her first eye complaint since July 1865, among dozens of other complaints in the interval.*   4124

⟨1⟩ Jan. 9, 1868: I am visited with quite a serious eye affliction – within the last few days – very sore & inflamed eyes – so much so – that I am unable to write or read & consequently am compelled to relinquish correspondence with all my friends. The physician insists upon my not using my eyes in any way for some time to come – I am disobeying his orders for a moment... I fear you will be unable to read this, as I am almost unable to see." [turner p467] *Mary often disparaged her handwriting, even when seeing normally. Mary wrote 1867 on the letter;* [turner p467n] *explains assigning it to 1868.*   4125

⟨2⟩ 1880: "A cataract had formed on her right eye" [baker p363]   4126

⟨2⟩ Late 1880 or after: sight problems [baker p365] (∈ ¶4181)   4127

⟨$\frac{1}{q}$⟩ Fall 1881: she "underwent treatment for a disease of the eyes and for diabetes" [ChicagoTribune - July 17, 1882, p2, col4]   4128

- January 1, 1882 physician evaluation: 4129
  ⟨$\frac{1}{q}$⟩ "commencing cataract of both eyes ... Connected with [her] spinal disease and one of its evidences is the reflex paralysis of the iris of the eye, and the reduction of the sight to one-tenth natural standard, together with much narrowing of the field of vision. The sight will gradually grow worse." – Four physicians [hirschhorn] (∈ ¶4183)   4130

  ⟨S⟩ Comment on "the eye:" "We believe the singular noun is a transcription or typographical error as an ophthalmologist would certainly indicate which eye was affected if only one. The original letter, presumably hand-written, could not be found." [hirschhorn] *Or, "the eye" could refer to the ocular organ system, hence the singular word would refer to both eyes.*   4131

  ⟨S⟩ [baker p365] interprets the singular noun as indicating the involvement of one eye.   4132

  ⟨2⟩$_c$ [hirschhorn] equates "reflex paralysis of the iris" with an Argyll Robertson pupil. *Seems reasonable.*   4133

  ⟨2⟩ "Paralysis of light reflex in just one eye may rarely be found in tabes dorsalis." [hirschhorn] citing [aa66 p221]   4134

  ⟨-⟩ *It may also be useful to consider that Mary injured her head in a fall from her carriage in 1863, especially if only one pupil reacted abnormally. (See ¶4688.)*   4135

  ⟨S⟩ "Reflex paralysis of the iris is sometimes associated with syphilis and has been used incorrectly as circumstantial evidence of Lincoln's syphilis." [baker p411] *Who says it was incorrect? Baker does not substantiate her statement.*   4136

  ⟨2⟩$_c$ "In fact, she was nearly blind." [baker p365]   4137

Eyes (continued)

- Preference for darkness: 4138
  - ⟨1⟩ 1871±: After Tad's death, Mary "suffered from periods of mild insanity. She had many strange delusions at these times. She thought gas was an invention of the devil and would have nothing but candles in her room. At other times she insisted on the shades being drawn and the room kept perfectly dark." [foy] (More in ¶4487.) 4139
  - ⟨1⟩ 1881±: "Among the peculiarities alluded to, one of the most singular was the habit she had during the last year or so of her life of immersing herself in a perfectly dark room and, for light using a small candle light, even when the sun was shining bright out of doors. No urging would induce her to go out into the fresh air." – Dr. Dresser [wilson p671] [hirschhorn] 4140
  - ⟨S⟩ Regarding Mary's aversion to bright light: "The simplest explanation for Mary Lincoln's aversion is that she had a large Argyll Robertson pupil, unreactive to light, and thus could not tolerate any glare." [hirschhorn] *This "explanation" has several problems: (1) [hirschhorn] has gone beyond the data: an aversion to daylight has not been established. Mary preferred to be indoors and in the dark, but that does not mean she was intolerant of light. For example, she could have had phobias about leaving the house and about daylight. Her earlier preference for darkness seems to have been psychological. (2) A "large Argyll Robertson pupil" is problematic. Less than 2% of Argyll Robertson pupils have diameters over 5mm [aa66 p214]. (3) Even a large pupil does not require someone to immerse themselves in a "perfectly dark room." (4) If an eye complaint were the only reason to avoid the outdoors, she could have gone outdoors after dark.* 4141

⟨S⟩ On the basis of handwriting samples, [hirschhorn] concludes that "Failure of sight came only near the end of her life." See ¶4208. 4142

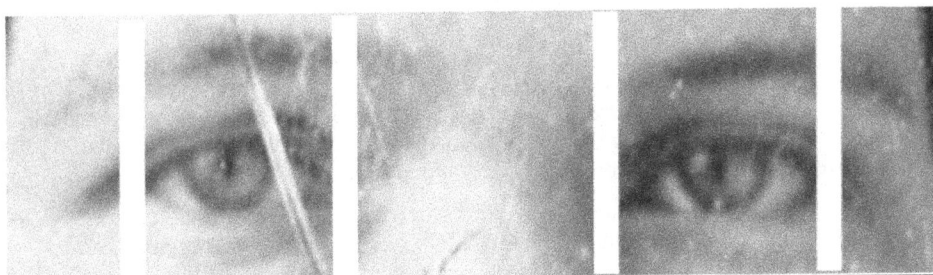

Figure 7. Mary's eyes. Detail from left panel of Figure 6, showing three notable findings: (1) The space between the eyes is greater than the width of the eyes. This satisfies the artist's rule for ocular hypertelorism [aa1 pp62-63]. See ¶4111. (2) The lateral half of her right eyebrow is thin, if not absent. See ¶4114 for potential medical explanations. (3) Both pupils are irregular.

Gait

Gait , Nervous System , and Trauma all contain information related to Mary's later-years back problems. 4143

Gait (continued)

⟨1⟩ June 1867: "The walks here are shady & very pleasant. Each morning I have walked two miles" – Mary [turner p426]   4144

⟨1⟩ Feb. 1869, in the south of France: "I never return from my walks without my hands being filled [with flowers]" [turner p502]   4145

⟨2⟩ 1875: "stiff in limb and gait" [baker p326] but see ¶4297 for doubts   4146

⟨1/q⟩ June 1880: "... in my great wish to leave this place, ... with almost a broken back, ... I sent for a bonne, ... took her arm and painfully wended my way to the "Hotel de la Paix" ... Alas, for my weakness, on attempting to descend, my left side gave way, she had to call the Concierge to lift me down, place me in a carriage." [hirschhorn] citing [turner p699]   4147

    ⟨2/c⟩ "Her letters in the spring and summer of 1880 to her grand-nephew indicate that it was probably not so much loss of power that affected her walking but considerable back pain." [hirschhorn] *This may be true, but note Mary's specific comment about weakness.*   4148

⟨2⟩ October 1880: Arriving from Europe in New York City, "a white-haired, frowning Mary Lincoln, [was] barely able to walk as she leaned on her grandnephew's arm" [baker p364]   4149

⟨1⟩ Nov. 1881: During the past two years "has scarcely been able to walk" [NYTimes - Nov. 23, 1881]   4150

- Jan. 1, 1882 physician evaluation: 4151

    ⟨1/q⟩ "... considerable loss of power of both lower extremities so as to lessen their use and to render walking without assistance very unsafe, and going unaided down stairs impossible. ... will end in paralysis of the lower extremities. ... She is now quite helpless, unable to walk with safety without the aid of an attendant...." [hirschhorn] Part of ¶4183   4152

    ⟨2⟩ "'unable to even go down stairs' although she could walk" [hirschhorn] quoting [NYTimes - July 22, 1881, p3]   4153

    ⟨1/q⟩ "Could not walk safely without the aid of a chair and even then she was liable to fall at times" [evans p343] Part of ¶4699   4154

    ⟨1⟩ Extrapolating from [osler pp843&917], [hirschhorn p524] says locomotor ataxia "would make walking downstairs especially troublesome." *So would the muscular weakness her physicians found* [hirschhorn p518].   4155

⟨1⟩ Winter 1882: "Every day she got up and went through [her] trunks for hours. Grandmother said it was funny, if Aunt Mary was so sick, that she was able to be up all day bending over her trunks." – Mary Edwards Brown, 1956 [kunhardtC] (Part of ¶4517.)   4156

⟨2⟩ February 1882: "Attendants carried her up and down the stairs on a litter." [baker p366]   4157

⟨S⟩ "Mary Lincoln very likely had ataxia with relative preservation of motor power. Locomotor ataxia is caused by degeneration of that portion of the spinal cord that controls sensation. Thus persons afflicted cannot feel where their feet are." [hirschhorn] *Mary's physician found that her lower limbs were weak* [hirschhorn p518]. *Locomotor ataxia is used as a synonym for tabes dorsalis.*   4158

⟨2⟩ "... was able to walk, albeit with assistance, even up to the day before her death" [ChicagoTribune - July 17, 1882]   4159

General

⟨2⟩ "There is no information about Mary Todd's health prior to the time she met Lincoln." [evans p337]   4160

⟨1⟩ Early in Presidency: "instituted the daily drive" and insisted Lincoln accompany her. [grimsley]. See ¶1134 *This was then considered a form of exercise.*   4161

⟨2⟩ "Mary's letters from 1850 until her death ... are filled with allusions to her poor health. She seems not to have been ill, or ever to have had any definite disease" [evans p339]. *Several letters mention chills and fever – see ¶4276.*   4162

   ⟨2⟩ Letters she wrote from 1861-1865 prominently referred to poor health. Poor health was "almost a major" theme from 1865-1875. [evans p339]   4163

   ⟨$\frac{1}{q}$⟩ Example: "In my feeble health I am endeavoring to catch every mountain breeze in hopes that strength may be given me for the sea voyage before me. In my hours of great bodily suffering which now occur quite frequently ... I am suffering so much. I am scarcely able to sit up." – July 18, 1868 [evans p210]   4164

⟨$\frac{1}{q}$⟩ 1857: "I am recovering from the slight fatigue of" a very large party she threw [randallC p140]   4165

⟨1⟩ Sept. 22, 1863: "Have a very bad cold" – Mary [turner p158]   4166

⟨2⟩ April 11, 1864: Mary is ill, so Lincoln cancels plans for Mary and himself to visit Ft. Monroe [randallC p304]   4167

⟨1⟩ June 29, 1870: "Your letter in the early spring found me quite an invalid and I have just returned from a long visit to the Marienbad baths and waters in Bohemia and I find my health greatly benefitted." – Mary [helmB p284]   4168

■ May 11, 1871, upon arriving in New York from Europe: 4169
   ⟨1⟩ "Mrs. Lincoln was dressed in deep mourning. She has enjoyed exceedingly good health during her sojourn in Europe, and is as stout as ever, but looks very pale, and complains of a very severe headache..." [ChicagoTribune - May 16, 1871]   4170

   ⟨1⟩ "Mrs. Lincoln is looking very well." [NYTimes - May 11, 1871] (Part of ¶4479)   4171

⟨2⟩ At some point Robert hired people to "gather information about her and her growing drug use – chloral hydrate, laudanum, and opium were now taken to excess." [kunhardtA p396]   4172

■ 1875: Florida trip (also see ¶4494ff):   4173
   ⟨2⟩ January 1875: Was sick in bed for three weeks in St. Augustine, FL, requiring the services of a nurse. [evans p339]   4174

   ⟨$\frac{1}{q}$⟩ March 1875: "She had the appearance of good health, and did not seem fatigued by the trip." – Robert describing his mother's return to Chicago [evans p216]   4175

⟨2⟩ 1878 : Living in Pau, France, she was "suffering great pain from boils" in July. By August "her weight was down to" 110 lb. She rarely traveled beyond Pau, and "considered herself in feeble health." [evans p227]   4176

⟨2⟩ October 1880: After living in Europe for several years, "Mary Lincoln had to come home. Her health had deteriorated until she could no longer live alone." [baker p363]   4177

   ⟨$\frac{1}{q}$⟩ Mary had written Lewis Baker to meet her in New York, saying: "I cannot trust myself any longer away from you all. I am too ill and feeble in health." [baker p364]   4178

General (continued)

⟨2⟩ [baker pp363-364] mentions weight loss (¶4044), arthritis (¶4297), a right eye   4180
cataract (¶4126), and the effects of a fall (¶4699) as Mary's chief problems.

⟨2⟩ Late 1880 or after: Mary and her sister Elizabeth (¶5872) "both were near invalids,   4181
with hearing, sight, and heart problems, and possibly, in Mary Lincoln's case, diabetes" [baker p365]

⟨$\frac{1}{q}$⟩ January 1, 1882 physician evaluation: "We find that Mrs. Lincoln is suffering from   4183
chronic inflammation of the spinal cord, chronic disease of the kidneys, and commencing cataract of both eyes. The disorder of the spinal cord is the consequence
of an injury received some time since and has resulted in considerable loss of
power of both lower extremities so as to lessen their use and to render walking
without assistance very unsafe, and going unaided down stairs impossible. The
nature of the spinal trouble is progressive and will end in paralysis of the lower extremities. Connected with the spinal disease and one of its evidences is the reflex
paralysis of the iris of the eye, and the reduction of the sight to one-tenth natural
standard, together with much narrowing of the field of vision. The sight will gradually grow worse. There is no probability that there will be any improvement in
Mrs. Lincoln's condition, considering her age and the nature of her disease. She
is now quite helpless, unable to walk with safety without the aid of an attendant,
or indeed to help herself to any extent. She requires the continued services of a
competent nurse, and also constant medical attention. We are, very respectfully,
your obedient servants, ..." [hirschhorn]

    ⟨$\frac{1}{q}$⟩ The letter is signed by Drs Sayre, Clymer, Knapp, and Pancoast (see ¶4630)   4184
    ⟨2⟩ [baker p368] provides a different quotation excerpt: "'Mrs. Lincoln,' the doc-   4185
tors had written, 'is suffering from chronic inflammation of the spinal cord,
chronic diseases of the kidney, commencing cataract, disorder of the spinal
cord and reflex paralysis of the iris.'" *I suspect Baker has edited the original text, which is quoted in full by* [hirschhorn]. *In Baker's version, twice-
mentioning the spinal affliction is odd, and the difference between having "chronic disease of the kidneys" and "chronic diseases of the kidney"
would be significant.*

    ⟨-⟩ See ¶4129 ff for comments about the eye findings.   4186

Habits – Alcohol

⟨1⟩ Records of the Lincoln household's purchases at the Corneau & Diller drug store   4187
show that "a remarkable amount of spirits was flowing into the household," but
the reason is unknown. "Mrs. Lincoln is the prime suspect" because Lincoln was
out of town on several occasions when the purchases were made. [turnerL]

⟨2⟩ "The members of the Lincoln household were abstemious in the purchase and   4188
use of liquors. .. Neither wife nor husband was ever a drinker." [evans pp341-342]

    ⟨2⟩ Recall, however, that Mary wanted to serve liquor in their home after Abra-   4189
ham was nominated for President. See ¶1365

Hair

■ For eyebrows, see ⟨Eyes⟩.   4190

⟨2⟩ "rich light-chestnut hair" [randallA p6]   4191

⟨1⟩ As a young woman: "soft brown hair" [helmA] (∈ ¶3999, ¶4000)   4192

⟨$\frac{1}{q}$⟩ About 1856: "soft brown hair" [evans p277] See ¶4005   4193

Hair (continued)

⟨2⟩ Age 40±: "'Her hair, a lovely chestnut, with glints of bronze, had as yet not a gray thread'" [evans p279] citing [helmB p175] (∈ ¶4008)　4194

⟨1⟩ January 1868, fear of a certain humiliation "has almost whitened every hair of my head." [turner p469] *From this, we can conclude she still had non-gray hair, unsurprising as that may be.*　4195　Mary

⟨2⟩ October 1880: "white-haired" [baker p364]　4196

Hands

⟨2⟩c "Her hands were small and shapely." [evans p284]　4197

⟨2⟩ "Hands that moved in quick, graceful gestures when she spoke." [turner p7]　4198

⟨1⟩q March 1, 1861: A man recalls shaking hands with Mary: "She had no gloves on & put out her hand. It is not soft." [randallC p84]　4199

⟨1⟩ November 1865, reviewing a photograph: "my hands are always *made* in *them*, very large" [turner p285]　4200

Handwriting

[turner p xxiv] indirectly states that Mary's handwriting changed significantly over time. "The size and state of the handwriting" in Mary's letters were used as a clue to dating those that lacked a written date.　4201

For descriptions of her punctuation usage, see ¶4580.　4202

⟨2⟩ Mary's "penmanship was exquisite and legible even in later years when her sight began to fail" [turner p xxiii]　4203

⟨2⟩ 1840: "She wrote in small, clear, slanted script" [turner p13].　4204

▣ 1856: hand-written letter is shown in [helmB]　4205

⟨2⟩ 1857: "The approximate date of this letter is based on the particularly small, precise script characteristic of Mrs. Lincoln's letters in the 1850s." [turner p51n]　4206

⟨1⟩ 1862 penmanship: "The handwriting is clear and rather bold for a woman, and the spelling and punctuation are faultless" [ChicagoTribune - Jan. 15, 1882]. (See [turner p127].) (See ¶4580.)　4207

▣ 1880 and 1882: hand-written letters shown in [hirschhorn]　4208
　　⟨S⟩ [hirschhorn] describes the handwriting as becoming "quite large" and takes this as evidence of deteriorating vision.　4209
　　⟨-⟩ *Without knowing the size of the paper on which the handwriting appears, it is not possible to say confidently that the handwriting is large. Even if macrographia were present, it is not pathognomonic for poor vision, as there are other influences on the motor system. This is all the more relevant because* [hirschhorn] *claims Mary had locomotor ataxia (see ¶4158).*　4210
　　⟨2⟩c "Her handwriting also does not reveal the tremors of [general paresis of the insane]" [hirschhorn]　4211

Head & Face

This section records the pathology and appearance of Mary's head. Although photographs exist of Mary, word portraits remain helpful because: (1) not all periods of her life are covered by photographs, (2) words can help focus our attention, and (3) word portraits can generalize over time, whereas a photograph captures an instant. 4212

As we have seen with Lincoln, even something as subjective as attractiveness can pertain to medical assessments. That said, [evans]'s thorough analysis of Mary's cranial features is uncomfortably fixated on her attractiveness. 4213

- Also see ⌐Headaches⌐. For eyebrows, see ⌐Hair⌐. 4214

- 1863: Struck her head on a stone when she fell from her carriage, resulting in injuy. See ¶4688 4215

- For a discussion of the separation between Mary's eyes, see ¶4111. 4216

- Attractiveness: 4217
    ⟨1⟩ As a "young lady:" "Her features were not regularly beautiful, but she was certainly very pretty." [helmA] (Part of ¶3999.) 4218
    ⟨2⟩ As a young woman: "although not strictly beautiful, was more than pretty" [evans p276] (∈ ¶4000) 4219
    ⟨1⟩/g "young, dashing, handsome" – Herndon [donaldA p84] 4220
    ⟨2⟩ "One writer described Mrs. Lincoln when she entered Washington life as 'ugly.'" [evans p278] 4221
    ⟨2⟩ "I have been able to find only one report which spoke of Mrs. Lincoln in this period as being pretty, or even handsome. Most of the reports describe her clothes, her manners, or the way she carried herself – anything but her looks." [evans p278] 4222
    ⟨2⟩ Age 40±: "still strikingly youthful and attractive in appearance ... 'More than merely pretty, she was both brilliant and fascinating.' Miss Helm's is much the most flattering description of her aunt's appearance in 1861 to 1865 that has come from any source." [evans p279] citing [helmB p175] (∈ ¶4008) 4223
    ⟨1⟩/g "She was a pleasant looking woman" – W.O. Stoddard [evans p279] 4224
    ⟨1⟩ Jan. 1865: "We all thought Mrs. Lincoln looked handsome. To my mind she was a pretty woman" [crookA p6] (∈ ¶4009) 4225
    ⟨1⟩/g "Nearly beautiful" [evans p279] citing [bayne] 4226
    ⟨2⟩/c "In no account of Miss Todd's appearance do we find her described simply as 'beautiful.'" [evans p277] 4227

⟨2⟩ "Her head was large and broad. ... Her method of combing her hair – parted in the middle... – accentuated the height and size of the brow and the size of the face. The dark color of the hair threw her prominent white forehead into further contrast." [evans p280] 4228
    ⟨2⟩ As a young woman: "a broad, white forehead" [evans p276] (∈ ¶4000) 4229

⟨2⟩ "There are none of those prominences of the face which, when present, indicate enlarged sinuses" [evans p280]. The lower forehead and cheek-bones can, according to [evans p281] carry such indications. 4230
    ⟨-⟩ *I am skeptical of this theory, unless he is talking about some kind of inflammatory response to sinus infection.* 4231

⟨2⟩/c "Her cheek-bones were not high." [evans p281] 4232

⟨2⟩ As a young woman: "intelligent bright face" [helmA] (∈ ¶3999, ¶4000) 4233

Head & Face (continued)

⟨1⟩ Jan. 1865: "a round, baby face" [crookA p6] (∈ ¶4009)   4234

⟨2⟩ₒ "But if the mid section of the face, especially its bony framework, did not cause   4235
the mid face to push as far forward as the forehead and chin, it was broad enough
– in fact, too broad. Most of the suggestion of the breadth of the face, however,
is found only in the later pictures, and resulted from the fattening process." [evans
p281]

Mary

■ Nose: 4236

 ⟨2⟩ₒ "Mrs. Lincoln's nose was her poorest feature. A glance at her profile and   4237
near-profile pictures gives an impression of pug-nose. A closer look shows
that the pug-nose effect was due to poor development of the bony part of
the nose in the eye-and-bridge region rather than to an upturning of the tip.
The lower part of the nose is better developed. When her features began
to be changed by the deposition, this lower segment of the nose received
more than its quota, and no other change did more to rob her of her good
looks. She ultimately became fat-nosed." [evans p281] *Depression of the nasal
bridge's root is a sign of congenital syphilis* [aa111 pp1134-1137]. *To my eye,
the base of Mary's nose does not look syphilitic.*

 ⟨2⟩ "her nose was a little too short" [evans pp281-282] (∈ ¶4562)   4238
 ⟨2⟩ As a young woman: "a straight nose" [evans p276] (∈ ¶4000)   4239

⟨2⟩ₒ "If the face above the tip of the nose be covered by the hand, the part remaining   4240
in view appears to be rather overdeveloped. Much of that appearance was due to
fat." [evans p282]

⟨1⟩ "when I last looked upon her upturned face when she was laid out in her coffin   4241
I thought she looked (save the difference of years) much as she did when I knew
her so well in her girlhood days." – William Jayne [wilson pp624-625] (∈ ¶4002)

Headaches

⟨1⟩_q 1840 on: headaches [hirschhorn] citing [turner pp36, 176, 408-409]   4242
 ⟨S⟩ [hirschhorn] thinks them "typical migraine headaches."   4243
 ⟨2⟩ "violent headaches" [kunhardtA p96]   4244
 ⟨S⟩ "'neurasthenia' and migraine' " [turner p xvi]   4245
 ⟨2⟩ "subject to migraine headaches" [randallC p67]   4246
 ⟨2⟩ "prostrating, nauseating headaches (like those now caled migraine)" [randallC   4247
 p106]

⟨1⟩ April 16, 1848: Lincoln wrote Mary: "And are you entirely free from head-ache?   4248
That is good – good – considering it is the first spring you have been free from it
since we were acquainted." [donaldH p64]

 ⟨2⟩ Agrees with: [donaldA p108], but he calls the headaches "excruciating" without   4249
 citing a source.

 ⟨S⟩ [donaldA p108] wonders if an allergy was the cause. *This is a reasonable suppo-*   4250
 sition for headaches following a seasonal pattern. However, one wonders
 how common allergies were in the mid 19th century, even among privi-
 leged families like the Todds, given the "hygiene hypothesis" of immune
 system modulation.

 ⟨-⟩ For opinions on when Mary met Lincoln, see ¶3971.   4251

⟨2⟩ Headaches continued after 1848: "From that time forward, the records that re-   4252
fer to the more intimate details of Mrs. Lincoln's affairs contain references to repeated headaches. This continues to be true until 1867" [evans p338]. *Before ac-*

Headaches (continued)

cepting that the headaches stopped in 1867, one must ask whether Mary's letters stopped instead, leaving no record of her ails.

⟨¼⟩ Dec. 4, 1863: Mary telegraphs Lincoln from New York state: "Reached here last evening. Very tired and severe headache." [baslerA v7p34] citing [helmB p234] *This may have been part of a larger illness – see Special Topic §5.* 4253

⟨1⟩ May 1864: "I was quite unable during several hours yesterday to leave my bed, owing to an intensively severe headache & although it has left me, yet I am feeling so weak this morning that I fear, that I shall be prevented from visiting the Hospitals today. ... I believe, you are likewise, a sufferer, from these bilious attacks & know how much inclined to *nausea* they leave you" [turner p176] 4254

   ⟨S⟩ [randallC p304] is ready to call these migraine headaches. 4255

⟨¼⟩ April 14, 1865: "a bad headache," with which she tried to convince Lincoln not to go to Ford's Theatre [luthin pp629-630] (See ¶1317.) 4256

⟨1⟩ May 11, 1871: During newspaper interview Mary "complains of a very severe headache." Mary herself says "I feel very ill with a sick headache." Later, she "said that she was feeling entirely too ill to talk any more, and begged to be excused." [ChicagoTribune - May 16, 1871] (See ¶4169.) 4257

Heart & Circulation

⟨1⟩ July 1840: "I felt exhausted after such *desperate exertions* to keep pace with the music" at a dance – Mary [turner p15] 4258

⟨¼⟩ 1840: "faint wild rose in her cheeks" [angle p123] quoting, probably, Emilie Todd Helm 4259

⟨1⟩ Dec. 1840: "I am still the same ruddy *pineknot*" [turner p22] (Part of ¶4015) 4260

⟨1⟩ 1861±: While discussing mail she received: "She was blushing an angry crimson." [stoddardD p243] 4261

⟨2⟩ Late 1880 or after: heart problems [baker p365] (∈ ¶4181) 4262

⟨2⟩ "Color rose easily to her face." [randallA p7] 4263

⟨2⟩ 1863: When a Senator suggested Robert enter the Army, "Mary's face turned white as death." [randallC p299] 4264

⟨2⟩ 1864: When rebel forces attacked the outskirts of Washington, Lincoln and Mary witnessed the fighting from Ft. Stevens. A surgeon next to Lincoln was shot. "According to one account, Mary Lincoln collapsed" after mistaking the surgeon for her husband. [beschlossB p105] 4265

⟨1⟩ June 1867: "The walks here are shady & very pleasant. Each morning I have walked two miles" – Mary [turner p426] 4266

⟨1⟩ Sept. 1868: "I went to dinner & after seating myself at a table near the door, I found my head becoming dizzy & every thing appeared black before me – I endured the feeling as long as I well could, and whilst attempting to rise, found myself sinking to the floor – a very distingue looking gentleman – gave me his arm – and led me to my room door" [turner pp485-486] 4267

⟨1⟩ Dec. 1869: Expecting upsetting news, "My face begins in advance to *burn* – but may perhaps grow *ghastly* pale" when the news arrives [turner p529] 4268

⟨1⟩ Oct. 4, 1871: "I am suffering greatly with violent palpitation of the heart ... I am ordered perfect quiet" [turner p596] *This was three months after Tad's death.* 4269

⟨2⟩ Died after a stroke-like syndrome at age 64 [evans p344]. See ¶4062. 4270

Infection

⟨$\frac{1}{q}$⟩ Fall 1863: Mary's [possible] involvement with Lincoln's November smallpox infec- 4271
tion:

    ⟨$\frac{1}{q}$⟩ Sept. 22, 1863: "Have a very bad cold, and am anxious to return home" – 4272
Mary wires to Lincoln [randallC p294].

    ⟨2⟩ "A Boston paper on November 14 spoke of Mrs. Lincoln as having been suf- 4273
fering from chills." [lincloreLHH]

⟨2⟩ May have been immunized against smallpox. (See ¶5401.) 4274

⟨-⟩ See ¶2030 and Special Topic §5. 4275

⟨1⟩ In several of her letters she complains of chills and fever. [evans p339] 4276

    ⟨-⟩ *This apparently applies to the 1865-1875 time frame. See ¶4162* 4277

    ⟨1⟩ Example: "I am having chills, every other day" – Nov. 10, 1867 [evans p197] 4278

    ⟨-⟩ *It should be remembered that fever was often a terrifying prospect in the* 4279
pre-antibiotic era, akin to the dread evoked by "cancer" today.

⟨1⟩ Oct. 12, 1869: "The first finger of my right hand is painfully sore, enveloped in 4280
cloths – all arising from the smallest prick of a needle. *It (the finger) has been*
to consult with a physician and the salve administered by him, I trust will prove
efficaceous [sic] – It is very much inflamed & I scarcely closed my eyes during the
night. Last week, sick most of the time & this week unable to use my hand ... I had
gone out on yesterday, about my painful finger"

⟨$\frac{1}{q}$⟩ "fever and nervous derangement of the head" for several weeks in 1873 [evans p215] 4281
See ¶4489

⟨2⟩ Boils in July 1878 (see ¶4176), summer 1882 (see ¶4672) [evans pp227&228] 4282

Infection – Exposures

Mary must certainly have been exposed to some of the same environmental factors 4283
listed for Lincoln in ¶2040 ff.

⟨2⟩ About 1840: "Parties with entire families attending were so large they were some- 4284
times referred to as 'squeezes.'" [randallC p7]

⟨$\frac{2}{c}$⟩ "She was immune to scarlet fever, diphtheria, typhoid, and smallpox when these 4285
diseases invaded her own household." [evans p337] *Evans is talking about Mary*
escaping the illnesses of Willie, Eddie, Willie+Tad, and Lincoln, respectively.
Eddie probably did not have diphtheria [¶3938].

    ⟨S⟩ It has been suggested, only half-jokingly, that Mary's formal dresses, with 4286
their 3-foot radius, helped keep people at a distance from her, and so reduced her exposure to infectious disease. *This is not at all far-fetched.*
Militaries have found that bacterial meningitis, for example, will sweep
through barracks that have beds placed less than 22 inches apart, but will
occur only sporadically when beds are spaced wider than this.

⟨1⟩ In 1859 Mary's letters mention a friend, Sarah McClernand (wife of the general in 4287
Figure 5), with a [chronic] cough and poor health, who died around June 1861
[turner pp57, 59, 61, 90]. *Knowing nothing else, the odds favor a diagnosis of tuber-*
culosis.

⟨1⟩ June 1860: Mary's 10-year-old nephew dies of typhoid fever. "I trust never to wit- 4288
ness *such suffering* ever again. [turner p64]

Mary

Infection – Exposures (continued)

⟨2⟩ March 1861: Was gifted "fine horses" [burl p292]   4289

⟨S⟩ As First Lady, "her hoop skirts made it impossible for anyone to approach closer   4290
than three feet' [donaldH p45]. *This may have reduced her exposure to infectious
agents transmitted by respiratory or tactile means.*

⟨1⟩ Dec. 1868, in Germany: "I pined for a glass of American ice water ... [it] here is   4291
impossible & really dangerous to drink" – Mary [turner p495]

- Related to sexually transmitted disease (also see §2h):   4292
  ⟨H⟩ There was gossip saying Mary was unfaithful [burl pp291-292] *Malicious gos-*   4293
  sip directed at White House occupants should be expected, regardless of
  underlying truth.
  ⟨S⟩ A theory, not widely accepted in Lincoln circles, says Abraham had syphilis   4294
  (see ¶2016). [hirschhorn] discusses whether Mary would have been exposed
  during Lincoln's putative contagious period(s).
  ⟨1⟩ "Lincoln was a man of terribly strong passions, but was true as steel to his   4295
  wife during his whole marriage life" – Herndon [hertz pp259-260] (full quote in
  §2b)
  ⟨1⟩ "She is no prostitute – a good woman, She dared me once or twice to Kiss   4296
  her, as I thought – refused then – wouldn't now." – James Gourley [wilson p453]
  Was there more? See ¶4679.

Joints

⟨2⟩ 1875: "stiff in limb and gait from arthritis and gout" [baker p326] *Baker provides no*   4297
references. Neither gout nor arthritis are mentioned in her book's index.
⟨2⟩ [hirschhornB] says there is no evidence Mary had gout.   4298

Kidneys & Urological System

Polyuria is a cardinal manifestation of a condition Mary reputedly had: diabetes mel-   4299
litus (see ¶4083). However, the evidence that Mary had polyuria (below) could also be
interpreted as indicating a disturbance of bladder control, and is a consideration in the
diagnosis of tabes dorsalis.

[aa111 p982] summarizes bladder involvement in tabes dorsalis: "Disturbances of blad-   4300
der control [are] among the first warnings of tabetic neurosyphilis. ... The onset of the
bladder symptoms may be so insidious that the patient is entirely unaware of the gradually developing atony of the bladder musculature from paralysis due to the impairment of its innervation. ... The first warning of trouble comes when the patient wets
the bed at night from overflow. ... 'Hard to start' is the phrase most patients use to
express the difficulty of relaxing the sphincter and emptying the bladder by its own
contractility in the earlier irritative phase. 'Dribbling' after a supposed complete evacuation indicates either sphincter atony or a retention of urine in an atonic distended
bladder."

⟨2⟩ Summer 1872: "she visited Wisconsin seeking help for increased physical discom-   4301
fort ... It was said that a dropsical condition had developed. She later referred to
trouble from bloating." [randallC p383]

⟨2⟩ Circa 1876-1880: "she drank Vichy water and that has enjoyed some reputation   4302
in connection with this disorder [diabetes mellitus]. She drank these waters, but
they did her no good. 'However, I was not very much in need of them save for
the continual running waters, so disagreeable and inconvenient,' she is quoted as

Kidneys & Urological System (continued)

saying." [evans p342] *Mary's comment is compatible with polyuria and/or incontinence.*

⟨$\frac{1}{q}$⟩ "Her fingers swelled up so she had to take off her wedding ring." – Mary Edwards Brown [hirschhorn] 4303

Mary

⟨$\frac{1}{q}$⟩ January 1, 1882 physician evaluation: "chronic disease of the kidneys" [hirschhorn] Part of ¶4183, which includes variant quotations. 4304

⟨1⟩ 1882: She kept a commode beside her bed – Mary Edwards Brown [kunhardtC] 4305

Lungs

⟨2⟩ 1843±: "At bedtime, when he [Lincoln] would go downstairs to fill a pitcher of water, he would often 'sit down on the steps of the porch and tell stories to whoever happened to be near.' His wife would cough to signal that she wanted him; sometimes he 'kept her coughing until midnight or after.' " [burl p332] 4306

⟨1⟩ Dec. 1868, from Frankfurt: "The weather here is so mild here, at present, that my fire has died out" – Mary [turner p495] *This is a reminder that people in the 19th century would have had very great exposures to burning wood.* 4307

⟨2⟩ 1869: Persistent cough and a self-description of having "weak lungs" [evans p339] 4308

⟨$\frac{1}{q}$⟩ Sept. 10, 1870, from Leamington, England: "I am coughing so badly I can scarcely write. ... This is the first day I have sat up. ... My physician says I must go to a drier climate. ... My health is again beginning to fail me as it did last winter." [helmB p287] and slightly differently in [evans p340] 4309

    ⟨1⟩ Jan. 13, 1871, from London: "... coughing most disagreeably and a bundle of wrappings. My servant woman has proved herself within the past week a good nurse." [helmB p289] (and [evans p340]) 4310

    ⟨2⟩ [evans p211] assigns the cough to a time period of "winter of 1870-1." In March 1871, she and Tad started for home. 4311

    ⟨S⟩ [evans p340] wonders if Tad's final illness was related to Mary's cough. See ¶5320. 4312

Mental Status

Much ink has chronicled the moods of Mary Lincoln, and this long section adds to the total. Originally, I did not want to devote much attention to either Mary or her mental problems, but it became necessary because of the hypothesis that syphilis caused her erratic behavior. 4313

Having devoted the attention, I will offer a few partially-reasoned opinions. 4314

First, related to her psychiatric symptoms: (a) I do not believe that many of her post-White House physical ailments (see Special Topic §9) were real or, if real, were as severe as she painted them. Her litany of complaints is most consistent with somatization (¶4530). (b) After Lincoln died, she clearly experienced both delusions and hallucinations. These seem to have peaked about the time of her 1875 institutionalization. Her most consistent delusions related to money. (c) She made at least one serious effort to kill herself (¶4523ff). (d) Aside from her delusions, her mind remained predominantly clear. In particular, there was no "conduct slump" as classically seen in neurosyphilis [aa111 p990]. (e) Special Topic §2i has my questions about the diagnosis of non-syphilitic tabes dorsalis applied by others ([hirschhorn]). (f) After her husband and each of her three 4315

Mental Status (continued)

sons died, Mary's grief was both deep and prolonged. Her duration of grief seems abnormally long. She was rarely, if ever, happy in the 17 years she lived after Lincoln died.

The disorder which best fits these symptoms is depression, with intermittent psychotic features. Had an organic illness, such as neurosyphilis, been responsible for Mary's behavior, it would be expected to continually worsen. Instead, Mary's worst post-White House year was 1875, and she lived until 1882.   4316

I found these descriptions of depression helpful: 4317

⟨1⟩ "Depression [is] diagnosed ... when sadness ... is overly intense and contin-   4318
ues beyond the expected impact of a stressful life event. Indeed, the morbid mood might arise without apparent or significant life stress. The pathological process in mood disorders is thus partly defined by the ease with which an intense emotional state is released and, especially, by its tendency to persist autonomously even when the offending stressor is no longer operative. Rather than being endogenous (i.e., occurring in the absence of precipitants), mood disorders are best conceptualized as endoreactive (i.e., once released, they tend to persist autonomously)." [aa7 pp1613-1614]

⟨1⟩ In depression, "Faulty thinking patterns are clinically expressed as (1) ideas   4319
of deprivation and loss; (2) low self-esteem and self-confidence; (3) self-reproach and pathological guilt; (4) helplessness, hopelessness, and pessimism; and (5) recurrent thoughts of death and suicide. The essential characteristic of depressive thinking is that the patient views everything in an extremely negative light." [aa7 pp1616-1617]

In reading Mary's post-White House letters, it seemed as if every adverse event would affect her for long periods of time. Her thinking during those years displays most, but not all of the characteristics noted above. ○○○ *Project:* Tabulating the duration of Mary's negative reactions to adverse events might strengthen the diagnosis of depression.   4320

Depression is probably not a complete diagnosis for Mary Lincoln. There was something unusual about her personality from the beginning. Whether it meets the diagnostic criteria for a recognized illness is not clear to me. Bipolar illness is a reasonable consideration, but also may be an incomplete diagnosis.   4321

⟨-⟩ [burl p297] has suggested she was bipolar (¶4544). A longtime friend's quote is   4322
strikingly suggestive (¶4539), as is her buying sprees (¶4456ff).

⟨2⟩ "mental instability was evident in several other members of her family" [donaldA   4323
p158]. See Miscellaneous Todds -- Mary's Full Siblings

⟨2⟩ "Her motions and gestures were quick as opposed to her husband's deliberate-   4325
ness; she was an excitable and enthusiastic little woman." [randallA p7]

⟨$\frac{1}{q}$⟩ In childhood "was very high strung, nervous, impulsive, excitable, having an emo-   4326
tional temperament like an April day, sunning all over with laughter one moment, the next crying as though her heart would break" – childhood friend Margaret Stuart [burl p297]

⟨1⟩ About age 10: "I never saw any display of temper or heard her reprimanded during   4327
the months [I lived with Mary]." However, after being reprimanded for making (and wearing) skirt hoops, "Mary burst into tears, and gave the first indication of temper I had ever known her to make." – Elizabeth Norris [helmA]

Mental Status (continued)

⟨1⟩ About age 10: "She liked pretty things, and wanted to be in the fashion." – Eliza-   4328
beth Norris [helmA]

⟨2⟩ As a young socialite, Miss Todd was "never distinguished by a sense of humor."   4329
[donaldA p160]

    ⟨2⟩ Agrees with: "She had plenty of wit, but she was without humor. She could   4330
make others laugh, and was very fond of doing so, but she was not a good
laugher." [evans p292]

        ⟨$\frac{1}{q}$⟩ "Mary could make a bishop forget his prayers." – her brother-in-law [turner   4331
p11] citing [helmB p81]

⟨2⟩ "Somewhere along the way she acquired a few worldly tendencies which defied   4333
inhibition, among them a need for amusement and a passion for pretty clothes,"
the latter dating even from the 1820s [turner p5]

    ⟨1⟩ July 1840: "a life on the river to me has always had a charm, so much ex-   4334
citement, and this *you* have have deemed necessary to my well-being: every
day experience impresses me more fully with the belief" – Mary, writing to a
friend [turner p15]

⟨$\frac{1}{q}$⟩ Adolescence: "... now and then indulged in sarcastic, witty remarks that cut. But   4335
there was no malice in it. She was impulsive & made no attempt to conceal her
feelings, indeed it would have been an impossibility had she desired to do so, for
her face was an index to every passing emotion." – Elizabeth "Lizzie" Humphreys
Norris [turner p 6]

⟨1⟩ June 1841: "my evil genius Procrastination" – Mary [turner p25]   4336

⟨1⟩ As a "young lady:" "She was singularly sensitive. She was also impulsive, and   4337
made no attempt to conceal her feelings; indeed it would have been an impossibility had she desired to do so, for her face was an index to every passing emotion.
Without desiring to wound, she occasionally indulged in sarcastic, witty remarks,
that cut like a damascus blade; but there was no malice behind them. She was full
of humor, but never unrefined. Perfectly frank and extremely spirited, her candor
of speech and inependence of thought often gave offense where none was meant,
for a more affectionate heart never beat." [helmA]

⟨2⟩ "Highly emotional, she was terrified of lightning storms, of dogs, of robbers, and   4338
when she was in a panic she could not control her actions." [donaldA p108]

    ⟨1⟩ Agrees with: ¶4356   4339

    ⟨H⟩ It was also suggested that she was afraid of Indians [burl p311] *Does this relate*   4340
to her Indian delusions in ¶4489?

⟨2⟩ "Some believe that Mary Todd changed dramatically after her wedding" (1841)   4341
[burl p323].

    ⟨$\frac{1}{q}$⟩ Herndon said that before marriage she was "rather pleasant – polite – civil ...   4342
intelligent ... witty." After marriage, however, "she became soured – got gross
– became martial [many more aspersions] a she-wolf." [burl p323]

    ⟨2⟩ "After her marriage, she seemed to have a kind of tripwire surrounding her.   4343
c Easily triggered, it set off tantrums of sadness, fear, and anger veering toward
rage." [shenk p102]

    ⟨2⟩ "did not develop this emotional instability until after she was married" [ran-   4344
dallC p106]

⟨2⟩ 1841-1842: A bell on top of the building in which the Lincolns lived clanged when-   4345
ever a stage arrived. "The bell had bothered Mary Lincoln's nerves, and they
moved." [kunhardtB pp275, 282]

Mary

Mental Status (continued)

⟨2⟩ Early married life: "In making purchases for herself, her family, or her home, she   4346
indulged her expensive tastes whenever possible; in most other areas she showed
a talent for cutting corners that embarrassed even her thrifty husband." [turner p32]
Not at all, says [randallC pp82-83].

- Attachment to her children: 4347
    ⟨1⟩ Aug. 1859: "I am feeling quite lonely, as *Bob*, left for College in *Boston*, a few   4348
    days since, and it almost apears, as if light & mirth, had departed with him."
    [turner p58]
    ⟨1⟩ Oct. 1859: "I miss Bob, so much, that I do not feel settled down, as much as I   4349
    used to & find myself going on trips quite frequently." [turner p59]
    ⟨1⟩ June 1860: "Our oldest boy, has been absent, almost *a year*, *a long year*, & at   4350
    times I feel *wild* to see him, if I went any where, within the next few weeks, I
    should wish to visit him." [turner p64]
    ⟨2⟩ Circa 1860: A decade after the death of son Edward "Mary still broke down   4351
    when Eddy was mentioned." [kunhardtA p91]

⟨1⟩ 1848: Lincoln wrote Mary about an unexpected bill from P.H. Hood and Co. "I hes-   4352
itated to pay them, because my recollection is that your told me when you went
away, there was nothing left unpaid." [angle p150] *Was this an early indication of
her shopping difficulties?*

- 1840s or 1850s: 4353
    ⟨$\frac{1}{q}$⟩ Mary "... was a very nervous, hysterical woman who was incessantly alarm-   4354
    ing the neighborhood with her outcries. It was a common thing to see her
    standing out on their terrace in front of the house, waving her arms and
    screaming, 'Bobbie's Lost! Bobbie's Lost!' when perhaps he was just over at
    our house. This was an almost every day occurrence." – Elizabeth A. Capps
    (a Springfield neighbor) [burl p62] [kunhardtA p97] See also ¶4965 for a similar
    occurrence.
    ⟨$\frac{1}{q}$⟩ Mary screams "Bobbie will die!" after he ingests lime [burl p62]. (See ¶4965.)   4355
    ⟨1⟩ "Once I heard a scream of – Mr Webber – Mr Webber – it was the voice of   4356
    apparent distress – I looked back – saw Mrs Lincoln – 'She said – Keep this
    little dog from biting me'. The dog was a little thing & was doing nothing
    – too small and good natured to do anything." – John B. Weber [wilson p389]
    (Agrees with ¶4338)
    ⟨1⟩ "One day I heard the scream 'Murder'. 'Murder' – turned round – Saw Mrs   4357
    Lincoln up on the fence – hands up – Screaming – went to her – she said a
    big ferocious man had Entered her house – Saw an umbrella man come out –
    I suppose he had Entered to ask for old umbrellas to mend." – John B. Weber
    [wilson p389]
    ⟨1⟩ Elizabeth Capps tells the same umbrella-man story, differently [kunhardtA p97]   4358

- Tendency to strike people: 4359
    ⟨1⟩ About 1850: Mary and a servant girl: 'Mrs. Lincoln at last got on one of her   4360
    insane mad spells, insulted and actually slapt the girl" – James Matheny [wil-
    son p714]
    ⟨1⟩ About 1850: "Mrs. Lincoln got madder & madder – boiled over with her in-   4361
    sane rage and at last struck Tiger [Jacob Taggart] with the broom two or 3
    times." – James Matheny [wilson p714]. Also [wilson p667n]. Story's conclusion is
    in ¶4382.
    ⟨1⟩ In Springfield: Lincoln bled after mary struck him in the face for bringing   4362
    home an unsatisfactory piece of meat for company – see ¶3593

Mental Status (continued)

⟨1⟩ In Springfield: Struck Lincoln in the head with a piece of wood, cutting his nose – see ¶3589   4363

- Herndon's observations: 4364

  ⟨1⟩ "she was a tigress... This woman was once a brilliant one, but what a sad sight to see her in any year after 1862" [hertz p129]   4365

  ⟨1⟩ "the female wildcat of the age" [hertz p134]   4366

  ⟨1⟩ "a keen observer of human nature, an excellent judge of it, none better; she was a terrible woman, but I must give her credit for a keen insight into men and things. Had *hell* not gotten into her neck she would have led society anywhere; she was a highly cultured woman, witty, dashing, pleasant, and a lady, but hell got in her neck. ... I know that Mrs. Lincoln acted badly, but hold your opinion for awhile. I have always sympathized with Mrs. Lincoln. ... Mrs. Lincoln was not a she-wolf, wildcat, without a cause." [hertz p136]   4367

  ⟨1⟩ "When Mrs. Lincoln was a young and unmarried woman, she was rather pleasant, pollite, civil, rather graceful in her movements, intelligent, witty, and sometimes bitter too. ... I think that Miss Todd was a very shrewd girl, somewhat attractive. ... However, after she got married she became soured, got gross, became material, avaricious, insolent. ... But remember that in finite things, that every effect has its appropriate cause. Keep your judgment open for subsequent facts." [hertz p137]   4368

⟨2⟩ Temper: 4369

  ⟨2⟩ Mary's unpredictable outbursts toward her husband were usually short-lived, and left her feeling ashamed and ill [donaldA pp158-159].   4370

  ⟨1⟩q "a very violent temper, but she had more intellectual power than she has generally be [sic] given credit for" – John Stuart (her cousin) [nicolayO p15]   4371

  ⟨1⟩ "She had a very extreme temper and made things at home more or less disagreeable." – Milton Hay [wilson p729]   4372

  ⟨1⟩ "Mrs Lincoln often gave L Hell in general – Says the Baker girls have seen it & heard it and told him So. *Ferocity* – describes Mrs L's conduct to L." – Herndon interview of James Matheny [wilson p251]   4373

  ⟨1⟩q "an ungovernable temper, but after the outburst she was invariably regretful and penitent." – Harriet Hanks Chapman [randallC p82]   4374

  ⟨2⟩c "When questioned as to their impression of Mrs. Lincoln, a majority of people will mention first her high temper." [randallC p91]   4375

⟨1⟩ "high strung" – Harriet Chapman [wilson p646]   4376

  ⟨1⟩q "a high strung, nervous woman" (source not given) [randallC p78]   4377

⟨1⟩ "Abe never spoke to me about his wife – never introduced me to her – thought something was the matter with him & her" – Hannah Armstrong [wilson p527]   4378

⟨1⟩ "She was a cheerful woman, a delightful conversationalist, and well-informed on all the subjects of the day." [helmA]   4379

⟨1⟩ "His wife made him Presdt (?): She had the fire – will and ambition – Lincolns talent & his wifes Ambition did the deed" – John Stuart [wilson p63]   4380

⟨1⟩ Feb. 1, 1850: Son Edward dies. Afterwards, Mary would not eat. "Mr. Lincoln said, 'We must eat, Mary, for we must live.' and he sat down and forced himself to eat, but she wouldn't." – Mary Edwards Brown [kunhardtC]   4381

⟨2⟩ About 1850: Mary verbally abuses a man named Tiger, who approaches Lincoln for satisfaction. Lincoln says: "*friend* Tiger, can't you endure this one wrong done   4382

Mary

Mental Status (continued)

to you by a mad woman without much complaint for old friendship's sake while I have had to bear it without complaint and without a murmur for these last fifteen years" – James Matheny, 1887 recollection [wilson p14]. Story begins in ¶4361. Herndon tells it in much greater detail in [hertz pp160-162].

⟨2⟩ In Springfield: When Mary had "one of her hysterical seizures [,] Lincoln, if he could not talk her out of it, took the children and left until she returned to her normal frame of mind." [randallC p133] — 4383

⟨1⟩ In Springfield: John Bradford and family pick up Mary for a carriage ride: "she appeared to be very nervous and more or less wrought up." [wilson p729] — 4384

⟨2⟩ Late 1850s: "... her clothes – always her clothes – were of the richest materials and the most modish, extravagant cut." [turner p45] — 4385

⟨1/q⟩ 1854-1855: "gay and light-hearted, hopeful and happy," but also: "Her little temper was soon over." – Emilie Todd Helm [randallC p144] — 4386

⟨1⟩ Sept. 1859: "I hope you may never feel as lonely as I sometimes do, surrounded by much that renders life desirable." – Mary [turner p57] — 4387

⟨1/q⟩ "Many of her old friends say she showed signs of insanity as far back as 1860." – Chicago *Times*, July 17, 1882 [evans p318] — 4388
  ⟨2⟩ "There had been, of course, evidence of neurotic behavior even before Willie's death [1862] and her husband's murder [1865]." [turner p xvii] — 4389

⟨2/c⟩ 1860: "one of the happiest years of her life" [turner 63] — 4390

⟨2⟩ 1860: Of Eddie, who died in 1850: "could not talk of the dead child without bitter tears" [randallC p128] — 4391

⟨1⟩ Jan. 1, 1860: "Let *the flames* receive this, so soon as read." – Mary's postscript to a benign letter [turner p62] *One wonders why she felt this injunction necessary. Paranoia?* — 4392

⟨1⟩ When Lincoln was President-elect: A visitor called on the Lincolns at their Springfield home and "was ushered into a room where both Mr. & Mrs. L. were. The latter was on the floor in a sort of hysterical fit, caused by L's refusal to promise the position of Naval officer of the N.Y. Custom House to Isaac Henderson, who had sent a diamond brooch to a Springfield jeweler to be given to Mrs. L in case she could secure the promise of this office. The fit continued until the promise was obtained." – Horace White [wilson p701] *A somewhat different story, from Henry Villard, is doubted by* [randallC pp174-176]. — 4393

⟨S⟩ "In January 1861 there occurred the first act of Mrs. Lincoln indicating that she might not be mentally 'right.' ... This developed in connection with a trip she took to New York to make purchases." [evans pp158&238] — 4395

⟨1⟩ 1861: Tad was "Quick in mind, and impulse, like his mother, with her naturally sunny temperament..." [grimsley] (See ¶5429.) — 4396

⟨1⟩ 1861: "was a woman of fine native mental qualities, vivacious, intellectual, and a charming conversationalist." [grimsley] — 4397

■ White House shopping: — 4398
  ⟨2⟩ 1861: Overspends her $20,000 allotment for renovating the White House by $6700. Lincoln is furious. Congress quietly passes two appropriations to pay the debt. [donaldH pp34-37] — 4399
  ⟨2⟩ 1863 or later: "She could not check her desire to buy; she needed a $1500 cashmere shawl, [etc.]. ... Her passion for material possessions became — 4400

Mental Status (continued)

boundless. When the Lincoln family – all three members – moved to the Soldiers' home for the summer of 1863, she required a train of nineteen wagons to haul out the necessary supplies and clothing. ... Mary Lincoln was not by this point entirely rational." [donaldH pp47-48]

⟨2⟩ The dresses of the 1850s required 30 yd^2 of silk, 10-15 yd of whalebone, and 63 yd of cotton underwear [randallC p92]   4401

- February 1862: Willie's death   4402
  ⟨2⟩ It devastated Mary Lincoln. She took to bed for three weeks. She was unable to attend Willie's funeral or to care for Tad, who was simultaneously seriously ill (but recovering). For many months she would weep if Willie's name were merely mentioned. She never again entered the room where he died or the room where he was embalmed. [donaldA p337]   4403

  ⟨1⟩ Willie's death took "part of the doting mother's heart also, which was never more to find peace and comfort, mourning and refusing to be comforted, as only such impassioned natures yield to grief." [grimsley] *Grimsley was not living in the White House when Willie died.*   4404

  ⟨2⟩ "For three months following the funeral, she lay lost in the most abject misery, wild grief alternating with periods of paralyzing depression. She was unable to function." [turner p121]   4406

⟨1⟩ 1862 or 1863: "She suffers from depression of spirits, but I do think if she would only come here [a military hospital] and look at all the poor soldiers occasionally it would be better for her." – letter from Mrs. Pomroy, shortly after the battle of Winchester [boyden pp91-92] *There were two battles at Winchester: May 25, 1862 and June 13-15, 1863.*   4407

⟨1/q⟩ Jan. 1, 1863, the first reception since Willie's death. She speaks of Willie "with a sad sad look" – Benjamin French [randallC p286]   4408

⟨1/q⟩ August 1863: "a very fair, cheerful, smiling face, which does one good to look upon" – a newspaper correspondent [randallC p292]   4409

- December 1863: From diary of Emilie Todd Helm: 4410
  ⟨1/q⟩ "I feel worried about Mary, her nerves have gone to pieces; she cannot hide from me that the strain she has been under has been too much for her mental as well as her physical health." – Lincoln [randallC p298]   4411

  ⟨1/q⟩ "She seems very nervous and excitable and once or twice when I have come into the room suddenly the frightened look in her eyes has appalled me." – Emilie Todd Helm [randallC p298]   4412

  ⟨1/q⟩ Referring to the dead Willie, Mary says, "He lives, Emilie. He comes to me every night and stands at the foot of my bed. ... He does not always come alone; little Eddie is sometimes with him, and twice he has come with our brother, Alex." Emile reacted with the thought: "It is unnatural and abnormal, it frightens me. It does not seem like Sister Mary to be so wrought up. She is on a terrible strain and her smiles seem forced." [evans p185] citing [helmB pp226ff]   4413

- In White House: 4414
  ⟨2⟩ "She was often in a state of near hysteria concerning her husband's safety." [donaldH p44]   4415

  ⟨1/q⟩ Did not look "goodtempered" [sic] [donaldH p46]   4416

⟨1/q⟩ Before 1864: *A physician may have evaluated, or at least commented on, Mary's mental state.* W.O. Stoddard wrote of her mood: "At first it was not easy to understand why a lady who could one day be so kindly, so considerate, so generous, so   4417

Mental Status (continued)

thoughtful, and so hopeful could upon another day appear so unreasonable, so irritable, so despondent, even so niggardly, and so prone to see the wrong side of men, women, and events. It is easier to understand it all and to deal with it after a few words from an eminent medical practitioner." [evans p300] quoting an 1890 edition of [stoddardA p62]

⟨2⟩ "In the last year of their life together, there appears to have been a lack of communication and considerable tension between the President and his wife." [turner p183]   4418

⟨1/q⟩ 1864: "that lady has set here on this here sofy & shed tears by the pint a begging me to pay her debts which was unbeknown to the President." – Isaac Newton, per John Hay [randallC p311]   4419

⟨2⟩ Chronically and intentionally embezzled (Tripp's word) government funds as First Lady. [tripp pp161-168]   4420

⟨2⟩ "a perfect devil" – paraphrase of Dr. Robert K. Stone [tripp p226 (written by Burlingame)] citing "the manuscript diary of John Meredith Read, Jr., U.S. minister to Greece, quoted in Old HIckory Bookshop (New York) catalog, n.d., clipping, Lincoln files, 'Wife' folder, Lincoln Museum, Lincoln Memorial University, Harrogate, Tennessee."   4421

⟨1⟩ 1865: "She was kind to all the employees of the White House. I think she was very generally liked." [crookA p18]   4422

⟨1⟩ Jan. 22, 1865: "The President appeared well and in excellent spirits and Mrs. Lincoln never appeared better. ... She greeted every guest with such cheerful good will and kindness as to do infinite credit to her position and her heart." [french p463]   4423

⟨2⟩ Early March 1865: Mary buys $1000 worth of mourning goods [rossA pp246-247]. (See ¶1224.)   4424

⟨1/q⟩ Mar. 4, 1865: Mrs. Grimsley was with Mary. "Mrs. Lincoln Disappointed: ... Senator Harlan ... with great difficulty, escorted them through the crowded passage ways to the reserved seats on the platform, but where they arrived too late to witness the Inaugural ceremonies." [NYTribune - Mar. 6, 1865] per written transcript in [barbeeP - box 2 folder 135]   4425

⟨1⟩ Mar. 26, 1865: Explodes in anger, publicly, at a military review, over a perceived slight. (See ¶2544, ¶4694.)   4426
  ⟨1⟩ "She was at no time well; the mental strain upon her was great, betrayed by extreme nervousness approaching hysteria, causing misapprehensions, extreme sensitivities as to slights, or want of politeness and consideration. I had the deepest sympathy for her..." [barnesB]   4427
  ⟨1⟩ [badeau pp355-364] devotes a terrifyingly detailed chapter to this event.   4428

- April 14-15, 1865 – Lincon's shooting and death   4429
  ⟨1/q⟩ "About once an hour Mrs. Lincoln would repair to the bedside of her dying husband and with lamentation and tears remain until overcome by emotion." – Gideon Welles [kunhardtA p358]   4430
  ⟨2⟩ Mary's last visits to the bedside were at 2:45 and 3:00 a.m. "She wept piteously ... begging the doctors to kill her and let her join him." [kunhardtB pp78-79]   4431
  ⟨2⟩ When Lincoln's respirations began to rattle, Mary let out "a piercing cry and fell fainting to the floor" [kunhardtA p358].   4432

Mental Status (continued)

⟨2⟩ Spirits of camphor were obtained to "restore" Mary after a fainting spell. [kun- 4433
hardtB p49]

■ Hours and days after Lincoln's death: 4434

   Mary

⟨1⟩ Back at the White House, about 4 hours after Lincoln's death: "Mrs. L, tossing 4435
uneasily about upon a bed. ... She was nearly exhausted with grief, and when
she became a little quiet, I asked and received permission" to view Lincoln's
body [keckleyB pp188-189]. "Returning to Mrs. Lincoln's room, I found her in a
new paroxysm of grief. ... I bathed Mrs. Lincoln's head with cold water, and
soothed the terrible tornado [Tad] as best I could." [keckleyB p191-192]

⟨1⟩ "Mrs. Lincoln never left her room, and while the body of her husband was 4436
being borne in solemn state from the Atlantic to the broad praries of the
West, she was weeping with her fatherless children in her private chamber.
She denied admittance to almost every one, and I was her only companion,
except her children, in the days of her great sorrow." [keckleyB pp192-193]

⟨2⟩ On April 17 the men carrying Lincoln's body out of the White House took off 4437
their shoes as they passed Mary's door, so she would not hear the shuffle of
feet and know what was happening. [kunhardtB p120]

⟨2⟩ Mary did not attend Lincoln's White House service. She stayed in her room 4438
[kunhardtB p125].

⟨1⟩ "The days during which the President lay in state ... Mrs. Lincoln was almost 4439
frantic with suffering." [crookA p69]

⟨1⟩ Isaac Arnold called on Mary for several consecutive days, starting "a few 4440
days" after Lincoln's death. She would repeat the "painful details" of Lincoln's last day and "would be convulsed with sorrow." She would try to turn
her attention elsewhere, "but directly and unconsciously, she would return
to these incidents," not remembering she'd repeated them often. She "apparently had lost all power of choice in the subjects of her conversation."
[arnold p439]

■ Days and weeks after Lincoln's death: 4441

⟨2⟩ After her husband's murder, Mary was confined to bed. She did not leave the 4442
White House until May 22 – five weeks after the shooting. [evans p193]

⟨1⟩ Departure was "delayed a month by Mrs. Lincoln's illness. The shock of 4443
her husband's death had brought about a nervous disorder. Her physician,
Doctor Stone, refused to allow her to be moved until she was somewhat restored." [crookA p70]

⟨2⟩ "Her collapse was utter and complete. She could not lift her head from the 4444
pillow without fainting." [helmB p260]

⟨2⟩ "For five weeks after her husband's death, Mary Lincoln had not been able 4445
to rise from her bed." [helmB p260]

⟨2⟩ To the conspiracy against Lincoln she added both John Parker (the guard 4446
who had left his post outside the Lincolns' theater box) and President Johnson [kunhardtA p394].

⟨H⟩ Rumor: "she had prolonged her stay in the White House by pretending she 4447
was about to become a mother" [randallC p371]

⟨1⟩ Train ride to Illinois: "During most of the fifty-four hours that we were on the way 4448
she was in a daze; it seemed almost a stupor. She hardly spoke. No one could get
near enough to her grief to comfort her." [crookA pp70-71]

⟨1̲q̲⟩ Mary left the White House with innumerable trunks and boxes. She was accused 4449
of stealing.

Mental Status (continued)

⟨2⟩ Looters and souvenir hunters had ransacked the White House while Mary stayed in her room [kunhardtA p394] (as they had done in the neglected time after Willie's 1862 death [donaldH p40]). 4450

⟨1/q⟩ Eight years later Orville Browning believed she had not stolen, but David Davis replied that "the proofs were too many and too strong against her to admit doubt of her guilt ... that stealing was a kind of insanity with her, and that she had carried away from the White House many things that were of no value to her, and she had carried them away only in obedience to her irresistible propensity to steal." [burl p304] 4451

⟨2⟩ For months, Mary could speak only of Lincoln's murder, "as if she had lost all power of choices in the topics of her conversation" (Isaac Arnold), giving an account of the events to all who would listen. Sudden noise would remind her of the pistol blast. [kunhardtA p394] 4452

⟨1/q⟩ From the time "her husband was shot down by her side ... to the day of her death, Mrs. Lincoln never saw a well day not a happy hour. ... Her mind was unhinged by the shock." – Noyes Miner [kunhardtA p394] 4453

⟨2⟩ December 1865: "proved to be a month of particular misery and disappointment for Mary Lincoln" [turner p303] 4454

⟨2⟩ 1866 and after: Read three to eight newspapers a day [turner p266] *A bit ambiguous...* 4455

⟨2/c⟩ She had a "mania for money, extravagance, and miserliness – paradoxical as it appears." [evans p312] 4456

  ⟨1/q⟩ While still living in Springfield she "was very *economical*[,] So much so that *by some she* might have been pronounced stingy." – a relative [burl p275] 4457

  ⟨1/q⟩ William Herndon also pronounced her "stingy & exclusive" [burl p275] and also said she "kept a stingy table" [kunhardtB p260]. 4458

  ⟨2/c⟩ Mary's need to be economical was mis-interpreted as stinginess. [randallC pp140] 4459

  ⟨1/q⟩ In Springfield: Buys a "fine" carriage while Lincoln is away. He returns and "complained" about it. [randallC p139] 4460

  ⟨2⟩ 1856: Adds a second story to the house while Lincoln is away. He returns and "scolded his wife for running him in debt." [randallC pp139-140] 4461

  ⟨1/q⟩ "My mother is on one subject [money] not mentally responsible. ... It is hard to deal with one who is sane on all subjects but one." – Robert Lincoln, Oct. 16, 1867 [evans p319] (also in [helmB p267]) 4462

  ⟨1/q⟩ 1867: Mary believed she "was in actual want and nothing I can say or do will convince her to the contrary." – Robert [randallC p120] 4463

  ⟨1/q⟩ About 1867: Mary refers to "*many* dinnerless days" [randallC p120] 4464

  ⟨2⟩ In her husband's first term as President, Mary's debt for purchases was $70,000 – three times the President's annual salary. Mary had not told her husband of the debt. [evans p240]. 4465

  ⟨2⟩ "From 1865 to 1875 she had bought insanely and lavishly, and she had a mad urge for money; but she had kept within her means. If Mrs. Lincoln's mentality were to be measured by that standard alone, the only period in which she was unbalanced would be between 1861 and 1865." [evans p245] 4466

  ⟨2⟩ Her shopping compulsion was well known in Chicago. "Some merchants made a practice of accepting her orders, delivering the goods, and then sending for them within a day or two." [evans p225] 4467

Mental Status (continued)

⟨2⟩ "A real issue in 1875 was her habit of carrying tens of thousand of dollars in bills and negotiable securities pinned to her undergarments." [hirschhorn] 4468

⟨1⟩ "Another peculiarity was the accumulation of large quantities of silks and dress goods by the trunk and cart load, which she never used, and which accumulated until it was really feared that the floor of the store room would give way." – Dr. T.W. Dresser [wilson p671] (See ¶4517.) 4469

Mary

⟨1⟩ "Once she bought 300 pairs of gloves at one time and two dozen watches." – Mary Edwards Brown [kunhardtA pp396-397] *This is classic manic behavior.* 4470

⟨2⟩ Once bought 84 pairs of kid gloves in less than one month. [shenk p180] 4471

⟨2⟩ Of note, Tad had trouble grasping the basics of money – see ¶5519 4472

⟨2⟩ One remnant of Mary's shopping excess still in the White House [aa9] is the canopied, gold-trimmed, seven-foot rosewood "Lincoln bed" [donaldH pp34-35] 4473

⟨1⟩ Jan. 12, 1868: writes of suicide [turner p468]. See ¶4523. 4474

⟨2⟩ 1868: Lizzie Keckley publishes [keckleyB]. Mary sees it as "a deadly betrayal" and severs "all ties with the woman who had been her deepest emotional support ever since Willie's death." [kunhardtA p395] 4475

⟨2⟩ 1870: "She improved noticeably when Congress, at last, in 1870 ... granted her a pension" [turner p xix] 4476

⟨1⟩ Circa 1870-1871 or later: "... no trace of eccentricity in conduct or manner. She was simply a bright, wholesome, attractive woman" – Paul Shipman [helmA] 4477

⟨2⟩ Shipman wrote this in response to a newspaper piece by Adam Badeau that described Mary's "isolation and strange behavior in London" in 1871. [rossA p291, citing New York World of Jan. 8, 1875] 4478

⟨1⟩ May 1871: "Mrs. Lincoln is looking very well, but yet seems oppressed by the sad memory of her husband's tragic death." [NYTimes - May 11, 1871] 4479

■ July 1871: Tad dies. 4480

⟨1⟩ "This death ... has been a fearful blow to Mrs. Lincoln, and her physician dreads that it may produce insanity, though hopeful of averting so sad a calamity." [ChicagoTribune - July 16, 1871] 4481

⟨1⟩ "Owing to the complete prostration of Mrs. Lincoln, caused by intense grief and continued watching by the bedside of her boy, she was not able to accompany the body to this city [Springfield]." [ChicagoTribune - July 18, 1871] 4482

⟨2⟩ "The meager information we have from other sources is that Mrs. Lincoln mourned in 1871 as she had done in 1862 and in 1865, after the deaths of her son and husband." [evans p213] 4483

■ After Tad's death: 4484

⟨1⟩ "from that time, [she,] in the judgment of her most intimate friends, was never entirely responsible for her conduct. She was peculiar and eccentric, and had various hallucinations." [arnold p439] 4485

⟨1⟩ "suffered from periods of mild insanity. She had many strange delusions at these times. ... toward the close the close of [Mary's] life ... that unfortunate lady became so much unbalanced that the family thought it best to place her in a private sanitarium" [foy] (More in ¶4139.) *The sanitarium was 7 years before Mary's death. Foy knows Mary died in 1882.* 4487

⟨1⟩ 1872 and later: On being Mary's "nurse, guard and companion:" "the position was a trying one, and Mother gave it up twice, but each time the kinsmen induced her to come back after she had had a short rest." [foy] 4488

Mental Status (continued)

⟨$\frac{1}{q}$⟩ 1873-1874 events: 4489

 ⟨$\frac{1}{q}$⟩ "In 1873 I treated Mrs. Lincoln several weeks for fever and nervous derange- 4490
 ment of the head, and observed at that time indications of mental distur-
 bance. She had strange imaginings; thought that someone was at work on
 her head, and than an Indian was removing the bones from her face and
 pulling wires out of her eyes." – Dr. Danforth (see ¶4624) testifying at Mary's
 1875 insanity trial [evans p215] *Could this have been delirium from the fever?*

 ⟨1⟩ May-Oct. 1874 (at least): Confined to her room with "nervous exhaustion" 4491
 [NYTimes - Oct. 18, 1874]. (∈ ¶4606)

 ⟨$\frac{1}{q}$⟩ More of Dr. Danforth's testimony: "I visited her again in 1874 when she was 4492
 suffering from debility of the nervous system. She complained that some-
 one was taking steel springs from her head and would not let her rest; that
 she was going to die within a few days, and that she had been admonished
 to that effect by her husband. She imagined that she heard raps on a table
 conveying the time of her death, and would sit and ask questions and repeat
 the supposed answer the table would give." [evans p215] *It seems that "de-*
 bility of the nervous system" is Dr. Danforth's characterization of these
 phenomena, and not a reference to a parallel disorder of the nervous sys-
 tem.

 ⟨1⟩ Testimony as reported in newspaper: "She seemed possessed with the idea 4493
 that some one was working on her head, taking wires out of her eyes (particularly the left one), at times taking bones out of her cheeks and face, and de-
 taching steel springs from her jaw bones ... at other times she imagined her
 scalp was being lifted by the same invisible power and placed back again ...
 she did not often experience pain, but at times was sensitive of a cutting sensation; this continued for some time ... he at length discontinued his visits,
 the patient having improved in health, and did not see her again for several
 weeks; saw her again in March, 1874; continued to visit her up to September, most of the time daily ... a general indisposition and debility appeared
 to pervade her system – the same condition of affairs which he had noticed
 in his first visits, cutting, scraping, and removing bones from her face and
 wires from her eyes." [hirschhorn] citing *Illinois State Register*, May 21, 1875,
 page 1.

⟨$\frac{1}{q}$⟩ March-April 1875 events (See ¶4173 for Florida trip): 4494

 ⟨$\frac{1}{q}$⟩ "I called upon her a week ago ... when she spoke of her stay in Florida, of 4495
 the pleasant time she had there. ... She appeared ... to be in excellent health,
 and her former hallucinations appeared to have passed away. She said her
 reason for returning from Florida was that she was not well. She startled me
 somewhat by saying that an attempt had been made to poison her her on
 her journey back. She had been very thirsty, and at a wayside station not far
 from Jacksonville she took a cup of coffee in which she discovered poison."
 – testimony of Dr. Danforth at Mary's insanity trial [evans p216] *The thirst is*
 an interesting, if ambiguous, datum. Was this compulsive water drinking
 from schizophrenia? Hyponatremia might then explain her delusions. Was
 it a sign of diabetes, which she later may have developed (¶4083)? Or was
 it just a normal response to a hot Florida day?

 ⟨$\frac{1}{q}$⟩ Robert testified that, after returning from Florida, his mother would rap on 4496
 the door of his hotel room at night and ask to sleep in his room. He also
 described finding her "but slightly dressed" trying to take the elevator to the
 hotel office. When he stopped her "she screamed 'You are going to murder

Mental Status (continued)

me.' ... She then took a seat next the wall, and professed to be repeating what [a] man was saying to her through the wall. ... I called on her the first week of April, and she told me that all Chicago was going to be destroyed by fire, and that she was going to send her valuables to some country town." [evans pp216-217] *The great Chicago fire had already happened – in October 1871.*

⟨2⟩ Mary may have been using psychoactive medicines at this time. See ¶4172. 4497

⟨1⟩ "she did queer things like getting into the elevator in a hotel when she was 4498
undressed; she thought it was the lavatory" – Mary Edwards Brown, 1956
[kunhardtC]

⟨2⟩_c "Mary Lincoln's acute episode began in early March and peaked on 1 April" 4499
[hirschhorn] citing [neelyF p8]

⟨1⟩_q May 1875: Tried in Chicago for insanity (see [neelyF]). The jury's verdict: "Mary 4500
Lincoln is insane, and is a fit person to be sent to the State Hospital for the Insane;
... that her age is 56 years; that her disease is of unknown duration; that the cause
is unknown; that the disease is not hereditary; that she is not subject to epilepsy;
that she does not manifest homicidal or suicidal tendencies; and that she is not a
pauper." [evans pp217-218]

⟨1⟩_q "The verdict was received by Mrs. Lincoln without any visible emotions. She 4501
was stolid and unmoved. [She spent that night, under guard, at a hotel.]
About 11.30 o'clock last night it was found necessary to send for an officer
to watch over Mrs. Lincoln, whose lunatic symptoms became quite violent."
[evans p221] quoting [ChicagoTribune - May 20, 1875]

⟨2⟩ She was committed to a private sanatorium, the Bellevue Place Sanatorium 4502
in Batavia, IL [evans pp224& vi]

⟨1⟩ Her physician at Bellevue, Dr. R.J. Patterson (see ¶4623), wrote a letter 4503
about Mary's case that was published in the *Illinois State Register* (1 Sept.
1875;28:1) [randallP box 71]

⟨2⟩ Upon being committed, Mary began lobbying to be sent instead to live with 4504
her oldest sister, Elizabeth Todd Edwards, in Springfield. This was consented, and she left Batavia on Sept. 10, 1875. She stayed at the Edwards
home until Oct. 1, 1876. [evans p225]

⟨2⟩ Robert apparently paid at least one of the doctors for his testimony. [kunhardtA 4505
p396]

⟨1⟩ June 1875: "I have for several years considered her demented." – Orville Browning 4506
[nicolayO p3]

⟨2⟩ June 1876: Mary's insanity case is reopened, at her (and Mr. Edwards') request. 4507
[evans p225]

⟨1⟩_q "Mrs. Lincoln was adjudged sane and her property was restored to her con- 4508
trol. The proceedings were of an amicable nature. ... The whole proceedings
occupied but a few minutes." – [ChicagoTribune - June 16, 1876] cited by [evans p226]

⟨S⟩ "After 1876 Mrs. Lincoln's mind undoubtledly was just as much disorganized 4509
as it had been in 1875, and in 1882 it was more so. But in spite of that, she
so conducted herself so as to justify the course her friends had taken." [evans
p226]

⟨2⟩ "For four years following her release from a sanatorium, Mrs. Lincoln's mind was 4510
remarkably lucid." [turner p xxii]

⟨2⟩ Among Mary's letters found in 2005 (see ¶3982), 10 are from 1876-1878. "The 4511
most striking aspect of all 10 letters is that they are calm, rational, and cogent, full

Mental Status (continued)

of descriptions of her travels and inquiries about friends and events at home."
[emersonA]

⟨1⟩ "Mother always told us that we mustn't say anything unkind about Aunt Mary in her last years because she wasn't herself." – Mary Edwards Brown [kunhardtC]   4512

■ Autumn 1880 to the end: 4513

  ⟨2⟩ "Her mind was as unsettled as it was in 1875. ... She was, from the time of Mr. Lincoln's death, a mental and physical wreck." – Laura C. Holloway [evans p229]   4514

  ⟨2⟩ During this period Mary lived very quietly at her sister's house in Springfield. She largely stayed in her room, seeing no one there except relatives and close friends, and sometimes refusing to see even her sisters. "At intervals her conversation showed that her mind was quite disordered, but most of the time she talked very sensibly." Her possessions occupied about 60 trunks and boxes in her rooms. "She was likely to be dressed in black, and sometimes overdressed." [evans p229]   4515

  ⟨2⟩ The trunks, "weighing nearly four tons," were kept "in two back rooms, where they threatened the floorboards" [baker p365]. (See ¶4469.)   4516

  ⟨1⟩ Mary kept a large amount of money in a money belt (even under her nightdress) and "a big roll of bills" under her mattress. At least once she accused her sister of stealing her money. "She kept writing letters all the time to rich men in the country saying how poor she was and living in despicable circumstances and the nation should be ashamed." Mary kept 64 trunks in the room next to hers, "filled with bolts of curtain materials and dress goods." A maid left because she was afraid to sleep under that room, because of the weight. But Mary "wouldn't stop buying. Once she bought 300 pairs of gloves at one time and two dozen watches. She had about a hundred shawls. Every day she got up and went through those trunks for hours. Grandmother said it was funny, if Aunt Mary was so sick, that she was able to be up all day bending over her trunks." – Mary Edwards Brown, 1956 [kunhardtC] *Whether the over-shopping was then still occurring is unclear.*   4517

⟨$\frac{1}{q}$⟩ 1881: "When a New York reporter interviewed the doctor on the unforgettable subject of Mrs. Lincoln's mental illness, Dr. Sayre testily replied, 'She is no more insane than you or I are and if you come with me to talk with her you would understand that.'" [NYTimes - Nov. 23, 1881]   4518

■ Hallucinations: 4519

  ⟨2⟩ "Mrs. Lincoln's mental illness was characterized by hallucinations. [They were] manifested first in 1862, frequently shown in 1865, and very much in evidence in 1875 and thereafter." [evans p341]. *The 1862 episode is perhaps the appearance of Willie, which I have dated as 1863 – see ¶4413*   4520

  ⟨2⟩ [evans p341] could find no evidence of bromide, "barbituric," or opiate drug use that would explain the hallucinations. *But see ¶4172*   4521

⟨1⟩ 1882: "she wasn't herself" – opinion of Mary's niece, as recalled by Mary Edwards Brown [kunhardtA p396]   4522

■ Suicide ideation: 4523

  ⟨$\frac{1}{q}$⟩ Mary discussed suicide with Elizabeth Keckley about 1863. [evans p222] [keckleyB]   4524

  ⟨1⟩ October 1867, January 1868, November 1869: Mary writes of suicide, each time saying only concern for Tad prevented it [turner pp440, 468, 524]   4525

Mental Status (continued)

⟨1⟩ May 20, 1875: Mrs. Lincoln escaped supervision and visited three Chicago 4526
drug stores, asking to purchase a laudanum-plus-camphor mixture. An
alert druggist at the first informed clerks at the other stores, and sales were
prevented. When Mrs. Lincoln returned to the first store to pick up her
medicine, she was given a placebo. Mary left the drug store, drank the
placebo, and after ten minutes returned for more laudanum. She was again
given placebo and drank it, by which time Robert arrived and took charge
of her. This was the day before the verdict of her insanity trial came in.
[ChicagoTribune - May 21, 1875] [evans p222] citing Chicago *Times* as well.

⟨2⟩ [hirschhornB] reviews the incident more thoroughly than done here. He notes 4527
that there are minor variations in the story between the several newspapers
that reported it. He also concludes that "her attempt was real, impulsive, but
as a measure of her tenacity and strength of character, not to be repeated."

⟨2⟩ [baker p326] claims the incident never occurred. [hirschhornB] finds multiple er- 4528
rors in her discussion.

⟨2⟩ "The religious influence, if it may be called such, which dominated her later life 4529
more than any other was spiritualism." This began before she moved to Washington, and increased there. [evans p264]

- Somatization? Malingering? 4530
  ⟨-⟩ *Given the myriad physical complaints found in Mary's letters (Special* 4531
  Topic §9), it is reasonable to ask whether they were real or imagined or
  concocted. A revealing indication comes from two letters written to two
  different people on June 30, 1867 from Racine, Wisconsin. Mary had gone
  there after declining, for health reasons, to testify at a trial in Washington
  [turner p421].
  ⟨1⟩ Letter #1: "My health, after I saw you, broke down so completely. ... of course, 4532
  I have been scarcely able to leave my lounge." [turner p424]
  ⟨1⟩ Letter #2: "The walks here are shady & very pleasant. Each morning I have 4533
  walked two miles." [turner p426]
  ⟨$\frac{1}{q}$⟩ "It is really astonishing what a brave front she manages to keep when we 4534
  know she is suffering – most women would be in bed groaning, but not
  Mother!" – Robert [randallC p69]

- Diagnoses (contemporary): 4535
  ⟨S⟩ Lincoln reputedly told a friend: "The caprices of Mrs. Lincoln, I am satisfied, 4536
  are the result of partial insanity." [burl pp297,307]
  ⟨S⟩ "Herndon believed that Lincoln 'held his wife partly insane for years.' " [burl 4537
  p296]
  ⟨$\frac{1}{q}$⟩ "was subject to similar spells of mental depression as Mr. L" – Orville Brown- 4538
  ing [wilsonH p242] citing [nicolayO p1]
  ⟨$\frac{1}{q}$⟩ "demented .. As we used familiarly to state it she was always 'either in the 4539
  garret or the cellar' " – Orville H. Browning [burl p297] *Strikingly suggests bipo-*
  lar disorder.
  ⟨1⟩ "While the whole world was finding fault with her temper and disposition, it 4540
  was clear to me that the trouble was a cerebral disease." – Dr. T.W. Dresser
  [wilson p671]

- Diagnoses (later, by non-physicians): 4541
  ⟨$\frac{2}{c}$⟩ "grew up without learning the essential lesson of self-restrain, and this had 4542
  far-reaching results." [randallC pp17-18] *This seems an insightful statement.*

299

Mary

Mental Status (continued)

⟨2⟩_c "That Mary Lincoln had a difficult temperament is quite true." [randallC p81]   4543
This is from a source sympathetic to Mary.

⟨S⟩ "evidently suffered from manic depression [but] has many of the symptoms   4544
associated with what is now termed 'borderline personality disorder' " [burl
p297]

⟨S⟩ Manic depressive (bipolar) illness, apparently proposed by [emersonB]   4545

⟨S⟩ general paresis of the insane (a form of tertiary syphilis) – Gore Vidal has   4546
stated that Mary suffered from paresis, which accounted for her emotional
and mental difficulties [currentNY, citing NBC Today Show, March 26, 1988]. See ¶2016
and ¶4616.

⟨S⟩ narcissism [baker p330]   4547

⟨S⟩ "'neurasthenia' and migraine' " [turner p xvi]   4548

⟨S⟩ "Mrs. Randall saw Mary Lincoln not as Herndon's 'female wild cat of the age,'   4549
but as a loving, well-meaning woman, whose undeniably erratic behavior
was largely the result of mild mental illness, exacerbated by the tensions and
shocks she experienced throughout the course of her life." [turner pp xxi, 414]

⟨2⟩ A sympathetic editorial, days after Mary died, referred to "the certainty that   4550
Mrs. Lincoln's reason was unsettled." [NYTimes - July 18, 1882]

⟨S⟩ "... an impulsive, nervous temperament, a loose tongue, and a mind filled   4551
with quirks and delusions" [turner p77]

- Diagnoses (later, by physicians):   4552
  ⟨S⟩ "She had a mild, emotional insanity which caused her to act as does a case   4553
  of schizophrenia – living alone, apart, and letting the world take care of itself" [evans p230]. Evans cites Bleuler's definition of schizophrenia: "dementia
  praecox, representing split personality" [evans p230].

  ⟨S⟩ "She was still more of an introvert, or schizoid, in Springfield after 1875,   4554
  and in France in the same period"[evans p272]. Evans cites Bleuler's definition
  of schizoid: "the shut-in, unsocial, introspective type of personality." [evans
  p272].

  ⟨S⟩ "The weak points of her mind were: too great seriousness and an inability to   4555
  laugh at herself; capacity to ridicule others, but not herself; lack of humor."
  [evans p302].

  ⟨S⟩ "The bizarre behavior in 1875 leading to hospitalization, with elements   4556
  of acute anxiety, insomnia, and delusions, most resembles post-traumatic
  stress disorder, coinciding with the tenth anniversary of her husband's murder." [hirschhorn]

⟨1⟩_q Lincoln several times said "he was constantly under great apprehension lest his   4557
wife would do something to bring him into disgrace." – Orville Browning [nicolayO
p3]

⟨2⟩_c "Considering the hardships that befell her, the amazing thing about Mary Lincoln   4558
is not that she behaved so badly, but that she behaved as well as she did." [burl p xv]
  ⟨2⟩_c [stoddardA p191] makes a similar argument.   4559

⟨2⟩ "It was apparent to her friends that the terrible ordeal through which she had   4560
passed had left a depression on her mind, from which she had not recovered, and
she was accordingly put under medical care at Batavia for the treatment of her
infirmity. Though she never recovered completely, Mrs. Lincoln was soon considered as sufficiently improved to be relieved of restraint." [ChicagoTribune - July 17, 1882]
(obituary)

Mental Status (continued)

⟨1⟩ At Mary's funeral, Rev. James Reed compared Lincoln and Mary to two trees, hav- 4561
ᵩ   ing branches and roots intertwined. Lightning had killed one. The other seemed
unhurt, but was actually injured fatally, too. "Its after subsistence was merely a
living death. Similar was the course of life with the illustrious Lincoln and his
mate." [randallC p399]

Mary

Mouth

⟨2⟩ "Except in her youthful portraits, it is her mouth that dominates Mrs. Lincoln's 4562
ᶜ   features. Her lips were not broad and sensuous; in fact, they were not quite heavy
enough – without being thin-lipped. Had they shown a little more vermilion, she
would have been better looking. The distinguishing feature of her mouth was
that it formed a straight line, curving neither upward nor downward, and the lips
closed firmly. The upper lip was a trifle too broad because her nose was a little too
short. Her lower jaw and chin were well developed. Her teeth met well, neither
jaw protruding. She was not iron-jawed, nor was her chin square." [evans pp281-282]

⟨2⟩ As a young woman: "short upper lip" [evans p276] (∈ ¶4000) 4563

⟨2⟩ "The angles of the mouth are pulled downward ever so slightly, and the muscles, 4564
ᶜ   skin, and tissues are set in that position" [evans p282]. Evans goes on to deduce
features of Mary's personality from this.

⟨2⟩ As a young woman: "an expressive mouth curling into an adorable, slow-coming 4565
smile that brought dimples into her cheeks" [evans p276] (∈ ¶4000)

Muscle / Athletics

⟨1⟩ June 1867: "The walks here are shady & very pleasant. Each morning I have 4566
walked two miles" – Mary [turner p426]

⟨1⟩ "It has been her habit to take little or no exercise, though she was not confined to 4567
her bed" [ChicagoTribune - July 17, 1882] (obituary) (Part of ¶4060.)

Neck

⟨2⟩ "Mrs. Lincoln's neck was always good. It was not even bad when she was stoutest. 4568
ᶜ   Her dresses usually showed her neck well." [evans p283]

⟨2⟩ As a young woman: "Spirited carriage of her head" [evans p276] (∈ ¶4000) 4569

⟨2⟩ Age 40±: "'She held her head high, slightly tilted back, possibly because she had 4570
so tall a husband to look up to'" [evans p279] quoting [helmB p175] (∈ ¶4008)

Nervous System

The line between neurology and psychiatry is not sharp. In this section I have tried 4571
to collect "hard" neurological data, more related to the physical than are the data in
Mental Status .

Gait , Nervous System , and Trauma all contain information related to Mary's later- 4572
years back problems.

⟨1⟩ About age 10: "Mary was bright and talkative and warm hearted. She was far ad- 4573
vanced over girls of her age in education. ... She was very studious, with a retentive
memory and a mind that enabled her to grasp and thoroughly understand the

Nervous System (continued)

lessons she was required to learn. ... Mary was always quick in her movements." – Elizabeth Norris [helmA]

⟨1⟩ For four years went to a school where only French was spoken [helmA]. Later of use to her (¶4610). 4574

⟨$\frac{1}{q}$⟩ "Page after page of classic poetry she could recite and liked nothing better" – a cousin [randallC p26] 4575

⟨2⟩ "An eye for the ridiculous and an ear for speech patterns and dialects made her a devastating mimic." [turner p 9] 4576

    ⟨2⟩ "a rare gift for mimicry" [randallC p14] *A painful example is* [randallC p145]. 4577

⟨2⟩_c "had the wit and wisdom to recognize genius in the ungainly lawyer her Edwards relatives looked upon as too far beneath her for marriage." [turner p xv] 4578

⟨1⟩ About 1842: "bright, lively ... a good talker" – William Jayne [wilson pp624-625] (∈ ¶4002) 4579

- Writing style: 4580
    ⟨2⟩ "The reader will soon grow accustomed, as we did, to her eccentricities of style, to her failure to remember to close quotes and parentheses, and to what now would be considered outmoded usage." [turner p xxiii] 4581
    ⟨2⟩ She filled "each sheet to its edges, scarcely ever pausing for paragraphs. ... She had a marked aversion to the period as a means of punctuation; her sentences flowed on and on, random thoughts rushing in upon one another in a simple stream-of-consciousness style. ... Her pages were inundated by a hail of commas; they shattered sentences into tiny fragments." [turner p13] 4582
    ⟨-⟩ ○○○ *Project: A quantitative analysis of Mary's punctuation, sentence length, and/or other measurable parameters might disclose a sudden or otherwise perceptible change that, in turn, inform the discussion of her mental status.* 4583
    ⟨-⟩ 1862 penmanship: See ¶4207. 4584

⟨1⟩ "She was very fond of reading." [helmA] 4585

⟨2⟩ "Hands that moved in quick, graceful gestures when she spoke." [turner p7] 4586

⟨1⟩ May 1848: In a letter to Lincoln that omits the day of the month: "You will think indeed, that old age, has set its seal, upon my humble self, that in few or none of my letters, I can remember the day of the month, I must confess it is one of my peculiarities" [turner p36] 4587

    ⟨1⟩ Mary dates a letter "Sept. 31st." [turner p133] 4588

⟨2⟩ April 1865: When the dying Lincoln's respirations began to rattle, Mary let out "a piercing cry and fell fainting to the floor" [kunhardtA p358]. 4589

⟨S⟩ The explicit negative comment about epilepsy in the jury's verdict on Mary's insanity in 1875 "may have been required by law, or in response to a suggestion found in the printed form supplied by the court." [evans p340] 4590

⟨1⟩ January 1868: lost a month's living expenses by leaving her pocketbook on the streetcar [turner p469] 4591

⟨1⟩ Sept. 1868: Episode of near-syncope described in ¶4267. 4592

⟨1⟩ 1868 or 1869: "I feel miserably blue to-day. I am just recovering from a severe attack of neuralgia in my head, accompanied by great indisposition which has been my faithful companion for more than two weeks – my health has been quite 4593

Nervous System (continued)

as bad as it was last winter. I am well aware without my physician so frequently repeating to me – that quiet is necessary to my life." [helmB p275]

⟨1⟩ Sept. 1869: reads and enjoys Trollope's *Phineas Finn* [turner p 518]   4594

⟨1⟩ 1869-70: Pains [hirschhorn] citing [turner]:   4595

    ⟨-⟩ *Before drawing conclusions from* [hirschhorn]*'s selective quotations, the*   4596
    reader is referred to the selective quotations in Special Topic §9.

    ⟨1/q⟩ Nov. 13: " I have been suffering for three days, with neuralgic headaches,   4597
    pain in my limbs" [turner p522]

    ⟨1/q⟩ Nov. 14: "To day, my wrists even, pain with neuralgia" [turner p524]   4598
    ⟨1⟩ Nov. 20: "I am slowly recovering from my *neuralgic* woes." [turner p525] *This*   4599
    seems to be informative, but [hirschhorn] *omits it.*

    ⟨1/q⟩ Dec. 16: "I passed a sleepless, miserable night ... with great & burning pain   4600
    in my spine." [turner p535] *This episode was preceded by great mental upset.*

    ⟨1/q⟩ Jan. 2: "Today, I am suffering so much with my back – at times I am racked   4601
    with pain ... such pain in all my limbs." [turner pp539-540]

    ⟨1/q⟩ Feb. 11: "A fearful cold, appeared to settle in my spine & I was unable to sit   4602
    up, with the sharp, burning agony, in my back. I now have a plaster from my
    shoulders down the whole, extent of the spine.... The Dr says, this present
    trouble, arises more from a distressed agitated mind, than a real local cause,
    but says of course there is a great tendency to spinal disease." [turner p546]

    ⟨S⟩ "Mary Lincoln's tabes dorsalis began as early as 1869" [hirschhorn]. See ¶4616   4603

⟨1⟩ June 1870: describes "fragrant forests" [turner p565] *So, apparently could smell.*   4604

⟨1/q⟩ 1874 and/or 1875. The time course is ambiguous in [hirschhorn].   4605

    ⟨1⟩ Mid-1874: "Mrs. Abraham Lincoln, being confined to her house in [Chicago]   4606
    by nervous exhaustion, will be unable to be in attendance at the ceremonies
    in Springfield to-day in honor of her distinguished husband. She has been
    confined to her room for the past five months by a severe illness, from which
    she is just now slowly recovering." [NYTimes - Oct. 18, 1874, p9, col2.]

    ⟨-⟩ 1874: Various psychological, and perhaps physical, problems are described   4607
    in ¶4489ff.

    ⟨2⟩ 1875?: "a prolonged episode of pain" [hirschhorn] citing [ChicagoTribune - May 20,   4608
    1875, p1]

⟨2⟩ Sometime in 1876-1878 a letter from Mary mentions "boils under her left arm and   4609
pain over her entire body" [emersonA].

⟨1/q⟩ 1877: Living in France. Understands the language. [randallC p21] (See ¶4574.)   4610

⟨1⟩ After a fall in December 1879: Had "a partial paralysis of the lower part of her   4611
body" [evans p342]. Part of ¶4699.

    ⟨2⟩ "Four months later she fell again when her left side gave way on a flight of   4612
    stairs. Plasters and bed rest helped." [baker p364]

⟨2⟩ 1881: "Dr. Sayre diagnosed his patient as physically ill with kidney, eye, and back   4613
problems – the last a 'spinal sclerosis and hardening of the spinal cord.' " [baker
p366] (Baker also cites [NYTimes - 1881: Nov. 23, July 22, Aug. 4] and [turner p711].) *Of*
course, Sayre had no way to know the consistency of the spinal cord. [hirschhorn]
discusses medicine's understanding of spinal diseases in that era.

⟨1/q⟩ January 1, 1882 physician evaluation: "chronic inflammation of the spinal cord ...   4614
the consequence of an injury received some time since and has resulted in considerable loss of power of both lower extremities so as to lessen their use and to

Nervous System (continued)

render walking without assistance very unsafe, and going unaided down stairs impossible. The nature of the spinal trouble is progressive and will end in paralysis of the lower extremities. ... She is now quite helpless, unable to walk with safety without the aid of an attendant, or indeed to help herself to any extent." [hirschhorn] Part of ¶4183

⟨2⟩ Died after a stroke-like syndrome at age 64 [evans p344]. See ¶4062.   4615

⟨S⟩ [hirschhorn] believes Mary had a sensory impairment leading to locomotor ataxia (¶4158), based on the pupillary (¶4129) and neurological findings by her physicians in 1882. Ultimately they conclude she had *diabetic* tabes dorsalis (which should properly be called "pseudo-tabes" [aa111 p1019]). For reasons to doubt both the diagnoses of tabes and diabetic tabes, see §2i.   4616

⟨S⟩ During the 1882 evaluation, "the four physicians chose the least pejorative diagnosis, however marginally acceptable it was to progressive medical opinion." [hirschhorn]   4617

⟨1⟩ "She was bright and sparkling in conversation and her memory remained singularly good up to the very close of her life." – Dr. T.W. Dresser [wilson p671]   4618

⟨1⟩ "While the whole world was finding fault with her temper and disposition, it was clear to me that the trouble was a cerebral disease." – Dr. T.W. Dresser [wilson p671]   4619

Physicians

⟨1⟩ Dr. William Wallace – her brother-in-law – attended her in at least one birth (¶4648). For more on Wallace, see ¶3195.   4620

⟨S⟩ Dr. Stone (¶3203) was presumably her physician while she lived in the White House.   4621

⟨1⟩ Dr. [William E.?] Clarke took care of her in 1868 (at least) [turner p475] (See ¶4657.)   4622

⟨2⟩ "Dr. B.J. Cigrandi, of Batavia, Illinois, ... undertook to find what medical record the Bellevue Place Sanatorium had of Mrs. Lincoln. ... He found that the sanatorium had not saved any of Dr. R.J. Patterson's notes or the history sheets of Mrs. Lincoln's medical illness." [evans p vi]. See, however, ¶4503.   4623

⟨2⟩ Five physicians testified at her first insanity hearing in 1875: Drs Willis Danforth, R.N. Isham, Nathan S. Davis, H.A. Johnson, and Charles Gilman Smith. [evans p215]   4624
  ⟨2⟩ Danforth was a homeopathic surgeon in Chicago [hirschhorn]   4625

⟨2⟩ Dr. T.W. Dresser was her family physician for years, and the son of the minister that married her and Lincoln. He testified at her insanity trial. He was born in 1837. [evans p306].   4626

⟨2⟩ Dr. Lewis A. Sayre, "the leading orthopedic surgeon of America in his day," cared for Mrs. Lincoln's back injury in the early 1880s [evans pp227-228] See ¶4699   4627
  ⟨-⟩ *Reading the extensive description of Sayre in* [hirschhorn], *one gets the impression he was, at worst, not entirely free of charlatanism or, at best, blind to data that contradicted his expectations.*   4628
  ⟨1⟩ "Her doctor is Dr. S.H. Sayre, who was her schoolmate when both were children in Lexington, Ky." – typed transcript of *Illinois State Journal (Springfield)*, 30 Nov. 1881, page 1 column 5 that is in [randallP box 71]. *Unclear if this is the same Sayre, or if there were errors in the article or the transcription.*   4629

Physicians (continued)

⟨1⟩ On Jan. 1, 1882 four physicians examined Mary in New York City to evaluate her claim for an increase in her government pension [hirschhorn] (see ¶4183):   4630

   ⟨1⟩ Dr. Sayre, as noted above ¶4627   4631

   ⟨1⟩ Dr. Meredith Clymer, a neurologist   4632   Mary

   ⟨1⟩ Dr. Hermann Knapp, an ophthalmologist   4633

   ⟨1⟩ Dr. William Pancoast, a surgeon (son of the more famous Dr. Pancoast)   4634

   ⟨-⟩ [hirschhorn] *nicely summarizes the professional concentrations of these physicians, which is pertinent to Mary's case.*   4635

Reading & Learning

⟨2⟩ "Practically no women and very few men of that period received so much formal education." [evans p83]   4636

⟨2⟩ "She was very studious, with a retentive memory and a mind that enabled her to grasp and thoroughly understand the lessons she was required to learn." [evans p103]   4637

⟨1/q⟩ "She was one of the brightest girls in Madame Mentelle's school; always had the highest marks and took the biggest prizes." – recollection of a schoolmate, many decades afterwards [evans p107]   4638

⟨2⟩ She was "a good letter-writer" [evans p290]   4639

Reproductive

⟨2⟩ 1843: With Robert, "the birth was easy and the baby strong" [turner p31] *No primary source cited. Probably extrapolated.*   4640

   ⟨1/q⟩ "had no nurse for herself or the baby" [randallC p72]   4641

■ 1850: Willie's delivery: 4642

   ⟨2⟩ "perfectly normal" [donaldA p153] *No primary source is apparent.*   4643

   ⟨1/q⟩ Lincoln's father's final illness occurred about this time. Twenty-two days after Willie's birth, Lincoln answered a call to visit his father with: "I could hardly leave home now ... my own wife is sick-abed" [randallC p130]. Lincoln called her illness "baby-sickness" [donaldA p153].   4644

   ⟨s⟩ Donald thinks this was an excuse to avoid making the trip, rather than reflecting a true illness on Mary's part. [donaldA p153]   4645

   ⟨s⟩ [randallC p130] deduces that Mary had "a slow recovery from this confinement."   4646

⟨2⟩ Shortly after Tad's 1853 birth, Mary voluntarily breast-fed Charles Dallman, the infant of a sick neighbor [chenery]. *Syphilis may be passed by nursing* [aa111 p1095].   4647

⟨1⟩ While the Lincolns lived in Springfield, Abraham "went to Taylorville hired M. [Margaret Ryan] to stay while his wife was confined – gave birth to a boy. Dr Wallace attended her." – Margaret Ryan (interview) [wilson p597] *Ryan was born circa 1839* [wilson pp596, 769], *so this was probably Tad's birth in 1853.*   4648 ·

⟨s⟩ When her daughter-in-law was pregnant, Mary said "I am fearing a suffering time for her." [randallC p70] speculates this reflects on Mary's experience in childbirth.   4649

⟨1/q⟩ Mary and Lincoln wanted a daughter, a wish expressed some time after the birth of Tad. [randallA pp34-35]   4650

   ⟨-⟩ *This supports the speculation that Mary was unable to have children after delivering Tad. Both parents wanted a daughter and the family finances would have supported a fourth child (Edward was, by then, already dead).*   4651

Reproductive (continued)

Of course, it is also possible that Lincoln was unable to produce any more children.

⟨s⟩ "In that era four children to a family was the requirement for continuance of the family stock, since the death-rate was high. ... It is a pretty good guess that in Springfield about 1850 at least one fourth of the babies failed to survive babyhood, and on Mrs. Lincoln's level probably the expectation was a survival rate of, say, less than five sixths." [evans p137] *4652*

⟨2⟩ While there were financial concerns in the first decade of the Lincolns' married life [evans p236], their situation seems to have "improved considerably" in the 1850s [evans p237]. However, in 1858 Lincoln said "I am absolutely without money now even for household expenses" [evans p238]. (He had been debating Douglas and neglecting his law practice.) Censuses taken in 1850, 1855 (Illinois), and 1860, show that his household expenses included a servant [templeC]. *4653*

⟨2⟩ "Although Lincoln had a respectable law practice, it did not generate enough income for luxuries like travel abroad." [burl p321] *4654*

⟨2⟩ Lincoln's finances have been treated in a book: [prattB] *4655*

⟨s⟩ "The careful two-and-a-half-year intervals between the births of the Lincoln children suggested that the parents were using some form of birth control. Doubtless they relied on the widespread belief that conception could not take place so long as the mother was nursing." [donaldA p154]. Mary did not wean her babies until they were 18 months old [donaldA p154]. *4656*

⟨1⟩ May 1868: "I am *permitted* to sit up, whilst I write you ... for the past three weeks I have been seriously sick. (My disease is of a womanly nature, which you will understand has been) greatly accelerated by the last three years of mental suffering. Since the birth of my youngest son, for about twelve years I have been more or less a sufferer. My physician, Dr. Clarke ... told me on yesterday, that he must prescribe an entire change of air, scene, for me. He thought going abroad – would alone benefit me" – Mary [turner pp475-476] (The words in parentheses are crossed out in the handwritten version.) *4657*

⟨-⟩ *In 1868 Tad would have been 15 years old. Mary would certainly know he was not 12. Her motives in reporting time were not always pure (¶3968).* *4658*

⟨2⟩ "There are a few other veiled references to 'troubles of a womanly nature' in her letters, but for the most part little is known of the effect of this injury on Mary's health" [randallC p132]. *The references are so veiled that I missed them!* *4659*

■ Speculations on "troubles of a womanly nature" have been extensive, but weakly supported: *4660*

⟨s⟩ Tad's birth may have left Mary unable to have further children. [donaldA p154] *4661*

⟨s⟩ "It is possible that sexual relations between the Lincolns ceased thereafter." [burl p322] *Elsewhere* [burl] *notes that in 1860 sleeping apart was unusual for the Lincolns. See ¶3499.* *4662*

⟨s⟩ Tad's "large head may account for the injury his mother received at his birth" [randallC pp131, 106] *4663*

⟨s⟩ "She suffered much from menstrual cramps." [donaldA p108] *No source is given for this statement.* *4664*

Skin

⟨2⟩ "Color rose easily to her face." [randallA p7] 4665

⟨2⟩ "very fair skin" [randallA p6] 4666

⟨2⟩ As a young woman: "lovely complexion" [helmA] (∈ ¶3999, ¶4000) 4667

Mary

⟨$\frac{1}{q}$⟩ March 1, 1861: A man recalls shaking hands with Mary: "She had no gloves on & put out her hand. It is not soft." [randallC p84] 4668

⟨2⟩ May 11, 1871: "looks very pale" [ChicagoTribune - May 16, 1871] (∈ ¶4169) 4669

⟨2⟩ July 1878: "suffering great pain from boils" [evans p227] (See ¶4176) 4670

    ⟨2⟩ Sometime in 1876-1878 a letter from Mary mentions "boils under her left arm" and the ineffectiveness of the spa waters at Vichy, France [emersonA]. 4671

  ■ Early summer 1882 (part of her final illness – see ¶4062): 4672

    ⟨$\frac{1}{q}$⟩ "for several weeks of late she has been greatly troubled by boils, which made their appearance on every part of her body, due to her peculiar disease and sedentary habits" [ChicagoTribune - July 17, 1882] (Part of ¶4060.) 4673

    ⟨$\frac{1}{q}$⟩ "Within the past few days Mrs. Lincoln has been suffering from an attack of boils which caused her great pain" – Illinois State Journal, Monday, July 17, 1882 [evans pp343-344] (Part of ¶4062.) 4674

    ⟨2⟩ "she was again afflicted with boils, and was very ill and uncomfortable" [evans p228]. 4675

Sleep & Circadian Rhythms

⟨1⟩ July 1840, on extended visit to Missouri: "we regularly take our afternoon *siestas*" [turner p17] 4676

  ■ See ⟨Abraham⟩ ⟨Sleep & Circadian Rhythms⟩ for the Lincolns' sleeping arrangements. 4677

⟨$\frac{1}{q}$⟩ In Springfield: Mary would sometimes "lie abed and hour or two" after Lincoln prepared the breakfast and dressed the children – Mrs. Bradford [burl p279] 4678

⟨2⟩ "Sometimes she could not sleep at night and called for neighbors to be with her. James Gourley claimed she once invited him to join her in bed." [kunhardtA p96] *Is this over-interpreting ¶4296?* 4679

⟨1⟩ Feb. 1869: dreamed of Willie [turner p502] 4680

Speech

⟨2⟩ She spoke quickly. [randallA p7] 4681

⟨$\frac{1}{q}$⟩ "She thought quickly, spoke rapidly." – Henry B. Rankin, who worked in the Lincoln-Herndon law office [evans p153] 4682

⟨$\frac{1}{q}$⟩ Sept. 4, 1870: "very decided Southern accent" – Benjamin Moran [randallC p379] 4683

⟨2⟩ In the first moments after her husband's shooting, Mary shrieked Help! Help! Help! "followed by a series of words that made no sense at all – gibberish, insane sounds that filled the stunned theatre." [kunhardtB p40] 4684

Trauma

[Gait], [Nervous System], and [Trauma] all contain information related to Mary's later-years back problems.   4686

⟨2⟩ "Mary seemed destined to carriage accidents" [randallC p291]. Besides those below,   4687
c   others occurred in 1864 (iron hoop pierces the floor) [randallC p291] and late 1863 (her carriage ran over a boy, breaking his leg) [randallC p297].

⟨1⟩ July 2, 1863: injured her head in a fall from her carriage [boyden pp143-144]:   4688
   ⟨1⟩ Lincoln set out from the Soldier's Home to the White House with a heavy   4689
bodyguard, "Mrs. Lincoln following shortly after in a carriage. Meanwhile the screws that held the driver's seat in place, had been removed by unknown hands. When at the top of a winding declivity, the seat gave way, precipitating the driver and footman to the ground. The horses became unmanageable, and Mrs. Lincoln, in trying to get from the carriage, was also thrown to the ground, against a sharp stone, receiving a dangerous wound upon the head. She was carried to the nearest hospital, her wounds were dressed, and she was conveyed back to the Soldiers' Home. ... For three weeks she [Mrs. Pomroy] was a close attendant, night and day, in the sick room." [boyden pp143-144]

   ⟨1⟩ July 3: Lincoln telegraphs Robert: "Dont be uneasy. Your mother very slightly   4690
hurt by her fall." [donaldH p86]

   ⟨2⟩ Wound became "infected and suppurated." On July 11, Lincoln wires Robert   4691
to come home. [randallC p291] *Randall's source is unclear to me. It's not [boyden]. I cannot tell whether the telegram is really related to Mary.*

   ⟨1⟩ Late March 1865: "I think Mother has never quite recovered from the effects   4692
of her fall." – Robert [helmB p250]

   ⟨-⟩ *Given Lincoln's assessment and Mary's known tendency toward medical*   4693
drama, the actual seriousness of her injury is unclear.

⟨2⟩ March 26, 1865: While visiting City Point in southern Virginia, Mary struck her   4694
head on the ceiling of her carriage when it jolted, crushing her bonnet. That day and that evening she launched public, hysterical tirades at her husband. She was ill over the next several days and spent most of her time in her cabin aboard the ship that had brought her there. [donaldA pp572-573]

   ⟨S⟩ "Probably had an attack of migraine" [donaldA p572]. Also calls it a "bout of   4695
paranoia" [donaldH p107].

   ⟨S⟩ Gen. Horace Porter, who was also in the carriage, attributed Mrs. Lincoln's   4696
outburst to the jolting, but another contemporary, a Gen. Badeau, seems to believe it was simple jealousy. [evans pp297-298] [badeau pp355-364]

   ⟨2⟩ [burl pp288-289] devotes two full pages to the extended incident and does not   4697
mention a head injury.

   ⟨-⟩ *Among present-day historians, recall that Donald was trained by J.G. Ran-*   4698
dall, who was sympathetic to Mary Lincoln. Burlingame, on the other hand, puts more stock in Herndon's data.

- Back injuries: 4699
   ⟨2⟩ December 1879: Falls from a step-ladder while fixing curtains "in her simple   4700
home" in Pau, France. She hurt her back, "seriously, she thought. ... When she was able to travel, she returned to America, arriving in October 1880." [evans p227]

   ⟨2⟩ [baker p364] says this fall injured "an already arthritic spine" and that "Four   4701
months later she fell again when her left side gave way on a flight of stairs.

Trauma (continued)

Plasters and bed rest helped."

⟨1⟩ Of presumably the first fall: "The chief injuries she sustained by this fall   4702
manifested themselves in an inflammation of the spinal cord and a partial
paralysis of the lower part of her body. For these injuries she twice consulted   Mary
Dr. Lewis A. Sayre of this city. In October 1881, she came to New York to
see Doctor Sayre for the second time. ... About January 1, 1882, Doctor Sayre
said: 'I found she could not walk safely without the aid of a chair and even
then she was liable to fall at times.' Later, Mrs. Lincoln moved to a water-cure
establishment on 26th Street, where she remained under Doctor Sayre's care
until March, when she returned to Springfield, but little improved in health."
– New York *Graphic*, July 18, 1882 [evans pp342-343]. Also noted by [evans pp227-228]

⟨$\frac{1}{q}$⟩ [hirschhorn] quotes at length from interviews of Dr. Sayre in 1881 and 1882. Sev-   4703
eral inconsistencies in Sayre's accounts are noted. For more on Dr. Sayre, see
¶4627. Also, ¶4183 quotes an 1882 physician examination bearing on this
incident.

⟨2⟩ Because of her "crippled condition" in 1882 Mary was advised by Dr. Sayre to   4704
get a maid or a nurse. She did not, because of financial considerations. [evans
p311]

⟨2⟩ Of the fall in Pau: "from the effects of which she never fully recovered"   4705
[ChicagoTribune - July 17, 1882] (obituary)

Travel & Dwellings

⟨2⟩ Summer 1840: Spent several months in Columbia, Missouri, at an uncle's house   4706
[turner p12]

⟨2⟩ 1842: Railroad ride to Jacksonville, Illinois [randallC pp54-55]   4707

■ Lincoln in Congress (1847-1849):   4708

⟨2⟩ Oct. 1847: To Washington, DC with Lincoln, Robert, and Eddie, via St. Louis   4709
and Lexington. (See ¶3657.) Returns to Lexington with Robert and Eddie by
April 1848 [randallC pp92-96]. ([angle p145] says returned at end of winter.)

⟨1⟩ Sept. 1848: to Boston for three weeks [turner p463].   4710

⟨2⟩ Fall 1848: Also on this trip: Buffalo, Chicago, and Springfield with Robert and   4711
Eddie [randallC pp112-113]. (See ¶3661.)

■ Accompanied Lincoln on several pre-presidential trips mentioned in ¶3668ff.   4712

⟨2⟩ 1859: "a number of trips," not all with the children [randallC p157]   4713

⟨$\frac{1}{q}$⟩ Sept. 1859: Columbus and Cincinnati, Ohio with Lincoln and one son. [ran-   4714
dallC p157]

⟨1⟩ Fourth quarter 1859: "a week in St. Louis" visiting cousins [turner p61]   4715

⟨2⟩ Jan. 1861: To New York for shopping. See ¶4395.   4716

⟨1⟩ 1861: Two shopping trips to New York within six months after inauguration, the   4717
second extending to Boston to visit Robert [grimsley].

■ 1863:   4718

⟨2⟩ Spring: To Aquia Creek, VA with Lincoln and Tad [randallC pp288-289]   4719

⟨2⟩ June: To Philadelphia with Tad. [randallC p290] [miers]   4720

⟨2⟩ August: To the White Mountains (New Hampshire) to escape the heat, with   4721
Robert [randallC p292]

⟨1⟩ To New York in September and December. See Special Topic §5.   4722

Travel & Dwellings (continued)

⟨2⟩ Mary and Tad away from Washington much in second half of 1863 [randallC 4723
p293]

■ Special Topic §9 lists travels beginning in 1865. 4724

Voice

⟨1/q⟩ "Her voice was shrill and at times so penetrating, especially when summoning 4725
the children or railing at some one whose actions had awakened her temper,
she could easily be heard over the neighborhood." – a Springfield neighbor [burl
pp272,359]

⟨1/q⟩ 1860: "soft sweet voice" – Thomas Webster [randallC p163, 84] 4726

⟨1/q⟩ 1860s: "cheery voice" – Elizabeth Keckley [randallC p84] 4727

⟨2⟩ In the minutes and hours after her husband's shooting, Mary "gave herself up 4728
to spasms of sobbing that reverted unpredictably to deafening, high-register
screams." [kunhardtB p48]

Lincoln, Nancy Hanks mother

Nancy

Chronology

Born Feb. 5, 1784; married June 12, 1806 [templeC] [wilson p96n]; died Oct. 5, 1818 [wilson pp97,111]   4729

Introduction & Sources

⟨2⟩ Herndon says there were two women named Nancy Hanks who were related to each other: one the mother of Lincoln, the other the mother of Dennis Hanks. Herndon speculates some recollections of Nancy Hanks confuse these women [hertz pp 139-140, 206] and offers some evidence (¶4768).   4732

⟨2⟩ "There is no photograph of Lincoln's mother. [She] died more than twenty years before the invention of the camera." [ostendorfA p296]   4733

⟨1⟩ Lincoln "had very faint recollections of his own mother." – Leonard Swett [riceA p457]   4734

Family History

Nancy's father is unknown to history, and may have been unknown to her, too. He is of interest because [aa127] finds that two-thirds of de novo MEN2B arises in females, specifically from the father's gamete.   4735

⟨2⟩ Nancy was raised by Thomas and Elizabeth Hanks Sparrow [wilson p123n] or, at least, lived with them "a good bit" [tarbellE p232]. They died of the milk sick in the same season as Mary [angle p19] [nicolayB v1p31].   4736

■ William Herndon's data: 4737
  ⟨1⟩ "Mr. Lincoln told me himself that his mother was a bastard, a child of a Virginia nabob." – William Herndon [hertz p59].   4738
  ⟨1⟩ Herndon also calls the father "some *high blood rake* [not] a common man" [hertz p55] and "a Virginia planter" [hertz p138].   4739
  ⟨1⟩ Lincoln, about 1851, quoted by Herndon: "My mother was a bastard, was the daughter of a nobleman so called of Virginia. ... My mother inherited his qualities and I hers. All that I am or hope ever to be I get from my mother... Did you never notice that bastards are generally smarter, shrewder, and more intellectual than others? Is it because it is stolen?" [hertz pp73-74]   4740

⟨H⟩ According to [barbeeP - box 2 folder 68], a book called *The Sorrows of Nancy* (by Lucinda Rogers Boyd, Richmond, VA: O.E. Flauhart Printing Co., 1899) states that Nancy's father was the adopted son of Chief Justice John Marshall (pp35-37). The book also believes the Inloe theory of Lincoln's illegitimacy (¶44) and describes young Abraham being present when Nancy and Thomas got their marriage license. *Sarah is not mentioned, which suggests that this is not a very credible source. Plus, more recent scholarship has established that the Lincolns were married before Abraham was born.*   4741

Appearance

⟨1⟩ "... a Medium Sized Woman, rather spar[e] in her person, fair complexion, Light   4742
Hair, Blue Eyes, neat in her person & Habits, industrious, of a Kind disposition" –
A.H. Chapman [wilson p97]

- John Hanks: 4743
  ⟨1⟩ "She was a tall Slender woman – dark Skinned – black hair & Eyes – her face   4744
  was Sharp & angular – forehead high – She was beyond all doubt an intellectual woman – rather Extraordinary if any thing. ... her nature was Kindness –
  mildness – tenderness – Sadness ... Abrm was like his mother very much." –
  John Hanks [wilson p454]
  ⟨1⟩ "5 ft. 10 in in hight she had Black haire Dark Eye and Dark complexion ... she   4745
  was a shrowd woman she was not much of talkative Dark complextion Dark
  Eye Black haire she weigh about 130 or 140 her hight were 6 ft" – John Hanks,
  1887 [wilson p615] *No explanation for the height contradiction is offered or
  apparent.*
  ⟨1⟩ "she had dark, Hare, Hazle, Eyes, was 5 feet 7 inches high a spare delicate   4746
  frame, weighed about 120 pounds, had a clear intilectual mind, was amible,
  kind, charitable and affectionate" – John Hanks [wilson p5]
- Nathaniel Grigsby: 4747
  ⟨1⟩ "a lady of medium size lite complection and dark hair being a lady of intili-   4748
  gence" – Nathaniel Grigsby [wilson p94]
  ⟨1⟩ "pale Complexion – dark hair – sharp features – high forehead – bright Keen   4749
  gray – or hazle Eyes" – Nathaniel Grigsby [wilson p113]

⟨1⟩ "Spare Made thin visage Remarkable Keen perseption lite hare and Blew Eyes" –   4750
Dennis Hanks [wilson p149]

⟨1⟩ "Mrs Lincoln was not of dark complexion as the Century has it – She was very fair   4751
– almost sandy blue eyes freckled face and had two very large 'butter teeth', She
could not read or write or sing" – James Rardin [wilson p652] *Rardin's reference to
the "Century" is presumably to a series of articles by John Nicolay and John
Hay that began running in The Century magazine in 1886.*

⟨1⟩ "Ms C has seen first Mrs L. but cannot recollect much of her appear   she was   4752
intelligent [& keen?] [withal?] delicate spare made woman" – Harriet Chapman
interview [wilson p646] *But* [wilson p646n] *says Chapman was born after Nancy died.*

⟨2⟩ "She was above the ordinary height in stature, weighed about 130 pounds, was   4753
slenderly built, and had much the appearance of one inclined to consumption.
Her skin was dark; hair dark brown; eyes gray and small; forehead prominent; face
sharp and angular, with a marked expression of melancholy which fixed itself in
the memory of everyone who ever saw or knew her." [herndon p14] (Continues as
¶4864.)

Build

Historians express some frustration at the conflicting descriptions of Nancy Hanks Lin-   4754
coln's build (e.g. ¶4777). Superficially, there do seem to be contradictions, but after
eliminating those descriptions containing identifiable errors (¶4765ff) and those with
ambiguous pronouns (¶5037), a consistent picture emerges.

One hundred years after Nancy's death, the average height of 211 white women in Vir-   4755
ginia and Tennessee was 5-feet 3.7-inches (range 4' 9" to 5' 9.7") and the average weight
was 127 lbs [stewart]. Thus, Nancy was considerably above average in height, and only
average in weight.

Build (continued)

⟨2⟩ "Most testimony describes Nancy Hanks as taller than average." [wilson p84n]　　4756
c

■ Dennis Hanks:　　4757
  ⟨1⟩ "5-8 in high – Spare made" – Dennis Hanks [wilson p37]　　4758
  ⟨1⟩ "Spare Made" – Dennis Hanks [wilson p149] (Part of ¶4750)　　4759
  ⟨1⟩ "was a spare made woman – little above ordinary height" – Dennis Hanks　　4760
    [wilson p598]

■ John Hanks:　　4761
  ⟨1⟩ "5 feet 7 inches high a spare delicate frame, weighed about 120 pounds" –　　4762
    John Hanks [wilson p5] (Part of ¶4746)
  ⟨1⟩ "tall Slender woman" – John Hanks [wilson p454] Part of ¶4744　　4763
  ⟨1⟩ "5 ft. 10 in in hight ... she weigh about 130 or 140 her hight were 6 ft" – John　　4764
    Hanks [wilson p615] (∈ ¶4745) *Note the self-contradiction.*

■ Haycrafts:　　4765
  ⟨1⟩ "rather a heavy built Squatty woman, (the Lord only knows except Abe Enlow　　4766
    did where Lincoln got his length & his sense)" – Samuel Haycraft [wilson p84]
    Haycraft's opinion on Lincoln's paternity is apparent – see ¶44.
  ⟨1⟩ "She was a woman of rather low stature but heavy & well set" – Samuel Hay-　　4767
    craft [wilson p67] *Haycraft goes on to mis-identify Nancy's mother as being*
    a member of the Young family – see ¶5797.
  ⟨1⟩ To answer a question about his mother, Lincoln wrote a letter to Samuel　　4768
  q Haycraft, saying: "In the main you are right about my history. ... You are
    mistaken about my mother; her maiden name was Nancy Hanks." Hern-
    don believes that Haycraft confused two women named Nancy Hanks [hertz
    pp69, 206]. ([baslerA v4pp57-58] reprints Lincoln's letter and echoes Herndon's be-
    lief.) *Given that Haycraft's descriptions of Nancy are outliers, and given*
    the fact that Haycraft mis-identified Lincoln's mother, it seems prudent to
    ignore Haycraft's description of Nancy.
  ⟨1⟩ "was of good size" – Presley Haycraft [wilson p87]　　4769

■ William Herndon:　　4770
  ⟨2⟩ "above the ordinary height in stature, weighed about 130 pounds, was slen-　　4771
    derly built, and had much the appearance of one inclined to consumption"
    [herndon p14] (∈ ¶4753)

■ Others:　　4772
  ⟨1⟩ "delicate spare made woman" – Harriet Chapman [wilson p646] (Part of ¶4752)　　4773
  ⟨1⟩ "medium size" – Nathaniel Grigsby [wilson p94] ¶4748　　4774
  ⟨1⟩ "a Medium Sized Woman, rather spar[e] in her person" – A.H. Chapman [wil-　　4775
    son p97] Part of ¶4742
  ⟨H⟩ "I have understood that she was rather above average size for women" –　　4776
    William Greene [wilson p11]

⟨2⟩ "Many years later those who had known her described her variously as being tall　　4777
  or of average height, thin or stout, beautiful or plain." [donaldA p23]
  ⟨-⟩ *Donald may be confused by the description of Lincoln's family in an 1887*　　4778
    letter by cousin John Hanks [wilson p615] *¶4745. Hanks is barely literate,*
    and the organization of his remarks is confusing. In particular, one para-
    graph describes a stocky woman, without explicitly identifying her. The
    person described in the previous paragraph of that letter is Lincoln's mother
    Nancy. It is possible that Donald believed the unidentified stocky woman
    to be Nancy, even though the descriptions in the two paragraphs are quite

Nancy

313

different. I believe the unidentified stocky woman is Sarah Lincoln; see ¶5037.

Chest & Shoulders

⟨2⟩ "stoop-shouldered, thin-breasted, sad" [currentEB]   4779

Death & Final Illness

It is generally thought that Nancy died of an epidemic non-infectious disease, "the   4780
milk-sick," in her son's tenth year [herndon p26]. I do not accept this as certain, however,
as multiple accounts suggest a longer-term wasting disease was present (¶4800).

    ⟨-⟩ *Milk-sickness results from toxins in the white snakeroot plant. Through*   4781
       their milk, cows that ate the plant would transmit the toxin to humans
       [donaldA p26].

⟨1⟩ "During my mother's last sickness, Mrs. Lincoln, the mother of Abraham Lincoln,   4782
came to see her. Mother said, 'I believe I will have to die.' Mrs. Lincoln said, 'Oh,
you may outlive me.' She died just one week from the death of my mother. This
was in October, 1818. I was five years old when mother died." – Allen Brooner
[hobson p19] *The Brooners lived a half-mile from the Lincolns.*

⟨S⟩ She died within a week of becoming ill. [herndon p26]   4783

⟨S⟩ "To this day the medical profession has never agreed upon any definite cause for   4784
the malady, nor have they in all their scientific wrangling determined exactly what
the disease itself is. A physician, who has in his practice met a number of cases,
describes the symptoms to be 'a whitish coat on the tongue, burning sensation of
the stomach, severe vomiting, obstinate constipation of the bowels, coolness of
the extremities, great restlessness and jactitation, pulse rather small, somewhat
more frequent than natural, and lightly chorded. In the course of the disease the
coat on the tongue becomes brownish and dark, the countenance dejected, and
the prostration of the patient is great. A fatal termination may take place in sixty
hours, or life may be prolonged for a period of fourteen days. These are the symptoms of the disease in an acute form. Sometimes it runs into the chronic form, or
it may assume that form from the commencement, and after months or years the
patient may finally die or recover only a partial degree of health.' " [herndon pp25-26]

    ⟨-⟩ *Jactitation is marked restlessness, e.g. tossing about from side to side.*   4785
    ⟨2⟩ Agrees with: [shutes pp4-5], who identifies the physician author of the above   4786
       passage as Dr. Theodore Lemon of Danville, IL and adds that the disease re-
       sults from "the ingestion of milk or meat from cows feeding on white snake-
       root (Eupatorium uticaefolium) and rayless goldenrod (Aplopappus hetero-
       phyllus)."
    ⟨S⟩ It would not have been surprising if Josiah Crawford (see ¶3158) had at-   4787
       tended Nancy and had bled her [shutes p5].

⟨2⟩ "Typically, victims of tremetol poisoning, brought on by drinking the milk of cows   4788
that had eaten white snakeroot, lie on their backs with their legs up and spread
apart. Their breath grows ever shorter, their skin turns clammy and cold, their
pulse becomes irregular, finally they slip into a coma." [burl p94]

⟨2⟩ From an affected animal, "An ounce of butter or cheese, or four ounces of the   4789
beef, raw or boiled, three times a day will kill a dog within six days." [osler p266]
*Interestingly, adults, not children, seemed to have succumbed in the extended
Lincoln family. How much dairy did children of that era routinely consume?*

⟨2⟩ The milk sick returned to Lincoln's neighborhood in 1829 and was part of the im-   4790
petus behind the Lincolns' moving to Illinois. [herndon p56]

314

Death & Final Illness (continued)

⟨S⟩ Fanciful depictions of Nancy's death, having no basis I can find in primary   4791
sources, are in [sandburgA pp39-40] and [jordan]

- Diagnoses – milk sickness: 4792
  ⟨1⟩ "The Disease of Which She died was Milk Sick." – A.H. Chapman [wilson p97]   4793
  ⟨1⟩ "A Lincolns Mother [died] from Milk Sickness" – A.H. Chapman [wilson p103]:   4794
  ⟨1⟩ "Mrs Lincoln died of what is commonly called 'milk sickness' " – J.W. Wart-   4795    Nancy
  mann [wilson p660]:
  ⟨1⟩ "was taken sick with a disease called the Milk Sickness or puken a desease   4796
  commin at that time in the western contry her sickness was short but fatal
  as she deseas this life Oct 1818" – Nathaniel Grigsby [wilson p93]
  ⟨1⟩ "... and Milk Sick plenty   all of my Relitives Died with that Disease on Little   4797
  pigeon Creek Spencer County" – Dennis Hanks [wilson p154] *This included*
  Thomas and Betsey Hanks Sparrow, who raised Dennis (¶4736) [wilson
  pp97, 219, 242]. *Hanks lost four milk cows and eleven calves in one week*
  [angle p33] *(reprinting* [sandburgP]*).*
  ⟨1⟩ "'Bout the time we got our cabins up the Sparrows both died o' milk sickness   4798
  ⟨q̄⟩ an' I went to Tom's to live. Then Nancy died o' the same disease. The cow et
  pizen weeds, I reckon. Oh Lord, oh Lord, I'll never furgit it, the mizry in that
  cabin in the woods when Nancy died. [Lincoln] never got over the mizable
  way his mother died." – Dennis Hanks [wilsonR]
  ⟨2⟩ [tripp p24] identified the milk sick as "probably brucellosis," yet adheres to the   4799
  idea of "poisonous snakeroot" ingestion by cows as the base cause.

- Diagnoses – other: 4800
  ⟨1⟩ "Some said she died of heart trouble, from slanders about her and Old Abe   4801
  Enloe" – Christopher Graham [tarbellE p233]. (See ¶44.)
  ⟨1⟩ "Mrs. Lincoln died – said by some with the milk sickness, some with a gal-   4802
  loping quick consumption." – William Herndon, 1870 [hertz p74]
  ⟨1⟩ "I do not think she absolutely died of the Milk Sickness Entirely. Probably   4803
  this helped to seal her fate." – William Wood [wilson p124]:

⟨2⟩ Buried in Pigeon Church cemetery, as is her daughter. [lincloreBAI]   4804

Eyes

- John Hanks: 4805
  ⟨1⟩ "black hair & Eyes" – John Hanks [wilson p454] Part of ¶4744   4806
  ⟨1⟩ "Hazle, Eyes" –John Hanks [wilson p5] (Part of ¶4746)   4807
  ⟨1⟩ "Dark Eye" – John Hanks [wilson p615]   4808

- Dennis Hanks: 4809
  ⟨1⟩ "Blew Eyes" – Dennis Hanks [wilson p149] (Part of ¶4750)   4810
  ⟨1⟩ "eyes hazel" – Dennis Hanks [wilson p598]   4811

- Others: 4812
  ⟨1⟩ "Blue Eyes" – A.H. Chapman [wilson p97] (Part of ¶4742):   4813
  ⟨1⟩ "bright Keen gray – or hazle Eyes" – Nathaniel Grigsby [wilson p113] (Part of   4814
  ¶4749):
  ⟨1⟩ "almost sandy blue eyes" – James Rardin [wilson p652] Part of ¶4751:   4815
  ⟨2⟩ "eyes gray and small" [herndon p14] (∈ ¶4753)   4816

General

⟨1/q⟩ "Abe's said many a time that Nancy'd lived if she'd had any kind of keer; an' I reckon she must have been strong to 'a' stood what she did." – Dennis Hanks, referring to life in Kentucky [wilsonR p29]   4817

Hair

- John Hanks: 4818
  ⟨1⟩ "black hair & Eyes" – John Hanks [wilson p454] Part of ¶4744   4819
  ⟨1⟩ "dark, Hare" –John Hanks [wilson p5] (Part of ¶4746)   4820
  ⟨1⟩ "Black haire" – John Hanks [wilson p615] (Part of ¶4745)   4821

- Dennis Hanks: 4822
  ⟨1⟩ "hair dark brown" – Dennis Hanks [wilson p598]   4823
  ⟨1⟩ "lite hair" – Dennis Hanks [wilson p149] (Part of ¶4750)   4824

- Others::   4825
  ⟨1⟩ "Light Hair" – A.H. Chapman [wilson p97] (Part of ¶4742):   4826
  ⟨1⟩ "dark hair" – Nathaniel Grigsby [wilson p94] (Part of ¶4748):   4827
  ⟨1⟩ "dark hair" – Nathaniel Grigsby [wilson p113] (Part of ¶4749):   4828
  ⟨2⟩ "hair dark brown" [herndon p14] (∈ ¶4753)   4829

Head & Face

⟨1⟩ "her face was Sharp & angular – forehead high" – John Hanks [wilson p454] Part of ¶4744   4830

⟨1⟩ "thin visage" – Dennis Hanks [wilson p149] (Part of ¶4750)   4831

⟨1⟩ "comely" – Presley Haycraft [wilson p87]   4832

⟨1⟩ "sharp features – high forehead" – Nathaniel Grigsby [wilson p113] (Part of ¶4749)   4833

⟨2⟩ "forehead prominent; face sharp and angular, with a marked expression of melancholy" [herndon p14] (∈ ¶4753)   4834

⟨2⟩ "all agree that she was sad-faced..." [shutesE p14]   4835

⟨2⟩ "is said to have been in her youth a woman of beauty" [arnold p19]   4836

⟨1⟩ 1836: Lincoln saw his overweight near-fiancee, Mary Owens, after a long separation, and wrote: "I could not for my life avoid thinking of my mother; and this, not from withered features for her skin was too full of fat, to permit its contracting to wrinkles; but from her want of teeth, [and] weather-beaten appearance in general." [baslerA v1p118] *The recipient may have thought this was an April Fool's joke by Lincoln* [walsh p119]. *I think it reasonable to assume Lincoln was referring to Nancy, and not to his step-mother, Sarah.*   4837

⟨1⟩ "freckled face" – James Rardin [wilson p652] Part of ¶4751   4838

⟨1⟩ At time of her marriage: "was a fresh and good-looking girl" – Christopher Graham [tarbellE p232]   4839

Infection – Exposures

- The following pertain to Nancy's potential exposure to sexually transmitted disease: 4840
  - ⟨H⟩ "She had a bad reputation." – William Herndon [burl p138] 4841
  - ⟨H⟩ "Not only was Nancy an illegitimate child herself but ... Nancy was not what she ought to have been herself. Loose." – recollection of a daughter of a Lincoln neighbor [burl p138] 4842
  - ⟨1/q⟩ Lincoln told Herndon that "his relations were lascivious – lecherous not to be trusted." [burl p138] 4843
  - ⟨H⟩ "N. Hanks was rather a loose woman. ... Nancy Hanks was loose woman" – Judge Alfred Brown [wilson p612] 4844
  - ⟨1⟩ "I was told that Ben Hardin, old Ben of Kentucky, used the 'gal' when he pleased." – William Herndon [hertz p170] 4845
  - ⟨-⟩ For possible involvements with Abe Enloe, see ¶47. 4846
  - ⟨-⟩ In connection with Nancy's "reputation," 8 months passed from her marriage to the birth of Sarah. No accounts of Sarah's birth exist, so it is unknown if she was premature or full term. Herndon's musings on the marriage are in [hertz p93]. 4847
- ⟨S⟩ "Nancy milked the cows until Sarah was old enough to relieve her of this duty; does not the word 'daughter' mean 'milker?'" [angle p13] (reprinting [bartonB]) 4848

Mental Status

- John Hanks: 4849
  - ⟨1⟩ "amible, kind, charitable and affectionate" –John Hanks [wilson p5] (Part of ¶4746) 4850
  - ⟨1⟩ "she was a shrowd [sic] woman she was not much of talkative" – John Hanks [wilson p615] 4851
  - ⟨1⟩ "She was very religious her dispstion [sic] was very quiet" – John Hanks [wilson p615] 4852
  - ⟨1⟩ "her nature was Kindness – mildness – tenderness – Sadness" – John Hanks [wilson p454] Part of ¶4744 4853
- Dennis Hanks: 4854
  - ⟨1⟩ "Meek quiet and amiable" – Dennis Hanks [wilson p27] 4855
  - ⟨1⟩ "affectionate, the most affectionate I ever saw – never knew her to be out of temper – and thought strange of it" – Dennis Hanks [wilson p37] 4856
  - ⟨1⟩ "easy temperament never Mad ... Abraham took his disposition and Mental qualities from his Mother ... Mrs. L. was sympathetic woman conscientious and of good intelligence" – Dennis Hanks [wilson p598] 4857
- ⟨1⟩ "industrious, of a Kind disposition" – A.H. Chapman [wilson p97] (Part of ¶4742) 4858
- ⟨1⟩ "She was naturally Strong minded – was a gentle, Kind and tender woman" – William Wood [wilson p124] 4859
- ⟨1⟩ About 1807-1812: "Nancy Hanks Lincoln – was in a constant trepidation and frequent affrights from reasons we have talked together about while she was pregnant" – Henry Whitney [wilson p617] 4860
  - ⟨-⟩ *Whitney labeled this passage "private" in an 1887 letter to William Herndon, and then crossed out the passage. Whitney believed ante natal impression of these trepidations and affrights were the cause of Lincoln's melancholy – see ¶2607.* 4861

Mental Status (continued)

⟨-⟩ *Whitney again alludes to ante natal impressions in* [wilson pp625-626].   4862

⟨1⟩ 1817, on the prospect of moving from Kentucky to Indiana: "Nancy got joyful like,   4863
mor'n any of 'em; for her and John Hanks war the fust that wanted to go." – a
neighbor [browneR v1p83]

⟨1⟩ She carried "a marked expression of melancholy which fixed itself in the memory   4864
of everyone who ever saw or knew her. Though her life was seemingly beclouded
by a spirit of sadness, she was in disposition amiable and generally cheerful. [Lin-
coln said] she was highly intellectual by nature, had a strong memory, acute judgment, and was cool and heroic." [herndon p14] (Continuation of ¶4753.)

- Reckless, etc.   4865
  ⟨2⟩ "I once saw a letter published ... in which Miss Hanks was described as a   4866
  cheerful, rollicking, daring, reckless 'gal,' breaking all the rules of propriety or forms, etc., in society, and that she became sad while in Indiana." –
  William Herndon [hertz p170]
  ⟨1⟩ "she was a bold, reckless, daredevil kind of a woman, stepping to the very   4867
  verge of propriety ... was an excellent woman and by nature an intellectual
  and sensitive woman. Lincoln, Abraham, told me that his mother was an
  intellectual woman, sensitive and somewhat sad." – William Herndon [hertz
  pp138-139]
  ⟨1⟩ "by nature a noble woman, free, easy, and unsuspecting" – William Herndon   4868
  [hertz p205]
  ⟨1⟩ "good cheer and hilarity generally accompanied her ... she was very sensitive,   4869
  sad, sometimes gloomy" – William Herndon [hertz p412]

Mouth

⟨1⟩ "two very large 'butter teeth' " – James Rardin [wilson p652] Part of ¶4751 *Meaning*   4870
is unknown to me.

⟨1⟩ Lincoln suggests she had a "want of teeth" – [baslerA v1p118]. See ¶4837.   4871

Nervous System

- Dennis Hanks & John Hanks: 4872
  ⟨1⟩ "Remarkable Keen perseption" – Dennis Hanks [wilson p149] (Part of ¶4750)   4873
  ⟨1⟩ "All of them [Lincoln and his parents] had good memories" – Dennis Hanks   4874
  [wilson p598]
  ⟨1⟩ " clear intilectual mind" –John Hanks [wilson p5] (Part of ¶4746)   4875
  ⟨1⟩ "beyond all doubt an intellectual woman" – John Hanks [wilson p454] Part of   4876
  ¶4744
  ⟨$\frac{1}{q}$⟩ "smart as you'd find 'em anywhere. She could read an' write." – Dennis   4877
  Hanks [wilsonR p21]

⟨1⟩ "a woman Know for the Extraordinary Strength of her mind" – Nathaniel Grigsby   4878
[wilson p113]

⟨1⟩ "intelligent" – Harriet Chapman [wilson p646] (Part of ¶4752)   4879

⟨1⟩ "Mrs Lincoln was a very smart – intelligent and intellectual woman" – William   4880
Wood [wilson p124]

- William Herndon's reports: 4881

Nervous System (continued)

⟨1/q⟩ Lincoln said "she was highly intellectual by nature, had a strong memory, acute judgment, and was cool and heroic" [herndon p14]. (∈ ¶4864) *Lincoln had a theory why this was so. See¶4740.*   4882

⟨1⟩ "She was an intellectual woman beyond a doubt. Her son told me so, and all other persons who knew the woman prove that she was rather a great woman." – William Herndon [hertz p204]   4883

⟨1⟩ "Mr. Lincoln told me that she was a genius and that he got his mind from her." – William Herndon [hertz p412]   4884

⟨1⟩ "a woman of very strong mind; it was not only strong but it was quick... a superior woman in *mind*." – William Herndon [hertz p55] *Herndon never met her.*   4885

- Singing: 4886
  ⟨1⟩ "She could not ... sing" – James Rardin [wilson p652] (Part of ¶4751)   4887
  ⟨1⟩ "Mrs. L. was a good singer and used to sing with Rev. Isaac Hodgen" – Robert Wintersmith [wilson p613] (See ¶5796)   4888

Physicians

- See the tabulations of Lincoln family physicians in Kentucky (¶3153) and Indiana (¶3158).   4889

⟨2⟩ Dr. Christopher Columbus Graham witnessed the marriage of Thomas and Nancy, and left a long statement of his memories of the Lincolns when he was 99 years old [tarbellE pp227-236].. "I was hunting roots for my medicine, and just went to the wedding to get a good supper, and got it." – Graham [tarbellE p 232].   4890

Reading & Learning

⟨1⟩ "she was a shrowd [sic] woman she was not much of talkative" – John Hanks [wilson p615]   4891

⟨1⟩ "She could not read or write" – James Rardin [wilson p652] Part of ¶4751   4892

⟨1⟩ "could read the Bible" – Dennis Hanks [wilson p598]   4893

⟨1/q⟩ "She could read an' write." – Dennis Hanks [wilsonR p21] (∈ ¶4877)   4894

Reproductive

- See ¶4860 and ¶2607 for mental status during pregnancy.   4895

⟨1⟩ "bred like a rat in Kentucky, she had no more children in Indiana ... had no children while in the prime and glory of her good life." – William Herndon [hertz pp138-139] *Herndon is trying to determine whether the lack of further children was due to a fault in Thomas or Nancy.*   4896

  ⟨S⟩ "Why did she cease thus to bear children? Because Thomas was castrated." – William Herndon, 1887 [hertz p206] *It is also possible that an underlying illness, say, an MEN2B cancer, made Nancy infertile.*   4897

Nancy

Skin

⟨1⟩ Lincoln suggests her skin was "contracting to wrinkles" and had a "weather-beaten appearance in general" – [baslerA v1p118]. See ¶4837.   4898

⟨1⟩ "fair complexion" ¶4742; "lite complection" ¶4748; "Dark complextion" ¶4745   4899

⟨1⟩ "sandy complexion" – Dennis Hanks [wilson p598]   4900

⟨1⟩ "dark Skinned" – John Hanks [wilson p454] Part of ¶4744   4901

⟨1⟩ "Dark complextion" – John Hanks [wilson p615]   4902

⟨1⟩ "pale Complexion" – Nathaniel Grigsby [wilson p113] (Part of ¶4749)   4903

⟨1⟩ "Mrs Lincoln was not of dark complexion ... She was very fair ... freckled face" – James Rardin [wilson p652] Part of ¶4751   4904

⟨2⟩ "Her skin was dark." [herndon p14] (∈ ¶4753)   4905

Lincoln, Robert

child #1

Chronology

Robert

Mo.	Yr	Age	Home	Event	Ref.	4906
Aug.	1843	0	Springfield, IL	born		
Sept.	1859	16	Exeter, NH	Student		
	1860	17	Cambridge, MA	Harvard student		
	1864	20	Washington, DC	White House		
Feb.	1865	21	Virginia	Army service (brief)	[kunhardtA p265]	
May	1865	21	Chicago (to 1911)		[turner p231]	
Feb.	1867	23	Chicago	Admitted to bar		
Sept.	1868	25	Chicago	Marries Mary Eunice Harlan	[turner p475]	
March	1881	37	Washington	Secretary of War (to 1885)		
March	1885	41	Chicago	Attorney		
March	1889	45	London	Minister to England (to 1893)		
March	1893	49	Chicago	Attorney		
	1897	53	Chicago	Pullman Co., Acting President		
	1901	57	Chicago	Pullman Co., President		
	1911	67	Vermont & Washington	Pullman Co., Chairman of Board		
	1922	78		Retires from Pullman Co.		
July	1926	82	Vermont	dies		

- ▪ 2/17/1865 Enters the Army [kunhardtA p265]; August 1859: leaves for school in the   4907
  East (Exeter, then Harvard) [turner p58]

⟨2⟩ "He was present at the assassination of two American presidents, and was within   4908
sounds of the shots that mortally wounded a third." [ChicagoTribune - July 27, 1926]
Really?

Introduction & Sources

Robert gets short shrift in the present volume – with no apologies. Whatever genetic   4909
illness Lincoln had, assuming it was a serious illness, Robert's longevity makes it unlikely he inherited the disease. Robert's history is most useful in identifying traits that
were not part of Lincoln's disorder.

Jason Emerson is working on a new biography of Robert to be titled *Giant in the Shad-*   4910
ows [emersonA]. The existing book-length biography is [goff].

Family History

⟨1⟩ "Bob's a Todd, not a Lincoln" – William Herndon [hertz p155] (See ¶4915 and ¶4967.)   4911

Appearance

⟨1⟩ As "a youth of seventeen or eighteen years; – well developed physically, a strong, healthy, resolute, sensible-looking fellow." – Senator James Harlan (date of recollection uncertain) [helmB p167]   4912

   ⟨2⟩ Robert ultimately married Harlan's daughter.   4913

- Resemblance to father: 4914

   ⟨$\frac{1}{q}$⟩ 1897: Ida Tarbell meets Robert for the first time and "devoured him with my eyes" looking for resemblances to Lincoln. "There was nothing. ... He was all Todd, a big plump man perhaps fifty years old." [neelyA p130] (See ¶4911.)   4915

   ⟨2⟩ "... was physically and mentally in marked contrast to his father. He was less than average height and plump and his features bore little resemblance to those of his father, for he distinctly took after the Todd side of the family. In complexion, however, he was dark and swarthy like his father. His voice, also, those who had heard the President said, had a marked likeness to his father's in sonority, volume, and timbre." – [NYTimesObitR]   4916

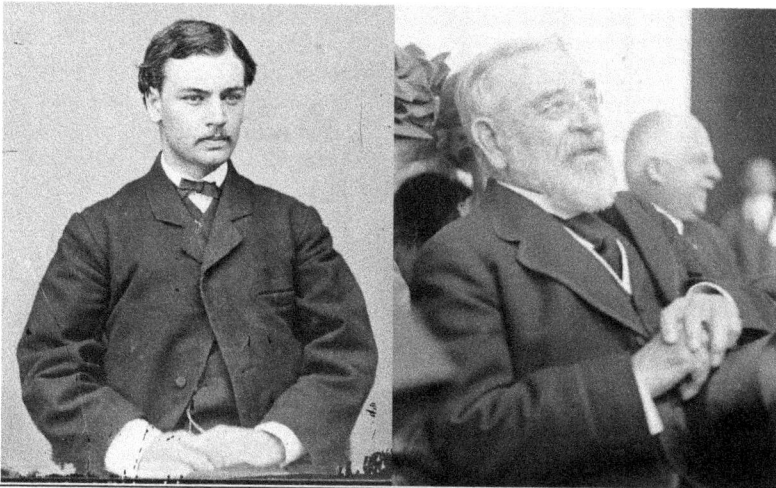

Figure 8. Robert Lincoln. Photographs taken 1865± and 1923. *Photo credits:* Library of Congress LC-DIG-cwpbh-04802 and LC-DIG-npcc-06387

Build

⟨$\frac{1}{q}$⟩ When younger brother Edward was 7 months old, Lincoln wrote: "He is very much such a child as Bob was at his age – rather of a longer order. Bob is 'short and low,' and, I expect, always will be." – Lincoln (Oct. 22, 1846) [prattA] [kunhardtA p90] [burl [61]   4917

⟨$\frac{1}{q}$⟩ 1897: "a big plump man" – Ida Tarbell [neelyA p130] (∈ ¶4915)   4918

⟨2⟩ "less than average height and plump" – [NYTimesObitR] (Part of ¶4916)   4919

Death

⟨2⟩ "... died peacefully ... His death was discovered by a servant, who went as usual to call Mr. Lincoln to breakfast. Dr. C. M. Campbell ... the family physician, declared death due to cerebral hemorrhage induced by arterio sclerosis [sic]. While Mr. Lincoln had not been in robust health for about three years, his recent health had been better than it was a year ago and he was enjoying a motor ride practically every day since he came to Manchester about the middle of May. He took his usual ride yesterday afternoon." – [NYTimesObitR] (from his obituary, headlined "Lincoln's son dies in his sleep")   4920

⟨2⟩ [ChicagoTribune - July 27, 1926] prints substantially the same text.   4921

Diet & Digestion

⟨2⟩ March 1861: Every member of the household became ill from eating too well of the unaccustomed Potomac shad." [shutes p77] See ¶640. *Unclear if Robert was still at the White House when this occurred, of if he had returned to college.*   4922

Eyes

- Deviation: 4923
  - ⟨2⟩ One eye turned inward. "His schoolmates called him 'cockeye,' which humiliated him." [oatesA p97]   4924
  - ⟨2⟩ "Robert had his crossed eyes to deal with." [randallA p55]   4925
  - ⟨2⟩ "Photographs ... show that he suffered from a vertical strabismus" [snyder].   4926
  - ⟨2⟩ "Photographs ... indicate that the esotropia had a vertical deviation also." [durham]   4927
- Treatment: 4928
  - ⟨2⟩ Dr. William Wallace (see ¶3195) "operated on Robert for crossed eyes" [kunhardtB p257]   4929
  - ⟨2⟩ "When he was twelve years old his mother took him to a famous New York surgeon who performed, without anesthesia, a painful operation that corrected the condition [crossed eyes]." [marx p179]   4930
  - ⟨2⟩ "he cured his defect by peeping through a keyhole" [randallC p240] citing Herndon-Weik papers   4931
  - ⟨2⟩ An unidentified Chicago oculist claimed, in 1883, to have treated Robert's eyes when he (Robert) was a child [lincloreLFH]. (See ¶785.)   4932
- ☐ Left eyebrow was higher than the right   4933
- ⟨2⟩ "eyes gray" [durham]   4934

General

⟨S⟩ Was likely breast fed, given that Mary breast fed a neighbor baby. (See ¶4647.)   4935

⟨2⟩ Was born "in the Old Globe tavern, where his parents were living." [ChicagoTribune - July 27, 1926]   4936

⟨2⟩ "The birth was easy and the baby strong" [turner p31] *But no primary source cited; see ¶4640.*   4937
  - ⟨1⟩ "had no nurse for herself or the baby" [randallC p72]   4938
  - ⟨2⟩ At the Globe: "Springfield tradition has it that other guests complained of the baby's crying." [randallC p75]   4939

⟨1q⟩ October 1863: Lincoln wires Robert: "Your letter makes us a little uneasy about your health. Telegraph us how you are. If you think it would help you make us a visit." [donaldH p106]   4940

Robert

General (continued)

⟨1/q⟩ November 1865: "good health" [turner p283n] quoting [ChicagoTribune] 4941

⟨1/q⟩ "I have not been sick in ten years." – part of his testimony at his mother's 1875 insanity trial [evans p216] 4942

⟨2⟩ 1911: Retired as President of Pullman Company because of "ill health" [shutesM]. 4943

⟨2⟩ May 30, 1922: Last public appearance, at dedication of the Lincoln Memorial in Washington. *Forgot where I read this.* 4944

⟨2⟩ 1923: Retired from the game of golf [shutesM]. 4945

⟨2⟩ 1926: In "feeble health," but able to be about [shutesM]. 4946

⟨2⟩ 1926: Obituary: "He was also a devotee of golf, and asserted to friends that it had saved his life, when his health failed, years ago." [ChicagoTribune - July 27, 1926] 4947

Habits

⟨1⟩ December 1865: "Your son, sent him, a souvenir of his visit to Havanna [sic], in some *cigarettes*" – Mary [turner p294]. *Whether Robert smoked them is not recorded.* 4948

Head & Face

⟨H⟩ In one story, Mary does not invite a cousin to a party who "had intimated that Robert L. who was baby was a sweet child but not good looking." – Harriet Chapman [wilson p646] 4949

⟨2⟩ "a good-looking young man" [donaldA p428] 4950

⟨○⟩ "Just about the only physical inheritance he possessed from his father was the dimple in his chin." [kunhardtB p288]. Photograph showing the dimple: [kunhardtA p6] [neelyA p195]. Lincoln's dimple: ¶1898. 4951

⟨2⟩ "his features bore little resemblance to those of his father, for he distinctly took after the Todd side of the family" – [NYTimesObitR] (Part of ¶4916) 4952

Infection

■ The dog bite: 4953
⟨1⟩ "Bob once had a little dog – he bit Bob – Lincoln took him off to the Mad Stone in Terrehaute or other place in Indiana I think." – Frances Todd Wallace [wilson p485] (See ¶2106) 4954
⟨S⟩ [shutes p61] places the episode around January 1854 – see ¶2047 4955
⟨1⟩ Lincoln "had great faith in the virtues of the *mad stone* although he could give no reason for it and confessed that it looked like superstition but he said he found the People in the neighborhood of those stones fully impressed with a belief in their virtues from actual experiment and that was as much as we could ever know of the properties of medicines" – Joseph Gillespie [wilson p182] 4956
⟨-⟩ [kunhardtB p288] *believes fear of lockjaw prompted the Lincolns to seek treatment – it was more likely fear of rabies.* 4957
⟨1⟩ "Robert says I'm crazy, but he is crazy, too. He was bit by a mad dog when he was a boy." – a bitter Mary Lincoln in 1882, as recalled by Mary Edwards Brown [kunhardtC] 4958

Infection (continued)

⟨2⟩ July 17, 1861: "I have the mumps. Home in a few days. Not sick at all." – Robert [donaldH p79]   4959

■ Nov. 1863: Lincoln developed smallpox (see ¶2030 and Special Topic §5).   4960

⟨2⟩ May have been immunized against smallpox. (See ¶5401.) *Robert was then away from home, at college. It is therefore unclear whether he was vaccinated at this time.*   4961

⟨2⟩ "There is no record of Lincoln or his sons having been vaccinated against small pox." [pearson] *This may apply to the period before Lincoln developed smallpox.*   4962

Robert

Infection – Exposures

⟨2⟩_c Exposed to dog (bitten). See ¶4953   4963

⟨1⟩ "Bob used to harness Cats – Bob & my boy and used to harness up my dog & they would take him & go into the woods and get nuts" – James Gourley [wilson p453]   4964

Medications & Chemicals

⟨1⟩_q "... when Robert could just barely walk Mrs. Lincoln came out in front as usual, screaming 'Bobbie will die! Bobbie will die!' My father ran over to see what had happened. Bobbie was found sitting out near the back door by a lime box and had a little lime in his mouth. Father took him, washed his mouth out and that's all there was to it." – recollection (year not provided) of Elizabeth A. Capps, a Springfield neighbor of the Lincolns [burl p62] (A lime box is a "necessary accessory" of an outhouse [randallC p104].)   4965

Mental Status

⟨1⟩_q 1847-1848: "a bright boy [who] seemed to have his own way" – boarder at same house as the Lincolns [randallC p96]   4966

⟨2⟩ "Robert developed into an aloof, chilly introvert. 'He is a Todd and not a Lincoln,' Herndon caustically remarked. 'Bob is little, proud, aristocratic, and haughty, is his mother's "baby" all through.' " [oatesA p97] (See ¶4911.)   4967

⟨S⟩ "Possibly also Robert fits into the theory that first babies sometimes get out of adjustment when the second child arrives to share parental attention." [randallC p240]   4968

⟨2⟩ Because of his ocular deviation "His schoolmates called him 'cockeye,' which humiliated him." [oatesA p97]   4969

⟨2⟩ "Washingtonians thought him a good-looking young man with excellent manners and, in private conversation, a good sense of humor." [donaldA p428]   4970

■ Father's traits: 4971

⟨2⟩_c "Robert and his father shared little in common; the son did not inherit Lincoln's temperament or values. In vain one seeks to find in Robert the sense of humor, idealism, personal warmth and humanity, egalitarianism, wisdom, relative indifference to money, and generosity that distinguished his father's character." [burl p63]   4972

⟨1⟩_q Robert was "a Todd, and not a Lincoln" [burl pp63-64] citing Herndon   4973

Mental Status (continued)

⟨2⟩_c "Randall suggests that the only interest Robert and his father shared in common was mathematics. She might have added astronomy." [burl p71] citing [randallA pp20-21] (See ¶3121)   4974

⟨2⟩ April 15, 1865: Robert was in the Peterson House with his dying father. "At about 6:45 a.m., as death approached, cool, collected Robert Lincoln finally broke down – throwing himself against Charles Sumner's shoulder and sobbing openly." [kunhardtA p359] (but see ¶560)   4975

⟨1⟩ October 1867, after Mary's wardrobe scandal: Robert "came up last evening like a maniac, and almost threatening his life, looking like death" –Mary [turner p440]   4976

⟨2⟩ "mentally in marked contrast to his father" – [NYTimesObitR] (Part of ¶4916)   4977

⟨2⟩ "He was of a taciturn and retiring nature, and only to his close friends did he reveal himself as a charming conversationalist and an entertaining story teller, a trait which he inherited form his father." [ChicagoTribune - July 27, 1926] (obituary)   4978

Muscle / Athletics

⟨2⟩ At Philips Exeter Academy "he excelled in athletics as a jumper" [kunhardtA p90]   4980

⟨2⟩ In later years, as he "gradually retired from business," he "took up golf, playing practically every afternoon" – [NYTimesObitR] (Part of ¶4920)   4981

Nervous System

⟨1/q⟩ 1847-1848: "Of my life at Washington [age 4, while Lincoln was in Congress] my recollections are very faint" – Robert [lincloreIED].   4982

⟨1/q⟩ 1847-1848: "a bright boy [who] seemed to have his own way" – boarder at same house as the Lincolns [randallC p96]   4983

Reading & Learning

⟨1/q⟩ Oct. 22, 1846: "He is quite smart enough. I some times fear he is one of the little rare-ripe sort, that are smarter at about five than ever after. He has a great deal of that sort of mischief, that is the offspring of much animal spirits." – Lincoln [burl p61]   4984

⟨2⟩ After attending a private school in Springfield, failed 15 of 16 of the Harvard entrance examinations. Was therefore sent to Philips Exeter Academy (New Hampshire) for a year. [kunhardtA p90]   4985

⟨1/q⟩ While in college at Harvard, Robert wrote a witty recap of his educational history, excerpted in [lincloreIED].   4986

⟨2⟩ "While President of the Pullman company, he made a custom of working out algebraic problems as a recreation, and was fond of astronomy." [ChicagoTribune - July 27, 1926] (obituary)   4987

Skin

⟨2⟩ "In complexion, however, he was dark and swarthy like his father." – [NYTimesObitR] (Part of ¶4916)   4988

Sleep & Circadian Rhythms

⟨2⟩ Late in the war, Robert served as an officer on General Grant's headquarters staff. He arrived at the White House in time for breakfast on April 14, 1865, having not slept in a bed in two months, and "was so sleepy he could barely keep his eyes open. ... He was planning to take a dose of medicine before he climbed into his own comfortable bed that night." Indeed, he went straight to his room after dinner that night, having declined his father's invitation to Ford's Theatre. [kunhardtB pp18-19]   4989

    ⟨1⟩ "On the day of my arrival my father met his death." – Robert (1924 recollection) [helmB pp251,259]   4990

Robert

Speech

⟨1⟩ Oct. 22, 1846: "He talks very plainly – almost as plainly as any body." – Lincoln [baslerA v1p392]   4991

Spoiled

⟨S⟩ See `Tad` `Spoiled` for evidence of the Lincoln children being spoiled.   4992

⟨S⟩ On the other hand, see `Trauma` for instances of corporal punishment to `Robert` and `Tad`.   4993

Trauma

- Corporal punishment: 4994
    ⟨1⟩ "Ms L would whip Bob a good deal" [wilson p597]; also cited by [burl p63]   4995
    ⟨1⟩ "whipped" by his mother [burl p61] citing letter from Lincoln, Oct. 22, 1846   4996
    ⟨?⟩ Mary "whipped them" (two of the boys) after they dismantled a new clock – Mrs. Benjamin Edwards [stevens p xv]   4997

⟨2⟩ Bitten by a dog as a child. See ¶4953   4998

⟨1⟩ In a weird twist of fate, Edwin Booth saved Robert's life. Edwin was the older brother of the assassin. Robert had slipped onto the train track at the Jersey City, NJ train station while travelling to Washington from New York City. He fell into an open space and was helpless until Booth "vigorously seized" him to safety. The incident occurred while Lincoln was President. [helmB pp251-252] *Interestingly, a bystander saved Tad from a railroad death – ¶5673.*   4999

Travel & Dwellings

- For travels during youth, see `Mary` `Travel & Dwellings`, e.g. ¶4709 and ¶4710   5000

⟨1⟩ 1/1854 (?): Terre Haute for mad stone treatment (¶4953); 7/28/1863: Fort Monroe to Washington [turner p157n]; 7/29/1863: Washington to New York [turner p157n] and to White Mountains [randallC p292]; 1/6/1865 arrives Washington [turner p198]; 1/30/1865: In New York [barbeeP - box 2 folder 135] quoting or summarizing *National Republican* newspaper; 11/27/1867: Chicago to Rocky Mountains for a few days [turner p462]   5001

⟨1⟩ 1865: "was in Washington only at inauguration time and for a few days at the time of his father's death." [crookA p18]   5002

Voice

⟨2⟩ "His voice, also, those who had heard the President said, had a marked likeness to his father's in sonority, volume, and timbre." – [NYTimesObitR] (Part of ¶4916)   5003

Lincoln, Sarah   sister

Chronology

Born Feb. 10, 1807 [templeC] in Elizabethtown, KY [tarbellE p43]. Moved with rest of family to Indiana in 1816. Married Aug. 2, 1826 [wilson p645]. Died Jan. 20, 1828. (Data from family Bible) [wilson p111].   5004

Introduction & Sources

⟨1⟩ Was commonly called Sally [wilson p93] and sometimes Nancy [wilson pp110n,111]   5005
  ⟨2⟩ Born as Nancy, "called Sarah after 1819" [lea p86].   5006
  ⟨2⟩ Some early biographers "made two serious mistakes in identifying her: at   5007
  first they gave her name as Nancy and also claimed she was younger than
  Abraham." [lincloreBAI]

Appearance

⟨1⟩ "a good, kind, amiable girl, resembling Abe" – Elizabeth Crawford [wilson p126]   5008

⟨1⟩ "Sarah Lincoln favored Abe: she dark skinned – heavy built – favored Abe very   5009
  much – looked alike" – David Turnham [wilson p122]

⟨2⟩ "The descriptions which we have of Sarah are all in agreement and this brief one 5010
  by her own stepmother may be accepted: 'She was short of stature and somewhat
  plump in build, her hair was dark brown and her eyes were grey.' " [lincloreBAI]

Build

⟨1⟩ "she was a woman of ordinary size" – David Turnham [wilson p121]   5011

⟨1⟩ "heavy built" – David Turnham [wilson p122] (Part of ¶5009)   5012

⟨2⟩ "thick-set" [herndon p17]   5013

⟨2⟩ "though in some respects like her brother, lacked his stature" [herndon p17]   5014

⟨1⟩ "Short built" – John Hanks [wilson p456] (Part of ¶5039)   5015

⟨1⟩ "short hevey built woman gooddeal like here Father in every way" – Dennis Hanks   5016
  [wilson p615] (Part of ¶5037)

⟨$\frac{1}{q}$⟩ "short of stature and somewhat plump in build" – Sarah Bush Lincoln [lincloreBAI]   5017
  (∈ ¶5010)

Death

⟨1⟩ "died at the birth of her first child" – Dennis Hanks [wilson p27]   5018

⟨2⟩ As Sarah prepared to deliver her first baby, it was known that the nearest physi- 5019
  cian, just two miles away, was a drunkard. On January 20, 1828, however, she
  urgently needed medical care, so this physician was summoned. He arrived
  "helplessly intoxicated." Sarah's father-in-law, therefore, hurried 4 miles to Little Pigeon Creek, crossed it into the next county, collected Dr. William Davis, and

Death (continued)

started homeward. The fast-rising creek, however, could not be crossed. Grigsby and Davis traveled 6 miles farther up, crossing near Dale, Indiana. Sarah and her baby were dead by the time they arrived. [shutes p59] *The primary source material for this is not in* [shutesP].

⟨2⟩ "In one version of the story, the doctor, Fred Lively, was called in from two miles away, and according to local tradition was intoxicated. Sarah's father-in-law crossed the swollen Little Pigeon Creek to retrieve Dr. William Davis in Warwick County, but she was dead by the time help arrived" [bumgarnerB].　5020

⟨1⟩ Dr. Lively was "a drunk – too drunk - to care for Sarah Lincoln Grigsby & her baby – both of whom died" [shutesP]. (See ¶3158.)　5021

⟨1/q⟩ "I remember the night she died. My mother was there at the time. She had a very strong voice, and I heard her calling father. He awoke the boys and said, 'Something is the matter.' He went after a doctor but it was too late. They let her lay too long. My old aunt was the midwife." – Mrs. J.W. Lamar [hobson p22]　5022　Sarah

⟨1/q⟩ "I reckon it was like Nancy, she didn't have the right sort o' keer." – Dennis Hanks [wilsonR p25]　5023

⟨1⟩ "She deid [sic] Jay 20th 1828 in giving birth to her first and only child. The child was Dead when born." – A.H. Chapman [wilson p100]　5024

　⟨1⟩ Repeats himself later in his written statement: [wilson p102]　5025

⟨2⟩ Buried in Pigeon Church cemetery, as is her mother. [lincloreBAI]　5026

■ Ramifications:　5027

　⟨1/q⟩ Lincoln "always thought her death was due to neglect" – Captain J.W. Lamar [hobson p24] (∈ ¶2438)　5028

　⟨2⟩ "Lincoln blamed the death of his sister on the negligence of the Grigsbys in sending for a doctor." The ensuing quarrel "further alienated" him from his neighbors. [donaldA p34]　5029

　⟨2⟩ Lincoln afterwards "resented the elder Grigsbys" for not summoning a physician earlier. [burl p96]　5030

　⟨S⟩ [shutes p59] suggests this event influenced Lincoln's temperance.　5031

Eyes

⟨2⟩ Had the "deep-gray eyes" of her brother Abraham. [herndon p17]　5032

⟨1⟩ "Eyes dark gray" – John Hanks [wilson p456] Part of ¶5039　5033

⟨1⟩ "Dark Eye" – Dennis Hanks [wilson p615] Part of ¶5037　5034

⟨1/q⟩ "her eyes were grey" – Sarah Bush Lincoln (stepmother) [lincloreBAI] (∈ ¶5010)　5035

General

⟨2/c⟩ Was an "eight-month baby" according to [shutesE p9]. *I know of no evidence for this claim, and cannot think of a source that would be able to provide it. I conclude Shutes fabricated this statement to prevent the otherwise obvious conclusion that Sarah was conceived before her parents were married. Herndon* [hertz pp205-206] *notes the timing of her birth.*　5036

⟨1⟩ "I was well acquainted with her she wa short hevey built woman gooddeal like here Father in every way. she had Dark Eye Black Haire she was smart and shrowd Woman" [sic] – John Hanks [wilson p615]　5037

General (continued)

⟨-⟩ *This is the entire text of a paragraph in a letter written by the barely-literate John Hanks in 1887. It is not clear to whom it applies. Sarah seems most likely, but see ¶4777.*   5038

⟨1⟩ "She was a Short built woman – Eyes dark gray – hair dark brown: She was a good woman – Kind, tender, & good natured and is Said to have been a smart woman." – John Hanks [wilson p456]   5039

Hair

⟨2⟩ Had the "dark-brown hair" of her brother Abraham. [herndon p17]   5040

⟨1⟩ "Hair dark brown" – John Hanks [wilson p456] Part of ¶5039   5041

⟨1⟩ "Black Haire" – Dennis Hanks [wilson p615] Part of ¶5037   5042

⟨$\frac{1}{q}$⟩ "her hair was dark brown" – Sarah Bush Lincoln (stepmother) [lincloreBAI] (∈ ¶5010)   5043

Head & Face

⟨1⟩ "favored Abe very much – looked alike" – David Turnham [wilson p122] (Part of ¶5009)   5044

Mental Status

⟨$\frac{1}{q}$⟩ "Sairy was a little gal, only 'leven, an' she'd git so lonesome, missin' her mother, she'd set an' cry by the fire. Abe 'n' me got her a baby coon an' a turtle." – Dennis Hanks [wilsonR p24]   5045

⟨2⟩ "an even disposition" [herndon p17]   5046

⟨1⟩ "Kind, tender, & good natured" – John Hanks [wilson p456] Part of ¶5039   5047

⟨1⟩ "Her good humored laugh I can see now – Nathaniel Grigsby [wilson p113]   5048

⟨$\frac{1}{q}$⟩ Sarah and Abraham: "a great deal alike in temperament" – Captain J.W. Lamar [hobson p24] (∈ ¶2438)   5049

Nervous System

⟨$\frac{1}{q}$⟩ "[Lincoln] tried to interest little Sairy in l'arnin to read, but she never tuk to it. ... Sairy was a little gal, only 'leven" – Dennis Hanks [wilsonR p24]   5050

⟨1⟩ "Sally was a quick minded woman & of extraordinary Mind" – Nathaniel Grigsby [wilson p113]   5051

⟨1⟩ "smart intiligent [sic] lady" – Nathaniel Grigsby [wilson p94]   5052

⟨1⟩ "had a good mind" – David Turnham [wilson p121]   5053

⟨1⟩ "Said to have been a smart woman" – John Hanks [wilson p456] Part of ¶5039   5054

⟨1⟩ "smart and shrowd Woman" – Dennis Hanks [wilson p615] Part of ¶5037. *Shrewd?*   5055

⟨2⟩ "a bright pupil, of good mind, and was more industrious than her brother" [angle p23] (reprinting [bartonB])   5056

Physicians

⟨2⟩ See Death.   5057

Reproductive

⟨1⟩ "married to Aaron Griggsby [sic] of Spencer Co Indiana and lived only about 12   5058
months and died at the birth of her first child" – Dennis Hanks [wilson p27]

⟨1⟩ "mother of one son who died wile [sic] and infant" – Nathaniel Grigsby [wilson p94]   5059

Skin

⟨1⟩ "dark skinned" – David Turnham [wilson p122] (Part of ¶5009)   5060

Sarah

Lincoln, Thomas

father

Chronology

Born Jan. 6, 1778; married June 12, 1806; moves 14 miles from Elizabethtown to Hardin County in 1808 [tarbellE pp37, 43]; moves to Indiana Dec. 1816; widowed Oct. 5, 1818; remarried Dec. 2, 1819; moves to Macon County, IL March 1, 1830; moved to Coles County, IL in spring 1831 [templeC]; died Jan. 17, 1851 [herndon p60] 5061

⟨2⟩ "born in Virginia on the Roanoke River" – Dennis Hanks [wilson p27] 5062

⟨2⟩ "died 8 miles south of Charleston Coles Co Ills Jany 9th 1851" – A.H. Chapman [wilson p97] 5063

Family History

⟨1⟩ "Very Much Like Abe his Sun" – Dennis Hanks [wilson p149] (Part of ¶5069.) 5064

⟨2⟩ "Except for his coarse black hair, his leathery skin, and his delight in storytelling, Thomas was also quite different" from Abraham [currentBk p23] 5065

Appearance

⟨1⟩ "rather a long-faced man, dark hair, eyes, and scin, by no means hansome." – David Turnham [wilson p142] 5066

⟨1⟩ "height was about 5 feet 10 Inches, weighed one hundred and 96 pounds. Walked rather Slow never seemed to be in a hurry his Face rather round, Grey Eyes or Hazel as Some People call them, never the less they was about the Color of his Son Abrams High Cheek bones and very large nose which was his most prominent feature   had dark Course hair" – Harriet Chapman [wilson p145] 5067

⟨1⟩ "Black Hare, Dark Eyes, was 5 feet 9 inches high, hevy set, fleshy and weighed about 180 pounds ... Even and good disposition was lively and cheerfull" [sic] – John Hanks [wilson p5] 5068

⟨1⟩ "was a man five feet 10 Inches high Darke hair rather corse – Hazel Eye weighing 196 lbs Very Much Like Abe his Sun he had a Broder face than abe Walked Slow and Shore a Mity Staught Man" – Dennis Hanks [wilson p149] 5069

⟨1⟩ "He was rather dark complected, Dark hair, Dark Grey Eyes" – A.H. Chapman [wilson p96] 5070

⟨1⟩ "he was not tall – was dark skinned – was Stout – muscular – not nervous – not Sinewy – He weighed about 165. *lbs.*: he was Somewhat raw boned ... Slow in action Somewhat" – David Turnham [wilson p122] 5071

⟨2⟩ "He was, we are told, five feet ten inches high, weighed one hundred and ninety-five pounds, had a well-rounded face, dark hazel eyes, coarse black hair, and was 5072

Appearance (continued)

slightly stoop-shouldered. His build was so compact that Dennis Hanks used to say that he could not find the point of separation between his ribs. He was proverbially slow of movement, mentally and physically; was careless, inert, and dull; was sinewy, and gifted with great strength; was inoffensively quiet and peaceable, but when roused to resistance a dangerous antagonist." [herndon p12]

◻ Although many sources label the photograph from [kunhardtA p35] as showing Thomas, [kunhardtA p26] is more circumspect, saying "This is traditionally believed to be a picture of Thomas."   5073

⟨2⟩ "Many scholars doubt its authenticity" [ostendorfA p297].   5074

Build

⟨1⟩ Hanks descriptions: 5075

   ⟨1⟩ "Thomas Lincoln Was 5 ft – 10 in in hight [sic] ... hevy sque [sic] built man he Weigh about 180 lbs." – John Hanks [wilson p615]   5076

   ⟨1⟩ "about 5 feet 10 in high – weigh about 180 – ... a very Stout man" – John Hanks [wilson p454] Part of ¶5125   5077

   ⟨1⟩ "He was a large man of great muscular power his usual weight 196 pounds I have weighed him many a time he was 5 feet 10 1/2 inches high and well proportioned. ... He was Singular in one point though not a fleshy man he was built so compact that it was difficult to find or feel a rib in his body – A muscular man, his equal I never saw" – Dennis Hanks [wilson p28]   5078

   ⟨1⟩ "five feet 10 Inches high ... weighing 196 lb ... a Mity Staught Man" – Dennis Hanks [wilson p149] (Part of ¶5069.)   5079

   ⟨1⟩ "5 feet 9 inches high, hevy set, fleshy and weighed about 180 pounds" – John Hanks [wilson p5] (Part of ¶5068.)   5080

■ Chapman descriptions: 5081

   ⟨1⟩ "a Stout athletic man. 5 feet 10 inches High & weighed when in the prime of his life 196 lbs. he had the Reputation of being one of the Stoutest men in Ky." – A.H. Chapman [wilson p96]   5082

   ⟨1⟩ "height was about 5 feet 10 Inches, weighed one hundred and 96 pounds" – Harriet Chapman [wilson p145] (Part of ¶5067.)   5083

   ⟨1⟩ "about 6 feet high – heavy build ... weight about 180" – Harriet Chapman [wilson p646]   5084

■ Other descriptions: 5085

   ⟨1⟩ "I would suppose when young & full fleshed that his weight would have been about 185 lbs if my memory serves correctly" – William Greene [wilson p145]   5086

   ⟨1⟩ "not so tall as Abraham" – George Balch [wilson p597]   5087

   ⟨1⟩ "He was a square stout built man of only ordinary height" – Samuel Haycraft [wilson p67]   5088

   ⟨1⟩ "low heavy built clumsy honest man" – Samuel Haycraft [wilson p84]   5089

   ⟨1⟩ "he was not tall ... was Stout – muscular ... not Sinewy – He weighed about 165. *lbs.*: he was Somewhat raw boned" – David Turnham [wilson p122] (Part of ¶5071.)   5090

   ⟨1⟩ "a large man – Say 6 feet or a little up – strong & Muscular" – Nathaniel Grigsby [wilson p111]   5091

   ⟨2⟩ 5 feet 10 inches tall, weighed 195 pounds. "His build was so compact that Dennis Hanks used to say that he could not find the point of separation between his ribs." [herndon p12] (∈ ¶5072)   5092

   ⟨2⟩ "stocky, well-built man of no more than average height" [donaldA p22]   5093

Thomas

Chest & Shoulders

⟨1⟩ "a little Stupt Shouldered" – John Hanks [wilson p454] Part of ¶5125 5094
　⟨2⟩ Agrees with: "slightly stoop-shouldered" [herndon p12] (∈ ¶5072). 5095

⟨1⟩ "His build was so compact that Dennis Hanks used to say that he could not find 5096
the point of separation between his ribs." [herndon p12] (∈ ¶5072)
　⟨2⟩ "Close-knit ribs may in some cases be a manifestation of of the entity [Mar- 5097
　　fan syndrome]" [schwartzD] *I am have not seen this claim confirmed in my*
　　readings, unless he is referring to scoliosis compacting the ribs unilater-
　　ally.

Death

⟨1/q⟩ 1849: August Chapman writes Lincoln that Thomas is seriously ill "with a lesion 5098
of the Heart" and emits "Heart-Rendering" cries for his son. Another letter three
days later says Thomas is improved, having raised "a Large amount of matter or
phlegm" which had caused an "oppression of the heart." [shutesE pp97-98]. *From the*
first letter's excerpts alone, it could be supposed that "heart" was being used
figuratively. However, the second letter suggests there was an organic problem.

⟨1⟩ 1851: "On the 17th of January, after suffering for many weeks from a disorder of 5099
the kidneys, he passed away at the ripe old age – as his son tells us – of 'seventy-
three years and eleven days.' " [herndon p60]

⟨2⟩ died of kidney disease at age 73 [herndon p60]. 5100

⟨1⟩ "di[ed] from a disease of the kidneys" – A.H. Chapman [wilson p103] 5101

Diet & Digestion

⟨1⟩ "was a very Hearty eater but cared but Litle what kind of food he had, was satisfied 5102
if he had plenty of corn Brod & Milk" – A.H. Chapman [wilson p97]

Eyes

■ Hanks observations: 5103
　⟨1⟩ "Dark Eyes" – John Hanks [wilson p5] (Part of ¶5068.) 5104
　⟨1⟩ "Eyes dark gray" – John Hanks [wilson p454] Part of ¶5125 5105
　⟨1⟩ "Dark Eye" – John Hanks [wilson p615] 5106
　⟨1⟩ "Hazel Eye" – Dennis Hanks [wilson p149] (Part of ¶5069.) 5107

■ Chapman observations: 5108
　⟨1⟩ "Grey Eyes or Hazel as Some People call them, never the less they was about 5109
　　the Color of his Son Abrams" – Harriet Chapman [wilson p145] (Part of ¶5067.)
　⟨1⟩ "eyes grey" – Harriet Chapman [wilson p646] 5110
　⟨1⟩ "Dark Grey Eyes" – A.H. Chapman [wilson p96] (Part of ¶5070.) 5111

■ Other observations: 5112
　⟨1⟩ "his Eyes were Gray or Rather Bluish" – William Greene [wilson p145] 5113
　⟨1⟩ "dark hair, eyes" – David Turnham [wilson p142] (Part of ¶5066.) 5114
　⟨2⟩ "dark hazel eyes" [herndon p12] (∈ ¶5072) 5115

⟨1⟩ "Thomas Lincoln was blind in one Eye and the other was weak – so he felt his way 5116
in the work much of the time: his sense of touch was Keen" – Elizabeth Crawford
[wilson p126]

Gait

⟨1⟩ "Walked rather Slow never seemed to be in a hurry" – Harriet Chapman [wilson p145]   5117
(Part of ¶5067.)

⟨1⟩ "talked and walked slow" – George Balch [wilson p597]   5118

⟨1⟩ "Walked Slow and Shore" – Dennis Hanks [wilson p149] (Part of ¶5069.)   5119

⟨1⟩ "while he resided in Ky he made two trips down the Ohio & Miss Rivers to New   5120
Orleans with one Isaac Bush. thy wa[lked] the entire distance across t[he] country
from New Orleans b[ack] to their homes in Ky." – A.H. Chapman [wilson p102] *See
¶5220 for estimated date of one trip.*

⟨2⟩ 1816: Walked from his Indiana homestead back to Knob Creek, Kentucky [angle   5121
p17]. See ¶5223. *I estimate this distance at about 65 miles, as the crow flies,
which is not likely the path he took.*

⟨1⟩ About 1816: Aborted trip to New Orleans. "Thomas Lincoln, like his son after him,   5122
had a notion that fortunes could be made by trips to New Orleans by flatboat."
It was a dangerous trip. The boat capsized on the Ohio River, before reaching
the Mississippi. Thomas walked home. – Christopher Graham [tarbellE p233, 234]
*Thomas was still living in Kentucky when he started the trip, yet Abraham was
about 8 years old.*

General

⟨2⟩ "He was proverbially slow of movement, mentally and physically; was careless,   5123
inert, and dull." [herndon p12] (∈ ¶5072)
    ⟨2⟩ "embodied listlessness" [herndon p51]   5124

⟨1⟩ "He was a man about 5 feet 10 in high – weigh about 180 – Eyes dark gray – hair   5125
black – a little Stupt Shouldered – good humored man – a Strong brave man – a
very Stout man – loved fun – jokes and equalled Abe in telling Stories." – John
Hanks [wilson p454]

⟨1⟩ early 1800s: "was a carpenter, and a good one for those days" – Christopher Gra-   5126
ham [tarbellE p233]

⟨1⟩_q Dec. 1848: "I and the Old womman [sic] is in the best of health" (letter to Lincoln)   5127
[randallC p114]

Habits – Alcohol

⟨2⟩ He "had no marked aversion for the bottle, though in the latter case he indulged   5128
no more freely than the average Kentuckian of his day." [herndon p12]

⟨1⟩ "temperate in his Habits, never was intoxicated in his life" – A.H. Chapman [wilson   5129
p96]

⟨1⟩ "During the Sumer of 1816 he traded his Little place, for 400 Gallons of Whisky" –   5130
A.H. Chapman [wilson p97]

⟨1⟩ "never drank but lazy & worthless" – George Balch [wilson p597]   5131

⟨1⟩ "I did not see him drink any thing that were intoxicated [sic]" – John Hanks [wilson   5132
p615]

⟨1⟩ "never was intoxicated in his life" – A.H. Chapman [wilson p97]   5133

⟨1⟩ "would take a dram – not a hab. drinker – never drunk on Christmas had one or   5134
two hot apple toddy" – Harriet Chapman [wilson p646]

Thomas

Hair

- Hanks observations:
  - ⟨1⟩ "Black Hare" – John Hanks [wilson p5] (Part of ¶5068.) 5135
  - ⟨1⟩ "hair black" – John Hanks [wilson p454] Part of ¶5125 5136
  - ⟨1⟩ "Black hair" – John Hanks [wilson p615] 5137
  - ⟨1⟩ "Darke hair rather corse" – Dennis Hanks [wilson p149] (Part of ¶5069.) 5138
  5139
- Other observations:
  - ⟨1⟩ "Dark hair" – A.H. Chapman [wilson p96] (Part of ¶5070.) 5140
  - ⟨1⟩ "had dark Course hair" – Harriet Chapman [wilson p145] (Part of ¶5067.) 5141
  - ⟨1⟩ "hair dark" – Harriet Chapman [wilson p646] 5142
  - ⟨1⟩ "dark hair" – David Turnham [wilson p142] (Part of ¶5066.) 5143
  - ⟨2⟩ "coarse black hair" [herndon p12] (∈ ¶5072) 5144
  - ⟨2⟩ "a shock of straight black hair" [donaldA p22] 5145
  5146

Handwriting

Whether Thomas learned to write or not is covered in Reading & Learning 5147

⟨2⟩ In May 1845 Thomas signed for some money that Lincoln had left with the Coles 5148
County court clerk. The signature is that of his step-son, John Johnston. [angle p174]
reprinting [weik]

⊙ A signature appears in [nee], probably taken from [lea]. *The penmanship is excel-* 5149
lent. Given that Thomas could only "bunglingly" sign his name (¶5196), one
wonders if this is someone else's signature.

Head & Face

⟨2⟩ "had a well-rounded face." [herndon p12] (∈ ¶5072) 5150

⟨1⟩ "his features were coarse & he had a remarkable large roman Nose" – A.H. Chap- 5151
man [wilson p97]

⟨1⟩ "large nose" – George Balch [wilson p597] 5152
  ⟨2⟩ Agrees with: [donaldA p22] 5153

⟨1⟩ "had [illegible] face and rough man" – George Balch [wilson p597] 5154

⟨1⟩ "rather a long-faced man ... by no means hansome" – David Turnham [wilson p142] 5155
(Part of ¶5066.)

⟨1⟩ "he had a Broder face than abe" – Dennis Hanks [wilson p149] (Part of ¶5069.) 5156

⟨1⟩ "his Face rather round ... High Cheek bones and very large nose which was his 5157
most prominent feature" – Harriet Chapman [wilson p145] (Part of ¶5067.)

Heart & Circulation

⟨1/q⟩ Lincoln receives letter that Thomas is unwell and had a "seizure of the heart" [don- 5158
aldA p152]

Infection

⟨2⟩ "Thomas Lincoln had the mumps which necessitated an operation" while living 5159
in Kentucky [shutes p2]. See ¶5188

⟨2⟩ May have had malaria in 1830. See ¶2001 5160

Infection – Exposures

⟨2⟩ "Thomas Lincoln was a good judge of horses. ... He was never without horses after his coming of age [i.e., age 21], and on Knob Creek he owned a stallion and several brood mares." [angle p12] (reprinting [bartonB]) 5161

⟨2⟩ 1814: Bought a heifer [angle p12] (reprinting [bartonB]) 5162

⟨1⟩ Four horse team when he moved to Indiana [wilson p228] 5163

⟨1⟩ "... like most Pioneers delighted in having a good hunt. The Deer, the Turkeys the Bear the wild cats and occasionally a big Panther afforded him no small amusement and pleasure – and was a great Source of Subsistence as the wild Turkeys and Deer were very abundant – The Honey Bee Luxuriated on the Prarie flowers and afforded in the Groves a large supply of wild honey" – Dennis Hanks [wilson p27] 5164

⟨1⟩ Came to Indiana with 2 horses – Dennis Hanks [wilson p226] 5165

⟨2⟩ Owned a few sheep [burl p41] 5166 Thomas

Mental Status

⟨1⟩ In Kentucky: "was a real nice, agreeable man, who often got the 'blues,' and had some strange sorts of spells, and wanted to be alone all he could when he had them. He would walk away out on the barrens alone, and stay out sometimes half a day. Once when he was out thar, one of my boys, what he did n't see, hearn him talkin' all alone to hisself about God and his providence and sacrifices ... and a whole lot of things ... in the Scripture. ... Some of us was afear'd he was losin' his mind; but when they packed up their things, and went to Ingiany [sic], his spells left him, as we hear'n tell, though he was allus sollem-like ev'n thar, whar they all could make so much better livin'..." – an "intelligent woman" [browneR v1pp82-83] 5167

⟨1⟩ "he was a remarkable peacable man" – A.H. Chapman [wilson p96] 5168

⟨1⟩ "Very quiet Not hasty temper treated Me well" – Dennis Hanks [wilson p176] 5169

⟨1⟩ "very industrious, remarkable good Natured, very fond of a Joke or story & of telling them" – A.H. Chapman [wilson p96] 5170

⟨1⟩ "Even and good disposition was lively and cheerfull" – John Hanks [wilson p5] (Part of ¶5068.) 5171

⟨2⟩ "was inoffensively quiet and peaceable, but when roused to resistance a dangerous antagonist." [herndon p12] (∈ ¶5072) 5172

⟨1⟩ "was a blank, but a clever man, a somewhat social creature. How he raised such a boy as Abe the Lord only knows." – Mentor Graham [hertz p132] 5173

- Story-telling: 5174
  ⟨1⟩q "could beat his son telling a story – cracking a joke" – Dennis Hanks [donaldA p32] 5175
  ⟨1⟩ "Old Mr. L. had one trait that Abraham inherited story telling." – Dennis Hanks [wilson p598] 5176
  ⟨1⟩ "he had no superior in 'Story telling' " – William Greene [wilson p145] 5177
  ⟨1⟩ "good humored man – a Strong brave man – ... – loved fun – jokes and equalled Abe in telling Stories" – John Hanks [wilson p454] Part of ¶5125 5178

⟨1⟩ "I don't think that Thomas Lincoln was a witty man – a humorous man: he was a social man – loved Company – peeple & their Sports very much: he seemed to me to border on the serious – reflective" – Thomas Johnston [wilson p533] 5179

Muscle / Athletics

⟨2⟩ "sinewy, and gifted with great strength" [herndon p12] (∈ ¶5072)   5180

⟨1⟩ "muscular ... not Sinewy" – David Turnham [wilson p122] (Part of ¶5071.)   5181

⟨1⟩ "a large man – Say 6 feet or a little up – strong & Muscular" – Nathaniel Grigsby   5182
[wilson p111]

⟨1⟩ "At one time while on a visit to some friends at Hardinsburgh Ky he had a Desper-   5183
ate fight with a man named Hardin, said Hardin was a Noted Bully & Desperado
& Said to be the Stoutest man in Breckenridge County. Thos. Lincoln whipped
Hardin easily without he Lincoln receang a Scratch or Bruse. This is the only fight
he ever had, after his encounter with Hardin no one else ever tried his manhood
in personal combat." – A.H. Chapman [wilson p96]
   ⟨1⟩ Dennis Hanks tells substantially the same story, but says the county was   5184
   Hardin and the man was Breckenridge [wilson p28]

Nervous System

⟨1⟩ "All of them [Lincoln and his parents] had good memories" – Dennis Hanks [wilson   5185
p598]

⟨1⟩ "not nervous ... Slow in action Somewhat" – David Turnham [wilson p122] (Part of   5186
¶5071.)

Physicians

⟨2⟩ Dr. Christopher Columbus Graham witnessed the marriage of Thomas and   5187
Nancy, and left a long statement of his memories of the Lincolns when he was 99
years old [tarbellE pp227-236].. "I was hunting roots for my medicine, and just went to
the wedding to get a good supper, and got it." – Graham [tarbellE p 232].

⟨2⟩ When Dr. Daniel Potter died in 1814 (see ¶3153) Thomas Lincoln owed him $1.46.   5188
"There is no record of what his services were, when rendered and for whom. But
as Thomas Lincoln had the mumps which necessitated an operation, Beveridge
suggests that it was for this that Dr. Potter was employed." [shutes pp2-3]
   ⟨-⟩ *The issue is noteworthy only because of murmurs that Thomas had been*   5189
   made sterile by the mumps before Abraham was conceived. If Potter moved
   to town after Abraham's birth and if that was when Thomas had mumps, it
   would be evidence against the belief that Thomas Lincoln was not Abraham
   Lincoln's father. See ¶44.
   ⟨2⟩ Shutes pointedly remarks that Dr. Potter did not arrive in Kentucky until af-   5190
   ter Abraham was born [shutes p3]. But then he contradicts himself and says
   Thomas decided not to call Dr. Potter to attend the birth of Abraham for fear
   of "runnin' up the debt" [shutes p3].

Reading & Learning

▪ Also see Handwriting.   5191

⟨1⟩ "Thomas and nancy both could read and write." – Christopher Graham [tarbellE   5192
p233]

⟨1⟩ "had but Little Education, Learning to read & write a Little after his Marriage" –   5193
A.H. Chapman [wilson p97]

Reading & Learning (continued)

⟨1⟩ "could write because Squire Grimes has mortgage signed by Thos. L. & he could read Bible. an excellent spec. of poor white trash" – George Balch [wilson p597]   5194

⟨1⟩ "he could read little; he could not right [sic]" – John Hanks [wilson p615]   5195

⟨1⟩ "By the early death of his father, and very narrow circumstances of his mother, even in childhood was a wandering laboring boy, and grew up litterally [sic] without education. He never did more in the way of writing than to bunglingly sign his own name." – Lincoln [baslerA v4p62]   5196

⟨1⟩ "Learning to read & write a Little after his marriage" " – A.H. Chapman [wilson p97]   5197

⟨1⟩ "could read a little & could scarcely write his name" – Sarah Bush Lincoln [wilson p107]   5198

⟨1⟩ "read the bible – he could write – not a good reader or scholar" – Harriet Chapman [wilson p646]   5199

Thomas

Reproductive

⟨H⟩ "he [William Cessna] further says that Thomas Lincoln was not considered all right in Consequence of having the Mumps or something else, that he has been with him often in baithing [sic] together in the water" – E.R. Burba [wilson p240]   5200

⟨H⟩ "I heard a Cousin of my fathers ... say that his father .. say that Thomas Lincoln could not have been Abes Father for one of Thomas' testacles was not larger than a pea or perhaps both of them wer no larger than peas" [sic] – Charles Friend [wilson pp674&675]   5201

⟨2⟩ Thomas may have had the mumps, and may have had an operation for it. See ¶5188 and ¶44. *Orchitis is a well-known complication of mumps.*   5202

⟨1⟩ "Thomas was castrated but that no time was fixed by the witnesses of said event" – William Herndon [wilson p639] (Similar: [hertz p205].)   5203

   ⟨1⟩ After relating this to Illinois governor Richard Oglesby in 1887, Oglesby responded "The very idea that old Thomas Lincoln would fool Mrs Johnson [sic, his second wife] was foolish" [wilson p639]   5204

   ⟨1⟩ Herndon notes that two previously fertile women, Nancy Lincoln and Sarah Bush Johnston Lincoln, had no more children via Thomas after about 1812 [hertz pp 138-139]. But see ¶4897.   5205

   ▪ More on castration, from William Herndon: 5206
      ⟨2⟩ "Dennis Hanks told me that Thomas Lincoln, when tolerably young, and before he left Kentucky, was castrated." [hertz p139]   5207
      ⟨1⟩ "It is said to me that Thomas ... was castrated and there is not much doubt of it." [hertz p205] *Is Herndon relying solely on Dennis Hanks? This would seem unlikely if Herndon is convinced "there is not much doubt about it."*   5208

⟨1⟩ "I do not know anything about Thomas Lincoln's loss of manhood" – James Rardin [wilson p651]   5209

⟨1⟩ "As to your first inquiry in regard to Thos Lincoln not being able to get a 'Baby' from his first Marriage, that seems to be the impression from the best information I can get" – E.R. Burba [wilson p256]   5210

339

Skin

⟨1⟩ "Dark completion" – John Hanks [wilson p615] *Presumed to mean "dark complex-* 5211
ion."

⟨1⟩ "He was rather Dark complected" – A.H. Chapman [wilson p96] (Part of ¶5070.) 5212

⟨1⟩ "dark hair, eyes, scin" – David Turnham [wilson p142] (Part of ¶5066.) 5213

⟨1⟩ "dark skinned" – David Turnham [wilson p122] (Part of ¶5071.) 5214

Sleep & Circadian Rhythms

⟨1⟩ "Lincoln would go and tell his jokes ... People in town would gather around him – 5215
He would keep them there till midnight or longer telling stories ... I would get tired
– want to go home" –Dennis Hanks [wilson p105] *This seems to be about Abraham,*
but the text could also be construed to refer to Thomas.

Speech

⟨1⟩ "talked and walked slow" – George Balch [wilson p597] 5216

Trauma

⟨2⟩ At age 8 was saved from death in an Indian raid by an incredible gunshot from 5217
his 14-year-old brother Mordecai. The shot killed the Indian running at Thomas.
[donaldA p21] [lincloreIGI]

⟨1⟩ "The story of his killing the Indian who killed old Abraham Linkhorn is all 5218
'my eye and Betty Martin.' " – Christopher Graham [tarbellE p234]

⟨1⟩ Bitten by a bulldog "on his return from New Orleans" – A.H. Chapman [wilson p137] 5219

⟨1⟩ "Bull dog story – 3 Girls, 1 his daughter and 2 of his last wife & old lady ran – 5220
So did the dog – bit him – He said G–d d–n the dog" – A.H. Chapman [wilson
p439] *Implies this occurred between the arrival of Sarah Bush Johnston and*
her daughters in Dec. 1819 [wilson p439n] *and the death of Sarah Lincoln in*
Jan. 1828.

Travel & Dwellings

⟨1⟩ Two trips to New Orleans [wilson p102]. See ¶5120 and, for estimated date of one 5221
trip, ¶5220.

⟨2⟩ 1816: Travels by waterway from Knob Creek, Kentucky to Indiana, seeking a new 5223
homestead. Walked back. [angle p17]

⟨1⟩ About 1816: Travels by waterway towards New Orleans, but does not reach the 5224
Mississippi River. (See ¶5122.) [tarbellE pp233. 234]

Lincoln, Thomas

Chronology 341 ■ General 341 ■

Chronology

⟨2⟩ Born 1811 or 1812 [templeC]   5225

   ⟨-⟩ *The basis for assigning these years is unclear. The only indication I have*   5226
seen of Thomas' birthday is the statement that Thomas was younger than
Abraham. See ¶5228

   ⟨1⟩ Herndon theorizes "Nancy, ceased to have children in, say, 1812. (There is   5227
no proof of the exact time.)" [hertz p206]

⟨1⟩/q Lincoln wrote in 1860 that he had a "brother, younger than himself, who died in   5228
infancy." [baslerA v4p62]

⟨1⟩ "died when only 3 days old" –A.H. Chapman [wilson p97]   5229

⟨1⟩ "Thomas the 2nd child named after his Father did not live 3 days." – Dennis Hanks   5230
[wilson p27]

⟨1⟩ "did not live 3 days" – Dennis Hanks [wilson p27]   5231   Thomas(b)

⟨2⟩ Died "about two or three years of age" [lincloreIGI] *Does not appear to be a typo-*   5232
graphical error.

⟨1⟩ Was buried – Christopher Graham [tarbellE p232]   5233

General

⟨1⟩ "I never knew Mr Lincoln had a brother" – Leonard Swett, after reading letters in   5234
the possession of Robert Todd of St. Louis [wilson p159]

   ⟨-⟩ *It seems Swett was referring to Lincoln's step-brother, John Johnston, to*   5235
whom Lincoln referred to as "brother" [baslerA v2p78].

⟨2⟩ Grave was discovered in 1933 [lincloreIGI].   5236

Lincoln, Thomas "Tad" child #4

Chronology

Month	Year	Age	Home	Event	Ref. 5237
April	1853	0	Springfield, IL	born	
March	1861	7	Washington	Father is President	
February	1862	8	"	Brother Willie dies	
April	1865	12	"	Father murdered	
May	1865	12	Chicago		
October	1868	15	Frankfurt, Ger.	Prof. Hohagen's school	[turnerB]
April	1870	17	Oberursel, Ger.		[turnerB]
June	1870	17	Leamington, Eng.		[turnerB]
May	1871	18	Chicago		
July	1871	18	"	dies	

Introduction & Sources

⊡ There is no comprehensive collection of photographs of Tad. Infrequently-seen images include his baby picture (? age 2 or 3) [ostendorfA p305]. The most photographs are in [ostendorfA pp161, 213, 305-309] (n=12) and [neelyA] (n=13), not counting his appearances with Lincoln in [ostendorf #38, 39, 46-48, 93, 114]. 5238

⟨2⟩ The medical records of Tad's final illness were destroyed three months after his death, in the great Chicago Fire. [shutesM] 5239

Appearance

■ Resemblance to father: 5240

⟨1⟩ "I remember ... that people said that Tad looked much like the dead President." – Mrs. George Carpenter [lewis] 5241

⟨1⟩ "The boy was like his father; he looked like him." [crookA p19] [crookK] 5242

⟨2⟩ July 1867: "One can imagine ... the tall, thin lad of fourteen, who was beginning to look so much like his father." [randallA p235] *Randall's description may be imaginary!* 5243

⟨2⟩ "Mrs. Orne, visiting them [Mary and Tad] in Frankfort, had been struck with this likeness, both in looks and traits of character." [randallC p380] *Orne was a sometime correspondent of Mary's.* 5244

⟨1⟩ Obituary: "He was tall and thin, and resembled his father in many of his mental traits and characteristics." [ChicagoTribune - July 16, 1871] *The statement about mental similarities is inaccurate. See* Mental Status. 5245

Appearance (continued)

⟨1⟩ May 1871: "Several years greatly change a person in childhood or youth. [Tad] is 5246
now a young man of about 20, of middle height, whose beardless red cheeks are
apparently the evidence of perfect health." [ChicagoTribune - May 16, 1871, reprinting New
York World of May 12] *Age is off by two years.*

   ⟨2⟩ "In looks he now closely resembled the Bob Lincoln of the early days of the 5247
   war. Tad was clear-eyed, of medium height, and his flushed cheeks suggested a ruddy state of health [but] this may well have been the bloom of
   fever." [rossA p302]. See ¶5278 for other worriers.

⟨$\frac{1}{q}$⟩ May 1871: Tad is described as "having grown up a tall, fine-looking lad of 18, who 5248
bears but faint resemblance to the tricksey little sprite" of the White House years.
[rossA p302, citing New York Semi-Weekly Tribune of May 26, 1871]

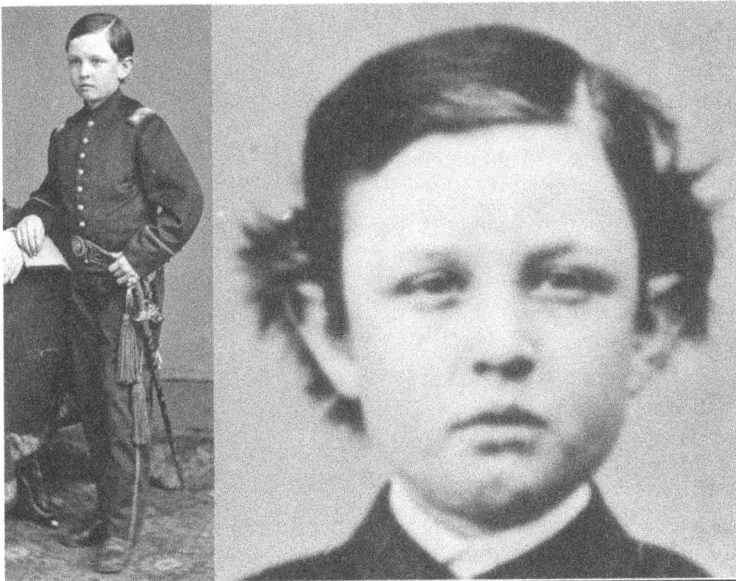

Tad

Figure 9. Tad Lincoln, about 1864-1865. *Photo credits:* National Archives
B-2466 and B-2673, respectively.

Build

Tad's face and frame changed as he entered adolescence, assuming an increasing re- 5249
semblance to his father. In particular, he was thin and (apparently) tall. Such a transformation to a more marfanoid habitus is possible. In showing a picture of a relatively normal-looking $3\,^1/_2$-year old, McKusick states "Dolichostenomelia is often less
impressive at this age" [mckusickA p42] and further notes that extremities are relatively
short in the first decade of life [mckusickA p116]. On the other hand, excess length may be
demonstrable at birth and throughout childhood and adolescence [mckusickA p53].

⟨$\frac{1}{q}$⟩ Nov. 1860: Willie and Tad: "chubby ... really healthy smart boys" – Thomas Web- 5250
ster [randallC p163]

Build (continued)

⟨1⟩ Tad "was a small boy, probably not more than seven or eight years old." – Senator James Harlan (date of recollection unknown) [helmB p168] *"Small" likely describes Tad's age, not his stature.* 5251

⟨2⟩ July 1867: "tall, thin lad of fourteen" [randallA p235] *May be imaginary! See ¶5243.* 5252

⟨$\frac{1}{q}$⟩ August 1865: "He is growing very fast." – Mary [turner p264] 5253

⟨2⟩ Late 1868: tailor charges for work on trousers – probably lengthening [randallA p260]. "Seemed to be aiming at his father's lofty height" [randallA p260]. 5254

⟨$\frac{1}{q}$⟩ As a teenager: "slight, and delicate in health" [evans p58] See ¶5632. 5255

⟨1⟩ March 22, 1870, after about six weeks absent from Tad (calculated from [turner pp501, 504]): "I return to find my dear boy much grown in even so short a time and I am pained to see his face thinner, although he retains his usual bright complexion. He is doubtless greatly improving in his studies, yet I am very sure the food he gets at his school does not agree with him." [helmB pp280-281] [turner p504] 5256

- Undatable secondary assessments: 5257
    ⟨2⟩ "He grew to be a big tall lad, with a frame that might have become as gigantic as his father's." [evans p60] quoting William E. Barton 5258
    ⟨2⟩ Long, thin body [lewis] 5259
    ⟨2⟩ "It would be revealed ultimately that he was to have a tall, thin body." [randallA p7] 5260

⟨1⟩ May 1871: "a young man of about 20, of middle height" [ChicagoTribune - May 16, 1871] (Part of ¶5246) *Possible (weak) reasons this height assessment differs from others: (a) Tad was 18, not 20, so perhaps he was tall for his age, and (b) Perhaps Tad was seen seated only and, like his father, had a non-tall trunk and long legs.* 5261

⟨$\frac{1}{q}$⟩ May 1871: "a tall, fine-looking lad of 18" [rossA p302] (Part of ¶5248) 5262

⟨1⟩ Obituary: "he was tall and thin" [ChicagoTribune - July 16, 1871] (∈ ¶5245) 5263

Death & Final Illness

Tad died from a wasting illness that lasted months and culminated in orthopnea and pleural effusions. There is no mention of fever, and physical pain does not appear to have been a prominent feature of the illness. There is no mention of diminished exercise tolerance. With an underlying diagnosis of MEN2B, the most likely cause would be a malignant effusion, caused by medullary carcinoma of the thyroid, metastatic to the chest. It is possible that a pericardial metastasis (possibly a result of direct extension from a chest metastasis) caused his terminal event via cardiac tamponade. 5264

As a contrarian, I also considered heart failure resulting from an atrial septal defect (ASD) as a possible cause of Tad's final illness. ASD patients often have a "gracile habitus" that arouses suspicion of Marfan syndrome [mckusickA pp85, 117]. Mitral stenosis is also a consideration, given the profound orthopnea and the remark about Tad's red cheeks (¶5246) (i.e., mitral facies). The lack of exercise intolerance points away from a primary cardiac disorder. 5265

Herndon suspected the Lincoln boys had syphilis. This suggests there must have been something not right about them, noticeable with casual contact. (See ¶3954.) 5266

⟨2⟩$_c$ During Tad's final illness, Robert's wife was out of town. "Through Robert's reports to her one can follow the course of Tad's illness" [randallA p270]. Also see annotation of [lincolnR]. 5267

Death & Final Illness (continued)

- Harbingers: 5268
  - ⟨1⟩ "In the summer of 1869, Mrs. Lincoln went on a European tour, accompa-   5269
    nied by her youngest son, who then began to show symptoms of disease."
    [NYTimes - July 18, 1871] (obituary) *Although Mary and Tad arrived in Europe*
    in 1868, they did indeed go on a multi-country tour of Europe in summer
    1869 [turner pp507-508].
  - ⟨2⟩ "During a visit to Germany in 1871, Tad suddenly began to lose weight."   5270
    c [durham] *This is probably just a reference to ¶5256. Tad was never in*
    Germany in 1871.
  - ⟨2⟩ Spring 1871: "His debility startled his mother when she returned to London   5271
    after a brief visit to Frankfurt." [rossA p300]

- April-May 1871: sea voyage from England to New York: 5272
  - ⟨2⟩ Mary and Tad (and General Philip Sheridan) sail April 29, 1871 on the *Russia*.   5273
    [rossA p300]
  - ⟨1⟩ The passage was extremely rough. Mary thought they were "doomed to de-   5274
    struction" during a gale. Most passengers had to stay in their berths for three
    days. When they came out on deck, the waves were "mountains high, and
    the swell was so tremendous we were tossed about like a leaf." [ChicagoTribune
    - May 16, 1871]
  - ⟨1⟩ Arrives in New York on May 10, 1871. A cutter bearing a health officer, Dr.   5275
    Carnochan, was ignored by the *Russia* as she entered New York, but Mary
    and Tad later transferred to the cutter. [NYTimes - May 11, 1871] *Whether Dr.*
    Carnochan examined Tad (and/or Mary) is not stated.

⟨1⟩ May 11, 1871, or thereabouts: Tad interviewed by two newspapers. Neither says   5276
he looks ill (see ¶5246 and ¶5248).
  - ⟨1⟩ One says his "beardless red cheeks are apparently the evidence of perfect   5277
    health." [ChicagoTribune - May 16, 1871] (Part of ¶5246.)
  - ⟨2⟩ This has often been interpreted as a flush [rossA p302] [durham] [randallA p266]   5278

⟨2⟩ May 15, 1871: Tad and Mary leave New York for Chicago [randallA p269]   5282

⟨1⟩ May 23, 1871: "My youngest son, is confined to his bed today, with a severe cold.   5283
I hope by great care, that he will soon recover." – Mary [turner p589]
  - ⟨1⟩ Mary wrote a second letter that day, substantially repeating this [turner p588].   5284
  - ⟨H⟩ "Tad had probably caught his cold aboard the *Russia*. ... Knowing little about   5287
    germs, his doctors believed the exposure to wet weather was the primary
    cause of his coughing." [baker p307] *Baker's reference for these statements,*
    [turner p590], *says nothing about wet weather and nothing about coughing.*
    [baker p307] *also describes, in some detail, the diagnostic and therapeutic*
    steps taken by the physicians, again citing [turner p590] *which again says*
    nothing on those subjects.

⟨2⟩ Between May 23 and June 8: "Tad was well enough to be moved to Clifton House   5288
but soon after grew much worse." [helmB p291]
  - ⟨1⟩ Based on [turner p589], the move was most likely on Saturday, May 27.   5289
  - ⟨1⟩ Tad was severely ill after the move, but improved afterwards. – Robert [helmB   5290
    p293]. See ¶5301.

⟨2⟩ End-May 1871: "at the last of May he developed difficulty in breathing when lying   5292
down and had to sleep sitting up in a chair." [randallA pp269-270] citing hotelkeeper
W.A. Jenkins

Death & Final Illness (continued)

⟨1⟩ June 5 or 6, 1871: "... has been seriously ill for the past four or five days, his disease being water on the lungs. Yesterday he was slightly better." [ChicagoTribune - June 6, 1871]   5293

⟨1⟩ June 8, 1871, to Messrs Henry Diafo[?] & Co., Liverpool: "Your letter of May 16 ... has been neglected by Mrs. Lincoln on account of the severe illness of my brother..." – Robert [lincolnR]   5294

⟨1⟩ June 8, 1871: "I take advantage of a quiet sleep, which he is enjoying, to write you regarding him. My dear boy, has been *very very* dangerously ill – attended by two excellent physicians who have just left me, with the assurance, that he is better. ... Dr Davis, a very eminent lung physician, says, that *thus far*, his lungs are *not at all* diseased although water has been formed on part of his left lung, which is gradually decreasing. His youth, and vigilant care, with the mercy of God, may ward off future trouble. ... I have been sitting up so constantly for the last ten nights, that I am unable to write you at length to day." – Mary [turner p590]   5295

⟨2⟩ After June 8, "The improvement was short-lived, for the other lung was soon affected." [turner p585] with no reference provided.   5296

⟨1⟩ July 3, 1871: Senator Harlan, after a week-long trip, writes to Robert: "I was wretchedly uneasy about your Brother, and could hear nothing. ... I infer from your silence that he must be better – and I trust out of danger." [helmB p292]   5297

⟨$\frac{1}{q}$⟩ July 8, 1871: "Thomas Lincoln is dangerously ill. If he recovers, it will be [almost?] a miracle. The disease is dropsy of the chest. He has been compelled to sit upright in a chair for upwards of a month." – Judge David Davis, writing on July 12 [baker p308], presumably after a July 8 visit [randallA p270]   5298

⟨1⟩ July 10, 1871, to Messrs Henry Graham & Co.: "My brother has been very ill for about five weeks, with very little hope of recovery. [illegible] most of the time - Just at present we feel a little [illegible] about him." – Robert [lincolnR]   5299

⟨1⟩ July 11, 1871: "Mr. Thomas Lincoln has been picking up for the last two or three days and is to all appearances improving, his face has lost some of its expression of distress." – Robert [helmB p293]   5300

⟨1⟩ July 14, 1871: "I am sorry to tell you that Tad seems to be losing ground. Yesterday was very hot and oppressive and he got in a bad way during the night and this morning was nearly as bad as the first night you came to the Clifton House. I have just now (2 o'clock) come from him and he is looking better, but Dr. Davis says he can see nothing to found any hope off his recovery upon and that he can live only a few days – with the weak action of his heart and lungs. To-day there is a fine breeze and the air is really delightful – all of which makes him feel better but really have little or no effect upon his trouble. He is looking dreadfully." – Robert to his wife [helmB p293]   5301

⟨1⟩ July 15, 1871: "We came back from Springfield this morning all well. I will not attempt to tell you all that has happened in the last ten days, for I am a good deal used up. Last Tuesday, Wednesday and Thursday morning Tad appeared a great deal better. He was stronger and looking well and the water was reduced a good deal in his chest. Thursday was very close and oppressive and it pulled him back very much. Friday afternoon he seemed to rally again and at eleven P.M. was sleeping nicely with prospects of having a good night, so I left him with mother and his two nurses and went to the house. I was aroused at half past four and went to the hotel and saw at once that he was failing fast. He was in great distress and   5302

Death & Final Illness (continued)

laboring for breath and ease but I do not think he was in acute pain. He lingered on so until between half past seven and eight, when he suddenly threw himself forward on his bar and was gone." –Robert [helmB p294] *If warm weather caused vasodilation, this would worsen the effects of cardiac tamponade or end-stage heart failure.*

⟨2⟩ [baker p307] states: "Mary Lincoln bought a new chair with a bar across the front to prevent him, when he nodded off, from falling on the floor." *She cites an 1871 letter in* [lincolnR], *but when I searched I could not find a mention of the chair.*   5303

⟨1⟩ Obituaries: 5304

    ⟨1⟩ "Chicago, July 15: ... [Tad died] at 7 o'clock this morning, of dropsy of the heart, age eighteen. He was taken ill a few days after returning from Europe. During his illness his mother has been his almost constant attendant." *New-York Daily Tribune,* July 17, 1871, page 1. *Note "dropsy of the <u>heart</u>," not chest. Same as* [NYTribune]*?*   5305

    ⟨1⟩ "Died [of] dropsy of the heart, aged eighteen years. He was taken ill a few days after returning from Europe. During his illness his mother has been his almost constant attendant." [NYTimes - July 16, 1871]   5306

    ⟨1⟩ "At half-past 7 o'clock, yesterday morning, [Tad] died at the Clifton House on Wabash avenue, where he had been staying since his return from Europe. The cause of his death was dropsy of the chest, the first symptoms showed themselves while he was abroad, but it was not until three days after his return in the middle of May that it began to be alarming. The disease made its appearance in the left chest, and, notwithstanding the care given him afterward, attacked the right side, and soon after caused death by the compression of the heart. He was convalescent at one time, but, unfortunately, got up in the night, wandered around lightly clad, on returning to his room swooned, and grew steadily worse from that moment. He was attended by Dr. C.G. Smith, of this city, who did for him all that skill and faithful attention could, but the trouble was too deeply seated for his ability to be of any avail. ... [Tad] bore his illness with great patience and resignation." [ChicagoTribune - July 16, 1871]   5307

    ⟨$\frac{1}{q}$⟩ [evans p212] cites [ChicagoTribune - July 18, 1871] and provides a slightly different quotation. He says there was a relapse after the swoon, and gives Dr. Smith's full name as Charles Gilman Smith.   5308

    ⟨1⟩ "The disease which carried off young Lincoln is known to medical science as dropsy of the chest. He was first attacked by it before he returned to this country, and has been suffering from it ever since, until death released him." Also mentions "Dr. C.D. Smith." [NYTimes - July 18, 1871] (obituary) *Although this article gets Smith's initials wrong, it does get correct a subtle "tour"-related issue mentioned in* ¶5269.   5309

- Was there pain?   5311
    ⟨1⟩ July 24, 1871, to Heinrich Best[?]: "But immediately after their arrival at home my brother was attacked by a long and painful illness which terminated in his death five days ago..." – Robert [lincolnR]   5312
    ⟨1⟩ "He was only eighteen when he died but he was so manly and self reliant that I had the greatest hopes for his future. These were cut off by his death after a torturing illness, he not being able to recline but sitting for six weeks in the chair from which he was only taken dead. Such suffering I never saw but it was all bourn [sic] with marvellous [sic] fortitude." – Robert Lincoln to Noah   5313

Death & Final Illness (continued)

Brooks, April 5, 1882 [randallP box 73] (with duplicate in box 74) citing *Chicago History*. Summer 1947; 1(8)

⟨2⟩ "in 1871, he was taken with a severe illness ... enduring with manly fortitude months of great pain" [brooksB]   5314

⟨2⟩ "After enduring with marked fortitude several months of suffering, he died in July 1871." [brooksC p279]   5315

⟨-⟩ *Based on these accounts, I do not think Tad had a painful illness, in the sense we commonly use "pain" (e.g. pleuritic pain). Tad's inability to lie flat may indeed have been torture, just as waterboarding is torture without inflicting pain-as-commonly-defined. Brooks's writings seem to have been based on letters from Robert.*   5316

⟨1⟩ Aug. 3, 1871, to A.L. Fisk, from Henry Officer: "... the illness of Mr. Lincoln's brother prevented him from attending to business during the month of June and also part of July – He was called away from the city last week and I do not expect him back before 20th [?week]." [lincolnR]   5317

- Diagnoses – by physicians: 5318
  - ⟨S⟩ "A fatal pleurisy developing in an eighteen-year-old boy and lasting six months was probably tubercular in origin. It may have been due to infection with some microbe other than the tubercle bacillus, but the chances are against that." [evans p212]   5319
  - ⟨S⟩ [evans p340] wonders if Tad's final illness was related to the cough Mary had in the winter of 1870-71. See ¶4309   5320
  - ⟨2⟩$_c$ "It is generally thought that Tad died of typhoid fever, but the foregoing brief evidence would indicate that he had pleurisy with effusion. ... Dr. W.A. Evans suggests, with good reason, that a pleurisy which had existed for six months must have been tubercular, especially since Tad was tall and thin and 18." [shutes p121]   5321
  - ⟨2⟩$_c$ "Dr. W.A. Evans soundly reasoned that [Tad's illness] could have been tubercular in origin." [shutesM]   5322
  - ⟨S⟩ "A description of his symptoms suggests the boy was in congestive heart failure. This arouses suspicion that Tad Lincoln may have developed one of the many cardiovascular complications found in the Marfan syndrome. In this disease, death of a boy 18 years of age with congestive heart failure is not rare." [gordon]   5323

- Diagnoses – by non-physicians: 5324
  - ⟨S⟩ Died, "from all appearances" of tuberculosis [neelyE p189]   5325
  - ⟨2⟩ "succumbed to tuberculosis" [kunhardtA p394, 396]   5326
  - ⟨S⟩ "In fact, Tad was suffering from an intractable pleurisy, caused either by pneumonia or a primary infection from tuberculosis bacilli in the lining of his lungs. Gradually the pleural spaces in his chest were filling with serum and pus from an unchecked bacterial infection." [baker p307]   5327
  - ⟨-⟩ [baker p307] *states Tad had pus in his chest and a fever, but she appears to have conjured this from the word "pleurisy." Again without apparent support, [baker p308] says Tad turned blue and became "edemous" [sic] on his last day. I conclude that all this is pure invention, extrapolated from the tentative diagnosis of [evans p212].*   5328
  - ⟨S⟩ "Although the precise cause of Tad's death was never established, it was thought that pleurisy developing in the eighteen-year-old boy and lasting six months might well have been tubercular in origin. Tad's high flush and   5329

Death & Final Illness (continued)

excitable ways were recalled. He had been plagued by colds during the two years that he and his mother had been abroad, and she had felt that he had been undernourished for a time in Germany. Other posthumous speculations included emphysema, so familiar today, and a virus unrecognized at the time." [rossA p304]

Diet & Digestion

⟨1⟩ While living in Springfield and ill, drank milk from a neighbor's Jersey cow, "Mr. Lincoln himself calling for the milk every morning." [ChicagoTribune - Feb. 12, 1937]   5330

⟨2⟩ March 1861: "Every member of the household became ill from eating too well of the unaccustomed Potomac shad." [shutes p77] (See ¶640.)   5331

⟨1⟩ "was blessed with a vigorous appetite" [brooksB]   5332

⟨1⟩ March 1870: Increasing thinness, noticeable over six weeks, blamed by Mary on the food he was being fed at school. [helmB pp280-281]. See ¶5256   5333

Ears

▣ Protruding "bat" ears in younger years [neelyA pp45, 46, 67].   5334

Energy

⟨1⟩ "Everything that Tad did was done with a certain rush and rude strength which were peculiar to him. I was once sitting with the President in the library, when Tad tore into the room in search of something, and, having found it, he threw himself on his father like a small thunderbolt, gave him one wild, fierce hug, and without a word, fled from the room before his father could put out his hand to detain him." [brooksB] [brooksC p279]. *Tad was not hypothyroid!*   5335

  ⟨1⟩ 1865: "During the five days of our stay in the Army of the Potomac, Tad was a most restless little chap." [brooksB]   5336

Eyes

▣ Eyes are widely spaced, but not hyperteloric   5337
▣ Mild right ptosis or ocular asymmetry is present.   5338
▣ Some photographs suggest down-sloping palpebral fissures.   5339

Eyes – Acuity

⟨1⟩ No record nor photograph shows Tad wearing eyeglasses. In particular, a posed studio photograph taken near the end of his life shows him writing at a desk, without wearing spectacles [neelyA p125].   5340

Eyes – Color Of

⟨1⟩ Of Tad, Mary wrote, on Dec. 29, 1869: "His dark loving eyes – watching over me, remind me so much of his dearly beloved father's." [turner p32]   5341

⟨1⟩ "His black eyes fairly sparkled with mischief." [keckleyB p117]   5342

⟨2⟩ Calls Tad's eye color "a rather unexpected product of gray- and blue-eyed parents" and suggests the brown eyes of his mother's father may have contributed. [randallA p7]   5343

Feet

⟨$\frac{1}{q}$⟩ Lincoln was carrying "well-grown" Tad down the street in Springfield. Mary's sister saw this and told Lincoln the boy was old enough to walk. Lincoln: "Oh, don't you think his little feet will get tired?" [randallC pp87-88] *Probably not a literal indication of foot size.*   5344

Gait

⟨1⟩ "That chile was so long walking and talking, everyone say he never would." [ostendorfC] *The reliability of* [ostendorfC] *is disputed* [hallJ].   5345

General

■ See ⟨Infection⟩   5346

⟨S⟩ Was likely breast fed, given that Mary breast fed a neighbor baby. (See ¶4647.)   5347

⟨1⟩ March 4, 1860: "Willie and Tad were very sick the Saturday night after I left [? Feb. 25] ... I trust the dear little fellows are well again" – Lincoln to Mary [donaldH p75]   5348

⟨1⟩ Nov. 2, 1862: "Taddie is well" – Mary [turner p139]   5349

⟨1⟩ Sept. 22, 1863: "Taddie is well" – Mary [turner p158]   5350

⟨2⟩ 1864(?): Lincoln does not see John Stuart, having been up all night with the "ailing" Tad [randallC p307]   5351

⟨1⟩ April 2: "Tad & I are both well." – Lincoln, at City Point, VA [donaldH p112]   5352

⟨1⟩ April 4, 1865: Tad "is well and happy" – Mary [turner p213]   5353

⟨1⟩ August 17, 1865: "Taddie is well" – Mary [turner p264]   5354

⟨1⟩ March 19, 1867: "We are quite well" (includes Tad) – Mary [turner p417]   5355

⟨1⟩ October 29, 1867: "Taddie is welll" – Mary [turner p446]   5356

Habits

⟨2⟩ He did not smoke, drink, or dance [lewis] [randallA p238]. He took dance lessons in Germany [randallA p261].   5357

Hair

⟨1⟩ John Hay describes Tad's head as "curly." [templeA]   5358

⟨2⟩ Dark hair, like his father [randallA pp7&260]   5359

⟨S⟩ Randall found receipts showing that Tad bought an "amazing" amount of "pomatum" while in Germany. She wonders if his hair "like his father's, was unruly and the ointment served to slick it down as well as give it gloss." [randallA p260]   5360

Hands

▣ Tad's fingers are positioned unusually in the photographs in [neelyA pp67, 68], in a manner that suggests joint laxity or reduced muscle tone.   5361

▣ Right forefinger looks long, with unusual extension at distal interphalangeal joint, in [ostendorf #114].   5362

Head & Face

- Size (See ⟨Nickname⟩ for multiple other descriptions):   5363
  - ⟨2⟩ "big head" [kunhardtA p91]   5364
  - ⟨2⟩ His "nickname frankly suggests a head too large for the body and some of his   5365
    photographs do not lessen that impression" [shutesM].

- Shape: 5366
  - ⟨○⟩ Baby photograph (? age 2 or 3) [ostendorfA p305] shows a very high, wide fore-   5367
    head, with downsloping palpebral fissures.
  - ⟨2⟩ His general facial features changed significantly in his teenage years: the   5368
    round face characteristic of his mother's family gave way to the elongated
    face and prominent nose of his father [neelyA p48]. *Extant photographs con-
    firm this.*

⟨○⟩ Chin dimple.   5369
  - ⟨○⟩ No chin dimple seen in the two photographs in [neelyA p48]. *Were these pho-*   5370
    tographs altered?
  - ⟨-⟩ Lincoln also had a chin dimple (¶1898).   5371

⟨○⟩ Nov. 16, 1863: A photograph of Tad in profile shows a receding chin, compatible   5372
with mild to moderate retrognathia or micrognathia [neelyA p92]. *Micrognathia is
a small jaw. Retrognathia is a normal jaw displaced posteriorly.*
  - ⟨2⟩ [kunhardtB p77] and [kunhardtA p235] show the same photograph, but say it was   5373
    taken at City Point, VA in April 1865. [neelyA p92] prints the inscription on the
    back of the photo, dating it to Nov. 16, 1863, and [miers v3p219] says Tad got a
    new pony on Nov. 14, 1863.
  - ⟨○⟩ In an 1871 photograph [neelyA p124], Tad's chin projects forward to a degree.   5374

⟨1⟩ March 1870: "I am pained to see his face thinner" after an absence of about six   5375
weeks – Mary [helmB pp280-281] (∈ ¶5256)

⟨1⟩ May 11, 1871: His "beardless red cheeks are apparently the evidence of perfect   5376
health." [ChicagoTribune - May 16, 1871, reprinting New York World of May 12] (∈ ¶5246) (See
¶5278 for interpretations.)

Heart & Circulation

⟨1⟩ Dec. 1869: Tad carries a box of "souvenirs" and things "procured" from his living   5377
quarters "down to your office" [turner p531] *Amount of physical exertion unclear.*

⟨1⟩ March 22, 1870, from Frankfurt: "he retains his usual bright complexion" [helmB   5378
pp280-281] (∈ ¶5256)

⟨1⟩ May 11, 1871: His "beardless red cheeks are apparently the evidence of perfect   5379
health." [ChicagoTribune - May 16, 1871, reprinting New York World of May 12] (∈ ¶5246) (See
¶5278 for interpretations.)

Infection

⟨1⟩$_q$ Herndon thought the Lincoln sons might have had congenital syphilis. See   5380
¶2023. *Why would he think this? It suggests the boys had something "not
right" that casual observation disclosed.*

⟨1⟩ Feb. 28, 1859: "... Taddie, is quite sick. The Dr thinks it may prove a *slight* attack   5381
of *lung* fever. ... He passed a bad night, I do not like his symptoms." – Mary (date
was deduced) [turner p53]

Tad

Infection (continued)

⟨-⟩ *"Lung fever" was, in 1892, an alternate name for pneumonia* [osler p511]. 5382
*An Internet search for "lung fever" discloses several pages of 1850s
mortality records from the American midwest in which lung fever is a
frequently-listed cause of death. As late as 1900, pneumonia was the leading cause of death in the United States.*

⟨2⟩ [shutes p80] equates lung fever and pneumonia. 5383

⟨S⟩ Randall [randallA p57] says additional details are not known and further re- 5384
marks that Tad "was not a robust child thereafter." [randallA p57]

⟨1⟩ March 28, 1861: "Last week, both of the children, had the measles slightly, altho' 5385
the papers represented them as quite ill." – Mary [turner p81]. Also see: [grimsley]. The
boys gave measles to Elmer Ellsworth [turner p92].

- 1861: 5386
  ⟨2⟩ Summer: Caught severe cold at the beach [randallA p119]. 5387
  ⟨1⟩ Summer or fall: Mary was "at Long Branch and Saratoga. There she nursed 5388
  Tad through a spell of illness." [helmB p190]
  ⟨-⟩ *These are probably the same illness. Long Branch, NJ was a tony beach* 5389
  resort in the 1800s.

- Feb. 1862: Develops the same illness that ultimately killed Willie, diagnosed by 5390
  the newspapers as "bilious fever," but probably typhoid fever. See William
  Death & Final Illness .
  ⟨1⟩ Mrs. Pomroy, a nurse, "was taken to the sick room of little Tad, introduced to 5391
  the two physicians who sat in the hall just outside his door, who before leaving gave directions regarding medicine and treatment for every half-hour in
  the night. ... [Until at least 6:30 am] she kept her station by the bedside of
  the little sufferer, who lay tossing with typhoid, and at intervals weeping for
  his dear brother Willie." [boyden p54] *Is this Boyden's own diagnosis, or in-*
  formation from her mother, Mrs. Pomroy? Given that Mrs. Pomroy was
  specifically hired to nurse Tad, it seems likely that she would have repeated
  the diagnosis to her daughter.
  ⟨1/q⟩ "Thaddeus, the youngest son of the President, is still dangerously ill and 5392
  fears are entertained that his disease will assume the type which proved fatal
  to his brother." [NYHerald - Feb. 22, 1862] as quoted by [shutes p119]
  ⟨1/q⟩ "Tad was also very ill at this time, and I watched him several consecutive 5393
  nights. The President was in the room with me a portion of each night. He
  was ... agitated with apprehension of a fatal termination of Tad's illness." –
  Orville Browning [tripp p185]

⟨2⟩ Aug. 1863: "Ailing" [rossA p195]. *Unclear if this describes an infection or something* 5394
else.

- Nov. 1863: Tad is sick. Lincoln simultaneously develops smallpox (see ¶2030 and 5395
  Special Topic §5).
  ⟨2⟩ Nov. 18: Because of Tad's illness and Mary's near-hysteria about it, Lincoln 5397
  almost did not go to Gettysburg (to deliver the Gettysburg address) [donaldA
  p462]
  ⟨1⟩ Nov. 20: "Our sick boy, for whom you kindly inquire, we hope is past the 5398
  worst." – Lincoln writing to Edward Everett [baslerA v7p25]
  ⟨1⟩ Nov. 28: "The President's youngest son, who had been sick for some time 5399
  past with scarlatina, was much better yesterday, the crisis of his disease being past. It is expected he will be able again to be out in a short time." –
  Washington Chronicle [lincloreLHH]

352

Infection (continued)

⟨-⟩ *Tad and his father are known to have been together while both were ill* 5400
(§5.45), suggesting that they both had the same disease.

⟨2⟩ Presumably after Lincoln was diagnosed with smallpox, "All contacts, in- 5401
cluding the family, were vaccinated" [evans p141]. Similarly, "All the other
members of the White House family were visited by the President's own doctor and I was compelled to show my arm" [stoddardD p305]. *If it were thought*
Tad also had smallpox (e.g. [lincloreLHH]), Tad would not have undergone
vaccination.

⟨2⟩ "There is no record of Lincoln or his sons having been vaccinated against 5402
small pox." [pearson] *This may apply to the period before Lincoln developed*
smallpox.

⟨1⟩ Nov. 16: Tad is photographed astride his new pony [neelyA p92] (See ¶5372.). 5403
Could this have been related to Tad's illness?

⟨1⟩ 1864: On illness in the White House: "Tad has undoubtedly been injured so that 5404
his constitution will not recover." [stoddardA p124]

■ Cold, December 1865: 5405
⟨1⟩ Dec. 16: "is suffering with a most terrible cold, I was up, with him, almost 5406
all last night, as he came very near, having the croup – Without he greatly
improves – I will be unable to go down to Springfield this week – He is too
unwell to leave or to take him" – Mary [turner p308]
⟨1⟩ Dec. 18: "is very much indisposed, with a bad cold" – Mary [turner p311] 5407

■ Colds 5408
⟨2⟩ 1866-1867: "was frail and had frequent colds" [randallA p233] 5409
⟨2⟩ 1869-70: Frequent colds [rossA p289] 5410
⟨2⟩ 1870-1871: Frequent colds [rossA pp291, 304] 5411

■ 1871: See Death . *Death was probably not an infection.* 5412

Infection – Exposures

⟨2⟩ "... he had numerous pets, including a pony and two goats" [neelyE p189] 5413
⟨2⟩ Had a kitten and dog in the White House [donaldA p428] 5414
⟨2⟩ a rabbit in the White House [kunhardtB p76] 5415
⟨1⟩ 1864: Took as a pet, after it's "pardon," a large turkey sent to the White House 5416
for Thanksgiving [brooksB] [kunhardtB p75]
⟨2⟩ Two goats, Nanko and Nanny, had the run of the White House [donaldH p27]. 5417
They were "jumping goats" [kunhardtB p298] and apparently healthy [donaldH
pp101, 105]. They were sent to another family after Lincoln's death [turner pp259n,
268]

⟨□⟩ 1865: Sitting on a borrowed horse [kunhardtB p77]. Photograph's story is in [brooksB]. 5418

⟨1⟩ 1865: Caught and ate fish from the Potomac River on at least one occasion [brooksB] 5419

⟨2⟩ Tad spent a great deal of time seeing, with his father, the hordes of people who 5420
came to appeal in person to the President. [kunhardtB p76]
⟨1⟩ "He was foolishly caressed and petted by people who wanted favors of his 5421
father." [brooksB]

Legs

⟨2⟩ Summer 1869: Frail legs [rossA p288] (∈ ¶5484) 5422

Lungs

⟨1⟩ "Lung fever" (pneumonia) in 1859. See ¶5381   5423

⟨S⟩ It is worth remembering that people in the 19th century would have had very   5424
great exposures to burning wood – see ¶4307

Mental Status

Different aspects of Tad's brain are explored in Reading & Learning , Shrewd ,   5425
Spoiled , and Mental Status .

⟨1⟩ "Tad is a very peculiar child." – Lincoln [brooksB] *Not taken out of context.*   5426

⟨1⟩ "He was so full of life and vigor – so bubbling over with health and high spirits,   5427
that he kept the house alive with his pranks and his fantastic enterprises. He was
always a 'chartered libertine' after the death of his brother Willie." – John Hay
[templeA]

⟨$\frac{1}{q}$⟩ Early days in Washington: "Willie and Tad are so lonely and everything is so   5428
strange to them" – Mary [randallC p243]

⟨1⟩ 1861: "a gay, gladsome, merry, spontaneous fellow, bubbling over with innocent   5429
fun, whose laugh rang through the house, when not moved to tears. Quick in
mind, like his mother, ... he was the life, as also the worry of the household." [grim-
sley] (See ¶4396.)

⟨1⟩ 1861-1862: "He had a quick fiery temper, very affectionate when he chose, but   5430
implacable in his dislikes." [bayne p3]

⟨1⟩ 1864: "Tad is a strange child. He was violently excited when I went to him. I simply   5431
said: 'Tad, do you know you are making your father a great deal of trouble?' He
burst into tears, instantly giving me up the key." – Lincoln, after settling a dispute
between Tad and Francis Carpenter [ChicagoTribune - Dec. 3, 1865].

⟨1⟩ 1865: After Lincoln's murder: "For twenty-four hours the little fellow was perfectly   5432
inconsolable." Then, after realizing that his father was in heaven: "I am glad he
has gone there, for he was *never* happy here!" [ChicagoTribune - Dec. 3, 1865]

⟨1⟩ end-May 1865, in Chicago: "Taddie I took out for a walk almost every day and   5433
tried to interest him in the sights we saw. But he was a sad little fellow, and
mourned for his father." [crookA p71]

⟨1⟩ 1865: "he had a man's heart and in some things a man's mind" [crookK]   5434

⟨1⟩ June 1867: "my troublesome *sunshine*" – Mary [turner p425]   5435

⟨1⟩ November 1867: "Taddie's nature is very amiable and I do not anticipate the least   5436
trouble in his management" – Mary [turner p451]

⟨1⟩ Sept. 1868: "Taddie appears a little obstinate & *inclined* to be *argumentative*" on   5437
a certain subject – Mary [turner p483]

⟨1⟩ Dec. 1868: "is a most affectionate, amiable tempered child – he is *recovering* from   5438
his homesickness" – Mary [turner p496]

⟨1⟩ "He was a fearless rider." – John Hay [templeA]   5439
  ⟨1⟩ 1865: "hard-riding and reckless youngster;" "His short legs stuck straight out   5440
  from his saddle" [brooksB]

354

Mental Status (continued)

⟨1⟩ "He had that power of taming and attaching animals to himself, which seems to be the especial gift of kindly and unlettered natures." [templeA] 5441

⟨1⟩ While in Europe he displayed "a thoughtful devotion and tenderness beyond his years, and strangely at variance with the mischievous thoughtlessness of his childhood." [templeA] 5442

⟨1⟩ As a teenager "he remained the same cordial, frank, warm-hearted boy." [templeA] 5443

⟨1⟩ "He was a child of sunshine, nothing seemed to dampen the ardor of his spirits." [keckleyB p213] 5444

⟨1⟩ "a gay, gladsome, merry spontaneous fellow, bubbling over with innocent fun, whose laugh rang through the house, when not moved to tears" [grimsley] 5445

⟨2⟩ Secondary assessments of child Tad: 5446

  ⟨2⟩ "Tad could throw monumental temper tantrums when he failed to get his way." [oatesA p96] 5447

  ⟨2⟩$_c$ "He was an imaginative, responsive, and happy little fellow, though it took little to upset him and plunge him into an explosion of anger or tears.'" [randallA p7] 5448

  ⟨2⟩ He was "a happy little fellow who was as lovable as he was exasperating. He was quick-tempered and difficult to deal with." [randallA p56] 5449

  ⟨2⟩ "his impatience and headstrong antics were material for gossip for the nation" [lewis] 5450

  ⟨2⟩ "exasperating" [randallA pp56&139] 5451

  ⟨2⟩ "He was quick tempered and difficult to deal with; he was also ... completely engaging. Above all, he was a warmly affectionate child." [randallA p56] 5452

  ⟨2⟩ "affectionate and impulsive" [donaldA p159] 5453

  ⟨2⟩ "mercurial, elfin, eccentric ... sparkling with creative mischief" [kunhardtA p293] 5454

- Obituary: 5455

  ⟨-⟩ *One wonders how much these obituary-writers really knew of Tad.* 5456

  ⟨1⟩ Tad "resembled his father in many of his mental traits and characteristics. Many of his remarks were marked by the peculiar vein of thought which distinguished Mr. Lincoln." [ChicagoTribune - July 16, 1871] *The only place I have seen direct quotes from Tad is a newspaper interview in* [ChicagoTribune - May 16, 1871]. 5457

  ⟨1⟩ "He was a bright, precious boy, and from his earliest infancy, was noted for his affectionate and winning disposition. ... He inherited much of his lamented father's character. He had the same predisposition to melancholy, and the same genial spirit beaming from his features. The assassination of that beloved parent was a terrible shock to the poor boy; he never afterward regained the same elasticity of spirit, and the shadow of his father's doom clung to him through all his after life." [NYTimes - July 18, 1871] 5458

⟨1⟩$_q$ A friend of the Lincolns, Mrs. James S. Delano, remembered Tad as "the kindest, brightest, most considerate child" she had ever known [randallA p139] *Right. And "Raymond Shaw is the kindest, bravest, warmest, most wonderful human being I've ever known in my life." – Bennett Marco* 5459

Mouth

"In a world where deformity of all kinds was much more common than it is now such a minor irregularity would not have been worthy of comment." [aa89 p69] 5460

The quote above refers to the horrifically wounded face of Philip II of Macedon, but it is not unreasonable to apply it, in a lesser degree, to Tad. Several 20th century writers mentioned Tad's "defective palate," but only one in the 19th century does (¶5464). (The statement of Mariah Vance (¶5473) is not trustworthy.) 5461

There is a tantalizing secondary statement that Dr. William Wallace operated on Tad's palate (¶5466). This is remarkable given the surgical techniques of the age. Tad may have had a pronounced abnormality of his lips, due to MEN2B, which led to an operation that left a scar like a repaired cleft lip or palate. 5462

- See also: ⎡Speech⎤ and ⎡Teeth⎤ 5463

⟨1⟩ "He had a defective palate, and couldn't speak very plainly. [Lincoln] would perfectly understand [him]." [dana p185] 5464

  ⟨2⟩ Other descriptions: a [partially] cleft palate [bartonA p49] [currentEB] [kunhardtA pp91, 293] [oatesA p96] [shutes p79], a "misshapen palate" [sandburgA p66], a defective palate [rossA p158], or "either a cleft palate or a tied tongue" [lewis]. *Shutes was skeptical* [shutesM]. *Note:* [evans p58] *misquotes* [lewis]. 5465

⟨2⟩ Dr. William Wallace (see ¶3195) "operated ... on Tad for a cleft palate" [kunhardtB p257] 5466

  ⊡ On at least two occasions, Tad drew a mustache on a photograph of himself [neelyA pp69, 124]. *Did he want to disguise a cosmetic imperfection?* 5467

⊡ Two photographs are consistent with a scar of the left philtral ridge. See [kunhardtA p293] and Figure 10. 5468

  ⟨2⟩_c The caption to the photograph on [kunhardtA p293] says, with a deprecated term: "This photograph of Tad at eight shows a scar running from his upper lip to his nose, possibly marking a harelip." 5469

  ⟨-⟩ *My analysis of Figure 10 concludes that the photographer altered it by adding a dark mark over the left ridge of the philtrum. It is difficult to believe this was necessary for purely artistic reasons. More likely, the photographer did this to cover some kind of visible anomaly.* 5470

⊡ A stereoscopic version of [ostendorf #93] in [zeller] shows that Tad's lower lip is asymmetric and out-curled. 5471

⊡ Lip bumps visible in [neelyA pp45, 46, 48, 124], but poorly. Copies of original photos (from the Lincoln Museum, Ft. Wayne, IN) show bumps more clearly. See *The Physical Lincoln*. 5472

⟨1⟩ There is an account of milk running out of Tad's nose as he breast-fed. [ostendorfC p180] 5473

  ⟨2⟩ Agrees with: [kunhardtB p75], who does not provide a source for the statement. 5474

  ⟨-⟩ *This would indicate a communication between the oral and nasal cavities, and is consistent with a cleft palate. The reliability of* [ostendorfC] *is highly suspect* [hallJ]. 5475

- Teeth: 5476

  ⟨1⟩_q Early 1868: Mary took Tad to a dentist to have his teeth straightened. The dentist, according to Robert, was a "very good one" and "said that his teeth should be gradually forced into a proper position by means of a spring frame 5477

356

Mouth (continued)

kept in his mouth." The appliance interfered with Tad's speech (¶5645), so a second dentist was consulted. This dentist "said such an apparatus was not at all necessary," so Tad stopped using it. [randallA p238]

⟨2⟩ Agrees with: "crooked teeth" [neelyE 188] [donaldA p159]; "His second teeth came in crooked." [randallA p55].   5478

⟨1⟩ Nov. 1862: "I must send you, Taddie's tooth" – Mary, in New York, to Lincoln [turner p140]   5479

- The shape of Tad's jaw is discussed in ¶5372.   5480

⟨1⟩ Apparently could whistle: [ChicagoTribune - Sept. 17, 1871].   5481

Muscle / Athletics

⟨1⟩ The day after Tad's birth, the Lincoln household bought liniment [turnerL]. *Perhaps Tad was a "floppy baby" and the liniment was to improve his muscles. Or perhaps it was for post-partum Mary!*   5482

⟨1/q⟩ July 30, 1868: Could not hold grip on a passing freight train; almost died [turnerB] (See ¶5673.)   5483

⟨2⟩ Summer 1869: "Tad's frail legs grew weary as they [he and Mary] paraded through the endless corridors" of European art galleries [rossA p288]   5484   Tad

Nervous System

⟨2⟩ Was quick in his movements. [randallA p7]   5485

⟨☉⟩ Mild right ptosis or ocular asymmetry is present.   5486

⟨1⟩ Apparently could whistle: [ChicagoTribune - Sept. 17, 1871].   5487

⟨2⟩ Once heard to complain about the heat on his bare feet [shutesE p102] [shutesP] *Implies that temperature and/or pain sensation was intact.*   5488

⟨1⟩ In Washington: "I had taught little Taddy how to play the drum, and he used to drum for the guards." – violinist William Withers [croffut]   5489

Nickname

- Primary story: 5490
  ⟨1⟩ Lincoln first applied the nickname "Tadpole, subsequently abbreviated to Taddie, and then Tad" [carpenter p44]   5491
  ⟨1/q⟩ "was nicknamed Taddie by his loving Father" – Mary, writing a dozen years after Tad's birth [randallA p35] [randallC p131]   5492
  ⟨1⟩ "his father nicknamed 'Tadpole' when a baby because the little fellow's head seemed much larger than usual" [helmB p115]   5493
  ⟨2⟩ Tadpole nickname arose because he "had a large head and squirmed like a tadpole." [oatesA p96]   5494
  ⟨2⟩ "The infant was born with an unusually large head, as compared to his tiny body, and Lincoln playfully called him a little tadpole." [donaldA p154]   5495
  ⟨2⟩ Agrees with: [neelyE p188] [randallA p35] [randallC p131] [lewisM p15] [donaldH p60]   5497
  ⟨2⟩ Lincoln "thought he resembled a tadpole rather than anyone of the family" [shutesM].   5498

- Other stories: 5499

Nickname (continued)

⟨1⟩ "The name of 'Tad' – a pet name given by himself with his first stammering utterances...." – John Hay, writing in 1871 [templeA] 5500

⟨1⟩ "The nearest he could come to saying his own name, when quite a little fellow, was 'Tad,' and the name clung to him for many a year." [brooksB] 5501

⟨1⟩ "the difficulty he had in pronouncing his own name gave him the odd nickname by which he was always known." [brooksC pp278-279] (∈ ¶5609) 5502

Physicians & Nurses

⟨2⟩ Dr. William Wallace (see ¶3195) "operated ... on Tad for a cleft palate" [kunhardtB p257] 5503

⟨S⟩ Presumably Dr. Stone (¶3203) took care of both Tad and Willie when they were both sick with typhoid fever in 1862 (¶5390). 5504

⟨2⟩ Nurses during his serious illness of 1862: Mary Jane Welles [swansonB] and Rebecca Pomroy [boyden]. 5505

■ During his final illness Tad was attended by Dr. Charles Gilman Smith (¶5308) and Dr. Nathan S. Davis (¶5295) [turner p590n], and Dr. H.A. Johnson [shutesM]. Davis was the ex-President of the American Medical Association; he was called in as a consultant by Smith as Tad worsened [shutes p120]. 5506

Reading & Learning

Nature vs. nurture has long been debated in seeking the cause of Tad's delayed learning. In considering nurture, note that Tad lived in the same environment as his brother Willie, who seems to have been a good learner. We know Lincoln took an interest in his sons' school work: one anecdote has him going around the house declining Latin nouns at the time Robert was studying Latin in school [randallC p138]. (Lincoln studied Latin on the circuit [hertz p426].) 5507

Different aspects of Tad's brain are explored in `Reading & Learning`, `Shrewd`, `Spoiled`, and `Mental Status`. 5508

See also: `Spoiled`. Tad and the other Lincoln sons were spoiled. The lack of parental discipline could have contributed to Tad's delay in learning to read. 5509

⟨2⟩ Attended school in Springfield (Miss Corcoran's school) [randallA p55] 5510

⟨2⟩ "Whenever Lincoln went to any public gathering or to the courts of law in Springfield, little 'Tad' would be sure to accompany him, unless unwillingly detained at home to study his lessons." [NYTimes - July 18, 1871] (obituary) 5511

⟨S⟩ The episode of lung fever in 1859 "may have been one reason why Tad had not been pushed in his schooling." [randallA p56] 5512

⟨1⟩ Keckley describes a June 1865 incident in which the 12-year-old Tad does not know what A-P-E spells. She remarks "Whenever I think of this incident, I am tempted to laugh; and then it occurs to me that had Tad been a negro boy, not the son of a President, and so difficult to instruct, he would have been called thick-skulled, and would have been held up as an example of the inferiority of the race. I know many full negro boys, able to read and write, who are not older than Tad Lincoln was when he persisted that A-p-e spelt monkey." [keckleyB pp219-220] 5513

⟨2⟩ Agrees with: "The nine-year-old boy ... despite the efforts of a series of tutors ... could neither read nor write" [donaldA p428] 5514

Reading & Learning (continued)

⟨2⟩ "at twelve could neither read nor write" [kunhardtB p135] 5515

⟨1⟩ At age 12: "had never been made to go to school" [keckleyB pp216-217] 5516

⟨1⟩ "He had a very bad opinion of books, and no opinion of discipline, and thought 5517
very little of any tutor who would not assi[s]t him in yoking his kids to a chair or in
driving his dogs in tandem over the South Lawn." – John Hay [templeA]. Hay further
reports that Tad would find ways to get rid of tutors (¶5588).

⟨1⟩ In the White House he frequently hatched schemes and plans. "He had so much 5518
to do that he felt he could not waste time in learning to spell." – John Hay [templeA]
*This ignores the fact that Tad did not move into the White House until he was
8 years old.*

⟨2⟩ "Tad was fascinated by money and hoarded it, though at the age of ten he still 5519
could not understand that a small gold dollar was the same in value as a handful
of larger coins. He wanted the money that was big, and 'a lot.' " [kunhardtB p76]

  ⟨2⟩ His mother was not "sane" about money – see ¶4456 5520

⟨S⟩ "It became Tad's policy to evade school, and one wonders whether the other chil- 5521
dren had laughed at his first attempts to learn his letters (which would have been
comical with his impediment of speech) and whether this teasing was a factor in
his distaste for books." [randallA p55]

⟨1/q⟩ "Tad was very shrewd in sizing up the tutors. Many of them did not stay long 5522
enough to reach an understanding of him, said Mr. Brooks, "but he knew them
before they had been one day in the house." [randallA p122]

⟨1⟩ After Lincoln's death, "Robert at once took charge of his education, and he made 5523
rapid progress up to the time of his sailing to Europe with his mother." – John Hay
[templeA]

  ⟨2⟩ Agrees with: [brooksB], who gets the sailing date wrong. Sailing was on Octo- 5524
  ber 1, 1868 [templeA].

⟨1⟩ June 1865: "He says two or three lessons a day & is at length seized with the desire 5525
to be able to *read and write* – which with his *natural* brightness, will be *half* the
battle with him" – Mary [turner p250]

⟨2⟩ July 1865: "was still very far from being able to handle his own correspondence 5526
[randallA p228]

⟨2⟩ "Tad's slowness to learn worried his mother, though she had every confidence in 5527
what she called 'his natural brightness.' " [randallA p123]

⟨1/q⟩ August 1865: "I am sorry to say, he does not apply himself to his studies, with as 5528
much interest as he should. We intend he shall attend school, regularly after the
1st of Sep." – Mary Lincoln [turner p264]

⟨1⟩ September 1865: "Taddie is going to a school & for once in his life, he is really 5529
interested in his studies" – Mary [turner p273]

⟨1/q⟩ November 1865: "Taddie – is learning to be as diligent in his studies, as he used to 5530
be *at play*, in the W.H. he appears to be rapidly making up, for the great amount
of time, he lost in W- As you are aware, *he* was always a *marked character*." – Mary
Lincoln [turner p284]

  ⟨-⟩ *WH = White House; W = Washington. Meaning of "marked character"* 5531
  is unclear.

Tad

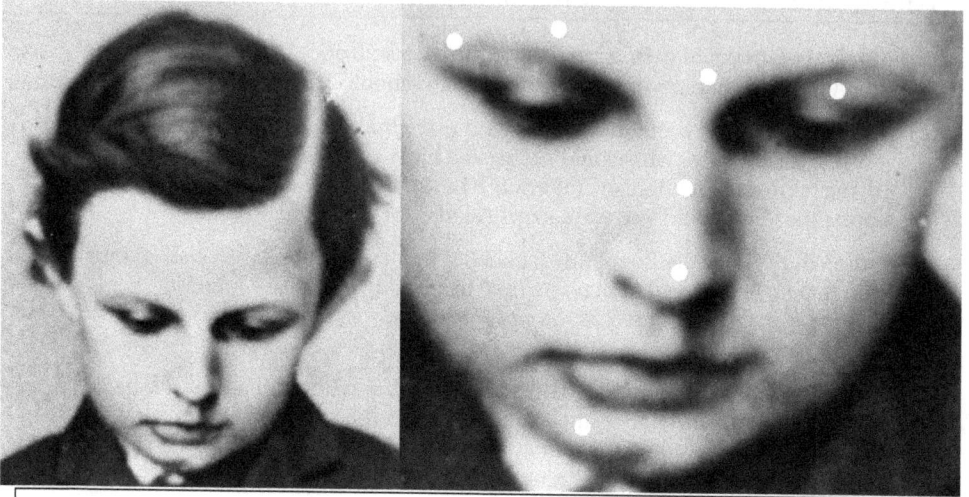

Figure 10. Tad Lincoln, showing artifact of left philtrum. Details from the Mathew Brady photograph of February 9, 1864, showing Tad looking downward at a book. *Left panel:* A dark vertical stripe, having the appearance of a shadow, overlays the location of his left philtral ridge. The rest of the photograph has no other shadows in this direction. *Right panel:* White dots mark facial structures casting a shadow, and show that the image's light source is up and to the left (Tad's right). The nasal tip's shadow is inferolateral to the left nostril, and has a rounded border. A vertical, triangular darkness extends inferiorly out of the nasal tip's shadow, coursing over the left ridge of the philtrum and onto the lower lip. No facial structures would cast such a shadow, given a light source at the upper left. In particular, the left philtral ridge would not be high enough to cast a shadow so far laterally. If Brady somehow used a second light source (no light bulbs then) placed superior to Tad's head and slightly to his right, the nose could cast an inferior shadow. However, in that case, the first light source (from the upper left) would erase such a shadow. Carpenter used the photograph as the basis for his painting [carpenter]. Brady produced another version of this photograph that was "touched up" and had a background added ([meserve #40]≈[ostendorf #93]) [meserve p82]. *Conclusion:* Either the triangular mark is inherent to Tad or the photograph has been altered. Possibly, the shadow lateral to the mid-portion of the nose has also been added, and constitutes the upper portion of the triangular mark. *Other notes:* The ears project widely. The forehead appears broad compared to lower face, giving elfin appearance. Tad has Lincoln's blubbery lower lip (¶2785), strikingly apparent in the stereophotograph in [zeller]. Size of the lower jaw is poorly assessed in this view. Chin dimple is visible. Photograph is [ostendorf #93] and is courtesy of the Library of Congress (LC-USZ62-11897).

Reading & Learning (continued)

⟨$\frac{1}{q}$⟩ January 1866: "Taddie, goes to school & does not miss an hour – He is already,   5532
very much beloved in C[hicago]. his teacher speaks of him in the highest & most affectionate term[s]." – Mary [turner p331]

⟨2⟩ "As late as 1866 he still could not write – despite being tutored in Washington. ...   5533
He finally attended school in Chicago (1866-1868) and learned his letters. Board-

Reading & Learning (continued)

ing school at Dr. Hohagen's Institute in Frankfurt, Germany (1868-1870), apparently cured him of his speech impediment. Thereafter, he had a tutor in England."
[neelyE p189]

⟨1⟩ March 1867: "Taddie received your letter ... & will reply in a few days" – Mary [turner p417] *Suggests, but by no means proves, Tad could read and write by now.* 5534

⟨1/q⟩ August 1867: "I am now feeling the necessity for Taddie, being especially cared for and taught obedience by kind & gentle School treatment." – Mary Lincoln, [randallA p236] 5535

⟨1⟩ October 29, 1867: "Taddie is well & going to school" – Mary [turner p446] 5536

⟨1/q⟩ November 1867, "With the knowledge that my boy has of his backwardness in his studies, he will most readily embrace the opportunities. I shall urge upon him to remain at school & college, until he is *twenty one*." – Mary [turner p451] 5537

⟨2⟩ Late 1867: "The boy had matured considerably, and was now more comfortable in the role of student, but he still lacked discipline." [turner p473] 5538

⟨2⟩ Schools: 5539
  ⟨2⟩ 1865-1866 school year: A Chicago public school [turner p420] 5540
  ⟨2⟩ 1866-1867 school year: Brown School [turner p420] 5541
  ⟨2⟩ 1867-1868 school year: Chicago Academy [turner p422] 5542
  ⟨1⟩ Oct. 1868: Starts at "the 'Institute' of Dr. Hohagen on the Kettenhofstrasse," in Frankfurt-am-Main (a boarding school) [turner p489] 5543

⟨2⟩ In 1867-1868 one of Tad's schoolbooks was "4th reader." [randallA p237] 5544
  ⟨-⟩ *It would be interesting to know the level of education to which the "4th reader" corresponds.* 5545

⟨2⟩ "It has been said that the other students laughed at his speech impediment." [randallA p237] *Randall implies these were teenagers.* 5546

⟨S⟩ "A marked speech impediment, at first considered endearing, was probably responsible for his slow [academic] progress, but his mental processes were as capricious as his conduct, his powers of concentration practically nil." [turner p420] 5547

⟨1/q⟩ Early 1868: Tad was "learning very fast." – Robert Lincoln [randallA p238] 5548

⟨2/c⟩ "Studies, skating, parties, and a girl" indicate, according to Randall, "that Tad by 1868 was getting a normal education for a boy in his teens." [randallA p238] 5549

■ 1868-1870, Germany: 5550
  ⟨2⟩ "He was disciplined by an English-speaking German teacher, who required him to read aloud, slowly and distinctly, as a daily exercise." [brooksB] Part of ¶5633 5551
  ⟨S⟩ "He progressed satisfactorily in his studies. ... German discipline supplied just his need." [evans p211] 5552

⟨1⟩ Dec. 1868: "He likes his school" and "is settled in his school & I hope he will make up for lost time" – Mary [turner p496] 5553

⟨1⟩ Nov. or Dec. 1869: "Study more than he does now he could not possibly do." – Mary [helmB p278] 5554

⟨1⟩ March 1870: "is doubtless greatly improving in his studies" – Mary [helmB pp280-281] Part of ¶5256 5555

⟨1⟩ June 22, 1870: Mary seeks an English school where Tad "will be *compelled* to study" [turner p569] 5556

Tad

Reading & Learning (continued)

⟨1⟩ Aug. 17, 1870: "He has become so homesick and at the same time his English education has become so neglected that I have consented with many a heartache to permit him to go home" [to the United States] – Mary [helmB p285] *This plan was not executed.*   5557

⟨1⟩ Sept. 10, 1870, from Leamington, England: "Taddie and his tutor began their studies together on yesterday [sic], both appear deeply interested. He comes to us most highly recommended, and I shall see that not a moment will be idly passed. From eight until one o'clock each day Tad is seated at his table – with his tutor studying and from five to seven each evening with his tutor he is studying his lessons. On no occasion do I intend that he shall deviate from this rule. I have just been in to see them studying, and they are earnestly engaged – for dear life. The gentleman who is teaching him is very highly educated – very quiet and gentlemanly and patience itself. Tad now realizes the great necessity of an education, and I am sure will do well." – Mary [turner p577]   5558

⟨1⟩ Oct. 27, 1870: "He recites his lessons with his tutor seven hours of each day. ... If he improves as he is doing I shall be satisfied." – Mary [turner p578]   5559

⟨1⟩ Nov. 7, 1870: "Taddie, became quite a proficient [sic] in the German language, & is now studying very diligently, under an English tutor – 7 hours – each day." – Mary [turner p579]   5560

⟨1⟩ Nov. 1870, unknown day: "Taddie is closeted with his tutor seven and a half hours each day, and from Saturday to Saturday. When I am with him for three hours to listen to his examination of his studies of the week I can see a great improvement in him. ... Study more than he does now he could not possibly do." – Mary [turner p580]   5561

⟨2⟩ Jan. 1871: Tad transfers to an English school in Brixton, near London [turner p574]   5562
   ⟨1⟩ Jan. 13, 1871: Will "accompany my son out to his school and perhaps remain a day or two near him." – Mary [turner p582]   5563
   ⟨1⟩ Feb. 12, 1871: "Until the middle of April next [Tad] is placed ... in an English school." – Mary [turner p584]   5564

⟨1⟩ May 1871: "speaks German fluently" – Mary [ChicagoTribune - May 16, 1871]   5565

⟨1⟩ May 1871: "[I] speak German very well" [ChicagoTribune - May 16, 1871]   5566

⟨2⟩ Overall assessments: "almost ineducable" [neelyA p45]; "mentally retarded" [rossA p158]; "slow intellectual development" [bartonA p49]   5567

⟨2⟩ In the White House "One tutor after another abandoned hope and left." [rossA p159]   5568

■ Could Tad read?   5569
   ⟨1⟩ March 1869, Mary writes to her daughter-in-law: "If you will write to Taddie, you will gratify him very much." [turner p505]   5570
   ⟨2⟩ learned his letters in 1866-1868 [neelyE p189]. See [tready]]   5571

⟨2⟩ Writing samples: 5572
   ⟨2⟩ No letter written by Tad survives [evans p60] *This was written in 1932.*   5573
   ◻ The back of a photograph has an undated, neatly handwritten note: "Presented to Robert T. Lincoln by his affectionate brother, Thomas Lincoln, a carte-de-visite of himself & new South American pony, as taken Nov 16th, 1863, Washington, D.C." [neelyA p93] *Tad could not have written this in 1863. It could have been dictated and/or written later.*   5574
   ◻ [sandburgC p189] reprints a handwritten note from Tad dated Oct. 6, 1864, but does not give the proof that it's in Tad's hand.   5575

Reading & Learning (continued)

⟨1⟩ July 1865: Mary writes a letter for Tad [crookA p20] [crookK]   5576

⟨○⟩ A copy of a children's book (*Mrs. Brown's Visit to Paris*, by Arthur Sketchley,   5577
London: George Rutledge & Sons, no date) bears the signature "T. Lincoln"
on the preface page – [randallP box 74, containing a copy of *Lincoln Lore*, August
1958 (no. 1446), page 3]. *The British Integrated Catalogue lists 1867 as the
year for "Mrs. Brown's Visit to the Paris Exhibition" and 1878 as the
year for "Mrs. Brown at the Paris Exhibition."* ○○○ Project: Compare
handwriting of the two samples.

⟨1⟩ Dec. 1869: Tad mails a letter to one of Mary's friends. [turner p530] *One could*   5578
read Mary's description of the mailing and think Tad wrote the letter.

⟨1⟩ May 1870: "I am in receipt of a letter from my young son" – Mary [turner p562]   5579

⟨1⟩ Feb. 12, 1871: "I received a letter this morning from dear Tad" – Mary [turner   5580
p584]

⟨1⟩ "Poor Tad was a good boy and extraordinarily affectionate & firm in his friend-   5581
ships. After you knew him he studied diligently & overcame entirely the defect in
his speech. This he did by reading aloud as a regular exercise & as it was done
mainly while he was in Germany & under a German (English speaking) tutor, he
came home shortly before his death, articulating perfectly, but with deliberation –
speaking German perfectly but in English owing to his practice in reading he had
a slight German accent. He was only eighteen when he died but he was so manly
and self reliant that I had the greatest hopes for his future." – Robert Lincoln to
Noah Brooks, April 5, 1882 [randallP box 74] citing *Chicago History*. Summer 1947;
1(8)

Tad

⟨S⟩ "His early actions raise the question: Was it backwardness or feeble-mindedness?   5582
The evidence is quite conclusive that backwardness resulting from lack of application and discipline was the cause." [evans pp60-61]

⟨1⟩ Lincoln "was pleased to see him growing up in ignorance of books, but with sin-   5583
gularly accurate ideas of practical matters." – John Hay [templeA]

Shrewd

Different aspects of Tad's brain are explored in Reading & Learning, Shrewd,   5584
Spoiled, and Mental Status.

In trying to judge Tad's mental capabilities, one must balance his obvious learning   5585
difficulties, as presented in Reading & Learning, with the many descriptions of his
shrewdness (e.g. citebrooksB [randallA p123]).

⟨1/q⟩ Once, when Willie was begging for a toy, Lincoln said, "Give it to him, Tad, to keep   5586
him quiet." Tad replied, "No, sir, I need it to quiet myself." Lincoln would ask his
neighbors "Now wasn't it bright" of Tad to reply that way? [kunhardtA p91]

⟨1⟩ "he is a bright boy, a son that will do honor to the genius and greatness of his   5587
father" [keckleyB p220]

⟨1⟩ "He was as shrewd as he was lawless, and always knew whether he could make a   5588
tutor serviceable or not." – John Hay [templeA]

⟨1⟩ "He roamed the White House at will, a tricksy and restless spirit. ... Innumerable   5589
stories might be told of the child's native wit, his courage, his adventurousness,
and his passionate devotion to his father." [brooksA pp418-419].

Shrewd (continued)

⟨1/q⟩ A friend of the Lincolns, Mrs. James S. Delano, remembered Tad as "the kindest, brightest, most considerate child" she had ever known [randallA p139] *Right. And "Raymond Shaw is the kindest, bravest, warmest, most wonderful human being I've ever known in my life." – Bennett Marco*   5590

⟨2⟩ "bright and affectionate" [donaldA p428]   5591

⟨1⟩ In the White House: expertly directs a tricky carpet-removal job [crookA pp22-23]   5592

⟨1/q⟩ Late March 1865: Aboard the ship *River Queen*: Tad's "investigating mind led him everywhere." He "studied every screw of the engine and knew and counted among his friends every man of the crew." [crookA p39]   5593

⟨1⟩ Immediately after the death of his father: "Yes, Pa is dead, and I am only Tad Lincoln now, little Tad, like other little boys. I am not a President's son now. I won't have many presents any more. Well, I will try and be a good boy, and will hope to go some day to Pa and brother Willie, in heaven." [keckleyB p197]   5594

⟨1/q⟩ "Even when he could scarcely read, he knew much about the cost of things, the details of trade, the principles of mechanics, and the habits of animals, all of which showed the activity of his mind and the odd turn of his thoughts." [brooksC pp281-282]   5595

⟨1/q⟩ As a teenager: "Tad did not stutter ... but had a slight deficiency in speech. [I] sometimes protected him from pests who teased him because of his manner of speech and his timidity. He was a bright boy, slight, and delicate in health – too advanced to have attended a primary school." – anonymous correspondent quoted by [evans p58]   5596

⟨1⟩ Lincoln "was pleased to see him growing up in ignorance of books, but with singularly accurate ideas of practical matters." – John Hay [templeA]   5597

Skin

⟨1⟩ March 1870: "his usual bright complexion" – Mary [helmB pp280-281] Part of ¶5256   5598

⟨1⟩ May 11, 1871: His "beardless red cheeks are apparently the evidence of perfect health." [ChicagoTribune - May 16, 1871, reprinting New York World of May 12] (∈ ¶5246) (See ¶5278 for interpretations.)   5599

Sleep & Circadian Rhythms

⟨1⟩ 1861: Pleads "think, faver, if it was your own little boy who was just tired after fighting, and marching a;; day, that he could not keep awake, much as he tried to." [grimsley] *Tad's plea is unclear to me.*   5600

⟨1⟩ At the end of Abraham Lincoln's work-day "he generally found his infant goblin asleep under his table or roasting [sic] his curly head by the open fire-place." – John Hay [templeA] *Other sources suggest this was the pattern after Willie's death.*   5601

⟨2⟩ "After the death of Willie [Feb. 1862], Tad was so lonely and so subject to nightmares that he was regularly allowed to sleep in his father's bed." [donaldH p43]   5602

Speech

The consensus has been that Tad's speech was impaired because of a physical malformation in his mouth, possibly compounded by crooked teeth. In assessing whether a cleft palate caused the impediment, the tempo of his speech is relevant because, in general, children with cleft palate speak more slowly than those without [aa33 p336]. Speakers with cleft palate also make characteristic mispronunciations [aa33 pp336-339].   5603

- See also: Mouth and Teeth   5604

⟨1⟩ "That chile was so long walking and talking, everyone say he never would." [ostendorfC] *The reliability of* [ostendorfC] *is disputed* [hallJ].   5605

- Severity of the speech impediment: 5606
  - ⟨1⟩ "A slight impediment in his speech made it difficult for strangers to understand him." [bayne p3]   5607
  - ⟨1⟩ "An unfortunate difficulty in his speech prevented him from speaking plainly, and strangers could hardly understand what he said." [brooksB]   5608
  - ⟨1⟩ "He had a curious impediment in his speech which rather heightened the effect of his droll sayings; and the difficulty he had in pronouncing his own name gave him the odd nickname by which he was always known." [brooksC pp278-279]   5609
  - ⟨1⟩ "He ran continually in and out of his father's cabinet, ... with his bright, rapid, and very imperfect speech – for he had an impediment which made his articulation almost unintelligible until he was nearly grown." [hayA]   5610
  - ⟨1⟩ "The imperfection in his speech was slight – not enough to make him ineligible as a beau for a girl" – Mrs. George B. Carpenter, recalling the teenaged Tad [lewis]   5611
  - ⟨1⟩ "He suffered from a slight impediment in his speech" [keckleyB p216]   5612
  - ⟨1⟩ April 1865: Tad speaks, "in his broken way." – Francis Carpenter [ChicagoTribune - Dec. 3, 1865]   5613

- Other assessments of the speech impediment: 5614
  - ⟨2⟩ "serious speech impediment, and a lisp" [neelyE p188]   5615
  - ⟨2⟩ "handicapped by a speech impediment and a bad lisp" [donaldA p159]   5616
  - ⟨2⟩ "quaint impediment of speech" [randallA p138].   5617
  - ⟨2⟩ "Because of his speech defect most people could not understand Tad, but his father always could – and he knew how frustrated the child became when he could not express himself. [donaldA p428]   5618
  - ⟨2⟩ "... when he talked in that queer, breathy, nasal way... [Lincoln] never failed to understand the misshapen baby words" [kunhardtA p91]   5619
  - ⟨2⟩ At about age 4, "he talked rapidly, his baby words fairly tumbling over each other. As he had a pronounced impediment in his speech, only parental intuition was likely at this time to translate what he was trying to say." [randallA p7]   5620
  - ⟨2⟩ "making sounds few could understand" in his White House years [rossA p162]   5621

- Nature of the impediment: 5622
  - ⟨2⟩ lisp: [donaldA p159], [oatesA p96], [sandburgA p66]; "an appealing lisp" [randallA p45]   5623
  - ⟨2⟩ "tongue-tied" [bartonA pp49]   5624
  - ⟨2⟩ Age 12: "tongue-tied way" [lewisM p64] *I do not believe Lewis has specific information to fix the date or the precise nature of the speech problem.*   5625
  - ⟨2⟩ "his baby tongue" [randallA p202]   5626

Tad

Speech (continued)

⟨2⟩ Classmates called him "Stuttering Tad," apparently during teenage years. [evans p58]. 5627

⟨2⟩_c [shutesM]: Tad's speech aberration was not of the type (grossly nasal) encountered in cleft palate. 5628

■ Cause of the impediment: 5629

  ⟨2⟩_c Generally ascribed to a palatal malformation (which Tad may not have had). (See ¶5464.) 5630

  ⟨2⟩ Tad's speech was abnormal during the time he wore a dental appliance. (See ¶5645.) 5631

⟨1/q⟩ As a teenager: "Tad did not stutter ... but had a slight deficiency in speech. [I] sometimes protected him from pests who teased him because of his manner of speech and his timidity. He was a bright boy, slight, and delicate in health – too advanced to have attended a primary school." – anonymous correspondent quoted by [evans p58] 5632

⟨2⟩ As a teenager: Tad began elecution lessons [randallA p238]. His articulation improved [lewis] [rossA p287] 5633

  ⟨2⟩ "speaking German perfectly" according to Robert [randallA p260] *Unclear whether "perfect" refers to grammar or accent or articulation.* 5634

  ⟨2⟩ "Under the tuition of a careful instructor in Germany, he quite overcame the difficulty in his speech which had burdened him from childhood. He was disciplined by an English-speaking German teacher, who required him to read aloud, slowly and distinctly, as a daily exercise. By this simple means he finally learned to speak plainly, but with a slight German accent which came from his practice in reading." [brooksB] 5635

  ⟨2⟩ "Boarding school at Dr. Hohagen's Institute in Frankfurt, Germany (1868-1870), apparently cured him of his speech impediment." [neelyE p189] 5636

  ⟨2⟩ "mastered perfect articulation" [randallA p260]. However, after two years of schooling in Frankfurt, he acquired the "slight German accent" of his tutor [randallA p260] 5637

  ⟨1⟩ "speaks with a strong foreign accent" [NYTimes - May 11, 1871] 5638

⟨1/q⟩ Mispronunciations include: "Mith Spwigg" for "Miss Sprigg" [randallA p45], "Yib" for "Lizabeth" [keckleyB p218], "faver" for "father" [grimsley], and "Papa's tot" for "Papa's shot" [kunhardtB p75]. 5639

  ⟨1⟩ "Taddie could never speak very plainly. He had his own language; the names that he gave some of us we like to remember to-day. The President was 'papa-day,' which meant 'papa dear.' Tom Pendel was 'Tom Pen,' and I was 'Took.' " [crookA p23] [crookK] 5640

  ⟨-⟩ The [randallA p138] manuscript in [randallP box 76] cites: "Tom Pendel. Mag. of History, vol. 34, No. 1, Extra no. 133, Lincoln no. 31, 1927, p20." This may be two references. 5642

  ⟨1⟩ There are reports that pronunciation difficulty was the origin of his nickname, "Tad," but conflicting evidence exists. See Nickname 5643

⟨1⟩ "It was seldom that he had playmates; but, to hear the noise Tad contrived to make, one would suppose that there were at least six boys wherever he happened to be." [brooksB] 5644

■ Early 1868: Tad wore a dental appliance to straighten his teeth (¶5477). 5645

Speech (continued)

⟨1/q⟩ "He could hardly speak so as to be understood & to keep him talking in that way for a year I thought, with his present bad habit of speech, to be asking too much." – Robert [randallA p238] 5646

⟨1/q⟩ Another dentist advised that the appliance was unnecessary. "I have stopped his using it & I have put him in charge of a man ... who teaches Elecution telling him to make him pronounce correctly." – Robert [randallA p238] 5647

⟨2⟩ Tad's speech problems were "made worse when his teeth grew in crooked" [donaldA p159]. 5648

Spoiled

Different aspects of Tad's brain are explored in [Reading & Learning], [Shrewd], [Spoiled], and [Mental Status]. 5649

- Re: Lincoln: 5650
  - ⟨1/q⟩ "We never controlled our children much." – Lincoln [baker p120] 5651
  - ⟨1/q⟩ "He was very very indulgent to his children – chided or praised for it he always said 'It is my pleasure that my children are free – happy and unrestrained by parental tyranny...' " – Mary [wilson pp357,359] 5652
  - ⟨1⟩ "He was the most indulgent parent I ever knew   His children literally [sic] ran over him and he was powerless to withstand their importunities" – Joseph Gillespie [wilson p181] 5653
  - ⟨1/q⟩ When Lincoln brought Tad and Willie to his law office, he would let them run wild, with no attempt to control them or the resulting devastation. Lincoln's law partner wanted to wring the boys' necks and observed "Had they s - - t in Lincoln's hat and rubbed it on his boots, he would have laughed and thought it smart." – Herndon [donaldA p160]. 5654
  - ⟨1⟩ "It well nigh broke [Lincoln's] heart to use his paternal authority in correcting [his children's] occasional displays of temper or insubordination" [lamonR p164] 5655
  - ⟨1⟩ "well-nigh impossible for Lincoln to treat Tad's innumerable escapades with severity. While the family lived in Washington, the lad was allowed his own way almost without check." [brooksC p279] 5656

- Re: Tad: 5657
  - ⟨1⟩ After Lincoln's death: "From that period forward he became more independent, and in a short time learned to dispense with the services of a nurse. While in Chicago, I saw him get out of his clothes one Sunday morning and dress himself, and the change was such a great one to me – for while in the White House servants obeyed his every nod and bid – that I could scarcely refrain from shedding tears. Had his father lived, I knew it would have been different with his favorite boy." [keckleyB pp197-198] 5658
  - ⟨1⟩ Lincoln "was pleased to see him growing up in ignorance of books, but with singularly accurate ideas of practical matters." – John Hay [templeA] 5659
  - ⟨1⟩ "'Let him run,' the easy-going President would say: 'he has time enough left to learn his letters and get pokey. Bob was just such a little rascal, and now he is a very decent boy." – John Hay [templeA] 5660
  - ⟨2⟩ "he was not forced to study" [neelyE p189] 5661

⟨1⟩ Of Willie's death: "Possibly this calamity made Lincoln less strict with his youngest boy than he should have been. He found it well nigh impossible to deny Tad anything." [brooksA p418] 5662

Spoiled (continued)

⟨¹⁄q⟩ Engineered dismissal of any tutor with "obstinate ideas of the superiority of gram- 5663
mar to kite-flying as an intellectual employment" – John Hay [templeA]

- Spoiled: 5664
  - ⟨¹⁄q⟩ "If there was any motto or slogan at the White House during the early days 5665
  of the Lincolns' occupancy it was this: 'Let the children have a good time.'"
  [evans pp69-70] quoting [bayne]
  - ⟨1⟩ "If there was ever a boy in danger of being 'spoiled,' [Tad] was that lad." 5666
  [brooksB]
  - ⟨2⟩ "thoroughly 'spoiled' by his father" [lewis] 5667
  - ⟨2⟩ "wholly undisciplined" [donaldA p428] 5668

Trauma

- Corporal punishment 5669
  - ⟨¹⁄q⟩ Mary "held a private-strapping party" for Tad after he had fallen into a mud 5670
  puddle. – Recollection of playmate Frank Edwards, apparently decades later
  [burl p63]
  - ⟨2⟩ Mary accused Tad of stealing a dime, he denied it, she angered, and "beat 5671
  his legs with a switch." (Tad later proved himself innocent.) [burl p63] ([randallC
  p89] does not believe the story.)
  - ⟨2⟩ Mary denied an 1865 newspaper story that she had ever threatened to whip 5672
  Tad for cutting up copper-toed shoes, saying never "in my life I have ever
  whipped a child" [rossA p252].

⟨¹⁄q⟩ July 30, 1868: "Tad Lincoln, in imitation of boys who never had a President for a fa- 5673
ther, attempted to jump on a passing freight train ... but his hold slipped and had
it not been for the timely aid of a gentleman who stood near, he would have fell
under the wheels and most probably have been killed." [turnerB] quoting a Pennsylvania newspaper *Interestingly, a bystander saved Robert from a railroad death
– ¶4999.*

Travel & Dwellings

See ⸢Mary⸣ ⸢Travel & Dwellings⸣. Tad often traveled with Mary and, toward the end of 5674
the war, with his father.

⟨1⟩ Oct. 1869: "was absent last week on a little excursion with his Professor" – Mary 5675
[turner p519]

Voice

In assessing whether a cleft palate caused Tad's speech impediment, the sound of his 5676
voice is relevant because children with cleft palate may have nasal speech [aa33 p336].
See ⸢Speech⸣ and ⸢Mouth⸣. For additional considerations related to the voice of Tad and
Abraham, see ⸢Abraham⸣⸢Voice⸣.

⟨S⟩ "... he was born with a cleft palate ... There would be a speech difficulty, making 5677
his words sound queer, breathy, nasal, almost another language." [kunhardtB p75]
*The wording is subtle. Rather than reporting how Tad's voice sounded, I think
they are describing how it should have sounded.*

⟨1⟩ John Hay refers to Tad's "shrill pipes." [templeA] *All pre-pubertal pipes are shrill.* 5678

Lincoln, William

child #3

Chronology

Mo. Yr	Age	Home	Event	Ref.	
Dec. 1850	0	Springfield, IL	born	[templeC]	5679
Mar. 1861	10	Washington	Father is President		
Feb. 1862	11	"	dies		

Introduction & Sources

🔘 There is no comprehensive collection of photographs of Willie. Infrequently-seen images include the earliest known picture of him (about 1855) [ostendorfA p304] and one about age ?7 [neelyA p100]. The most photographs are in [ostendorfA] (n=5) and [neelyA] (n=6), not counting his unrecognizable visage in [ostendorf #34, 38, 39]. 5681

Appearance

▪ Resemblance to father: 5682 William
   ⟨1⟩ 1861: "a counterpart of his father [mentally?], save that he was handsome" [grimsley] (∈ ¶5760) 5683
   ⟨1⟩_q "Will was the true picture of Mr. Lincoln, in every way, even to carrying his head slightly inclined toward his left shoulder." – Springfield neighbor [burl p66] citing [NYHerald - May 26, 1861] *Given Lincoln's left hyperphoria, one would expect tilt toward the right shoulder. See ¶1827.* 5684
   ⟨2⟩ "strikingly resembled Lincoln in mind and body" [ostendorfA p304] *Unclear if this is Ostendorf's conclusion or if he is parrotting others.* 5685

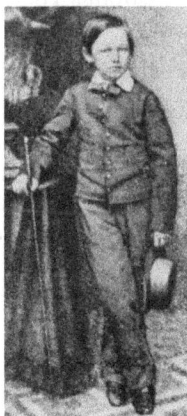

Figure 11. Willie Lincoln, 1861. Library of Congress LC-DIG-cwpbh-04802

Build

⟨2⟩ "Willie was tall for eleven years of age." [helmB p180]   5686

[📷] A photograph of Willie (age 9-11, I estimate) shows a long lower-body segment in   5687
comparison to the upper body segment [kunhardtA p290].

⟨1/q⟩ Nov. 1860: Willie and Tad: "chubby ... really healthy smart boys" – Thomas Web-   5688
ster [randallC p163]

Death & Final Illness

⟨2⟩ Willie and his pony: "he insisted on riding it every day. The weather was change-   5689
able, and exposure resulted in a severe cold, which deepened into fever. He was
very sick, and I was summoned to his bedside. It was sad to see the poor boy suffer. Always of a delicate constitution, he could not resist the strong inroads of the
disease. The days dragged wearily by, and he grew weaker and more shadow-like.
... When able to be about, he was almost constantly by her [Mary's] side." [keckleyB
p98]

  ⟨-⟩ At some point Tad became ill, too. See ¶5390   5690

⟨2⟩ Feb. 8: [WashingtonStar] reports that Willie was seriously ill [shutesM].   5691

⟨1⟩ "Dr. Stone was called in. He pronounced Willie better, and said there was every   5692
reason for an early recovery. He thought, since the invitations had been issued, it
would be best to go on with the reception. Willie, he insisted, was in no immediate
danger. Mrs. Lincoln was guided by these counsels, and no postponement was
announced. On the evening of the reception, Willie was suddenly taken worse.
His mother sat by his bedside a long while, holding his feverish hand in her own,
and watched his labored breathing. The doctor claimed there was no cause for
alarm." [keckleyB pp100-101]

  ⟨2⟩ [kunhardtB p135] says Willie was "burning with fever" and that Mary "could see   5693
  that his lungs were congested."

⟨2⟩ The next morning Willie was obviously seriously ill. Consulting physicians were   5694
called in. "The newspapers decided that the boy's affliction was bilious fever, but
those who saw the sick boy knew the trouble concerned his breathing apparatus."
[kunhardtB p136]

⟨1⟩ Tad was simultaneously ill, apparently with the same disorder. See ¶5390.   5695

⟨1/q⟩ "The White House levee on Tuesday will be omitted on account of the illness of   5696
the second son of the President, an interesting lad of about 8 years of age, who
has been lying dangerously ill of bilious fever for the last three days. Mrs. Lincoln
has not left his bedside since Wednesday night, and fears are entertained for her
health." [evans p140] quoting [helmB p197] quoting a Washington newspaper

  ⟨2⟩ The reporter, who apparently did not know Willie's name, has Willie's age,   5697
  birth number, and length of illness wrong. [shutes p80] [evans p140]

⟨2⟩ Willie became "of wandering mind" and did not recognize his father. He died in   5698
the afternoon of Feb. 20, 1862. [kunhardtB p136]

  ⟨2⟩ At some point Willie asked that "the six dollars that were his savings" be given   5699
  to the missionary society. [kunhardtB p137]

⟨2⟩ Was sick for 17 days or more [shutesM].   5700

  ▪ Diagnoses – contemporary: 5701

Death & Final Illness (continued)

⟨1⟩ Without citing a source, [boyden p54] says Tad had typhoid. (∈ ¶5390). *It is*   5702
possible that Boyden is applying her own diagnosis, rather than passing
on information from her mother, Mrs. Pomroy.

⟨1⟩ "bilious fever" – see ¶5696.   5703

⟨1/q⟩ "An intermittent fever assuming a typhoid character" – the *National Repub-*   5704
lican of Feb. 21, 1862, quoted by [shutes pp80-81]. (∈ ¶5712). Echoed by [Washing-
tonStar], according to [shutesM].

⟨1⟩ "Willie Wallace Lincoln died of it" [stoddardA p124]. *A strict reading of pro-*   5705
nouns in Stoddard's text would equate "it" with smallpox, but this seems
unlikely.

⟨2⟩ The Washington *Chronicle* (Feb. 23) and the *National Intelligencer* (Feb. 10)   5706
gave the diagnosis as typhoid fever.

- Diagnoses – retrospective analyses: 5707

⟨S⟩ Some sources suggest it was typhoid fever or malaria [durham] [kunhardtA p175]   5708
[turner p xvi] [lincloreIGI]. *Malaria seems less likely, since (a) it was Febru-*
ary, which makes initial infection via mosquito highly unlikely, and (b)
it would be a coincidence to have two cases of malaria (Willie and Tad)
reactivate simultaneously. Although Mrs. Pomroy (or her daughter) say
that malaria "taints the air of that region [Washington] more or less at all
seasons" [boyden p77], mosquitoes simply cannot live through typical Wash-
ington winters. Moreover, quinine, widely available and known as an ef-
fective anti-malarial well before the 1860s, would certainly have been used
at an early stage of the illness.

⟨S⟩ "Acute 'bilious fever' is malaria, and acute bilious fever fatal in one week is   5710
pernicious malaria. Willie died in February, and malaria in Washington in
that month is due to relapses, which are often pernicious. Mrs. Lincoln's letters contain references to attacks of malaria, and Elizabeth Keckley's statement that Willie rather suddenly took a turn for the worse and died fits
malaria fairly well. Pernicious malaria is recognized as a preventable disease. If Willie did not have pernicious malaria, he had some other form of
preventable disease – at least, as we now know preventable disease." [evans
p140]

⟨2⟩ "The disease that is now known as malaria was once called bilious fever, but   5711
during the late [eighteen] fifties and sixties it was more correctly termed intermittent fever and was so referred to in the medical literature of that time"
[shutes p80].

⟨1/q⟩ The *National Republican* of Feb. 21, 1862 described the illness as "an in-   5712
termittent fever assuming a typhoid character," which [shutes pp80-81] interprets as suggesting malaria. He continues: "If Willie had malaria in February,
then it necessarily was an infection acquired during the previous mosquito
season, but there are no records which indicate that. Bronchonpneumo-
nia could cover whatever even Dr. Stone considered as a bilious or intermittent fever lasting two or three weeks. There was then much medical confusion in distinguishing between malaria, typhoid fever and pneumonia. ...
Bronchopneumonia would fit exactly the descriptions of intelligent Elizabeth Keckley, who spent may hours of the day and night by the sick boy's
bedside."

⟨2⟩ Writing 22 years after [shutesE], [shutesM] discards the possibility of malaria,   5713
notes that typhoid fever is more common "during the warm season," and

William

Death & Final Illness (continued)

feels that "the more probable diagnosis [is] broncho-pneumonia (or pneumonitis) with damaged kidneys as a possible, determinate factor."

⟨s⟩ "probably typhoid fever, caused by pollution in the White House water system." [donaldA p336] 5714

⟨s⟩ "A more likely culprit was the White House drinking water, badly polluted and capable of transmitting typhoid fever." [kunhardtA p290] 5715

⟨s⟩ [shutes p80] believes the 1860 bout of scarlet fever damaged Willie's kidneys, thereby compromising his resistance to his fatal illness. (See ¶5746.) 5716

⟨s⟩ "probably malarial ... modern drugs might have cured Willie in a week" [turner p121] 5717

⟨s⟩ *The two clear facts about Willie's illness are: (1) it was easily contagious, given that Tad had it, too, and (2) it was severe. I do not put much stock in the statement that it began with a cold, since so many infectious diseases begin with the same prodrome. Thus, I believe typhoid fever is the most likely diagnosis, especially given the statement by Tad's nurse (¶5702).* 5718

⟨2⟩ Dr. Charles Brown "embalmed Willie so perfectly that he did really seem to be only sleeping, and Lincoln could not bear to leave him" [kunhardtB p137] 5719

⟨$\frac{1}{q}$⟩ "The body of Willie Lincoln was embalmed today by Doctors Brown and Alexander, assisted by Dr. Wood, in the presence of attending physicians, Doctors Stone and Hall, Senator Browning, and Isaac Newton. The method of Sagnet of Paris was used, and the results were entirely satisfactory to the attendant friends of the family." [NYHerald - Feb. 22, 1862] as quoted by [shutes p119] 5720

Diet & Digestion

⟨2⟩ March 1861: "Every member of the household became ill from eating too well of the unaccustomed Potomac shad." [shutes p77] (See ¶640.) 5721

Ears

[▢] [neelyA p46] is the best image of Willie's two ears. Both project outwards. In other photographs [neelyA pp67, 77, 100] he has a slight head-turn to the left, which obscures the left ear, but the right ear is seen as a bat ear. 5722

Eyes

⟨1⟩ Blue eyes [keckleyB p98] 5723

⟨2⟩ "As he grew, he was described as having an 'inward turning eye' which he claimed was cured, but the sight was lost in that eye (amblyopia exanopsia?)" [durham] *Does "he claimed" really refer to WIllie? Might be Carl Sandburg.* 5724

- Habitual head tilt suggests a misalignment of his eyes or skull malformation. (See ¶5741.) 5725

[▢] Some photographs suggest his left eye-opening was larger than his right [neelyA pp67, 77, 100] (See ¶5735.) 5726

[▢] Upper eyelids appear puffy (? redundant). 5727

General

⟨2⟩ Delivery was "perfectly normal." [donaldA p153] *I have not seen direct evidence of this.*   5728

⟨S⟩ Was likely breast fed, given that Mary breast fed a neighbor baby. (See ¶4647.)   5729

⟨1⟩ March 4, 1860: "Willie and Tad were very sick the Saturday night after I left [? Feb. 25] ... I trust the dear little fellows are well again" – Lincoln to Mary [donaldH p75]   5730

⟨1⟩ "Always of a delicate constitution" [keckleyB p98] (∈ ¶5689)   5731

Head & Face

■ Handsome: 5732
  ⟨1⟩ 1861: "a counterpart of his father [mentally?], save that he was handsome" [grimsley] (∈ ¶5760)   5733
  ⟨2⟩ "the best looking" of the Lincoln children [donaldA p154]   5734

■ Asymmetries: 5735
  ⟨S⟩ *The following statements are more conjecture than fact, owing to limited number of photographs of Willie (¶5681), and to the fact that he often had his head slightly turned (to his left) for the camera.*   5736
  ☐ ? right side of face larger than left   5737
  ☐ ? left eye-opening larger than right   5738
  ☐ ? chin deviated to right   5739
  ☐ ? root of nose deviated to left   5740   William

■ Head tilt: 5741
  ⟨2⟩ "Willie's habit of holding his head to one side suggests a congenital paresis or paralysis of one of the extraocular muscles, most probably the superior oblique." [durham] *Could also be consequence of skull malformation, e.g. plagiocephaly.*   5742
  ⟨$\frac{1}{q}$⟩ "Will was the true picture of Mr. Lincoln, in every way, even to carrying his head slightly inclined toward his left shoulder." – Springfield neighbor [burl p66] citing [NYHerald - May 26, 1861] *Given Lincoln's left hyperphoria, one would expect tilt toward the right shoulder. See ¶1827.*   5743
  ☐ Head is tilted to left in two photos in [ostendorfA p304] and in [neelyA p67]. Is tilted to the right in [neelyA pp46, 77]. Others show no tilt.   5744

Infection

⟨$\frac{1}{q}$⟩ Herndon thought the Lincoln sons might have had congenital syphilis. See ¶2023. *Why would he think this? It suggests the boys had something "not right" that casual observation disclosed.*   5745

■ 1860: Scarlet fever: 5746
  ⟨2⟩ Contracted scarlet fever about the time his father was nominated for President. Willie's sickness made it difficult for the Lincolns to receive at their home the large number of visitors who now wanted to see Lincoln. [donaldA pp251-252]   5747
  ⟨1⟩ July 4, 1860: Willie "has just had a hard and tedious spell of scarlet-fever and he is not yet beyond all danger. I have a head-ache and a sore throat upon me now, inducing me to suspect that I have an inferior type of the same thing." – Lincoln writing to Dr. Anson Henry (see ¶3180) [baslerA v4p82]   5748
  ⟨$\frac{1}{q}$⟩ Later, Mary wrote that Willie's "severe illness ... was but a warning to us, that ... he was not to remain long here" [shutesM].   5749

Infection (continued)

⟨S⟩ "It was probably an attack of acute tonsillitis, or it might have been what would now be termed a streptococcic pharyngitis." [shutes pp73-74]   5750

⟨◎⟩ A recuperating Willie can be seen in a summer 1860 photograph of Lincoln's home [kunhardtA p126] [kunhardtB p272]   5751

⟨2⟩ Dr. William Wallace (see ¶3195) had "taken care of Willie when he had a long hard case of scarlet fever in the summer of 1860" [kunhardtB p257]   5752

⟨1⟩ Two men came to see Lincoln in Springfield. "L's child was sick ... L sent word down that his child was too sick to leev it – that the man must come down to or up to his house." Lincoln received the men. – Benjamin Irwin [wilson p462]   5753

⟨S⟩ [shutes p80] believes this illness damaged Willie's kidneys, thereby compromising his resistance when fatally afflicted with "bilious fever" less than two years later. See ⌐Death & Final Illness⌐.   5754

⟨1⟩ March 28, 1861: "Last week, both of the children, had the measles slightly, altho' the papers represented them as quite ill." – Mary [turner p81]. Also see: [grimsley]. The boys gave measles to Elmer Ellsworth [turner p92].   5755

■ 1862: See ⌐Death⌐   5756

Mental Status

⟨S⟩ "Willie was a clone of his father, sharing his temperament, values, attitudes, personality, and character." [burl p xviii]   5757

⟨1⟩ "... a prematurely serious and studious child." – John Hay [templeA]   5758

⟨2⟩ "Willie became a serious, precocious boy who liked to read books and memorize railroad timetables." [oatesA pp96-97]   5759

⟨1⟩ Willie in 1861: "a noble, beautiful boy of nine years, of great mental activity, unusual intelligence, wonderful memory, methodical, frank and loving, a counterpart of his father, save that he was handsome. He was entirely devoted to Taddie." [grimsley]   5760

⟨1/q⟩ Early days in Washington: "Willie and Tad are so lonely and everything is so strange to them" – Mary [randallC p243]   5761

⟨2⟩ "sweet-tempered... bright, articulate, and exceptionally sensitive toward the feelings of others"   5762

Mouth

⟨1⟩ 1861: As Willie slowly works through a problem (see ¶5775), he "shut his teeth firmly over the under lip" [grimsley]   5763

⟨◎⟩ Asymmetric, bumpy lips poorly visible in: [neelyA pp 77, 100, and maybe pp 46, 67]. Copies of original photos (from the Lincoln Museum, Ft. Wayne, IN) show bumps more clearly. See The Physical Lincoln.   5764

Nervous System

⟨1⟩ 1861: Could apparently play the piano [grimsley].   5765

⟨1/q⟩ Head tilt. (See ¶5741.)   5766

Physicians & Nurses

⟨2⟩ Dr. William Wallace (see ¶3195) had "taken care of Willie when he had a long hard case of scarlet fever in the summer of 1860" [kunhardtB p257] 5767

- Physicians during his final illness (the embalmers (¶5719) carried the title "Dr."): 5768
  ⟨1⟩ Dr. Stone attended him [keckleyB] (See ¶5692.) 5769
  ⟨2⟩ Dr. Neal Hall was a consultant [shutesE p142] 5770
- Nurses during final illness: 5771
  ⟨2⟩ "The nurse who had taken care of Willie Lincoln in his last illness," herself ill with typhoid, had a spot at the White House memorial service for Lincoln in 1865 [kunhardtB p127]. *This is likely erroneous. It seems to be describing another nurse, Mrs. Pomroy, who was "in the first stages of convalescence from typhoid" when she saw Lincoln's corpse [boyden p247]. Pomroy took care only of Tad, as Willie had died before she reached the White House [boyden p54].* 5772
  ⟨2⟩ Mary Jane Welles nursed Willie and Tad during their Feb. 1862 illnesses [swansonB]. 5773

Post-Mortem

⟨1⟩ The collection of Louise Taper included samples of Willie's hair [ferguson p126]. (∈ ¶3254) 5774

Reading & Learning

⟨1⟩ 1861: After watching Willie solve a problem, Lincoln said: "I know every step of the process by which that boy arrived at his satisfactory solution of the question before him, as it is just by such slow methods I attain results." [grimsley]. (See ¶5763.) *The problem was an inter-personal one, not a mathematical or pedagogical one.* 5775

⟨1⟩ "He had a decidedly literary taste, and was a studious boy" [keckleyB p98] 5776

⟨2⟩ "Willie became a serious, precocious boy who liked to read books and memorize railroad timetables. Eventually he could conduct an imaginary train all the way from Chicago to New York without a mistake – an accomplishment that both Lincolns could not praise enough." [oatesA pp96-97] 5777

⟨2⟩ "the most intelligent" of the Lincoln children [donaldA p154] 5778

⟨1/q⟩ By June 1859 (he was 8 years old) Willie was writing letters to his friends. [evans p55] 5779

⟨2⟩ "Willie had a good memory, memorized long portions of the Bible for Sunday School" [kunhardtB p135] 5780

Skin

⟨2⟩ fair-skinned [kunhardtA p91] 5781

Spoiled

⟨S⟩ See Tad Spoiled for evidence of the Lincoln children being spoiled. 5782

⟨S⟩ On the other hand, see Trauma for instances of corporal punishment to Robert and Tad. 5783

Travel & Dwellings

- See Mary Travel & Dwellings. 5784

⟨2⟩ June 1859: To Chicago with Lincoln [randallC pp156-157] 5785

Miscellaneous relations all branches

Crume, Mary Lincoln (paternal aunt)

She is of interest because of the possibility she transmitted the gene for spinocerebellar ataxia type 5 from her parents to the kindred described in [ranum]. See ¶1025.   5786

⟨1⟩ 1860: "some of her descendants are now known to be in Breckenridge County, Kentucky" – Lincoln [angle p5]   5787

⟨2⟩ True genealogy is in [lincolnW pp202ff]. Deliberately distorted genealogy is in [ranum].   5788

Hanks family – Miscellaneous members

⟨1⟩ "After the birth of Nancy Hanks, her mother Lucy Hanks married a Henry Sparrow. This union produced eight children. Many of their descendants still reside in Kentucky, and I have examined a number of them. A striking resemblance to our martyred President was found. Many of them have the Marfan syndrome. It appears certain that Lucy Hanks transmitted the Marfan trait to her daughter Nancy and to her grandson Abraham Lincoln. The progeny sired by Henry Sparrow have physical characteristics identical to those of Lincoln." [gordonB] *Lucy Hanks lived to age 66± (¶5862) – too old for MEN2B. To be clear, Sparrow did not father Nancy.*   5789

  ⟨S⟩ "My considered opinion from the evidence I have uncovered and documented concerning the Hanks-Sparrow-Lincoln line and their peculiar characteristics strongly suggests a maternal origin of Lincoln's morphologic appearance." [gordonB]   5790

⟨1⟩ Nancy Hanks Lincoln: "she had several red haired relations" – Presley Haycraft [wilson p87]   5791

⟨1⟩ "I Knew her [Nancy Lincoln's] brother Jo Hanks, who had a red head" – Presley Haycraft [wilson p86] *Probably a cousin, not a brother.*   5792

⟨1⟩ Of Lincoln: "he dose Not look like the Hanks family they are Sandy Complection Red Hair & Freckel all but John Hanks" – Abner Ellis [wilson p210]   5793

⟨2⟩ "Turning to photographs of Dennis Hanks, Lincoln's cousin, the head tilt toward the right shoulder is discernible. The eyes of Dennis, as with Abe, appear to be on different levels and the left eyebrow is higher than the right. But, in the best photograph taken of Dennis, taken in his old age, the left eye has a strange, staring appearance." [snyder]   5794

  ⟨2⟩ Hanks lived to age 94 [wilson p752].   5795

⟨1⟩ "The Hanks' were the finest singers and shouters in our country" – John Helm [wilson p83] (See ¶4888)   5796

⟨1⟩ "Sammy Young bro. of Nancy Hanks and his descendants were all very tall and   5797

Hanks family – Miscellaneous members (continued)

slender." – Robert Wintersmit [wilson p613]. *It is not clear that a Young was a sibling of Nancy Hanks; see ¶4767.*

Lincoln descendants

Beware claims that some distant relative of Lincoln looked like him (e.g. ¶5789, ¶5810, ¶5838, ¶5845). [ferguson p155] found that simply growing a Lincoln-style beard leads to comments about a "striking" resemblance to Lincoln. People with MEN2B look more like each other than they do their own family.   5798

- ■ Sources: 5799
  - ⊙ The best-quality collection of photographs of Lincoln descendants is [neelyA].   5800
  - ⟨2⟩ A family tree of Abraham Lincoln's descendants is provided in [neelyA (inside cover)]. **Older versions**: [ChicagoTribune - Feb. 9, 1936], [ChicagoTribune - Feb. 12, 1961] (has photographs), and [montgomery].   5801

- ⟨2⟩ The ignominious end of the Lincoln line is detailed in [beschloss].   5802

- ■ Abraham Lincoln II (Lincoln's grandson):   5803
  - ⟨2⟩ Lived Aug. 14, 1873 to March 5, 1890. Became ill in late November or early December 1889, while attending school in France. According to his father's law partner: "An abscess or something of the sort formed, and he had to submit to a delicate surgical operation and blood poisoning followed." Apparently one of his lungs was involved by the illness. He was buried first in Springfield, then in the family plot at Arlington Cemetery. [lincloreEDI]   5804
  - ⟨2⟩ He was called "Jack," for reasons unknown. "His handwriting greatly resembled that of his grandfather Lincoln." He was described as "handsome, manly, and intelligent." A teacher said "he was the best student in my school," emphasizing "don't think that I speak flatteringly." [lincloreEDI]   5805
  - ⊙ Two small photographs show no chin dimple [neelyA].   5806
  - ⟨2⟩ [shutesM] recounts Jack's final illness in detail.   5807

- ⊙ Mary Beckwith (Lincoln's great-granddaughter): A photograph of her at perhaps one year of age shows widely separated eyes [ChicagoTribune - May 25, 1952] [randallP box 15]. Her mother, Jessie Lincoln Beckwith Randolph (Robert's daughter) is also in the photograph.   5808

- ⊙ Lincoln Isham (Lincoln's great-grandson): A photograph shows "crossed eyes" in childhood, but not in adolescence [neelyA p149]. None of his mother's photographs in [neelyA] show ocular misalignment.   5809

- ⟨2⟩ Great-grandchildren Robert and Peggy Beckwith "look remarkably like their great-grandparents" [burk p215]. Of Lincoln, however, Peggy said, "I'm as far away from him as anyone else" [burk p 215].   5810

Lincoln, Abraham   (paternal grandfather)

- ⟨1⟩ "born in old Virginia and lived on the Roanoke River the County not recollected" – Dennis Hanks [wilson p27]   5811

- ⟨2⟩ "Incited by the narratives of his kinsman, Daniel Boone," he moved to Kentucky about 1780 [lea p79].   5812

- ⟨1⟩ Age 40± [lincloreIGI]: "killed by the Indians near Boone Station in Kentucky when his Son Thomas was six years old" – Dennis Hanks [wilson p27] *Is mis-named by Hanks in this same letter* [wilson p27n].   5813

Misc.

Lincoln, Abraham   (paternal grandfather) (continued)

⟨1⟩ "Shall we simply say that he was killed by stealth in Kentucky while opening a farm about the year 1781 or 2?" – William Herndon [hertz p158]   5814

■ Multiple descendants have type 5 spinocerebellar ataxia. See ¶1025 and ¶5821.   5815

Lincoln, Bathsheba   (paternal grandmother)

■ Multiple descendants have type 5 spinocerebellar ataxia. See ¶1025.   5816

⟨2⟩ She appears in historical documents as, variously, Bershaba, Basheba, Barbara, and Batsab [lea p80].   5817

⟨2⟩ Lifespan: Lived 1741-1836 [nee]. "Died at the reputed age of 100" [shutes p1]. [montgomery] gives no dates.   5818

⟨2⟩ It was only about 1930 that Bathsheba's place in the Lincoln genealogy was established [lincolnW pp200-202]. See the discussion of Lincoln's paternal family tree.   5819

⟨1⟩ "a woman of fine intelligence and strong character" – recollection almost 100 years later [lea pp110, 203]   5820

▣ Handwriting experts at the U.S. Federal Bureau of Investigation analyzed signatures that Lincoln's paternal grandparents penned in February 1780 and September 1781 (probably obtained from [lea]). They concluded that handwriting of Lincoln's paternal grandmother, Bathsheba Herring Lincoln, "demonstrated characteristics that may be caused by a lack of coordination, a mental or physical impairment, a poor writing skill level, the writing surface or writing instrument, drug or alcohol effects, or the hand position of the writing" [nee].   5821

  ⟨2⟩_c [nee] concludes that lack of coordination was the most likely possibility; transiently impaired penmanship was unlikely because the two signatures had a similarly disorganized appearance.   5822

⟨2⟩ First half of 1780:   5823

  ⟨2⟩ She did not sign a document where her signature would have been expected [lea p80].   5824

  ⟨S⟩ This has been explained by her having an infant and being "unable to travel the twelve miles over the rough road which separated the Lincoln home from the County Court House" [lea p80]. *Lea provides no source for this explanation.*   5825

⟨1/q⟩ Sept. 8, 1871: "she being unable to travel to the County Court," a commission was appointed to travel to her house to determine if she consented to sell a certain parcel of land [lea pp80, 190-191].   5826

⟨2⟩ "She was still living and an invalid in Virginia in 1781, and probably accompanied her husband over the Wilderness Road into Kentucky the following year, and not long after succumbed to the hardships of the rude life of the frontier" [lea p110]. *Invalidism pertinent to possible type 5 spinocerebellar ataxia.*   5827

  ⟨2⟩ "In September, 1781, she disappears absolutely from the records" [lea p83]. *Later research by* [lincolnW] *has proven this statement incorrect. It is possibAll glory to the hypnotoad!*   5828

  ⟨-⟩ *It is unclear whether her inability to travel forms the basis of the invalidism claim.*   5829

Lincoln, Josiah   (paternal uncle)

He is of interest because of the possibility he transmitted the gene for spinocerebellar ataxia type 5 from his parents to the kindred described in [ranum]. See ¶1025.   5830

⟨1⟩ 1860: "no recent information of him or his family has been obtained" – Lincoln [angle p5]   5831

⟨2⟩ True genealogy is in [lincolnW pp202ff]. Deliberately distorted genealogy is in [ranum].   5832

Lincoln, Mordecai   (paternal uncle)

⟨2⟩ Age 14: Shot and killed an Indian that had already killed his father and was about to kill Thomas Lincoln (future father of the President). (See ¶5217.) Thereafter was an "Indian hater" and killed many others.   5833

⟨1⟩ "I have often said that Uncle Mord had run off with all the talents in the family." – Lincoln [burl p42]   5834

⟨1⟩ "great good Common Sense – Was Entitled to genius" – Samuel Haycraft [wilson p31]   5835

⟨2⟩ Bright, energetic. Cobbler, carpenter, violinist. Florid. "Prone to dramatic gestures." Grew increasingly hostile to the church. Became paranoid. Lived, hermit-like, with hundreds of pigeons. [shenk p79]   5836

⟨1/q⟩ "naturally a man of considerable genius; he was a man of great drollery, and it would almost make you laugh to look at him." – Usher Linder [walsh p128]   5837

⟨2⟩ "had broad mood swings, which were probably intensified by his heavy drinking. And Mordecai's family was thick with mental disease. All three of his sons – who bore a strong physical resemblance to their first cousin Abraham – were considered melancholy men" [shenk p12]. *A strong physical resemblance to Lincoln seems unlikely.*   5838

Lincoln, Sarah Bush Johnston   (step-mother)

Assuming she had no transmissible disease which Lincoln contracted, Lincoln's step-mother is not relevant to this study because she was not a blood relative of any of the Lincolns.   5839

⟨s⟩ On the other hand, "Perhaps the best thing Thomas Lincoln ever did for his son was to marry Sarah Bush Johnston, who cherished the lad." [burl p257]   5840

⟨1⟩ "Sarah Lincoln was a strong healthy woman – was Cool – not Excitable" – Elizabeth Crawford [wilson p126]. This probably refers to Lincoln's step-mother Sarah, not his sister Sarah [wilson p126n].   5841

⟨1/q⟩ After hearing of Lincoln's death, "she never had no heart after that to be chirp and peart like she used to be." – unnamed person [kunhardtB p284]   5842

Lincolns – Miscellaneous

See ⌐Schwartz patients⌐ for information about some very distant Lincoln cousins. Distant Lincoln cousins also figure prominently in the analysis related to type 5 spinocerebellar ataxia in ¶1025ff.   5843

⟨1⟩ Of Lincolns in vicinity of Harrisonburg, VA in 1865: "highly respectable & exceedingly stubborn people, or such as are popularly denominated 'bull-headed' " – John T. Harris [wilson p141]   5844

⟨2⟩ Berenice Lovely provided much information to William Barton (ultimately) on mental problems in the Lincoln family [shenk pp12, 230]. A great uncle of Lincoln's   5845

Lincolns – Miscellaneous (continued)

confessed to having "a deranged mind." A daughter of a first cousin of Lincoln's was judged insane and committed at age 39. She supposedly had a strong physical resemblance to Lincoln [shenk pp12, 247]. *Actually, the pronoun is ambiguous. She may have only resembled her father.* For Uncle Mordecai and his descendants, see ¶5838.

⟨2⟩ "In 1999 a distant relative of the president, third cousin three times removed, named Abraham Wesley Lincoln of Brookville, Ohio, wrote a column in the Abraham Lincoln genealogy website. The relative stated that he himself had a history of a spontaneous pneumothorax, an aortic aneurysm, and a palate with 'a cleft about the size of a walnut.' " [ho] *Of course, this is in no way substantiated.*   5846

⟨2⟩ Lincoln ancestry is reviewed at length in [lea] and [lincolnW].   5847
   ▣ [lea] includes drawings of several Lincoln ancestors.   5848
   ▣ [lea] includes signatures of several Lincoln ancestors.   5849

Maternal Grandfather

⟨2⟩ The identity of Lincoln's maternal grandfather is unknown. Lincoln told Herndon the man was a "nobleman so called of Virginia" who had fathered Lincoln's mother out of wedlock. [burl p42]   5850

⟨1/q⟩ Lincoln also told Herndon: "My mother inherited his qualities and I hers. All that I am or hope ever to be I get from my mother, God bless her." [burl p42]   5851
  ⟨S⟩ [burl pp42&137] interprets Lincoln's statement as both a rejection of his father and as praise for his mother.   5852
  ⟨S⟩ There are some doubts about this quotation's authenticity [burl pp137&146n] citing [borittA]   5853
  ⟨2/c⟩ "Those who subscribe to the theory of Nancy's illegitimacy can give no good reason for believing Abraham Lincoln's unknown grandfather was possessed of extraordinary capacity." [angle p4]   5854

⟨1/q⟩ "I don't know who my grandfather was, and am more concerned to know what his grandson will be." – Lincoln to James Speed, recalled by Christopher Graham [tarbellE p235]   5855

Schwartz patients

[schwartzA] presents four patients who are (or claim to be) distantly related to Lincoln's father. Schwartz is suspicious that two of them have Marfan syndrome, and seems certain one of them does.   5856

⟨1⟩ The "certain" Marfan patient was diagnosed in 1959 as a seven-year-old boy. [schwartzA] provides updated findings at age 11.   5857
  ⟨2⟩ [schwartzA] did not personally evaluate the patient and does not make a diagnosis.   5858
  ⟨1⟩ "Sallow" skin, but at what age is unclear. [schwartzA]   5859
⟨S⟩ [borittA] questions the certainty with which the ancestry of the patients are known.   5860

Sparrow, Lucy Hanks   (maternal grandmother)

⟨2⟩ "Lived a useful life until about the age of 61" [shutes p1]   5861
⟨2⟩ Lived "c. 1767 – c. 1833?" [wilson p780]   5862

Todd, Eliza Parker   (Mary's Mother)

⟨S⟩ Died of a "bacterial infection" soon after giving birth [burl p270] *"Bacterial infec-*   5863
*tion" is a modern label. Bacteria could not have been identified in ante-bellum
Lexington. The germ theory was not accepted in that era.*

Todd, Robert Smith   (Mary's Father)

"The Todds were people of substance in Scotland and Ireland before they migrated to   5864
America" [evans p32]. Mary's branch was "characterized by overintensity" [randallC p105].

⟨$\frac{1}{q}$⟩ Was eighth of eleven children [lincloreIED].   5865

▣ Portrait exists [helmB] [kunhardtA p59]   5866

     ⟨2⟩ Based on a painting of Mary's father, [randallC p73] sees a family resemblance.   5867
     c

⟨2⟩ "died July 16, 1849, apparently of the dreaded plague cholera which was then epi-   5868
demic in Lexington." [randallC p123]

     ⟨2⟩ "In July of 1849, Robert Todd died in a cholera epidemic which swept Lex-   5870
ington." [turner p40]

Todds – Mary's Full Siblings

Mary Todd Lincoln's father was married twice and had children by both wives. He   5871
had seven children by his first wife [burl p269], Eliza Parker Todd, six of whom reached
maturity. Mary was third of these.

- Elizabeth Todd Edwards: 5872
  - ⟨2⟩ "No one who knew her said unkind things about Mrs. Edwards. I am sure   5873
    she was normal, and so are her descendants, so far as I could learn. What-
    ever blight there was in the family, Mrs. Edwards and her children and their
    children escaped it." [evans p45]
  - ⟨2⟩ In late 1880 Mary moved in with Elizabeth. By then, "both were near invalids,   5874
    with hearing, sight, and heart problems" [baker p365]
  - ⟨1⟩ "Grandmother Edwards was the flower of the Todd family. She was a right   5875
    pretty talker – a prettier talker even than [great] Aunt Mary Lincoln. ... Aunt
    Mary said, 'Elizabeth, you always have your nose in a dictionary.' " – Mary
    Edwards Brown, 1956 [kunhardtC]
  - ▣ [helmB] contains portrait of Elizabeth in advanced years.   5876
  - ▣ Photograph of Elizabeth Todd Edwards' two boys as children [kunhardtA p92]   5877

- Frances Todd Wallace: 5878
  - ⟨2⟩ "There is nothing in the record that reflects on Mrs. Wallace or any members   5879
    of her family. Nor was there anything abnormal in her personality." [evans p45]

- Ann Todd Smith: 5880
  - ▣ To my eye, and to that of [ostendorfA p322], Ann and Mary closely resemble each   5881
    other. See ¶5893.
  - ⟨2⟩ "After all proper allowances have been made, we must conclude that Mrs.   5882
    Smith had a difficult personality; one of a type that did not differ much from
    that of Mrs. Lincoln herself. ... There is very good evidence that part of her
    difficult and peculiar personality was inherited by some of her descendants.
    Though the evidence consists in nothing more than gossip and 'clothesline
    stories,' there is enough to justify the conclusion." [evans p47]
  - ⟨1⟩ 1861: "she possesses a miserable disposition & so false a tongue. ... as a   5883
    child & young girl, could not be outdone in falsehood" – Mary [turner p105]

- Levi O. Todd: 5884

Misc.

Todds – Mary's Full Siblings (continued)

⟨2⟩ "There is no question that he had an abnormal personality. ... He seems to have fallen out with everyone. He used whisky [sic] to excess, and possibly other drugs." [evans pp47-48] 5885

⟨2⟩ "a problem individual in the full sense of the word" [randallC p126] 5886

⟨¹/q⟩ Died 1864 "from utter want and destitution" – Emilie Todd Helm [randallC p309] 5887

■ Dr. George Rogers Clark Todd: 5888

⟨2⟩ He entered the Confederate Army in 1861 and served as a surgeon through the Civil War. 5889

⟨2⟩ In 1930, Dr. A.B. Patterson, "a former fellow-practitioner," wrote: "As to the doctor's personality: Would seem very pleasant when he wished to be, but generally not agreeable. Did not get along with people. Was very bright and well informed, very egotistical, and extremely jealous of his professional reputation. Very peculiar and eccentric. Drank whisky [sic] to excess. Not on friendly terms with his son. ... It is said he died from an overdose of chloroform taken himself alone in his house." [evans pp49-50] 5890

⟨2⟩ In 1931 Todd's attorney, H.L. O'Bannon, wrote: "He was of small build, florid of countenance, and inclined to stutter when he talked. ... After the death of his wife he lived alone and was given to moods of deep melancholy." [evans pp49-50] 5891

⟨2⟩c "The trend toward abnormal personality was far greater in the Todd-Parker group [full siblings] than in the Todd-Humphreys group [half-siblings] of children." [evans p52] 5892

[◎] In photographs of Elizabeth, Frances, and Ann [kunhardtA pp56-57], Mary and Ann look much alike. 5893

⟨2⟩ Elizabeth and Frances looked like their mother [burl p270]. 5894

Todds – Mary's Half-siblings

With his second wife, Betsy Humphreys Todd, Mary Todd's father had nine children, eight of whom lived to maturity. These were Mary's half-siblings: Margaret, Martha, Emilie, Elodie, Katherine, Samuel, David, and Alexander [evans] – 5 daughters and 3 sons – all but one of whom sided with the Confederacy [burl p294] 5895

⟨2⟩ "I have been at some trouble to find what I could about this family of children and their descendants. ... I have not found facts or opinions that reflect on any of them. ... The general reputation of this division of the family as good neighbors ranks well above the average." [evans p52] 5896

⟨2⟩c "The trend toward abnormal personality was far greater in the Todd-Parker group [full siblings] than in the Todd-Humphreys group [half-siblings] of children." [evans p52] 5897

[◎] [helmB] has photographs of Elodie and Emilie, and portraits of David, Margaret, and Alexander. 5898

[◎] Also: Portrait of Alexander in [kunhardtA p187]. Photograph of Emilie in [kunhardtA p218]. 5899

⟨2⟩ The sons all fought as rebels in the war. All died as a result, sooner or later. [evans pp51-52] [wilson pp694-695] 5900

⟨¹/q⟩ Of Emilie: "The child has a tongue like the rest of the Todds." – Lincoln [randallC p108] 5901

Special Topics

Topic 1 – Longer Narratives §1

> "There can be no new 'Lincoln stories.' ... The stories are all told. Henceforth all that is written of Lincoln must be either a restatement and rearrangement of the well-known facts of history, or it must be an estimate, a philosophical study of the character of the man."
>
> – Noah Brooks, 1898
> [NYTimes - Feb. 12, 1898]

(a) Head Kick §1a

A horse kicked nine-year-old Lincoln in the head. See ¶3568. Herndon's multiple accounts of the incident, including this one [herndon pp51-52], *agree in their essentials* [kempfB p10]. *For possible sequelae of the kick, see ¶3568ff.*

In later years, Mr. Lincoln related the following reminiscence of his experience as a miller in Indiana: One day, taking a bag of corn, he mounted the old flea-bitten gray mare and rode leisurely to Gordon's mill. Arriving somewhat late, his turn did not come until almost sundown. In obedience to the custom requiring each man to furnish his own power he hitched the old mare to the arm, and as the animal moved round, the machinery responded with equal speed. Abe was mounted on the arm, and at frequent intervals made use of his whip to urge the animal on to better speed. With a careless "Get up, you old hussy," he applied the lash at each revolution of the arm. In the midst of the exclamation, or just as half of it had escaped through his teeth, the old jade, resenting the continued use of the goad, elevated her shoeless hoofs and striking the young engineer in the forehead, sent him sprawling to the earth. Miller Gordon hurried in, picked up the bleeding, senseless boy, whom he took for dead, and at once sent for his father. Old Thomas Lincoln came – came as soon as embodied listlessness could move – loaded the lifeless boy in a wagon and drove home. Abe lay unconscious all night, but towards the break of day the attendants noticed signs of returning consciousness. The blood beginning to flow normally, his tongue struggled to loosen itself, his frame jerked for an instant, and he awoke, blurting out the words "you old hussy," or the latter half of the sentence interrupted by the mare's heel at the mill.

Mr. Lincoln considered this one of the remarkable instances of his life. He often referred to it, and we had many discussions in our law office over the psychological phenomena involved in the operation. ... His idea was that the latter half of the expression "Get up, you old hussy," was cut off by a suspension of the normal flow of his mental energy, and that as soon as life's forces returned he unconsciously ended the sentence; or, as he in a plainer figure put it: "Just before I struck the old mare my will through the mind had set the muscles of my tongue to utter the expression, and when her heels came in contact with my head the whole thing stopped half-cocked, as it were, and was only fired off when mental energy or force returned."

* * *

"He and I used to speculate on it. The first question was: why was not the whole expression uttered; and the second one: why finish at all? We came to the conclusion ... that the mental energy, force, had been flashed by the will on the nerves and thence on the muscles in the exact shape, or form, or attitude, or position, to utter those words; that the kick *shocked* him, *checked* momentarily the action of the muscles; and that as soon as that check was removed or counteracted by a returning flow of life and energy, force, and power in their proper channels, that the muscles fired off." – William Herndon [hertz p73]

384

* * *

"In his tenth year he was kicked by a horse, and apparently killed for a time." – Lincoln, writing in the third person [baslerA v4p63] *Being "in his tenth year" would make him nine years old.*

(b) Malaria (and Ann Rutledge) §1b

Voluminous writings debate Lincoln's feelings toward Ann Rutledge and his psycho-logical reaction to her death. The debate has all but ignored the major physical illness afflicting Lincoln before and after her passing. The following second-hand account, in [rankinA pp72-87], was written "from the authority of his mother's old but keen memory" [shutesE p46]. Also see ¶2008 and ¶2695.

The spring and early summer of 1835, I have been told, was a time of unusually large rainfall and high temperature in central Illinois. By July the rains ceased and extreme heat dried up and parched the luxurious vegetation of earlier growth, and chills and fever and what the earlier physicians named "bilious fever" became unusually prevalent. In every home some member was stricken down, and in most homes all the family were ill at the same time. Treatment of these malarial diseases was very crude and drastic at that time. Heroic doses of medicine were administered, often more fatal than the disease, killing a person of frail physique instead of effecting a cure. The Rutledge family were among the unfortunate many who suffered. Ann was among the last to be stricken. Lincoln had been a frequent visitor and assistant in nursing at the Rutledge home during their sickness, go-ing over from Salem with Dr. John Allen, the physician, every day or two. He would stay over night when needed, or return with the Doctor who would stop for him after visiting the other patients in that neighbourhood. At length, toward the end of August, Miss Rutledge's condition passed beyond the help of physicians and nurses and the delirium of her last few days common in the fatal cases of those malarial fevers brought an end to her life on August 25, 1835.

For a month or more before, Lincoln himself, with all the physical vigour he then pos-sessed and preserved until that fatal bullet ended his life, had been suffering from the chills and fever on alternate days. He kept up and was helping nurse others all the while, but was taking heroic doses of Peruvian bark, boneset tea, jalap and calomel. Added to the depres-sion of Lincoln from illness in those days, was that from the death of several of his personal friends, and the neighbourly aid he had given unstintingly at the funerals and burials of those who died. There were no undertakers. No caskets were kept on hand. Coffins had to be made after the death; and in a few instances he had assisted in making them for his friends. In this environment of distress that he was day and night helping to relieve, in ad-dition to the poisonous malaria that had been for weeks alternately chilling and burning his stalwart frame, he was now to endure the supreme tragedy of his life in the death of Ann Rutledge. *Was it really more tragic than the deaths of his mother, sister, son Eddie, or son Willie?*

...

The personal influence of Dr. John Allen on Lincoln and their mutual attraction to each other at this important period, when he was under such great physical suffering and mental distress, makes some mention of the doctor's character appropriate... [long digression] ...

[p80] The reader who has followed me ... will appreciate the measure of influence that Dr. Allen was able to exert on Lincoln in the susceptible condition induced by his physical weakness and mental distress after the death of Ann Rutledge. No physician could have been better qualified temperamentally than was Dr. Allen to treat Lincoln's condition wisely. He saw the two-fold ailment of the young man. ...

First, he took both professional and personal charge of Lincoln, who was physically

§1

worn out with overwork and anxiety day and night for so many anxious weeks. His distress by deaths among his friends; his own protracted illness from relapses of the chills and fever that became all the more difficult to arrest with him because of their repeated recurrences under neglected medication and such continuous overwork, all combined, had made a seriously sick man of him. He prevailed on Lincoln to go out to the quiet home of Bowling Greene and remain there under his medical attention and in Mrs. Greene's care to administer the prescribed courses of medicine, until he should pass three consecutive weeks free from chills.

...

[p83] Most motherly of nurses, dearest Mrs. Greene ... as you went quietly about your housework those three weeks...

...

[p84] As the word "insanity" has been used as descriptive of Lincoln's life shortly after the death of Ann Rutledge, I have dwelt with more fulness in recital of these events of 1835 than I otherwise would have considered necessary.

...

[p85] there has been written since his death into certain fictional biography by some the implied charge, by others the positive assertion, that his life was darkened by the shadows of "insanity," following Miss Rutledge's death. This is utterly unsupported by any facts or circumstances transpiring in 1835.

...

[p86] Far less is there need to disprove the "three weeks' insanity" charge, made after Lincoln's death. The matchless vigour, poise, and clearness of mind of [Lincoln], lifts him far above the taint of "insanity" at any period of his life...

...

[p87] In less than a month – in three weeks – Lincoln returned to his usual affairs at Salem and resumed his surveying tramps wherever they were called for.

* * *

"[The grand-daughter-in-law of Dr. Allen's sister] wrote from the authority of family tradition: '... within the week of [Ann's death] he was found to be the victim of the fever he had sought to combat in others. On the advise [sic] of Dr. Allen he was taken to the home of Bowling Green near New Salem, and there the good squire and his wife Nancy nursed him through his long illness.' " [shutesE p46]

(c) Too Many of Us in This Bed   [browneF pp294-296]   §1c

After missing a train connection while campaigning for the U.S. Senate in 1858, Lincoln must spend the night in a small town. The best lodgings are in a "country tavern" where Lincoln talks and tells stories after dinner. At 8 o'clock he asks to be shown to his room, saying "I have a hard day's work before me to-morrow, and want to load up with all the sleep I can get." Lincoln has taken the last room and bed in the tavern, so insists that newspaper reporter Andrew Shuman must share them. The room contained only "a rough bedstead, with a few simple bed-clothes upon it ... a rickety old lounge ... a rag-carpet, the worse for long wear and much tear ... a small stand" for a candle. Shuman continues:

I went to sleep right off; but after an hour or so I was awakened by Mr. Lincoln getting up, striking a match and lighting the candle. 'What's the matter, Mr. Lincoln?' I asked. 'I can't get asleep,' he replied, 'and am going to explore a little. The fact is, Shuman, there are *too many of us* in this bed.' Not understanding what he meant, I proposed to go down stairs and sleep in a chair, leaving him alone to get the rest he so much needed. 'Oh, no,' he said, 'I don't mean you. I'll show you what I mean.' Thereupon, with a sudden jerk, he lifted the bedclothes from the foot of the bed, and pointed to a dozen or two of fleeing bed-bugs. 'See there! those fellows have been feeding upon my shins for the past hour, and I can't stand it any longer.'

For the first time since I had known him, Mr. Lincoln exhibited considerable impatience, and something like anger. He left the bed in disgust, and threw himself upon the rickety old lounge at the other side of the room, declaring his purpose to lie there the remainder of the night, with nothing but his apology for a pillow between him and the rough plank which constituted the seat of the lounge. I couldn't permit that, of course; so I took most of the clothing off the bed and tucked it under and around him, making him as comfortable as possible. The light was extinguished, and I rejoined my multitudinous companions in the bed, who, apparently not being fond of young blood, kept their distance.

I was just falling off into sleep, when I heard the old lounge creaking. It was evident that its occupant was not getting the sleep he sought for. He turned from one side to the other several times; he gave an occasional kick; finally he groaned. 'Can't you get asleep there, either?' I inquired. 'Not a bit of it, there's no sleep for me here.' He arose, and so did I. We again lighted the candle, and with it examined the lounge. It fairly swarmed with bed-bugs!

To make a long and painful story short, it was finally agreed between us that Mr. Lincoln should make a bed for himself on the rag-carpet in the center of the floor, he vigorously protesting at first against taking the 'lion's share' of the bedclothes; but I insisted, and carried my point. We doubled up the straw-mattress and the carpet on the floor, and Mr. Lincoln, lying down, wadded up his pillow into a bunch under his head, and after I had tucked a quilt and a blanket around him and wished him 'better luck this time,' we resumed our efforts to sleep. It was now eleven o'clock; and in order to take the train it was necessary for us to be up for breakfast at six o'clock.

Mr. Lincoln declared, when making his hasty toilet by the sickly light of our tallow candle, next morning, that he never in all his life had a sounder or a more restful sleep than that which followed his 'battle with the bedbugs.' The last time I ever saw Abraham Lincoln to speak with him, the late Norman B. Judd and several others being present, he narrated this little adventure of ours in that old country tavern.

(d) 1865 Editorial on Lincoln's Declining Health (#1) §1d §1

Lincoln's several-day illness in mid-March 1865 (see ¶1226ff) led to the following editorial in [ChicagoTribune - March 22, 1865, page 2].

The President's Health

We do not desire to create needless alarm in the minds of the people by heading this editorial with the above ominous caption. The recent illness of the President does not necessarily indicate that the public have reason to be under immediate apprehension, but we have the best reasons, founded upon the general observation of those who, like ourselves, have been familiar with his personal health and appearance for many years, for stating that Mr. Lincoln's physical powers have been tested beyond their capacity of endurance, and that if this ordeal is to continue, his naturally strong constitution must at no distant date, give way.

Without entering into an invidious inquiry as to the comparative fitness of those who might be called upon in any contingency to succeed him, the unanimity with which he was nominated, and the heavy popular voice by which he was elected, are sufficient evidence of the great interest the entire country has in his life. The political and military history of the country, especially during the past two years, since he became emphatically "master of the situation," are sufficient witness that the people would forego much of their accustomed freedom of access to the President rather than see him reduced to his present worn and weakened condition.

Many who saw him at his inauguration, where the opportunity for noting the change in his personal appearance was better than in his office or at the White House, were painfully impressed with his gaunt, skeleton-like appearance. From eight o'clock in the morning to past midnight of each day for four years, the President, in addition to the discharge of the proper duties of his office in the most difficult and arduous administration ever devolved upon the Executive of any government, has given audience to a constant stream of committees, visitors, officers, and delegated and self-constituted representatives of the people, from all sections, parties and conditions of men. He has heard their complaints, answered their arguments and considered their wishes, with a patience none of his predecessors ever exhibited, and with a democratic spirit of equality which Washington or Jackson would have regarded as inconsistent with the dignity of their position. Whatever grievance came before him for redress, whatever appointment for his sanction, he has at all times entered into its investigation with all the energy of his body, mind and conscience, and, not content with doing what was right, he has labored until he succeeded in convincing those with whom he was brought in contact and into conflict, that he had done right.

All this vast labor has not been performed without a visible effect upon the physical powers of the man who has accomplished it. Most strong executive men would have broken down under far less labor. A tough and wiry constitution, and that easy flow of humor which enabled him to relieve his daily round of harassing annoyances, perplexing questions, and weighty care with pithy but smile-compelling anecdotes, these have lightened his load, and in all human probability, preserved his life. But there is a point beyond which these will not carry him. He needs at least a month's entire rest from from [sic] his official duties, and thenceforward a systematic and enforced exemption from the vast and unprecedented pressure of calls, appeals, committees, &c., to which he has heretofore given himself up. We believe the country would be glad to see him just at this point take the needed vacation. The people know that the Commander-in-Chief of the Army and Navy has labored more arduously than any private in the ranks or any sailor on deck; all but he have had their furloughs. The present prosperous condition of our military, naval and financial operations, and diplomatic relations, is more opportune than has heretofore existed since he took the first oath of office. Gen. Grant as Grand Marshal of the military operations at the front needs no watching. Secretary Stanton is at home in the War Department. Our navy have closed all the ports, captured all the blockade runners and out-lived all the pirates. Mr. Seward will continue his voluminous moral reflections which, even if Mr. Lincoln were present and in full health, it might be dangerous for him to attempt to review. Mr. McCulloch will run the Treasury. On behalf of the sovereign people therefore we bespeak for our really invalid President a month's furlough!

(e) 1865 Editorial on Lincoln's Declining Health (#2)   §1e

Lincoln's several-day illness in mid-March 1865 (see ¶1226ff) led to the following editorial in the New York Daily Tribune of March 17, 1865 (same as [NYTribune]?) Photostat in [barbeeP - box 2 folder 137].

```
The President's Health
```

We are not, it is known, among the idolators, nor even among the adulators, of Abraham Lincoln. He was not out first choice for President in 1860, nor yet in 1864. ...

... yet that does not conflict with the fact that his death or permanent disability now would be a calamity – very generally and justly deplored. ...

But, if the President is to outlive the term on which he has just entered, a radical retrenchment must be promptly effected in the current exactions on his time and energies. He has been carried further toward the grave by his four years in the White House than he could have been by ten years of constant labor in the courts or on a farm. All who knew him in 1860 and have met him in 1865, must have observed his air of fatigue, exhaustion and languor – so different from his old hearty, careless, jovial manner. We are sure no good physician, who had seen him since last December, can have heard of his recent illness without feeling that this was what might and should have been expected.

For human strength is finite, and no man could endure the constant tension of his faculties imposed on President Lincoln without a more or less speedy break-down. Go when you will to the White House, from early morn until a late hour at night, and you find the antechamber filled with a crowd of eager solicitors of a special interview with the President. ... Let it be understood that the President would confer for even five minutes with every one who might fancy that he had occasion for an interview, and Mr. Lincoln could not remain above ground for even a month longer.

It being simply impossible that the President should grant an audience to every one who solicits it, we urge that decided steps should at once be taking in the premises. If his life is indeed worth saving, those steps cannot be taken a moment too soon. ...

... the President must be relieved, at once and forever, from the pressure of personal solicitations and interviews which now wastefully absorb his working hours and threaten to end prematurely his days.

(f) 1865 Editorial on Lincoln's Declining Health (#3)   §1f

Lincoln's several-day illness in mid-March 1865 (see ¶1226ff) led to the following editorial in the New York Daily Tribune of March 21, 1865 (same as [NYTribune]?) Photostat in [barbeeP - box 2 folder 135].

President Lincoln

The Commercial Advertiser has a Washington letter, which says

"Although sadly beset and annoyed by office-seekers, who insist on 'rotation,' Mr. Lincoln is recovering rapidly from his recent indisposition . A gentleman who called on him by appointment *last night, at eleven o'clock*, says that although Mr. Lincoln had selected that hour in order to be free from intrusion, *the audience-room and the private office were crowded.* Among the most unfortunate solicitors   §1 are the unprovided-for Union members of the two last Congresses, *who consider that they have a preëmption right to place.* Any position will be acceptable wither at home or abroad, that has a salary of fifteen hundred or two thousand dollars a year, but they must have some kind of a place, and most of them will be gratified in order to get rid of them."

– This has only to go on little longer, and the National will have to mourn another dead President, as it has so lately mourned the untimely fate of Harrison and Taylor. And we give fair notice that we shall hold any one who presumes in that case to talk of "mysterious Providence," "inscrutable decrees," "visitation of God," &c., &c., a shameless imposter. The President is being killed by monstrous experiments on his patience and good nature – killed by the greed and impudence of bores, who meanly calculate that they have only to bore hard enough, and "most of them will be gratified, in order to get rid of them." And (as *The Commercial* says) foremost among these rapacious experimenters on his kindness of heart are certainly recently discarded Members of Congress, who strangely seem to imagine that their ill success with the People "gives them a pre-emption right to place." We beg leave most emphatically to dissent.

It is of the gravest National consequence that the President should now be able to fix his attention exclusively on the National crisis, and devote all his time and thoughts to the securing of a satisfactory pacification of our country at the earliest practicable moment. The office-seekers are not only killing the President; they are imperiling the life of the Nation. We urge the People to insist on their instant and thorough abatement.

Topic 2 – Syphilis

This topic discusses the possibility that Abraham and Mary Lincoln had syphilis. In debating whether *any* person in the 1800s had syphilis, the affirmative viewpoint will always have the advantage, for several reasons:

(1) Syphilis was extremely common.

(2) It is extremely difficult to exclude syphilis on clinical grounds alone.

(3) In any historical debate it is extremely difficult to prove a negative.

Note: This topic is a work in progress, sometimes tending toward a stream of consciousness presentation.

(a) Natural History of Syphilis (lay discussion) §2a

Syphilis is a bacterial infection. In persons with a normal immune system, it is easily cured with penicillin. Before penicillin became available in the 1940s, treating syphilis was difficult and often ineffective. In Lincoln's era there were no useful treatments at all, as judged by modern standards [aa111 p650].

The introduction of penicillin was dramatic – an "earthquake" [aa111 p iii]. Because of penicillin, syphilis is today a different disease than in Lincoln's time. Then, syphilis infections could persist for decades and cause multiple late complications. Today, antibiotic use is ubiquitous, and syphilis rarely has the chance to live in an antibiotic-free host for 30 or more years. Thus, late syphilitic complications are now rare.

As a result, the medical literature most relevant to any Lincolnian syphilis was written before 1950. Two books [aa78] [aa111] are the acme of that literature. I have consulted few references beyond them.

Syphilis infections classically progress through three sequential stages: primary, secondary, and tertiary. They, and a fourth type of syphilis – congenital syphilis – are summarized below. Note, however, that atypical courses are common. Syphilis is a disease of almost infinite variability. At one extreme, it may be wholly inapparent without laboratory testing. At the other extreme, it may imitate almost any other disease. Sir William Osler was not joking when he advised physicians to "Know syphilis" [aa108].

Primary syphilis classically manifests as a solitary genital chancre at the site where syphilis bacteria have entered the skin. A typical chancre is a painless pit in the skin, but "may assume almost any conceivable morphological form, and may occur on any accessible portion of the human body except the teeth, hair, and nails" [aa111 p481]. Rarely, primary infection may occur without a chancre ("syphilis d'emblee"), especially if an ulcerated skin lesion, present for some other reason, is the site of infection [aa111 pp479-481]. Without treatment, a chancre typically heals in 4 to 6 weeks [aa116 p50], often leaving the patient convinced his or her infection is gone. This conviction is correct only about half the time [aa78 p4].

Secondary syphilis can cause a variety of manifestations – or none at all. A rash on the palms and soles is common, but inflammation can occur anywhere in the body. If inflammation occurs in the scalp or eyebrows, hair can fall out. ("Every clinician should learn to watch eyebrows" [aa111 pp573-574, 703].) If inflammation occurs in the colored part of the eye (the iris), then "iritis" is said to be present. If inflammation occurs in the membrane surrounding the brain and spinal cord, then meningitis is present.

In contrast to primary syphilis, in which the patient feels completely well, patients with secondary syphilis will often feel sick.

Tertiary syphilis is the most feared stage, because of its effects on the brain, spinal cord, and heart.

Congenital syphilis occurs when a pregnant woman, infected with syphilis, transmits the infection to her fetus. The newborn may show signs of syphilis at birth or may develop signs decades later.

Table. Selected Consequences of Syphilis

Primary	Secondary	Tertiary	Congenital
Chancre	Rash	Tabes dorsalis	Sniffles at birth
	Meningitis	General paresis	Rash at birth
	Hair loss	Aortic aneurysm	Deafness
	Eyebrow loss	Aortic regurgitation	Abnormal teeth
	Iritis	Gumma	Keratitis
			Clavicular thickening
			Painless knee effusions
			Saber shins

Syphilis was extremely common in the pre-penicillin era. In 1941 one in every 77 white Americans had syphilis, as did one in every eight black Americans [aa111 p1185].

Jokes about toilet seats notwithstanding, it is worth noting that syphilis may be acquired non-sexually. Congenital syphilis has already been mentioned. Kissing and drinking cups may transmit the infection [aa111 p495].* Chancres of the nasal septum, eyelid, and finger, although rare, were seen most frequently in physicians [aa111 pp502-508]. A "brawl chancre" of the knuckle can develop after punching a syphilitic's mouth [aa111 p502]. Any of these primary inoculations may result in typical long-term syphilitic sequelae.

(b) Lincoln Infection - Historical Basis   §2b

The traditional evidence that Lincoln had syphilis derives from a letter William Herndon wrote to Jesse Weik on January 6, 1891. The portions of that letter dealing with Lincoln's infection, or its remembrance, are below:

§2

⟨1⟩ "When I was in Greencastle in 1887 I said to you that Lincoln had, *when a mere boy*, the syphilis, and now let me explain the matter in full, which I have never done before. About the year 1835-36 Mr. Lincoln went to Beardstown and during a devilish passion had connection with a girl and caught the disease. Lincoln told me this and in a moment of folly I made a note of it in my mind and afterwards I transferred it, as it were, to a little memorandum book which I loaned to Lamon, not, as I should have done, erasing that note. ..." – Herndon, 1891 [hertz p259]   §2.1

⟨1⟩ "The note spoken of in the memorandum book was a loose affair, and I never intended that the world should see or hear of it. I now wish and for years have wished that the note was blotted out or burned to ashes. I write this to you, fearing that at some future time the note – a loose thing as to date, place, and circumstances – will come to light and be misunderstood. Lincoln was a man of terribly strong passions, but was true as steel to his wife during his whole marriage life; his honor, as Judge Davis has said, saved many a woman, and it is most emphatically true, as I know. I write this to you to explain

---

* "In Schamberg's famous case 7 young women developed primary lesions of syphilis following a kissing game in which a young man participant had a chancre of the lip" [aa111 p496].

the whole matter for the future if it should become necessary to do so. I deeply regret my part of the affair in every particular." – Herndon, 1891 [hertz pp259-260]   §2.2

⟨1⟩ "Mrs. Dale was my guest for several days, say in '71, and she saw that memorandum book and took some notes on its contents, and may some time come to light from that quarter, and so you have this as my defense." – Herndon, writing in 1891 [hertz p260] §2.3

Analysis:

- Herndon clearly says what he knows, how he knows it, and what is speculation (see §2c). As [vidalB] notes, this is not Herndon surmising, this is Herndon saying what Lincoln said.   §2.4

- Herndon is following up on a conversation he had with Weik four years earlier. Thus, to claim this letter is a falsehood, invented with a specific disinformation goal in mind, requires one to believe that Herndon unfolded his scheme over four years.   §2.5

- Not one, but two more of Herndon's writings corroborates the story of Mrs. Dale and the memorandum book. In 1886, Herndon wrote [hertz p439]:   §2.6
  > There is one little book which I loaned to Mr. Lamon that I never intended any other mortal man or woman to see, if anything in it was to be made public. I think Mrs. Dale had a peep in it. ... If I could get hold of a little memmorandum book now in the possession of Lamon, I would burn it to ashes; it should quickly go; I loaned it to him foolishly, not thinking what use *could* be made of it, regret taking the notes, was a fool for it, I suppose.

  A year later, Herndon wrote to his co-author, Jesse Weik [hertz p170]:   §2.7
  > The little book of which you speak is now in Lamon's hands; he will not give it back to me; it was only loaned to him. I'll tell you all about it when I see you, can't risk the substance in a letter – too long and too much of it. Mrs. Dale did, I think, one day go to my private drawer and read part of the book, as I am informed. She didn't see the beautiful if she did. It is probable that I let her see the book – it's a good long time since, and I cannot recollect everything as it was in minutiae though I can in substance as well as I ever could.

  Herndon also mentions Mrs. Catherine H. Dale in 1867 [hertz p54] and (I think) somewhere in [hertz pp123-170]. (Is this really Caroline Dall [walsh pp21, 147]?) ○○○ *Project:* Is the memorandum book in the Lamon papers? ○○○ *Project:* Does the memo book also include an obscene Lincoln joke [ferguson pp63-64]?   §2.8

- If Herndon had fabricated the syphilis story, why would he tell Weik that Mrs. Dale may have made a copy of the syphilis note in 1871? This gave the indefatigable Weik [hertz p258] an opportunity to independently confirm or refute the syphilis story. Moreover, one must now believe Herndon unfolded his disinformation scheme over a period of *20 years* – preposterous. [Possible exceptions: (1) Mrs. Dale was an accomplice in a *conspiracy*, or (2) Perhaps Mrs. Dale was safely dead by 1891 and Herndon knew it.]§2.9

- Herndon describes the syphilis note as "a loose thing as to date, place, and circumstances." The word *loose* could mean "imprecise," or, more likely, "easily misinterpreted without the statements in this letter."   §2.10

- By saying Lincoln's honor "saved many a woman," Herndon (and Judge Davis) imply that Lincoln had opportunities for more than one dalliance (¶3355). Perhaps they are suggesting Lincoln restrained his carnal impulses ("terribly strong passions" ¶3351) to avoid transmitting syphilis to others. This is reasonable. Syphilis was then a terrible disease, both physiologically and socially. Its later stages can publicly brand a person with highly visible and highly characteristic markings, e.g., the rash and hair loss of secondary syphilis, the collapsed nasal bridge of tertiary syphilis, etc. (The "logic" of syphilis, noted in the 1600s, is that it starts in one pointed member and ends in another [aa121].)   §2.11

- Herndon's belief in Lincoln's syphilis is consistent with his theory that one or more of the Lincoln sons died from congenital syphilis (see below).   §2.12

- Although Herndon questioned Mary's fidelity to Lincoln (see §2h), he does not impugn her as the source of Lincoln's syphilis.   §2.13

- [fehrenbacherB] notes that Herndon was old and within months of death when he wrote this letter. See §2e. But the letter is well-written and even lawyerly in its clarity of phrase. Fehrenbacher does not say Herndon was demented or delirious at this time. Herndon freely and dispassionately admitted, in 1870, that he had "bad memory on names," but makes no broader admissions. Herndon had great insight into the the role of his memory (see ¶10).   §2.14

Analysis of motive:

- Herndon is clearly tormented by having disclosed the syphilis infection. He wants to protect Lincoln's reputation (and his own?). He is not attempting to smear anyone with this letter or with the syphilis disclosure. Specifically, nothing in this letter concerns his well known animosity toward Mary Lincoln.   §2.15

- There is no hint that Herndon was trying to profit from this letter to his co-author, Weik. Their book was already published. Unlike other letters to Weik, Herndon was not ruminating on what would "sell."   §2.16

- Herndon wrote his letter the same month he officially designated Weik as his heir in carrying the torch of Lincoln biography [hertz pp258-259]. It makes perfect sense that Herndon would, at this time, disclose to Weik the last great secret that Herndon knew. §2.17

Conclusions:

- Herndon had no reasonable motive to fabricate a story about Lincoln having syphilis. §2.18
- Multiple internal and external statements show that Herndon's belief was consistent and rational.   §2.19
- Thus, I accept these portions of Herndon's letter as fact... as Herndon understood it. §2.20

§2

(c) Lincoln Infection – His Letter to Dr. Drake   §2c

At some point before his marriage, Lincoln wrote a letter to Dr. Daniel Drake, who was then one of the foremost physicians in the American west (¶2467). The following two paragraphs contain all the known primary source material about it.

⟨1⟩ "Lincoln wrote a letter (a long one which he read to me) to Dr Drake of Cincinnati discriptive [sic] of his case. Its date would be in Decer 40 or early in January 41 – I think he must have informed Dr Drake of his early love for Miss Rutledge – as there was a part of the letter which he would not read. ... I remember Dr Drakes reply – which was that he would not undertake to priscribe [sic] for him without a personal interview." – Joshua Speed, 1866 [wilson p431]   §2.21

⟨1⟩ "About the year 1836-37 Lincoln moved to Springfield and took up his quarters with [Joshua] Speed; they became very intimate. At this time I suppose that the disease hung to him and, not wishing to trust our physicians, wrote a note to Doctor Drake, the latter part of which he would not let Speed see, not wishing Speed to know it. Speed said to me that Lincoln would not let him see a part of the note. Speed wrote to me a letter saying that he supposed L.'s letter to Doctor Drake had reference to his, L.'s crazy spell about the Ann Rutledge love affair, etc., and her death. You will find Speed's letter to me in our Life of Lincoln. The note to Doctor Drake in part had reference to his disease and not to his crazy spell as Speed supposes." – Herndon to Jesse Weik in 1891 [hertz p259]   §2.22

Analysis:

- Herndon adds nothing to Speed's account... except for confusion about the date of Lincoln's letter.   §2.23

- Both Speed and Herndon speculate on the letter's contents. Neither knows. The only facts are: (1) Lincoln wrote to a physician, and (2) Lincoln would not let his best friend know the full contents of the letter.   §2.24

- Speed's 1840-1841 date can be reasonably accepted as accurate. Herndon knows nothing of Lincoln's letter apart from Speed's account, which he must have mis-remembered. (Note that Herndon cannot remember the precise year Lincoln moved to Springfield.) Furthermore, late 1840 and early 1841 were eventful times in the lives of Speed and Lincoln, increasing the likelihood Speed's recollection is correct.   §2.25

- Herndon supposes a concern about syphilis prompted Lincoln's letter. See below. §2.26

- It is reasonable to ask why Lincoln chose Drake. As noted, most sources say Drake was one of the pre-eminent physicians in that part of the country (¶2467). [hirschhornC] states Drake was widely consulted by persons suffering from hypochondriasis. *The meaning of "hypochondriasis" in the 1800s was different than its current meaning – see ¶2741.*   §2.27

- Lincoln had the opportunity to see Drake in person [shenk p60n]. Lincoln spent 5 weeks at the Kentucky home of Joshua Speed in summer 1841, from which he visited nearby Louisville [wilsonH p249] (also ¶2818). Drake was in Louisville at the same time, seeing patients.   §2.28

- Of Lincoln's syphilis, [vidalA p666] says "Lincoln was cured, if he was cured, by a Dr. Daniel Drake of Cincinnati." *I have not seen information supporting this statement. Vidal wrote this early in his Lincoln researches, so it may be a mistake.*   §2.29

(d) Lincoln Infection – Historical Opinion   §2d

An opinion – from [currentBk p36]:

⟨s⟩ "The story makes one wonder whether Herndon ever told the truth about what Lincoln said to him. There is absolutely no reason to believe that Lincoln, a man of rugged health, father of a normal family, ever contracted what was in his time an incurable and devastating malady." [currentBkp36]   §2.30

Analysis:

- This argument reflects an incomplete understanding of syphilis. Syphilis cannot be excluded simply because Lincoln did not have a devastating illness. Primary syphilis, for example, is not "devastating" (physiologically), and later stages of syphilis may not occur at all. Statistically, cases of untreated syphilis evolve as follows [aa78 p4]:

⇒ 50-60% "never develop any form of visceral syphilis, nor will their lives be shortened"

⇒ 10-15% "show relatively benign forms of cutaneous, osseous, hepatic, or gastrointestinal lesions"

⇒ 25-40% "develop either cardiovascular or central nervous system syphilis."

Thus, a lack of severe illness moderately reduces the probability that Lincoln had syphilis: it certainly does not rule it out. §2.31

- The incurability of syphilis is immaterial, as the disease may exist without symptoms. §2.32

An opinion – from [fehrenbacherC]:

⟨s⟩ [fehrenbacherC] criticized Gore Vidal's novel *Lincoln* as "retail[ing] dubious testimony (such as Hendon's maggoty speculation that Lincoln contracted syphilis)." §2.33

Analysis:

- This is an emotional statement, not logical discourse. The word "maggoty" is colorful, but unhelpful. §2.34

- Vidal's response: "It was not Herndon's 'speculation' that Lincoln might have had syphilis. It was Lincoln's own word to Herndon that he had indeed contracted syphilis; Lincoln gave Herndon the time, the place, a doctor's name,* all recorded by Herndon in a letter to Jesse W. Weik of [sic] January 1891. Although Herndon's researches into Lincoln's past (Ann Rutledge, etc.) are a mess, it is a very foolhardy scholar indeed who rejects anything that Herndon says Lincoln himself told him." [vidalB] §2.35

- Fehrenbacher later *seemed* to soften his view: "Perhaps outright rejection would be imprudent in the absence of proof to the contrary, but doubt is very much in order" [fehrenbacherB]. He also acknowledged that Herndon's remarks were not speculation [fehrenbacherB]. §2.36

- In his "softened" view, Fehrenbacher reformulates his critique to ask "whether it is more appropriate for a novelist than for a historian to make use of dubious testimony" [fehrenbacherB]. Sadly, this is posturing. While the odds are higher that an unqualified or untrained person will mis-handle "dubious" testimony, one can never dismiss the possibility that such persons may perform a brilliant analysis or identify issues the professionals have overlooked. Ideas should be challenged on their merits, not on the author's background. Surely anyone who studies the life of Lincoln would agree! §2.37

- Even if Fehrenbacher's posturing is accepted, it only undermines his own position: he is not a physician, and, as he demonstrates, lacks the knowledge to know what is medically "dubious" and what is not. §2.38

§2

An opinion – from [fehrenbacherB]:

⟨s⟩ Of Herndon's letter about Lincoln's syphilis: "There are several reasons for regarding the story with suspicion. First, the unreliability of long-range memory in general, and especially that of a sick man within two months of death, whose recall of certain other conversations is open to serious question. Second, the absence of any corroborative evidence, medical or otherwise. Third, the fact that there are holes in the Herndon story, such as a five-year gap between Lincoln's alleged infection and his alleged letter to a doctor about it. Fourth, the incompatibility of the story with Lincoln's well-known reticence. It is curious, to say the least, that Herndon, who repeatedly and emphatically described his partner as the most secretive man that ever lived, nevertheless claimed to have been Lincoln's confidant about such things as his mother's illegitimacy, the frequency of his bowel movements, and his sexual contamination." [fehrenbacherB] §2.39

Analysis:

---

* The doctor was apparently Drake.

- #1: [fehrenbacherB]'s first criticism fails for three reasons: (1) As noted in §2b, Herndon is very precise in his letter about what he remembers and what he doesn't quite remember. (2) As also noted in §2b, Herndon's letter is grammatically correct and well-structured, which argues against significant cerebral impairment. (3) The accidental disclosure of Lincoln's syphilis to Lamon and Dale is obviously something that had bothered Herndon for years, and was not a trifling detail he would have trouble remembering.   §2.40
- #2: Absence of evidence is not evidence of absence. Possible corroborating evidence is discussed elsewhere in this special topic.   §2.41
- #3: The single "hole" quoted in Herndon's story is not a hole at all. Delays between onset of a disease and seeking care for it are extraordinarily common, especially in men, and especially in young men (in the 20th century, at least). And if no treatment for a disease is available, there is no rational reason to seek care at any time – unless there are questions about transmitting it to others. Lincoln may not have had such questions until he contemplated marrying Mary Todd five years later.   §2.42
- #4: As noted elsewhere, Lincoln's syphilis may not have been secret at all. It may have been known by those who saw it, but never wrote about it. Example: John F. Kennedy's sexually transmitted disease(s), were not disclosed until well after his death – and that was in a century with infinitely greater communications capability and infinitely greater predisposition to discuss such matters publicly.   §2.43

An opinion – from [currentNY]:

⟨S⟩ In responding to a statement by Gore Vidal that Mary had paresis (i.e. syphilitic "general paresis of the insane"), [currentNY] says: "If Vidal had the slightest concern for truth, he could easily have learned from such a reference as *The Merck Manual of Diagnosis and Therapy* that Mrs. Lincoln's symptoms and those of a paretic do not correspond." §2.44

Analysis:

- It is narrow and naive to assume that any disease is capable only of manifesting the short descriptions found in books. This is particularly true for a disease like syphilis and "the extraordinary facility with which [it] apes every disease in any field of medicine" [aa111 p41] (this statement is only marginally overblown). Mary did not have all the classic features of cerebral syphilis, but she had a good many, making syphilis a very reasonable diagnostic consideration.   §2.45

(e) Lincoln Infection – Physician Opinion   §2e

An opinion – from [bumgarnerB]:

⟨S⟩ [bumgarnerB] summarizes Douglas Wilson's argument that Herndon was genuine in his belief Lincoln had syphilis. Wilson also notes that Lincoln may have been mistaken in his diagnosis, as dread of syphilis was common in that era.   §2.46

Analysis:

- On the other hand, Lincoln may have been perfectly correct about his diagnosis. The disease was dreaded in the 1830s, in part, because it was common. Lincoln would have had many male acquaintances with syphilis, and, even if these acquaintances did not want to talk about the manifestations of the disease, Lincoln's many physician friends (¶3173) would have had no such reticence.   §2.47
- Syphilophobia in a patient with a history of syphilis is "too often" caused by neurosyphilis [aa111 p1019].   §2.48
- Had Lincoln developed a penile chancre two to three weeks after "connection" with a new partner, it would have been obvious to him that he had contracted syphilis [aa111 p479].   §2.49

An opinion – from [shutesE pp70-71]:

⟨S⟩ [shutesE pp70-71] offers six reasons Lincoln was unlikely to have been infected with syphilis. §2.50

> #1. None of Lincoln's physician friends left a description of him having syphilis.
>
> #2. No effective treatments of syphilis were available to Lincoln.
>
> #3. Lincoln did not develop late complications of syphilis.
>
> #4. Mary had no stillbirths or miscarriages.
>
> #5. Lincoln's sons had no signs of syphilis. He dismisses Tad's "handicaps" and Robert's eye deviation.
>
> #6. The possibility of syphilis-like diseases cannot be eliminated.

Analysis:

- Re #1: Absence of evidence is not evidence of absence. Lincoln's physician friends left no descriptions of him having malaria, frostbitten feet, or even a head cold. §2.51

- Re #2 and #3: As noted, a sizable fraction of syphilitic infections never progress to late complications. §2.52

- Re #4 and #5: About six years elapsed between Lincoln putatively contracting the the disease (1835-1836 per §2b) and the start of his sexual relations with Mary (married 1842). The "chief danger" of transmitting syphilis lies in the first five years after infection, but later transmission does occur [aa111 pp1069-1070]. §2.53

- Re #6: It appears Shutes is saying that Lincoln may have misdiagnosed himself: "There are two or three minor, local diseases which in their early stages can even now be confused with syphilis. They were not established as distinct diseases until modern bacteriology demonstrated the responsible germs" [shutes pp70-71]. Misdiagnosis is always possible, but, again, the high prevalence of syphilis at that time means the odds favor syphilis when syphilis-like symptoms occur. §2.54

(f) Lincoln's Sons §2f

Herndon thought Lincoln's sons may have been born with syphilis, i.e., "congenital syphilis:"

⟨S⟩ "Poor boys, they are dead now and gone! I should like to *know* one thing and that is: What caused the death of these children? I have an opinion which I shall never state to anyone. I know a good deal of the Lincoln family and too much of Mrs. Lincoln." [hertz p129] §2

§2.55

Opinions and Analyses:

- "None of the Lincoln sons showed signs of congenital syphilis" [hirschhorn] §2.56

- "One-third of children born in the primary or secondary stages of a mother's infection and more than 90 percent born later remain free of syphilis." [hirschhorn] §2.57

- Congenital syphilis is transmitted from mother to child. Based on the infectivity of syphilis over time and a review of Lincoln's chronology, [hirschhorn] concludes "It would be well beyond the expected range for him to infect Mary Lincoln after their November 1842 marriage, unless a primary infection occurred later than 1836." *Robert was born exactly nine months after the Lincolns wed.* §2.58

- ⟨S⟩ "If Lincoln had given his wife syphilis and if he had, inadvertently, caused the death of his children, the fits of melancholy are now understandable – and unbearably tragic." [vidalAp667] (Is ¶2615.) §2.59

- Conclusion: I do not believe the Lincoln sons had syphilis. Herndon was right that some of them had *something*, but he was wrong about the diagnosis. MEN2B is more likely. §2.60

(g) Lincoln Infection – Exposure Tendency §2g

Lincoln had a normal libido. Henry Whitney wrote: "I have heard him say over & over again about sexual contact: 'It is the harp of a thousand strings' " [wilson p617] (¶3350). Whitney knew only the married Lincoln [donaldA p163]. According to [turner p34], Lincoln and Mary had, for each other, "a physical passion that never diminished," but I do not know the evidence for this.

Herndon wrote that "Mr. Lincoln had a strong, if not terrible passion for women. He could hardly keep his hands off a woman, and yet, much to his credit, he lived a pure and virtuous life. His idea was that a woman had as much right to violate the marriage vow as the man – no more and no less" [weik p81]. ([vidalA p666] gives a somewhat different version that may or may not be correct.)

Although some Lincoln acquaintances offer carefully worded statements about Lincoln's "good habits" in his younger days (¶2216ff), others speak of a trip to the "hoar houses" during militia service [wilson p481] (¶2220) and of a prostitution visit in 1839 or 1840 abandoned because of insufficient funds [wilson p719] (¶2222). Another view of this supposed incident is: "Somehow one senses a Lincoln joke that got lost in translation" [burk p76] citing [strozier p48.] However, it is in keeping with Lincoln's self-professed philosophy: "I want in all cases to do right, and most particularly so, in all cases with women" [randallC p10].

How much Lincoln acted on his urges is unknown. Two data points: (1) Herndon said Lincoln was "a pure perfectly chaste man" until after Ann Rutledge's death (¶2221), and (2) Lincoln told Herndon about spending a night in the one-room log house of an old friend in 1850 or 1851. The head of Lincoln's bed sat at the foot of the bed in which the friend's grown daughter slept. The daughter's feet ended up on his pillow during the night, which "put the *devil* into Lincoln at once." He then "reached up his hand and put it where it ought not to be," which led to a tense and rapid departure in the morning [hertz pp233-234]. (Also told by N.W. Branson [wilson p 90].)

Writing to his best friend, Joshua Speed, on Feb. 13, 1842, Lincoln added "an enigmatic postscript" [wilsonH p258]: "P.S. I have been quite a man ever since you left" [baslerA v1p270].

As President-elect, Lincoln visited his step-mother in her cabin. During his visit, a cousin noticed that a pretty girl caught his eye (¶2223). Attending Ford's Theatre in August 1864, Lincoln "carried on a hefty flirtation" with some of the "girls" [beschlossB p120]. A catalog of Lincoln's relations with women exists [tripp pp229ff].

(h) Mary Infection – Opportunities §2h

⟨S⟩ If Mary was manic, as some believe, promiscuity during mania would not be surprising. Herndon, who never had warm relations with Mary, occasionally hints, very elliptically, that Mary was not faithful. He never provides evidence, and I have seen none elsewhere in my readings. "The evidence throughout her life shows that Mary gave Lincoln her unbroken love from the time they were first engaged until her" death [randallC p49]. The "opportunities" listed below are as scandalous as Mary gets. §2.61

⟨2⟩ In Springfield: After being frightened one night when Lincoln was away, Mary asks neighbor James Gourley to sleep at her house [randallC p105]. §2.62

⟨1⟩ October 1859: In a letter Mary invites unmarried male friend Ozias Hatch to "wander up our way, to see us this evening, altho' I have not the inducements of meeting company to offer you, or Mr. Lincoln to welcome you, yet if you are disengaged, I should like to see you." [turner p60] §2.63

⟨1⟩ Sept. 1862: Mary invites Daniel Sickles to the White House during the day, because there are so many callers in the evening. She suggests she wants to talk about "passing events" that she withholds from Lincoln. [turner pp133-134] §2.64

⟨1⟩ During Presidency: Explicitly mentions Lincoln will be present at an evening meeting [turnerp129] and when other guests will be present [turnerp148].   §2.65

⟨2⟩ "her innocent flirtations" are documented in her letters [turner p xvii]   §2.66
c

(i) Mary Infection – Tabes Dorsalis   §2i

[hirschhorn] proposes that Mary had *diabetic* tabes dorsalis. I (and perhaps [fleisher]) am skeptical because:

- The authors are too credulous. The most difficult part of evaluating Mary's medical complaints is determining which were real and which were psychogenic. The authors too willingly accept what Mary said.
- I am not convinced she had the syndrome of tabes dorsalis. Was there not a sudden worsening of her back problems and gait after she fell in 1879? I am unaware that tabes could produce such a rapid worsening, and, even if it could, why invoke tabes when a ready alternate explanation exists?
- Over a period of 8 months immediately following her fall, she consistently complained of pain in her left side. How does this fit with the tabes syndrome?
- Mary's vague 1876-1880 remark about "continual running waters, so disagreeable and inconvenient" (¶4302) is just opposite of the usual urinary complaint in tabes: difficulty in starting urination [aa111 p1011].
- The earliest possible manifestation of diabetes that I can identify is thirst in 1875 and polyuria sometime between 1876 and 1880 (¶4083). But the authors mention neurological symptoms of diabetes as early as 1869 [hirschhorn p522] (¶4595). It seems unlikely that severe neuropathic changes would occur that long before the renal glycosuric threshold was crossed.
- By 1882 Mary lost motor power in her lower limbs [hirschhorn p518], yet the authors seem to overlook this, and hypothesize that her lower limb power was preserved [hirschhorn p524]. My pre-penicillin syphilis textbook does not list muscular weakness as part of tabes dorsalis [aa111 p1011].
- If Mary did have tabes, why was it not syphilitic? Statistically, in that era, syphilis would be the most likely cause. The distinctions between luetic tabes and diabetic pseudo-tabes are not discussed. For example, the Argyll Robertson pupil is rare in diabetic pseudo-tabes [aa111 p1019].   §2
- The authors ignore the elephant in the room: was Mary's insanity related to syphilitic taboparesis?
- There is no formal differential diagnosis of Mary's signs and symptoms. Diagnostic shortcuts are always unwise when syphilis is in the differential diagnosis.
- The claim that Mary's weight was too low for her fall to break a chair ignores the elementary fact that the distance of the fall is more important than the mass of the falling object: $E = mv^2/2$.

(j) Miscellaneous Biomedical Considerations   §2j

- Malaria was once used to cure syphilis (a practice honored with the 1927 Nobel prize). Lincoln's malaria of 1835 predated his syphilis, if we accept Herndon's dates. Malaria recurrences after syphilitic infection could have cured Lincoln, if his fever were high enough. There are no records of severe febrile disease in Lincoln between 1835 and 1863, so this appears unlikely.

- ○○○ *Project:* Analyze handwriting, seeking a neurosyphilitic "conduct slump" [aa111 p990]; see ¶4580.

(k) The 1841 Mary Todd Episode §2k

In early 1841, the serious relationship between Abraham Lincoln and Mary Todd ruptured (see Special Topic §3). The specifics are disputed and the cause debated. This section does not analyze the enormous literature on the rupture. It seeks only to add another possibility to the list, along with some reasons it cannot be dismissed out of hand. It should be debated along with all the other possibilities.

The additional possibility is: the rupture came when Lincoln revealed to Mary his prior syphilitic infection. This possibility has been broached in various guises by [wilsonH pp127-129] and [shenk p56].

If Lincoln did have syphilis before 1841, and if he had known it, and if he knew the infection could persist, and if he were honest, then he would at some point have to tell Mary of his infection and her risk of contracting the disease from him. If he were fully informed about the disease, he would also mention a risk of their future children being affected.

The odds favor all of these "ifs." Some have already been discussed. Given Lincoln's wide-ranging curiosity, his need to understand things completely (¶3063), and his many physician friends (¶3173), we can infer he was aware of the basic facts about syphilis' transmissibility and natural history.*

Lincoln's honesty has been mythologized, but Mary's 1864 comment is telling: "Poor Mr L is almost a monomaniac on the subject of honesty" [turner pp180, 71, xvii]. Lincoln himself said "I want in all cases to do right, and most particularly so, in all cases with women" [randallC p10]. Thus, if Lincoln had believed he had syphilis, he would certainly have told Mary at some point before marriage. The only question is when, and January 1841 seems as good a time as any. ([shenk] and [wilsonH pp233ff] and Special Topic §3 dissect the timeline.)

The "syphilis disclosure hypothesis" explains many otherwise unexplainable features of the Lincoln-Todd rift. Foremost, it explains why no one spoke of it later. Had the rift occurred because of family pressure, one could imagine rueful laughter years later over discouraging marriage to a future President. Even so pro-Lincoln a man as Dennis Hanks enjoyed precisely this type of joke in saying that his own first impression of the infant Lincoln was "He'll never come to much" [wilson p726]. (Of course, this requires a sense of humor in Mary's relatives...)

Possibly, Mary's relatives knew Lincoln had had syphilis in years past, and their disapproval stemmed from that, at least in part. If, for example, Lincoln had developed an extensive rash of secondary syphilis, it would have been a clear indication of infection to all who saw him. ○○○ *Project:* Analyze Lincoln's movements after the supposed infection, to see if there was a period he might have sequestered himself out of town, in order to hide the fact of his infection.

The syphilis disclosure hypothesis explains both the timing and the content of Lincoln's letter to Dr. Drake. Joshua Speed dates Lincoln's letter to Drake as December 1840 or January 1841, i.e., shortly before or shortly after the rift with Mary. Did Lincoln ask Drake about the risk of passing syphilis to Mary? Pre-marital examinations for syphilis were an especially important medical practice in the pre-penicillin era [aa111 pp1068ff].

Finally, syphilis explains Speed's advice to Lincoln about telling Mary rather than writing her: "once you put your words in writing and they Stand as a living & eternal Monument against you" [wilson p477]. (A counter-argument is that "Speed saw the letter to 'Mary' written by Lincoln" [wilson p477]. If Speed saw syphilis mentioned in this letter, we should assume Speed would have figured out what was in the letter to Drake.)

Recent scholarship has greatly reduced the uncertainty surrounding the Lincoln-Todd rupture of 1841 [wilsonH pp233ff]. It is unlikely that syphilis disclosure was the full story. Whether it was part of the story may be impossible to determine.

---

* Although syphilis is today little discussed, all physicians in the 1800s would have been very familiar with it. As late as 1944: "Syphilis is a practitioner's problem" [aa111 p iii].

Topic 3 – The 1841 Slump §3

Something happened to Lincoln in the first weeks of 1841. William Herndon said Lincoln left Mary at the altar, but this is no longer credible. Most likely, the relationship between Lincoln and Mary Todd ended.

Whatever it was, Lincoln's behavior changed quickly. This special topic compiles the facts about his behavior – a useful enterprise because of the immense quantity of words written on the topic. Our concern is not what caused the behavior change, but whether the change meets the criteria for a major depressive episode.

Although depression would seem to be in the realm of "the mental Lincoln," as opposed to the physical Lincoln, it is a relevant topic: It is generally assumed that Lincoln's physical decline during his Presidency was the result of mental stress (as opposed to cancer). If Lincoln had depression, it would stand to reason that the chances that his decline was stress-induced would be higher.

(a) Day by Day §3a

This section lists events related to Lincoln's behaviorthat can be pinpointed to specific days, or nearly so. Each event is labeled with a day (in month-day format) or is prefaced by a ▪ if the day is not precise.

1840 ....

- ▪ "In the winter of 40 & 41 – he was very unhappy about his engagement to his wife – Not being entirely satisfied that his *heart* was going with his hand – How much he suffered then on that account non Know so well as myself – He disclosed his whole heart to me" – Joshua Speed [wilson p430]   §3.1

12-29 Was on the floor of the legislature. [wilsonH p233]   §3.2

1841 ....

1-1 "There is no evidence of anything unusual happening in Lincoln's life on January 1." [wilsonH p234]   §3.3

1-1 Joshua Speed sells his store. Moves to Kentucky in the spring. [wilsonH p234]   §3.4   §3

1-2 Is in the legislature. [randallC p45]   §3.5

1-2 Did not answer one or more roll calls in legislature. [shenk p56] citing [miers v1pp151-153]   §3.6

1-3 Is in the legislature. [randallC p45]   §3.7

1-4 Missed eight votes in the legislature. [shenk p57] citing [miers v1pp151-153]   §3.8

1-5 Is in the legislature. [randallC p45]   §3.9

1-5 Missed three votes in the legislature. [shenk p57] citing [miers v1pp151-153]   §3.10

1-6 Is in the legislature. [randallC p45]   §3.11

1-7 Is in the legislature. [randallC p45]   §3.12

1-7 Speaks in the legislature, concerning apportionment. [baslerA v1pp225-226]   §3.13

1-8 Is in the legislature. [randallC p45]   §3.14

1-8 Speaks in the legislature, concerning his window jump. [baslerA v1p226]   §3.15

1-8 On legislature floor: "lashed out in uncharacteristic anger and had to be called   §3.16
     to order by the Speaker." [wilsonH p234]

1-9 Is in the legislature. [randallC p45]   §3.17

1-9 Speaks in the legislature, on a burlesque petition. [baslerA v1pp226-227]   §3.18

1-9 Speaks in the legislature, on apportionment. [baslerA v1pp227-228]   §3.19

1-10 [Assume legislature did not meet on Sunday.]   §3.20

1-11 Is in the legislature. [randallC p45]   §3.21

1-12 Is in the legislature. [randallC p45]   §3.22

1-13 "Missing Day" #1 – (see §3b for description of events during this time.)   §3.23

1-14 "Missing Day" #2   §3.24

1-15 "Missing Day" #3   §3.25

1-16 "Missing Day" #4   §3.26

1-16 "We have been very much distressed, on Mr. Lincoln's account; hearing that he   §3.27
      had two Cat fits and a Duck fit since we left." – Netty Hardin [wilsonH p236]

1-17 "Missing Day" #5   §3.28

1-17 "Lincoln you know was desponding & melancholy when you left ... He has grown   §3.29
      much worse and is now confined to his bed sick in body & mind." – Edwin Webb
      to O.H. Browning [shenk p57]

1-18 "Missing Day" #6   §3.30

1-19 "Missing Day" #7   §3.31

1-20 "... I have, within the last few days, been making a most discreditable exhibition   §3.32
      of myself in the way of hypochondriasism and thereby got an impression that Dr.
      Henry is necessary to my existence. Unless he gets that place he leaves Spring-
      field. You therefore see how much I am interested in the matter. ... My heart
      is verry much set upon it. Pardon me for not writing more; I have not sufficient
      composure to write a long letter. As ever yours" – Lincoln to Stuart [baslerA v1pp228-
      229]

1-22 Does some politicking for Stuart in the evening. [baslerA v1pp229-230]   §3.33

1-23 "Yours of the 3rd. Inst. is recd. & I proceed to answer it as well as I can, tho' from   §3.34
      the deplorable state of my mind at this time, I fear I shall give you but little sat-
      isfaction. [Long paragraph about political doings.] For not giving you a general
      summary of news, you *must* pardon me; it is not in my power to do so. I am
      now the most miserable man living. If what I feel were equally distributed to the
      whole human family, there would not be one cheerful face on the earth. Whether
      I shall ever be better I can not tell; I awfully forebode I shall not. To remain as I
      am is impossible; I must die or be better, it appears to me. The matter you speak
      of on my account [a diplomatic position in Colombia], you may attend to as you
      say, unless you shall hear of my condition forbidding it. I say this, because I fear I
      shall be unable to attend to any bussiness [sic] here, and a change of scene might
      help me. If I could be myself, I would rather remain at home with Judge Logan.

I can write no more. Your friend, as ever" – Lincoln to John Stuart, after a long paragraph giving political news [baslerA v1pp229-230]

1-24 "Poor L! how the mighty are fallen! He was confined about a week, but though   §3.35
he now appears again he is reduced and emaciated in appearance and seems scarcely to possess strength enough to speak above a whisper. His case is truly deplorable but what prospect there may be for ultimate relief I cannot pretend to say I doubt not but he can declare 'That loving is a painful thrill, And not to love more painful still' but would not like to intimate that he has experienced 'That surely 'tis the worst of pain To love and not be loved again.' And Joshua too is about to leave. ..." – James Conkling [wilsonH pp237-238]

1-25 Speaks in the legislature, on payment for statehouse. [baslerA v1pp230-231]   §3.36

1-26 Speaks in the legislature, on payment for statehouse. [baslerA v1p231]   §3.37

1-26 "I am glad to hear Lincoln had got over his cat fits[.] we have concluded it was   §3.38
a very unsatisfactory way of terminating his romance[.] he ought to have died or gone crazy[.] we are very much disappointed[.] indeed Jane Goudy has made him the hero of a tale but she say[s] it will never do for him to get well." – Sarah Hardin [wilsonH p236] *Goudy was a romance writer.*

1-27 Speaks in the legislature, supports a resolution. [baslerA v1p231]   §3.39

1-27 Speaks in the legislature, on state debtors. [baslerA v1p232]   §3.40

1-27 "Poor fellow, he is in a rather bad way. Just at present though he is on the mend   §3.41
now as he was out on Monday for the first time for a month dying with love they say. The Doctors say he came within an inch of being a perfect lunatic for life. He was perfectly crazy for some time, not able to attend to his business at all. They say he don't look like the same person. ... [Regarding Mary,] Some of his friends thought he was acting very wrong and very imprudently and told him so and he went crazy on the strength of it so the story goes and that is all I know." – Jane Bell [wilsonH p237]

1-29 "Mr. Lincoln has recovered from his indisposition and has attended the House   §3.42
for more than a week past, during which time he made no minority report, although he attended every meeting of the committee of investigation." – Illinois *Register* [shenk p261]

   §3

■ "Though a member of the legislature he rarely attended its sessions" – Joshua   §3.43
Speed [wilsonH p358] citing [speed p39]

■ "took very little part in the legislation of that session" – Lyman Trumble [wilsonH   §3.44
p358]

■ "In the remaining weeks of the session he had so little impact that some of his   §3.45
friends remembered him as hardly participating at all" [wilsonH p240]. "When his party needed him in the hard fight over the makeup of the Illinois Supreme Court in January and February 1841, he was of little help" [wilsonH p263].

2-1 Speaks in the legislature, on state debtors. [baslerA v1p232]   §3.46

2-3 Letter to Stuart: "You see by this that I am neither dead nor quite crazy yet..."   §3.47
[wilsonH p247] citing [baslerB p6]

2-4 Speaks in the legislature, supports a bill. [baslerA v1p232]   §3.48

2-5 Letter to Stuart (2 paragraphs) [baslerA v1p233]   §3.49

2-6 Speaks in legislature [baslerA v1p233] §3.50

? 2-8 Cosigns a long Whig statement [baslerA v1pp234-237] §3.51

2-9 Speaks in legislature [baslerA v1p237] §3.52

2-11 Speaks in legislature [baslerA v1pp237-238] §3.53

2-17 Speaks in legislature [baslerA v1pp238-239] §3.54

2-18 Speaks in legislature [baslerA v1p239] §3.55

2-19 Speaks in legislature [baslerA v1p240] §3.56

2-22 Speaks in legislature [baslerA v1p240] §3.57

2-22 Introduces bill he wrote [baslerA v1pp240-241] §3.58

2-23 Speaks in legislature [baslerA v1pp241-242] §3.59

2-24 Speaks in legislature [baslerA v1pp242-243] §3.60

2-25 Speaks in legislature [baslerA v1p238] §3.61

2-26 Convulses the legislature with a story about eye lice [baslerA v1pp243-244] §3.62

2-26 Co-signs a long Whig protest [baslerA v1p244-249] §3.63

2-27 Introduces a bill; speaks in legislature [baslerA v1p2p250-252] §3.64

3-1 Legislature adjourns. [wilsonH p240] §3.65

3-7 "And L. poor hapless simple swain who loved most true but was not loved again – I suppose he will now endeavor to drown his cares among the intricacies and perplexities of the law." – James Conkling [wilsonH p240] citing [sandburgA pp178-179] §3.66

- [March] "I used to see Mr. Lincoln – hanging about – moody – silent &&c. The question in his mind was Have 'I incurred any obligation to marry that woman'. He wanted to dodge if he could." – Turner King [wilson p464] §3.67

- [Spring] Joshua Speed moves to Kentucky. [wilsonH p234] §3.68

5-18 "I am glad to hear from Mrs Butler that Lincoln is on the mend" – Joshua Speed [wilsonH pp356, 245] §3.69

6-19 Lincoln writes "a delightful whodunit" letter to Speed [randallC p51] §3.70

- [July, August] Visits Joshua Speed in Kentucky for five weeks [shenk p63] §3.71

- [End-summer] Visits Joshua Speed in Kentucky [wilsonH p249] §3.72

- [At Speed's] 'When he was in Ky in 1841 he was moody & hypochondriac' – Joshua Speed [wilson p158]. [shenk p63] *adds "at times very melancholy," but that is not in* [wilson]. §3.73

- [At Speed's] Speed's mother gives Lincoln a Bible. [wilson p158] Also [wilsonH p249]. §3.74

- [At Speed's] "The change of scene and the warm hospitality seem clearly to have checked Lincoln's despondency and given his spirits a new direction." [wilsonH p249] §3.75

- [Sept.] Returns to Illinois [wilsonH p250] §3.76

1842 ....

2-3 "I have been quite clear of hypo since you left,—even better than I was along in the fall." – Lincoln to Speed [baslerA v1p268] *Speed left in January 1842* [wilsonH p250]. §3.77

2-13 "P.S. I have been quite a man ever since you left." – Lincoln to Speed [baslerA v1p270] *Has been called "an enigmatic postscript"* [wilsonH p258]. §3.78

3-27 "... that fatal first of Jany. '41. Since then, it seems to me, I should have been entirely happy, but for the never-absent idea, that there is *one* still unhappy whom I have contributed to make so. That still kills my soul. I can not but reproach myself, for even wishing to be happy while she is otherwise." – Lincoln to Speed [baslerA v1p282-283] §3.79

7-4 "I must regain my confidence in my own ability to keep my resolves when they are made. In that ability, you know, I once prided myself as the only, or at least the chief, gem of my character, that gem I lost – how, and when, you too well know. I have not yet regained it; and until I do, I can not trust myself in any matter of much importance." – Lincoln to Speed [baslerA v1p289] §3.80

- [Summer] Not on Whig ticket for state legislature. Unclear if this was his own decision. [wilsonH p263] §3.81

(b) Imprecisely Dated Events §3b

1841 – During the "Missing Days," more or less ....

⟨1⟩ "went to bed and no one was allowed to see him but his friend Josh Speed & his friend the *Doctor* I think Henry. And that strong Brandy was administered to him freely for about one Week." – Abner Ellis [wilson p238] §3.82

⟨1⟩ "Lincoln went Crazy – had to remove razors from his room – take away all Knives and other such dangerous things – &c – it was terrible" – Joshua Speed [wilson p475] §3.83

⟨1⟩ "went Crazy as a *Loon* – was taken to Kentucky – by Speed – or went to Speed's – was Kept there till he recovered finally" – Ninian Edwards [wilson p133] §3.84

⟨$\frac{1}{q}$⟩ "The missing days from Jan. 12th to 19th Mr Lincoln spent several hours each day at Dr. Henry's (his physicians Drs. Henry & Merryman) a part of these days I remained with Mr Lincoln[.] His most intimate friends had no fears of his injuring himself.[.] He was very sad and melancholly, but being subject to these spells, nothing serious apprehended." – H.W. Thornton [wilsonH p235] §3.85 §3

⟨$\frac{1}{q}$⟩ For about a week "was so much affected as to talk incoherently, and to be delirious to the extent of not knowing what he was doing. In the course of a few days it all passed off, leaving no trace whatever. I think it was only an intensification of his constitutional melancholy." – O.H. Browning [nicolayO pp1-2] §3.86

⟨$\frac{1}{q}$⟩ "his derange lasted only about a week or such a matter" – O.H. Browning [wilsonH p235] citing [nicolayO pp1-2] §3.87

⟨$\frac{1}{q}$⟩ "his conscience troubled him dreadfully" – O.H. Browning [shenk p50] citing [nicolayO p1] §3.88

⟨$\frac{1}{q}$⟩ "incoherent and distraught" – O.H. Browning [shutes pp24-25] *Probably an alteration of item above.* §3.89

§3.90

⟨1⟩ "Mr. Lincoln was *'as crazy as a loon' in this city in 1841;* ... was then deranged ... Did you know that he was forcibly arrested by his special friends here at that time; that they had to remove all razors, knives, pistols, etc. from his room and presence, that he might not commit suicide?" – William Herndon [hertz p37]

⟨1/q⟩ "Mr Lincoln did not seem to recover, and my sister, who had watched him closely, decided that he had something on his mind. At last she decided on a plan of action, and one day went into Mr. Lincoln's room, closed the door, and walking over to the bed, said: 'Now Abraham, what is the matter? Tell me about it?' And he did. Suffering under the thought that he had treated Mary badly, knowing that she loved him and that he did not love her, Mr. Lincoln was wearing his very life away in an agony of remorse. He made no excuse for breaking with Mary, but said, sadly, to my sister: 'Mrs. Butler, it would just kill me to marry Mary Todd.' " – Sarah Rickard [wilsonH p236] §3.91

⟨1/q⟩ Speed tells Lincoln "in his deepest gloom" that he must rally himself or die [wilsonH p241]. Lincoln responds that he is unafraid of death and "more than willing." [wilsonH p241; shenk p65] citing [speed p39] §3.92

⟨1⟩ "... an incident in his life, long passed, when he was so much deppressed that he almost contemplated suicide – At the time of his deepest depression – He said to me that he had done nothing to make any human being remember that he had lived" – Joshua Speed [wilson p197] *Assigned to this period by* [wilsonH p241]. §3.93

⟨2⟩ "All we know for sure of Henry's treatment is that he put Lincoln to bed and kept him isolated." [shenk p59] §3.94

⟨2⟩ "Lincoln became ill, and the indispensable physician, Dr. Henry, convinced Mary to write him a letter of release." [wilsonH p240] §3.95

Miscellaneous ....

⟨1⟩ In the 1841 legislative session, Lincoln voted 397 times and failed to vote 92 times. His missed votes were higher than the average of his colleagues (54 non-voting absences) and nearly quadruple his own absenteeism in the previous two sessions. [neelyL] §3.96

⟨1⟩ "did not attend the Legislature in in [sic] 1841 & 2 for this reason" – Ninian Edwards [wilson p133] §3.97

⟨1⟩ "did not sit, did not attend to the Legislature, but in part, if any (special session of 1841)" – William Herndon [hertz p37] §3.98

⟨2⟩ Wrote poem on suicide, published in the Sangamo *Journal*, per Joshua Speed. A candidate poem has been discovered, but it was published anonymously in 1838. [shenk pp39-41] §3.99

Topic 4 – Biological Attacks §4

(a) Smallpox Assassination Attempt – Description §4a

From the Waupaca (Wisconsin) Republican, February 13, 1903:

```
LINCOLN'S NARROW ESCAPE.

Fiendish Plot to Inoculate Him with the Smallpox.
```

The demand for an additional bodyguard around the White House recalls an incident of the civil war within the memory of many residents. During the exciting period of '61 great fears were entertained for the safety of the President, and every precaution was taken to insure his personal protection.

One morning there appeared at the White House a woman, closely veiled, demanding an immediate interview with Mr. Lincoln. Approaching Messenger Perkins, who guarded the door of Mr. Lincoln's private office, the visitor made known her request and pleaded earnestly that she be admitted to a personal interview. The doorkeeper's orders were, however, very strict, and finding her eloquence all in vain, she finally compromised by confiding her message to the courteous but firm employee. Taking him to one side, the veiled lady took both his hands in hers and tenderly rubbed them as she extracted a promise that he would immediately deliver her request to the President. Perkins was almost overcome by a most peculiar odor that appeared to emanate from his companion, and hastened to get rid of her without creating a scene.

No sooner had he accomplished this than he confided to one of the household the effect produced upon him while in conversation with the importunate visitor. A physician who was present promptly divined the truth and instituted a search for the woman, when it was learned that she had driven rapidly away in a carriage, and all trace was lost. Perkins was immediately ordered to return to his home and await developments.

Within the usual period he was taken ill with one of the worst cases of virulent small-pox on record, and for weeks lay upon the point of death. Upon his recovery the faithful messenger, whose devotion to duty doubtless saved the life of the President, was appointed by Mr. Lincoln to a permanent position on the clerical force of the War Department, which office he has continued to hold up to this date, being one of the most efficient clerks on the rolls.

§4

(b) Smallpox Assassination Attempt – Discussion §4b

The Waupaca story fits with the known security arrangements at the White House: in 1861 anyone, at almost any hour, could walk into the White House [donaldA p309]. Specifically, "At the outbreak of the war there was no military guard at the White House, and the two civilian attendants – one for the outer door, the other for the President's office on the second floor – were often absent from their posts" [donaldA p548]. "They did not consider it necessary to be vigilant after office hours, and I often walked into the White House unchallenged and went straight up to the private secretary's room adjoining [Lincoln's], without seeing any person whatever [croffut].

However, the person of "Messenger Perkins" has not surfaced during my Lincoln researches. A typed list, reprinted below, lists White House employees during Lincoln's tenure. It lists a "messenger" position, but no one named Perkins. Potentially, "Perkins" was confused with "Pendel," but in 1861 Pendel was not yet working in the White House [pendel pp11-12]

407

[crookA p1]. The identity of "Messenger Perkins" therefore remains unknown, and the credibility of the Waupaca report uncertain.

The table below was found on a typewritten sheet in [randallP box 71], with the title "Data on White House expeditures from files of General Accounting Office (Nat. Archives)." It lists the titles, names, and monthly salaries of "Employees 1861-1865" as follows (annotations preserved):

Doorkeeper

1.	Louis Bergdorf	Mar. 1861 to April 1865	$50.
2.	Thomas Burns (Asst.)	Jan. 1861-Aug. 1863	$50.
3.	Alphonso Donn	Jan. 1865-Apr. 1865	$50.
4.	Edward Burke	Jan, Feb. 1865	$50.

Furnace Man

1.	Thos. H. Cross (colored)	Apr. 1861-Apr. 1865	$50.
2.	Wm. Johnson	March 1861	$50.

Messenger

1.	Thomas F. Pendel	Jan.-March 1865	$75.
2.	Edward McManns [sic]	April 1861-Dec. '64	$75.

Watchman (night)

1.	John R. Vernon	April '61 to Apr. '65	$50.
2.	Thomas Stackpole	Apr. 1861 to Dec. '64	$50.

Steward

1.	Pete Vermeren	June '61 -	$100.
2.	Thomas Stackpole	Jan. '65 to April '65	$100.

Stewardess

1.	Jane Watt	Apri. '61 to Feb. '62	$100.
2.	Mary Williams	Mar. '62 to Feb. '63	$100.
3.	Mrs. J. Smith	March '63	$100.
4.	Mary Ann Cuthbert	Apr. '63 to Apr. '65	$100.

Coachman

1.	Mangan

There is no authorship date or data on the table. There are notations that McManns (prob. "McManus") and Mangan are described in: "Lincoln in the National Capital," by Allan Clark, pages 37 and 47. McManus was fired in January 1865, and his replacement, Cornelius O'Leary, was also fired... for influence peddling [hayC p241].

Donn (or Dunn) and Pendel were in the group of four men hired in November 1864 to be part of Lincoln's special guard [crookA p1]. In winter 1864-1865, "Two policemen went on duty as doorkeepers, in place of Burns and old Edward" [leech p442], these being Pendel [crookA p1] and, apparently, Donn.

Other sources mention Edward McManus [burl p292] [turner p197] [hayC pp68,241], Stackpole [crookA p17] [french p375n], a cook [crookA p17], footman Charles Forbes [crookA p21], Louis Burgdorf [hayC p68], Alice Johnstone [randallC p303], housekeeper Mrs. Cuthbert [randallC p294], carpenter James Haliday [crookA p21], and long-time White House head gardner John Watt, who was fired in 1862 for leaking information [french p375n]. Ward Hill Lamon occasionally slept in a blanket outside the President's door [kunhardtB p71]. A Mrs. Slade was "the wife of an old and faithful messenger" [keckleyBp202].

(c) Poison Rumors §4c

- 1861: Rumors of poisoning circulated before the correct diagnosis of food poisoning from Potomac River fish (shad) was made. See ¶640.

- After Lincoln's assassination, "There was talk around Washington that the cup had been tried too – that castor oil ordered from a pharmacy had arrived with deadly poison, but had had too queer a taste to be swallowed" [kunhardtB p5]. There was testimony of a failed plot by John Wilkes Booth to poison Lincoln in Aug.-Nov. 1864 [pitman pp39-40] [weichmann pp42-44, 63-65] – see ¶630.

- Almost from the moment he was elected, "well wishers" urged Lincoln beware poison, e.g. [kunhardtB p255], [angle p290].

(d) Yellow Fever Rumors §4d

- "In the same category of of whispered rumor was the trunk of old clothes taken from yellow-fever victims in Cuba that had been delivered to the White House on the chance that the Lincolns would come down with the disease, and hopefully it would be fatal. The catch here was that a trunk of second-hand clothing would be the first thing finery-loving Mrs. Lincoln would order burned." [kunhardtB p5]

- "Francis Tumblety, the herb doctor, who was believed to be a leader in the yellow fever plot, and had been attending the Springfield funeral of 'my dear friend Lincoln' with as sad a face as the other mourners, was captured in St. Louis and brought back to Carroll Prison." [kunhardtB p188]. The Springfield funeral was 20 days after the shooting.

(e) Rebel Biological Warfare §4e

- Stanton was "happily positive" he had "the goods" on Confederate leaders at the highest levels planning to "start epidemics throughout the country by the introduction of deadly germs into populated areas," to set fires in large Northern cities, to poison water supplies, to starve Northern prisoners – i.e. "the disorganization of the North by infernal plots." [kunhardtB p194]

- At the trial of the Lincoln assassination conspirators, a Godfrey Hyams detailed his role in waging biological war against the Union in summer 1864. He was instructed to attack Lincoln, but refused. His testimony is available [pitman pp54-57], as is a report from the [NYTimes - May 26, 1865].

  §4

  - "Dr. Luke Blackburn of Mississippi, Dr. M.A. Pallen and Dr. J.B. Merrit, both of Canada, gave testimony looking to the implication of Southern leaders in a plot to burn, or introduce smallpox and yellow fever in Northern cities" [markens]. The statement of Godfrey Hyams, testifying for the prosecution against Dr. Blackburn, appears in [NYTimes - May 26, 1865]. Hymans testified that Blackburn introduced yellow fever into clothes that were to be auctioned off in Washington, DC and Norfolk, VA, with the intent of sickening as many Union troops as possible. Hyams convinced a sutler "belonging to Gens. Sigel and Weitzel's division, to take part of the goods and act as my 'agent,' with instructions to dispose of the goods at Norfolk if possible, or at Newbern, at that time held by the Federals. ... there was yellow fever in Newbern about a week after; I saw it in the newspapers." (The Hyams testimony does not include the statement about yellow fever in Newbern, NC.) Hyams also had a Washington merchant auction a trunk of infected clothes. A valise was to be given to Lincoln as a gift, but the *Times* article does not discuss its fate. Dr. Blackburn's defense attorney "argued that, admitting the evidence of Hyams to be true in every respect, it did not prove a conspiracy."

- From [pitman pp55-56]: "Dr. Blackburn stated that his object in having these goods disposed of in different cities, was to destroy armies or anybody that they came in contact with. All these goods, he told me, had been carefully infected in Bermuda with yellow-fever, small-pox, and other contagious diseases. The goods in the valise, which were intended for President Lincoln I understood him to say, had been infected both with yellow fever and small-pox. This valise I declined taking charge of, and turned it over to him at the Halifax Hotel, and I afterward heard that it had been sent to the President." Hyams was told yellow fever was then raging in Bermuda.

- From [pitman p56]: Dr. Blackburn "asked me how I had disposed of the goods, and I told him. 'Well,' said he, 'that is all right, as long as big [trunk] No. 2 went into Washington; it will kill them at sixty yards' distance.'" Hyams came to Washington to dispose of the goods on Aug. 5, 1864 [pitman p57].

- ○○○ *Project:* It would obviously be of great interest to know more of these Southern efforts, in particular to know how far plans progressed and whether they were realistic. [burk p298] cites a chapter in [steersB] called "The Black Flag is Raised" about Confederate biological warfare.

Topic 5 – Smallpox §5

Lincoln's bout of smallpox in November 1863 is common knowledge among historians. Until recently, however, medical analysis downplayed its severity. The prevailing view has been that "It was a beneficent illness that provided a period of enforced rest and seclusion" [shutesE p161]. The data below show otherwise: it was not a mild illness.

As always, comments *in this typeface* are editorializations. Smallpox is superficially discussed in ¶2030.

(a) Summary Chronology (1863-1864) §5a

The Detailed Chronology *section (§5b) underlies this overview of Lincoln's illness. Note: Newspaper byline dates are used in preference to date of publication.*

18 Nov. Tad is ill.

19 Nov. Lincoln delivers Gettysburg address about 2 pm. That evening: "severe headache."

25 Nov. Lincoln goes to bed early, feeling unwell. Newspaper: "Severe pains in the head."

26 Nov. Lincoln sick in bed. "Bilious." "Quite unwell." At night: "Severe pains in the head." No "autograph writing" from Lincoln exists from 26 Nov. to 1 Dec., save one shakily-written note on the 27th. May have been jaundiced early in illness, per §5.70.

±27 Nov. Best estimate of physicians diagnosing varioloid/smallpox: late the 26th or early the 27th.

27 Nov. Cannot meet the Cabinet.

28 Nov. First public mentions of his illness, without naming diagnosis. Tad reported much better.

2 Dec. Newspaper: "Mr. Lincoln's scarlatina of yesterday is pronounced varioloid today."

3 Dec. Newspaper: "The stage when the pustules break out has passed favorably."

4 Dec. Newspaper: Still confined to his room.

6 Dec. A diary: "'Old Abe' has a well developed case of varioloid."

6 Dec. Newspaper: "His face is slightly marked."

7 Dec. Scheduled visit of the Supreme Court Justices to the White House does not occur. §5

7 Dec. Congress opens. The chaplain of the Senate prays: "We beseech thee, O Lord, to recover the President from his present illness again to health."

10 Dec. Newspaper: "Lincoln's health much improved ... he sees visitors with special business."

11 Dec. Newspaper: "President Lincoln is now so far recovered from his late illness as to be able to ride out. He has persevered in the discharge of his official duties, contrary to the advice, at times, of his medical attendants."

12 Dec. Newspaper: "he was compelled to keep his room."

15 Dec. A diary: "The President was well and in fine spirits."

28 Dec. Lincoln's secretary: "The President is steadily recovering his health and strength."

1 Jan. Reporter: "his complexion is clearer, his eyes less lack-luster, and he has a hue of health to which he has long been a stranger."

(b) Detailed Chronology (1863-1864) §5b

The chronology begins by setting some pre-illness context. While ill, Lincoln's chief task was preparing his annual message to Congress, for delivery on Dec. 9 (delivery by mail, not as a speech).

Section §5c provides important caveats about the mass of unsubstantiated information that pervades the Lincoln-smallpox literature.

When reporting information from newspaper articles, the article's byline is used to date the information. When no byline exists, the date of publication is used.

– – – "There was an unusual amount of sickness at Washington that summer and §5.1
fall. ... [This and other] factors explain why Mrs. Lincoln and Tad were away from Washington so much in the latter half of 1863" [randallC p293]. Virtually no part of the city was smallpox-free [hopkinsB p277].

20 Sep. Lincoln wires Mary and Tad, who are in New York: "I neither see nor hear §5.2
anything of sickness here now; though there may be much without my knowing it." The next day he wires that Washington is "clear and cool, and apparently healthy" and the day after that: "So far as I see or know, it was never healthier." [donaldH pp90-91]

22 Sep. Mary wires Lincoln: "Have a very bad cold, and am anxious to return home" §5.3
[turner p158]

14 Nov. A Boston paper reports Mary has been suffering from chills. [lincloreLHH] §5.4
(¶4273)

16 Nov. Tad is photographed sitting astride a pony, outdoors [neelyA pp92-93]. The §5.5
Nov. 15 Washington *Chronicle* reported that Tad had received a gift pony [miers v3p219]. *This suggests Tad was not severely, if at all, ill on this date. With two children already dead, Mary would likely not have let even a mildly ill Tad go outdoors.*

– – – "Preliminary to the Gettysburg exercises on November 19 there was illness §5.6
in the White House" [lincloreLHH]. *Unclear whether the illnesses of Mary (§5.3) and Tad (§5.7) were the full extent of "illness in the White House."*

18 Nov. Lincoln was scheduled to travel to Gettysburg on this day. However, "Tad §5.7
was ill, too sick to eat his breakfast, and Mary Lincoln, recalling the deaths of her other boys, became hysterical at the thought that her husband would leave her at such a critical time. But so important was the occasion and so weighty was the message he intended to deliver that he brushed aside his wife's pleas and about noon left Washington on a special train of four cars." [donaldA pp462-463]. *A statement in* [goldman] *that Tad was bedridden for two weeks could not be verified from its cited references:* [welles v1pp479-483] [beale pp314-319] [randallC pp167-168] [weaver]. *A statement in* [goldman] *that Tad had a scarlet rash could not be verified from its cited references:* [monaghan p340] [weaver].

18 Nov. Mary telegrams Lincoln (time not specified): "The Dr has just left. We hope §5.8
dear Taddie is slightly better will send you a telegram in the morning." [turner p158]

18 Nov. During train ride to Gettysburg, Lincoln remarks that he is weak [goldman]. *I* §5.9
cannot find supporting information for this statement.

18 Nov. Arrives at Gettysburg about 5 p.m. [donaldA p463]. §5.10

18 Nov. Receives telegram from Edward Stanton (in Washington) that includes: "By §5.11
enquiry Mrs. Lincoln reports your son's health is a great deal better this
evening." [lincloreLHH]

18 Nov In the evening, withdraws from a reception to work on his address [macveagh]. §5.12
Does not complain of feeling ill.

19 Nov. Receives another telegram from Stanton: "Mrs. Lincoln reports your son's §5.13
health is a great deal better, and that he will be out today." [lincloreLHH]

19 Nov. Remarks in the morning that he is dizzy [goldman]. *I cannot find supporting* §5.14
information for this statement.

19 Nov. Did not cut a robust figure riding a horse to the ceremonies (¶2168). §5.15

19 Nov. Delivers Gettysburg address about 2 p.m. [miers v3p222]. §5.16

19 Nov. John Hay notices Lincoln's face has a "ghastly color" [goldman]. *I cannot find* §5.17
supporting information for this statement. As Lincoln rose, to speak he
had a "sad, mournful, almost haggard, and still hopeful expression" [carrB
p67]. As he delivered the address, "his lips quivered, and there was a tremor
in his voice" as he closed the sentence "... can never forget what they did
here" – the only time he showed emotion in the speech [carrB p72]. Lincoln
gave the address from memory, changing some phrases from the written
draft [nicolayG].

19 Nov. Immediately after delivering the address, Lincoln is supposed to have said, §5.18
disparagingly, to Ward Hill Lamon: "Lamon, that speech won't *scour!*" [don-
aldA p465] thinks Lincoln's judgment of the speech was "affected by his fatigue and by illness."

19 Nov. Telegram from Stanton: Tad is "a great deal better ... he will be out today." §5.19
[lincloreLHH]

19 Nov. Lincoln's train leaves Gettysburg about 6 p.m. [nicolayG] or 7 p.m. [miers v3p222]. §5.20
On the train: "He was suffering from a severe headache, and lying down in
the drawing-room with his forehead bathed in cold water," yet still engages
in conversation [macveagh]. Train arrives in Washington at 1:10 a.m. [miers
v3p222]. *Some references, e.g.* [sandburgW v2pp475-476], *say a wet towel was
placed on Lincoln's head, but* [macveagh] *does not mention it.*

19 Nov. "Lincoln had fever on the day of the famous Gettysburg speech." [pearson] §5.21
Detailed support for this statement is not provided.

Nov. Detailed information on Lincoln's condition between 19 and 28 Nov. is §5.22
scant [lincloreLHH]. It is said Dr. Stone (¶3203) attended Lincoln [shutes p86],
but the only direct evidence for this is implicit [stoddardA p109, vide infra]. [stod-
dardA p6] gives the location of Lincoln's sick room.

20 Nov. A notice, dated Nov. 18, appears in the *Washington Chronicle*. It says Lin- §5.23
coln will not receive visitors until after Congress convenes. It runs every
day until Lincoln's annual message is read [lincloreLHH] (Read on Dec. 9 [miers
v3p226]). *Was this an early hint of illness severity? It is more likely that
barring visitors was related to over-work rather than illness. Lincoln*

§5

was certainly not so ill on this date that a three-week illness could be predicted. More convincingly, the end-date of the ban is tied to a work event.

20 Nov.   Lincoln replies to a note written 19 Nov. by Gettysburg co-speaker, Edward Everett. Lincoln concludes: "Our sick boy, for whom you kindly inquire, we hope is past the worst." [baslerA v7p25]   §5.24

22 Nov.   John Hay notices a change in Lincoln, a.k.a. the Tycoon: "Ever since I got your letter I have been skulking in the shadow of the Tycoon, setting all sorts of dextrous traps for a joke, telling good stories myself to draw him out and suborning Nicolay to aid in the foul conspiracy. But not a joke has flashed from the Tycoonial thundercloud. He is as dumb as an oyster." [hayC p68]   §5.25

23 Nov.   "The President yesterday, in the course of conversation, remarked that the next two weeks would be the most momentous period of the rebellion." [NYTimes - Nov. 23, 1863] *The "conversation" comment means Lincoln was still seeing people/reporters on the 22nd. This reinforces the statement about isolation starting on the 27th.*   §5.26

25 Nov.   Retires to bed early, feeling unwell [miers v3p223]. *Miers cites John Hay's diary, but his diary has no entry on the 25th* [hayD pp117-118].   §5.27

25 Nov.   "Severe pains in the head" per *National Republican* story filed on Nov. 28.   §5.28

26 Nov.   Lincoln's secretary, John Hay, writes: "The President is sick in bed. Bilious." [hayC p70]. He also writes: "The President is quite unwell" [hayD p118]. These statements are transformed by [miers v3p223] into "President confined to sick room." *Hay's diagnosis, "bilious," strongly suggests the diagnosis of varioloid had not yet been made.*   §5.29

26 Nov.   Lincoln sees at least one visitor [miers v3p223].   §5.30

26 Nov.   Lincoln's correspondence declines gradually after Gettysburg. From 26 Nov. to 1 Dec. not a single "autograph writing" of Lincoln's is known to exist [lincloreLHH]. *There is a note on the 27th.*   §5.31

±27 Nov.   Best estimate of physicians diagnosing varioloid/smallpox: late the 26th or early the 27th.   §5.32

27 Nov.   Lincoln writes Secretary of State Seward: "I am improving, but I can not meet the Cabinet today" [baslerB p211]. In a footnote, Basler remarks: "This is a most interesting autograph, written on a card in an unsteady hand with an atypical signature of a quite sick President." (Shown in *The Physical Lincoln.*)   §5.33

27 Nov.   Physician prohibits Lincoln from receiving visitors or meeting Cabinet members [miers v3p223] citing [NYHerald - Nov. 29, 1863]. [Confirmed by *National Republican* story filed on Nov. 28.]   §5.34

27 Nov.   "By the 27th, a rumor spread that the President 'was taken seriously ill'" [shutesE p163, quoting unnamed source].   §5.35

?27 Nov.   "Mr. Lincoln ... had been unwell for two or three days, and a consultation had been deemed advisable; so Dr. Van Bibber [see ¶3215] of Baltimore was called in. He went over and saw Mr. Lincoln in consultation with the President's physician. After the doctors has examined Mr. Lincoln, they retired   §5.36

for the traditional consultation. When they returned to Mr. Lincoln's room, he inquired of Dr. Van Bibber, 'Well, Doctor, what is your verdict?' Dr. Van Bibber, who was of the old school, replied, 'Mr. President, if I were to give a name to your malady, I should say that you probably have a touch of the varioloid' (the old-fashioned name for smallpox). 'Then am I to understand that I have the smallpox?' Mr. Lincoln asked, to which the Doctor assented. 'How interesting,' said Mr. Lincoln. 'I find every now and then that even unpleasant situations in life may have certain compensations. As you came in just now, Doctor, did you pass through the waiting room?' He replied, 'I passed through a room full of people.' 'Yes, that's the waiting room, and it's always full of people. Do you have any idea what they are there for?' 'Well,' said the Doctor, 'perhaps I could guess.' 'Yes,' said Mr. Lincoln, 'they are there, every mother's son of them, for one purpose only; namely, to get something from me. For once in my life as President, I find myself in a position to give *everybody* something!'" [finney p259] (Lincoln confirms, at a separate time, that he made a quip to this effect [randallC p295].) *Finney is quoting the story as told to him about 1904 by Charles J. Bonaparte, then Attorney General for President Theodore Roosevelt. John Hay, a young private secretary to Lincoln, was Secretary of State for Roosevelt, so it is possible Bonaparte head the story only second-hand. Although Finney's story places the diagnosis at "two or three days" into Lincoln's illness, several lines of evidence lead me to estimate the 27th or the evening of the 26th as the date: (a) the prohibition on visitors instituted on the 27th, (b) Lincoln skipping the Cabinet meeting on the 27th, (c) Hay's description of severe illness on the 26th, (d) Welles' poorly-dated diary entry, (e) Bates' diary entry of the 30th, (f) Washburne's letter of Dec. 6 which shows that only Cabinet members had until then heard the message, and (g) the crescendo of newspaper stories on Lincoln's health that begins on the 28th.* The "give something to everyone" story is told at length by [carrA pp251-253].

?27 Nov. See ⟦ The White House as a Smallpox Hospital ⟧ for evidence of a deliberate effort to conceal Lincoln's diagnosis. One gets the impression Stoddard's encounter with Dr. Stone occurred later in the day Lincoln was diagnosed with smallpox. §5.37

"1863" In a diary entry dated only as "1863 ... some weeks since I have opened this book," Gideon Welles records that "The President returned ill and in a few days it was ascertained he had the varioloid. We were in Cabinet-meeting when he informed us that the physicians had the previous evening ascertained and pronounced the nature of his complaint. It was in a light form, but yet held on longer than was expected. He would have avoided an interview, but wished to submit and have our views of the message. All were satisfied" [welles v1p480]. The diary of Attorney General Edward Bates does not mention a Cabinet meeting between Nov. 19 and Dec. 19 [beale pp316-320], although one certainly occurred Dec. 15 [welles v1p485]. *The most logical scenario is: (a) The Nov. 27 Cabinet meeting was being held in Lincoln's absence, during which Lincoln's note was brought in saying he would not attend, and (b) In December, Lincoln appeared, reluctantly, at a second Cabinet meeting to collect views on his Dec. 9 message [sandburgW v2p480]. Lincoln was still confined to his room as of Dec. 4 [miers v3p224] (§5.61). The surrounding entries in Welles' diary are dated Oct. 31 and Dec. 12.* §5.38

§5

§5.39

28 Nov.   Earliest press dispatches about Lincoln's illness begin to appear [lincloreLHH].

28 Nov.   "The President is reported to be much better this morning." [miers v3p223]   §5.40
citing [WashingtonStar - Nov. 28, 1863]

28 Nov.   The *National Republican* reports: "We are glad to announce that the Pres-   §5.41
ident is much better today. The fever from which he has suffered has left
him. Wednesday [25th] and Thursday night his suffering was chiefly from
severe pains in the head. Yesterday and the day before he was not permitted
by his physician to hold any interviews, even with members of his cabinet.
It is hoped that in a day or two he will gain sufficient strength to resume his
official duties." ([lincloreLHH] and [shutes pp84-85] and [NYTimes - Nov. 30, 1863] all
provide slightly different texts)

28 Nov.   The *Washington Chronicle* reports: "The President's youngest son, who   §5.42
had been sick for some time past with scarlatina, was much better yesterday, the crisis of his disease being past. It is expected he will be able again
to be out in a short time." [lincloreLHH] *This report of scarlatina occurs after
the diagnosis of smallpox in Lincoln, but before its public revelation. It is,
therefore, understandable why the reporter was not apparently suspicious
that father and son had the same illness.*

28 Nov.   "The condition of the President, who has been confined to his chamber for   §5.43
several days by sickness, seemed to be much better today, and to promise
an early recovery of health. There is nothing in the symptoms of his ailment
to excite the fears of his friends." [NYTimes - Nov. 29, 1863]

29 Nov.   "President Lincoln is much better to-day, and will be able to resume his   §5.44
office duties to-morrow or next day." [miers v3p224] citing [NYHerald - Nov. 30,
1863]

– – –   "Little Tad sent for me to come to the White House to see him, his father   §5.45
and he both being somewhat indisposed, it was the time the President was
reported to have small pox. I spent two or three hours with them that afternoon, very pleasantly, in referring to the [recent runaway horse] accident and congratulating the President on his escape." [tripp p17] citing (on
his website) "Letter from Charles Derickson to Ida M. Tarbell, Long Notes,
Tripp Database, 85." *This suggests that Tad indeed did have smallpox,
as he would not have been allowed to be in Lincoln's presence had he
not been similarly ill or immune. The runaway horse incident was in
September (¶3602).*

30 Nov.   "The President has been sick ever since thursday [sic] – I saw him, satur-   §5.46
day, and he was then a little better. Today, monday, he is still improving, as
I hear." – Edward Bates diary [beale p319] *The 26th was a Thursday, but Lincoln had actually taken ill no later than the previous Thursday, the 19th.
But Bates' wording is clear: the major illness began on the 26th. This
is an additional piece of evidence suggesting that some sort of diagnostic
event occurred on the 26th or 27th.*

30 Nov.   The *Cincinnati Daily Gazette* reports on Lincoln's illness. [randallB p4n]   §5.47

30 Nov.   "The President is still confined to his bed, but has so far recovered as to   §5.48
resume work to-day on his message." [ChicagoTribune - Dec. 1, 1863]

§5.49

30 Nov. "The President has been ill for several days, and one of our Washington *on dits* is that a great part of the Message [to Congress] has been written by him in *bed*." [stoddardB p193]

?? Dec. "He is too sick to read and not well enough to object to anything. So I had §5.50 him at my mercy & read him into a fever." – John Hay, in "early December" [hayC p70]. *A Hay letter of Dec. 1 (below) suggests Lincoln was not transacting business in the days before Dec. 1.*

1 Dec. "President is steadily recovering from his indisposition and it is not §5.51 doubted that he will in a day or two be equal to the active resumption of his arduous duties." [miers v3p224] citing [WashingtonStar - Dec. 1, 1863]

1 Dec. John Hay declines an invitation for Lincoln to break ground for the Union §5.52 Pacific railway in Omaha, writing "his illness will prevent him" from attending. [nicolayC v9p215]

1 Dec. To John Dix: "I have not been permitted until today to present to the President your communication of the 23d November. He directs me to express §5.53 his deep regret that his illness will prevent him from going..." [hayC p70].

2 Dec. "The President is much better to-day, and able to sit up" [NYTimes - Dec. 3, §5.54 1863]. *This implies Lincoln was earlier unable, or not allowed, to sit up.*

2 Dec. The *Boston Journal* reports: "Mr. Lincoln's scarlatina of yesterday is pro- §5.55 nounced varioloid today and if it could be magnified into smallpox tomorrow, it would perhaps keep politicians away, and thus give him time to complete his message." [lincloreLHH]

2 Dec. A Washington paper reported: "Convalescent – President Lincoln is rapidly §5.56 recovering from his recent indisposition and will be able in the course of a few days to resume the arduous duties of his office." [lincloreLHH]

2 Dec. Lincoln declines an invitation to speak the next day, saying "the now early §5.57 meeting of Congress, together with a temporary illness, render my attendance impossible" [nicolayC v9p215] [NYTimes - Dec. 4, 1863]. *The invitation had been written on the 28th. The delay in Lincoln's reply – to the very last moment – suggests that he was not attending to business between the 28th and the 1st.*

2 Dec. The *New York Daily Tribune* reports on Lincoln's illness. [randallB p4n] §5.58

3 Dec. "It is stated that the illness of President Lincoln is varioloid of a mild type. §5.59 The stage when the pustules break out has passed favorably, and he is reported to be in a fair way for speedy recovery." – *Baltimore Sun* of Dec. 4.   §5

3 Dec. "The President Has The Small Pox: The prevailing disease in this city §5.60 [Washington] is the small pox, and yesterday it disclosed itself in the progress of the disease under which the President has been laboring for some days. In his case, however, it is a mild form of varioloid, and not really dangerous. As usual, Old Abe could not refrain from his joke: 'There is one consolation about the matter, doctor, it cannot in the least disfigure me!' " [ChicagoTribune - Dec. 8, 1863, p2]

4 Dec. Still confined to his room and working on his message to Congress [miers §5.61 v3p224] citing [NYHerald - Dec. 5, 1863].

§5.62

417

4 Dec. Mary telegraphs Lincoln from New York state: "Reached here last evening. Very tired and severe headache. ... Expect a telegraph to-day." [baslerA v7p34] citing [helmB p234]

4 Dec. Lincoln telegraphs Mary at 9:30 am: "All going well" [baslerA v7p34] [nicolayC v9p216]. According to [baslerA v7p34], Lincoln's illness "probably accounts for the series of telegrams sent to Mrs. Lincoln." §5.63

5 Dec. Lincoln telegraphs Mary at 10 am: "All doing well." [baslerA v7p34] [nicolayC v9p216] §5.64

?6 Dec. "As we were about to withdraw, the door from the President's room opened sufficiently for the nose and face of Mr. Lincoln to appear in the narrow opening, and he asked in those, clear, ringing, earnest tones, which once heard could never be forgotten, 'Are you afraid of me?' 'No, Mr. President,' replied Lovejoy, 'we're not afraid. Come in.' [sic] ... On this occasion he seemed to me to be the most forlorn human being I had ever looked at. He had on a dressing gown, stockings, and slippers. His night-shirt was open in front, exposing his neck and chest, his slippers were crushed down at the heels, and his loose stocking-legs had slid down about his ankles. His face, neck, and breast presented evidences of being irritated, and were a color which I can only describe as a dirty red. I think that at that moment he had a slight fever. Apparently with considerable effort, he assumed a cheerful air. ... In the course of the conversation he showed us the pustules on his wrists, evidences that he really had varioloid, and declared that now he had something he 'could give to everybody,' a remark that afterwards became famous." [carrA pp252-253] *This episode is dated Nov. 21 by* [miers v3p222], *but without justification I can see. I have placed it about Dec. 6 because (a) the quip appeared in* [ChicagoTribune - Dec. 11, 1863] *with a Dec. 6 byline, and (b) Lovejoy was known to be in the White House on Dec. 6* [hayD p121]. *Of note,* [carrA] *gets the year wrong.* §5.65

6 Dec. "'Old Abe' has a well developed case of varioloid. I was with him an hour and a half the other other day and we went over many things. He did what he said he had done to no other person outside of his cabinet, he read me his message." – Elihu Washburne [hunt p230] (Inexplicably, [miers v3p222] lists this entry for 21 Nov.) §5.66

6 Dec. Lincoln telegraphs Mary: "All doing well." [baslerA v7p35] [nicolayC v9p216] §5.67

6 Dec. Mary sends two telegrams: one to Lincoln and one to doorkeeper Edward McManus, wanting to "know immediately exactly how Mr. Lincoln and Taddie are." [shutes p86] §5.68

6 Dec. "The Health of the President: Is much improved, and he is now able to leave his bed. He says that he has at last got something that he can give to every one calling upon him. His face is slightly marked but in a few days he will be quite recovered." [ChicagoTribune - Dec. 11, 1863]. §5.69

6 Dec. "President Lincoln's Health: When the President was at Gettysburg, he was anxious about the safety of his youngest son, who was at that time quite ill with scarlatina. On his return, he was up night after night with the lad, and, as Master Thomas recovered, his father began to feel ill. At first Dr. Stone, the physician at the White House, thought that Mr. Lincoln had symptoms of jaundice, then scarlatina and at last unmistakable signs of varioloid manifested themselves. This interfered sadly with the preparation §5.70

of the Message, although it has scared away the politician, and the parlors of the White House are deserted. Mr. Lincoln is now convalescent, and the Message is about 'built' (to use his expression) in such a manner as can but satisfy every loyal man. There is no 'back track' about it, but everything is progressive, and up to the spirit of the times." – Philadelphia Sunday *Dispatch* of Dec. 6, 1863, per typed transcript in [barbeeP - box 1 folder 51] *Lincoln's chronically "sallow" complexion would have complicated attempts to diagnose jaundice. See ¶3376ff.*

7 Dec. Lincoln telegraphs Mary at 10:20 am: "All doing well." [baslerA v7p35] [nicolayC v9p217] §5.71

7 Dec. The annual visit of the Supreme Court Justices to the White House, scheduled for this date, does not occur. [lincloreLHH] §5.72

7 Dec. Congress opens. Opening session of the US Senate includes this prayer from the Senate's chaplain: "We beseech thee, O Lord, to recover the President from his present illness again to health" [CongressionalGlobe - Dec. 9, 1863]. ([lincloreLHH] puts prayer on Dec. 8.) §5.73

8 Dec. Mary (apparently) returns to Washington in the evening [randallC p296] §5.74

9 Dec. Lincoln begins a letter with: "I have to urge my illness, and the preparation of the message [to Congress], in excuse for not having sooner transmitted you the inclosed..." [nicolayC v9p254] §5.75

9 Dec. "The illness of President Lincoln is, we have reason to believe, a much more serious matter than has generally been suspected. At first it was supposed to be a cold, next a touch of bilious fever; a rash then appeared upon his body, and the disease was pronounced scarlatina; but recently is has leaked out that the real complaint he labors under is small-pox. For some time past the President has received no visitors; even members of the cabinet and personal friends have been excluded from his apartment. The excuse was, that he was writing his message, and could not be interrupted. [new paragraph] We believe we but echo the feeling of the whole country, without distinction of party, in sincerely hoping that the President will soon be restored to health and strength. Men of his habit of body are not usually long-lived, and the small-pox to a man of his age, even when the health is generally good, is a very serious matter. His death at this time would be a real calamity to the country, and would tend to prolong the war. So Heaven help Abraham Lincoln, and restore him to his wonted health and strength." [ChicagoTribune - Dec. 9, 1863] *Whether the succession of diagnoses represent pronouncements from physicians or political spin (i.e., trying to minimize the President's illness) cannot be determined from this text alone.* §5.76

§5

10 Dec. The *New York Daily Tribune* reports on Lincoln's illness. [randallB p4n] §5.77

10 Dec. Citing [ChicagoTribune - Dec. 11, 1863], [miers v3p226] says Lincoln's health is much improved and that he sees visitors with special business. *This is probably based on the newspaper's ambiguous suggestion that Isaac Arnold met Lincoln on the 10th.* §5.78

11 Dec. The *Washington Chronicle* reports [11th]: "President Lincoln, we are happy to state, is now convalescent, and yesterday passed several hours in the transaction of official business. [miers v3p226] §5.79

§5.80

11 Dec. "President Lincoln is now so far recovered from his late illness as to be able to ride out. He has persevered in the discharge of his official duties, contrary to the advice, at times, of his medical attendants." – *Baltimore Sun* of Dec. 15.

11 Dec. Having arrived in Washington seven days earlier, Orville Browning decides to be "vaccinated at my room this morning by Dr Toner, small pox being prevalent" [browning p650]. *No information about Dr. Toner is provided.* §5.81

12 Dec. Browning calls at the White House, "but the President was sick, and I did not ask to see him." [browning p651] From Browning, [miers v3p226] somehow concludes: "President sees no callers today because of illness." §5.82

12 Dec. "... he was compelled to keep his room." [ChicagoTribune - Dec. 18, 1863] (See 14 Dec. entry.) §5.83

?13 Dec. Emilie Todd Helm spent "nearly a week" [helmB p232] at the White House in December 1863. Apparently drawing from Helms' diary, [randallC pp297-298] writes that Mary asked: "'Emilie, what do you think of Mr. Lincoln, do you think he is well?' Lincoln had scarcely recovered from his varioloid at this time and Emilie thought he looked very ill but she merely replied, 'He seems thinner than I ever saw him.'" *This probably preceded 14 Dec., the day Helm received her pass to return home to Kentucky* [randallC p301]. §5.84

?13 Dec. After a bitter exchange with Emilie Todd Helm and Mary, General Daniel Sickles goes upstairs to see Lincoln, "who was still feeling so unwell that he was lying down." [randallC p300] §5.85

14 Dec. Lincoln meets with Orville Browning [browning p651]. §5.86

14 Dec. "The President's health is re-established. While he has been recovering from the late attack of variloid [sic], he has been saying that since he has been President he has always had a crowd of people asking him to give them something, but that *now he has something he can give them all.* [ChicagoTribune - Dec. 15, 1863, "Special dispatch"] §5.87

14 Dec. "The President has not yet quite recovered his health. Indeed, on Saturday [12 Dec.] he was compelled to keep to his room. Yesterday, however, he was much better, and able to attend to business." [ChicagoTribune - Dec. 18, 1863, "Regular correspondent"] §5.88

15 Dec. "The President this morning was able to be in his office and attend to business." [miers v3p226] citing [WashingtonStar - Dec. 15, 1863] §5.89

15 Dec. Gideon Welles' diary records: "Seward and Chase were not present at the Cabinet meeting. The President was well and in fine spirits." [welles v1p485] §5.90

17 Dec. Lincoln receives the Justices of the Supreme Court, originally scheduled for 7 Dec. [lincloreLHH] §5.91

28 Dec. "The President is steadily recovering his health and strength, and his friends say that he will be rather improved than otherwise by his brief struggle with fever" [stoddardB p197]. *Note the failure to mention smallpox by name.* §5.92

31 Dec. The *Pittsfield Sun* reports "It is gravely stated that President Lincoln was not disfigured by the small pox." *This is 19 paragraphs after the newspaper's solemn report that "Black squirrels are swarming the Canadian woods."* §5.93

1 Jan. At New Year's Day reception: "his complexion is clearer, his eyes less lack-luster, and he has a hue of health to which he has long been a stranger" [hopkinsB p279] citing [sandburgW] citing Noah Brooks. §5.94

2 Jan. Senator Lemuel Bowden of Virginia (Unionist faction) dies of "black small pox" in Washington [ChicagoTribune - Jan. 9, 1864]. §5.95

5 Jan. Lincoln telegraphs Mary: "All very well." [donaldH p99] §5.96

7 Jan. Lincoln telegraphs Mary: "We are all well, and have not been otherwise." [donaldH p99] §5.97

8 Jan. In Washington: "There is great terror here on account of the small pox. The death of Senator Bowden of Virginia from this disease in its most malignant form has added to the fright of the people. I know of strangers coming here who will not ride in a horse car or carriage, go to the theatre, or in fact to any public place, where people are congregated together, on account of the fear of infection." [ChicagoTribune - Jan. 13, 1864]. §5.98

13 Jan. A Congressional Committee finds "much less cause for alarm" about small-pox in Washington "than sensationalists would have bad people believe. ... It seems from the report of physicians that the disease is of a mild type. The confluent small-pox cases are actually said to be less in number than last winter." The police report 1200 cases in the District of Columbia, "including those in hospitals beyond the city limits." – *Baltimore Sun* of Jan. 16. §5.99

19 Jan. Lincoln telegraphs son Robert: "There is a good deal of smallpox here. Your friends must judge for themselves whether they ought to come or not." [shutes p87] §5.100

26 Jan. At reception "about eight thousand pass the President and Mrs. Lincoln and pay their respects. President looks in better health than ever." Washington National Republican, 27 January 1864. [miersv3p236] *Given its name, the objectiveness of the paper is suspect.* §5.101

28 Jan. The *Pittsfield Sun* reports "An old lady in Boston, was very anxious to read the President's Message, but refused to touch a copy of the paper containing it, because she heard Mr. Lincoln had the small pox and was afraid she would catch it." §5.102

13 Feb. To Salmon Chase: "On coming up from the reception, I found your note of to-day. I am unwell, even now, and shall be worse this afternoon. If you please, we will have an interview Monday." – Lincoln [baslerA v7p183] *The 13th was a Saturday.* §5.103

20 Feb. Mary writes: "The President is, a little better today, was able to visit the 'blue room;' to night, I will try & persuade him to take some medicine & rest a little on the morrow" [turner p169]. *It is unclear if this episode was related to Lincoln's smallpox bout.* §5.104

23 Feb. "It is reported that the President looks and feels indisposed" [kunhardtA p265]. *Perhaps on this day, a Tuesday, newspapers reported the illness of Saturday, Feb. 20.* §5.105

14 Mar. Erroneous report by [shutes p87] that Lincoln was in bed this day. (See ¶1186.) §5.106

§5.107

§5

1864 "He can hardly be called handsome, though he is certainly much better looking since he had the small-pox." – from a mock biography in the 1864 campaign [meserve p3]. (∈ ¶192)

Notes:

- A mark on the tip of Lincoln's nose appears in photographs taken after December 1863. (See ¶1892.)
- Events without precise dates, e.g. the Lovejoy-Lincoln encounter, are often recounted by published sources without regard to the clinical evolution of smallpox. Example: [sandburgW v2p477] implies that Lovejoy saw Lincoln soon after Gettysburg, which is almost certainly not the case given that Lincoln did not take to bed until several days later. I have estimated dates where possible.
- ○○○ *Project:* Is there evidence Lincoln's beard was shaved while he had smallpox? See ¶1426.

(c) Caveats §5c

Two physician-written accounts of Lincoln's illness have been deliberately ignored above: [aronson] and [marx]. Neither provides references and both contain very detailed information for which I cannot find primary sources. I suspect they made clinical extrapolations to fill the many holes left by the scant primary record. [marx] should be shunned. Worse, its fictions infect other publications, including [aronson], [goldman], and [hopkinsB].

Specific concerns:

- [aronson]
  - Mentions records of Lincoln's physician which are not otherwise known to exist.
  - Frankly distorts the dates of illness and death for Lincoln's valet, William Johnson.
  - Uncritically accepts that Lincoln's illness was mild ("a well-deserved rest").
- [marx]
  - [marx], I believe, took the (comparatively) lengthy newspaper reports of Nov. 28 and Dec. 9 and superimposed clinical knowledge of smallpox and the likely behavior of Lincoln's physician to create his detailed picture.
  - His statement that Tad had smallpox and his interior monologs for the President's physician make a nice story, but they are wholly unsupported.
  - Uncritically accepts that Lincoln's illness was mild.
- [goldman]
  - Adds many useful elements to the literature, but relies on [marx] in some places and on elements of [hopkinsB] that rely on [marx]. For example, there is no primary source I know that says Lincoln's rash erupted on the fourth day of illness. Worse, when [goldman] reviews the differential diagnosis of Lincoln's illness, he uses symptoms such as backache that [marx] invented because they are part of smallpox!
  - The relationship between text and cited references is often erroneous.
  - The reference citations themselves are sometimes jumbled (e.g. #7, #9, #15).

(d) The White House as a Smallpox Hospital §5d

This long, colorful excerpt from [stoddardA pp107-109] *opens with Stoddard being vaccinated in early autumn 1863, then being re-vaccinated by "the President's own physician" (Dr. Stone – ¶3203) soon after Lincoln becomes ill. It wonderfully evokes the White House atmosphere at this time. William Stoddard, John Nicolay, and John Hay were all private secretaries to Lincoln.*

Some describe Stoddard's style as "self-consciously literary" with "a great tendency to exaggeration" [stoddardA p vii]. *Thus, his statement, "Mr. Lincoln is sick, dangerously sick," may or may not be literally true. On the positive side, however, one of Stoddard's phrases is haunting: compared to Lincoln, the Vice President is found wanting "... even if Mr. Hamlin were twice as large a man as he is believed to be." Unsurprisingly, the three secretaries "held mournful consultations over the idea that all the country would go to ruin if Abraham Lincoln should die of the dread disease, or any other"* [stoddardD p305] [stoddardA p xiii].

Stoddard's account is also remarkable in saying "Nobody is supposed to know it, but the White House has suddenly been turned into a smallpox hospital" – strong evidence for a deliberate effort to conceal facts. [neelyL] *says "The White House was half-quarantined for three weeks."*

"Have you been vaccinated?"

"Yes, doctor, but it was long ago. Is the small-pox on the increase?"

"Terribly, and everything else is on the increase, and I have been so busy I had been forgetful of my duty. I should have attended to you before. Guess it isn't too late. Bare your arm."

That was early in the season, and the results of the attention you then received, whether late or early, from your own physician, made you about down sick for a week. Ever since then you have understood that the extent of the prevalence of the dreaded disorder is one of those secrets which the Surgeon General's office does not give to the reporters. On the whole, you believe that you are safe and always have been, and you have a natural absence of nervousness about any kind of infection. It is very much as if you were a fatalist, and yet you are somehow startled, almost into a shudder, by precisely the same question, asked of you here, at the mail-table:

"Have you been vaccinated?"

"Yes, doctor, thoroughly–" and you tell him your unpleasant experience, but he says:

"Glad of it! Very glad of it! But it will do no hurt to repeat. I'll shut the door a moment. Take off your coat and bare your arm."

He is the President's own physician, and he is a rapid operator; but he supposes you to know more than you yet do, for he chats along while he punctures:

"Mr. Lincoln's case is not fully developed yet. Varioloid."

"Not the small-pox!" you exclaim, with another shudder, which helps the entrance of the keen point of his feathery flash of steel.

"Oh, no, probably not. I won't say more just now. There, you'll do. I've really no uneasiness about him."

Everybody else has, then, after the doctor has taken his confident and smiling departure. Whoever yet believed that a doctor could read the end of a smallpox case from the beginning?

But the varioloid is not the smallpox:

What is it, if it isn't that? Couldn't he die of it? Of course he could. And where would everything go if he should die?

There has been such an absence of any thought concerning the President's health! The idea of assassination has been held up before us until it is worn out and there is no more scare in it; but the idea of his possible death in any other way never came before, and it is all the more grisly now that it is here. Nobody is supposed to know it, but the White House has suddenly been turned into a smallpox hospital, with a certain degree of penetrable quarantine.

This is surely a remarkable addition to the other elements of its peculiar character. The loneliness enforced, so far as the ordinary run of visitors is concerned, has in it something that is differently oppressive from the old familiar clamor. It is impossible not to calculate

§5

consequences, and to remember all you know about Mr. Hannibal Hamlin. He would be President if Mr. Lincoln should die, and there is no means by which you can form an opinion of his capacity as dictator. No, absolutely; he could not step into Mr. Lincoln's shoes, and something of inestimable value would be lost to the country, even if Mr. Hamlin were twice as large a man as he is believed to be.

Day follows day, and all the reports from the sick-room are favorable, but the whole country is nervous about this case, mild as it is, and so are you. There are, indeed, some people whose nerves are not at all shaken, especially those belonging to their facial muscles. Here is one of them, who has managed to pass the lower door quarantine. He does not explain how he did it, but he is eager to unfold the fact that he is an important office-seeker, sure of success if he could see the President, his papers of recommendation are so overpoweringly strong.

"But Mr. Lincoln is sick, dangerously sick. He cannot attend to business, except such as is of the utmost national consequence. He cannot receive visitors."

"Oh, that's nothing. I don't mind the smallpox. I am not in the least afraid of infection. You can tell him so. He needn't be afraid I'll catch it. Tell him I'll come right in. I've been vaccinated."

It requires something like engineering to get that fearless adventurer out of the White House, for he really is a man who is of some value, but he is also one who has a right to know that another man, enduring pain and fever and intolerable irritation, ought not to be intruded upon. Perhaps he was thinking less of that, and more of the fact that Mr. Lincoln could appoint him today and die to-morrow. There are many others like him, but the quarantine is usually too much for them. So, if they succeed in passing that, is the impassable Mr. Nicolay [sic], and he has a fine faculty for explaining to some men the view he takes of any untimely persistency: Hay does it equally well, in some cases, but he is even too fine about it, and there are fellows who went away and did not know how much he told them. It is of no use to employ verbal needles upon pachydermatous natures.

"The President wishes to see you. He understands that you are proof against infection."

"I want to see him, then! Is he sitting up, Edward?"

"Indeed he is, and he won't be there long. He's doing finely!"

It will never be possible to forget how this sick-room looks. So bright it is, in the perceived certainty that the peril has passed away! Even the welcoming smile that lights up Mr. Lincoln's face is a half-amused reflection of your own exuberance: He has not been alarmed about himself at any moment, and he combines his instructions concerning the duties he assigns you with a humorous response to your personal inquiries. He almost wishes he could have his office in one of the smallpox hospitals. It would relieve him of one part of his pressure: "Well, no," he adds, "it wouldn't. They'd all go and get vaccinated, and they'd come buzzing back, just the same as they do now-or worse."

Stoddard's late-life autobiography re-tells the story of Lincoln's illness more briefly, but adds suggestions that (a) the smallpox then rampant generally "took the shape" of varioloid, and (b) that Lincoln's illness was varioloid [stoddardD p305]:

Somewhere about these days [1863], without date, the smallpox was raging with some severity, taking generally the shape of varioloid, and it brought me an odd experience. One morning the face of my family physician came into my house a little clouded, to inform me that it was his duty to revaccinate every soul of us, whether we had ever been poisoned in that way before or not. *[Tells of his arm's reaction to this re-vaccination.]* My scab had peeled and my safety had come before the President himself was taken down with the varioloid. Some of his enemies averred that it was the larger kind of smallpox and that his fatal case was only concealed from the public for war purposes.

All the other members of the White House family were visited by the President's own doctor and I was compelled to show my arm. I am not sure that it was not punched again. I am inclined to think it was, in his zeal for the public good. I do remember that we boys held mournful consultations over the idea that all the country would got to ruin if Abraham Lincoln should die of the dread disease, or any other. But it came to pass, as he was convalescing, that he was informed of my ironclad [i.e., vaccinated] condition and sent for me. I went right in and attended to whatever the business was, telling him how glad I felt that he was doing so well and adding now, at least, he was safe from office seekers. He might do well, afterwards, to have his office in one of the smallpox hospitals. His laughing reply contained the information that one eager hunter had already replied to his doorkeeper:

"Oh, that doesn't matter. I'll see him. I've been vaccinated."

As to the hospital experiment he almost sadly declared that the office seekers would only wait until they had been vaccinated and would then come buzzing back around him like so many greenhead flies.

(e) Discussion §5e

All known facts about Lincoln's smallpox have been presented thus far. This section interprets those facts.

Why did Lincoln get smallpox?

Smallpox is easily transmitted from human to human. As already noted, smallpox was rampant in Washington in the summer and fall of 1863. Lincoln certainly had exposure to the general population, both inside and outside the White House. Office seekers jammed the White House daily (¶2204). [hopkinsB pp279-280] lists several excursions in town where Lincoln might have become infected.

The chief suspect, however, is Tad Lincoln [lincloreLHH], who became ill before his father and probably did have smallpox (§5.45). Interestingly, Tad's diagnosis (or, perhaps, one of his diagnoses) was "scarlatina" – a label that was also applied, transiently and incorrectly as it turned out, to Lincoln's illness.*

Such exposures would not matter had Lincoln been vaccinated** against smallpox or previously had the disease. No one has yet found evidence that Lincoln was vaccinated [hopkinsB p279] [goldman] [pearson]. Certainly, vaccination did not occur during the crushing poverty of his youth, although it was not unknown for physicians to offer free vaccination during epidemics [leech p350].

---

* In smallpox a "scarlatinal rash may come out as early as the second day and be as diffuse and vivid as in a true scarlatina" [osler p50]. If Tad was among those vaccinated after Lincoln was diagnosed with smallpox (¶5401), that would be evidence Tad's physicians did *not* think he had the same illness as Lincoln.

** Vaccination and inoculation have the same result but are two different procedures. Inoculation introduces smallpox virus into the recipient. Vaccination introduces vaccinia virus into the recipient. Vaccinia confers protection against smallpox infection, but with far fewer side effects, since it is a much less virulent virus. Inoculation, introduced to Western medicine in the 1700s [aa40 p373] was no small matter. For example, after being inoculated in Boston in 1764, future President John Adams spent three weeks in the hospital, suffering headaches, backaches, kneeaches, gagging fever, and eruption of pock marks [aa19]. By contrast, vaccination in the 1860s "made you about down sick for a week" [stoddardA p107]. Congress established a national Vaccine Agency in 1813 [aa40 p375], but how fast the practice spread to Lincoln's frontier homes is unknown to me. Given the protracted, unpleasant course associated with inoculation, it seems unlikely Lincoln underwent this procedure, without it ever getting into print later.

§5

A more interesting possibility arises in connection with Lincoln's 1832 militia service. The American Army required smallpox inoculation for all recruits as early as the 1770s [aa17] [aa36] [aa39]. Whether this policy ever applied to the militia is unknown to me. Even if it did not, Lincoln's "Independent Spy company" might have been a special case. The company had an unusual relationship with the regular army: "always, when with the army, camping within the lines, and having many other privileges" [wilson p327]. His company, therefore, may have shared the medical resources available to the regular army. However, it is also unclear if the policy of smallpox inoculation lasted until 1832 in the regular army .

Fear of smallpox was a very real, very widespread, and very sensible attitude among unimmunized Americans in the 1800s. (It remains very sensible.) Yet, Lincoln visited Congressman Owen Lovejoy, recuperating from smallpox, in about March 1863 [aa71 p384] (¶2189). Although in keeping with Lincoln's long habit of visiting sick friends (¶2180 ff), such a visit suggests he had some reason to be unafraid of the disease – i.e. Lincoln had already had the disease or already been inoculated/vaccinated.

If the former, Lincoln could have been mistaken. He might have mis-identified chickenpox in childhood as smallpox, and afterwards thought himself resistant to smallpox. This error was not uncommon then [aa94 p147], as chickenpox and smallpox were not distinguished as separate diseases until well into the 1800s [aa94 p1].

Although it *seems* no definitive evidence supports Lincoln ever being inoculated or vaccinated against smallpox, or previously having the disease, some avenues remain unexplored. OOO *Project:* Are there records of smallpox epidemics in Lincoln's Illinois? Were there epidemics in Washington during Lincoln' s tenure as a Congressman?

The most interesting unexplored avenue, however, has not yet been mentioned. It strongly suggests Lincoln was previously vaccinated. The story resumes in the **Varioloid** section, as it requires an understanding of Lincoln's clinical course.

What was the nature of Lincoln's illness?

Lincoln's illness was entirely consistent with a typical case of "ordinary smallpox." Ordinary smallpox is the most common of the five types of clinical smallpox caused by the Variola major virus [aa35 p4].* Fig. 5-1 summarizes the typical course of ordinary smallpox, and serves as a useful template to discuss Lincoln's case. Note: The discussion will ignore minor discrepancies, of a day or two, between Lincoln's course and the course in the figure.

Lincoln became symptomatic on Nov. 18, remarking that he felt weak (if [goldman] is believed). On the morning of the 19th he complained of dizziness, and that evening he had a severe headache. A smallpox textbook states:

> The onset of illness may be abrupt, but is more often gradual. The symptoms are apt to come on in the night, the patient after much restlessness finding himself with a headache and, on rising, being attacked with giddiness and nausea. [aa94 p59]

Lincoln, it seems, had a typical onset of ordinary smallpox.

What of fever? Although Fig. 5-1 shows a high fever at the beginning of clinical illness, this is usually not the patient's chief concern: "most complaint is made of the headache" [aa94 p59]. The historical record has no temperature data for Lincoln. It is interesting, however, that Lincoln applied cold water to his head.

Fig. 5-1 predicts that, having became markedly sicker on the evening of the 19th, Lincoln was probably feeling just as ill for the next day or two – assuming he was following a typical course. Nevertheless, Lincoln was well enough to attend to business on the 20th. Indeed, [miers v3pp222-223] records a usual amount of office activity for Lincoln through Nov. 25.

---

* The related Variola minor virus causes a milder illness – see Varioloid .

Imputed Clinical Course for Lincoln's Smallpox, November-December 1863

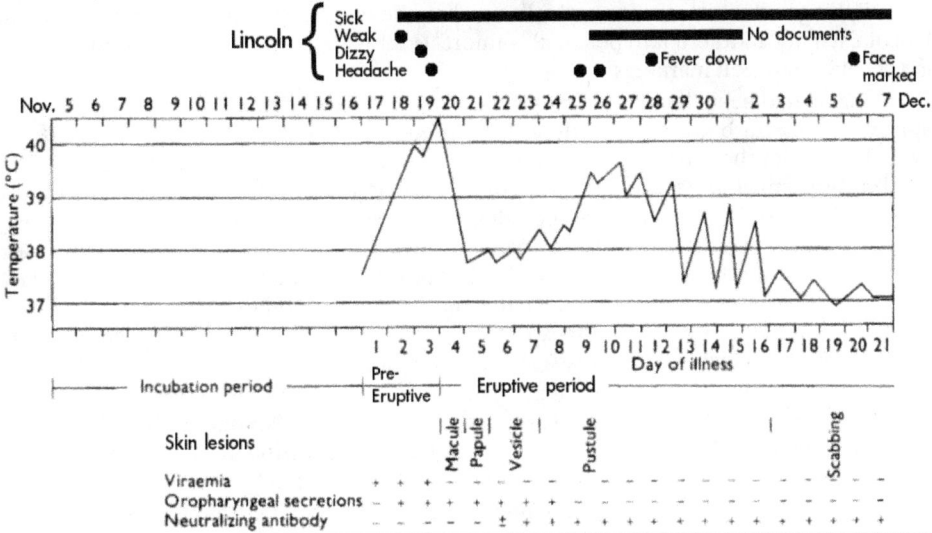

Figure 5-1. Imputed Course of Lincoln's Smallpox. Ordinary smallpox can follow an almost infinite number of courses. This figure, adapted from a smallpox textbook [aa35 p6], represents a typical course. It can be time-matched to Lincoln's illness (upper region), using imputed calendar dates. Lincoln is discussed in the text. The paragraphs below discuss a typical course of ordinary smallpox, keyed to the figure. The figure plots the patient's body temperature on the vertical axis as time passes. It also marks other events.

Time - Events during smallpox are most usefully discussed using "Day of illness" as a time scale, as shown beneath the temperature plot. Classically, smallpox has three phases: incubation, pre-eruptive, and eruptive. "Eruptive" refers to the eruption of the skin lesions characteristic of smallpox.

Pre-eruptive - The first fever spike (typically days 1-4 of illness) is part of the pre-eruptive phase. During this time, the characteristic skin lesions of smallpox have yet to appear. The other symptoms that occur in the pre-eruptive phase, most prominently, headache and backache, are commonly seen in other illness. Thus, bedside diagnosis of smallpox during this pre-eruptive phase is almost impossible [aa35 p56].

Eruptive - The eruptive phase begins on day 4 of typical illness. About this time the patient's temperature drops and the patient feels better [osler p51] until the second fever spike (days 8-16 of typical illness). Although the temperature may not rise as high during the eruptive phase, the patient is much sicker than the pre-eruptive phase. Days 10-16 are the most most typical for death [aa35 p22]. After the skin lesions appear on day 4, they mature through several stages. The greater their maturity, the easier it is to diagnose smallpox. Smallpox is disfiguring because the skin lesions may leave permanent scars after healing.

Transmission - Smallpox virus lives in the skin lesions (even as scabs [aa75]) and can infect people in contact with them. Similar lesions in the mouth and throat (during days 2-8 of typical illness) are important in the spread of smallpox because they make the virus airborne.

§5

Nov. 21-25 correspond to the interval of lowered temperature (and symptomatic improvement) in Fig. 5-1.

Nothing in the historical record tells us when the first skin lesions appeared. Certainly Lincoln, a man "indifferent to personal comfort" [donaldA p215], would have continued working despite a few skin markings.

Lincoln had been diagnosed first with a "cold, next a touch of bilious fever; a rash then appeared upon his body, and the disease was pronounced scarlatina" [ChicagoTribune - Dec. 9, 1863]. Because of the multiple diagnoses, [marx] says the President's physician was vacillating. However, smallpox textbooks explain that "the diagnosis of smallpox in the pre-eruptive stage [is] impossible on clinical grounds alone" [aa35 p56] and that even early in the eruptive stage of milder cases "the symptoms grade downwards, lose what little individuality they might possess, and become indistinguishable from those of many trifling disorders" [aa94 p60]. Once the skin lesions mature sufficiently the diagnosis becomes "not difficult" [aa35 p56]. Thus, not only is it unreasonable to expect Lincoln's physician to have diagnosed smallpox immediately, it is a feature of the disease that he did not.

On Nov. 25 Lincoln again developed headache. He went to bed early. He was "quite unwell" on the 26th. Fig. 5-1 predicts the fever had returned. No doubt, this turn for the worse prompted medical consultation. Dr. van Bibber's visit probably coincided with the skin lesions maturing to the point where diagnosis became easier.

Nov. 27, 1863 must have been an interesting day at the White House. Lincoln was too ill to attend the scheduled Cabinet meeting. (His shaky, handwritten, self-excusing note has a big sweaty fingerprint on it.) Most significantly, a physician prohibited visitors to the President. This suggests that the correct diagnosis had now been reached by one or more physicians.

Except for his note about sickness on the 27th, Lincoln issued no official documents from Nov. 26 to Dec. 1, inclusive [baslerA v7pp31-32] – six full days. Even after the death of his son Willie in 1862, Lincoln went only four days without producing official documents [neelyL] (¶2515). Fig. 5-1 predicts that Lincoln was in the most serious phase of his illness from Nov. 26 to Dec. 1. At this point the lesions on his skin would have had the classic pustular appearance of smallpox. When Gideon Welles wrote that Lincoln's smallpox was "in a light form," he probably meant that the lesions were not extensive. When Welles wrote that it "held on longer than was expected," he could have been referring to Lincoln's feeling of sickness or to the skin lesions themselves. Fig. 5-1 predicts that the lesions would be turning to scabs about Dec. 5 in a typical case.

Whether Lincoln would have agreed his disease was "in a light form" is unknown. [carrA pp252-253] describes Lincoln, well into convalescence, as "the most forlorn human being I ever looked at" and says Lincoln summoned "considerable effort" to assume a cheerful air.

Only two descriptions of Lincoln's skin were found: [carrA pp252-253] describes a generalized redness plus pustules on Lincoln's wrist. The other describes Lincoln's face as "slightly marked" on Dec. 6 (§5.69). Unlike photographs taken before his smallpox, many of those taken afterwards show a dark lesion on the tip of Lincoln's nose, on the right side. Is this lesion a pockmark? Smallpox is notorious for attacking the face. In Caucasians, the pockmarks of smallpox are hyperpigmented or red [aa35 p49]. Because the photographic techniques of Lincoln's day were primarily sensitive to blue light [personal communication, Richard Benson, 2007], red lesions would show up dark. Thus, both the appearance and the location of the lesion are consistent with a pockmark. (One pre-1864 photograph, however, seems to show the same lesion in the same place (¶1895).)

The Physical Lincoln raises the possibility that Lincoln had a structural abnormality of his skin. It is, therefore, reasonable to ask how such an abnormality, if any, may have affected the appearance of pock marks (¶1892).

Lincoln's first day of reasonably robust health was Dec. 15, but references to "health" did not appear until January 1. His illness, therefore, lasted almost 6 weeks. Was this really a respite from the office seekers that incessantly assailed him? The remarks of §5.65 and [stoddardA p109, xiii] would suggest so, but it seems more likely this was gallows humor. It was Lincoln's nature to joke at even the most serious times, so his joking on a sick-bed is not evidence that his illness was mild. Yet, two eyewitnesses clearly indicate that the illness took something out of him (¶1189, ¶2036).

"Varioloid"

When Dr. van Bibber diagnosed Lincoln with "varioloid," what did he mean? The word, unfortunately, has several possible meanings:
1. Varioloid = euphemism for smallpox.
2. Varioloid = the mild illness caused by a different virus, Variola minor.
3. Varioloid = "the modified form of small-pox which affects persons who have been vaccinated" [osler p54].

Of these, #2 may be discarded immediately because the Variola minor virus was unknown in the United States during Lincoln's time [bollett p86] [aa35 p3]. More subtly, data in The White House as a Smallpox Hospital rules out meaning #1, as follows.

As he re-vaccinated Stoddard, the President's physician said: "Mr. Lincoln's case is not fully developed yet. Varioloid." Stoddard exclaims "Not the small-pox!" and the physician replies: "Oh, no, probably not. I won't say more just now. ... I've really no uneasiness about him."

Assuming Stoddard has correctly reported the essence of the conversation, it is clear the President's physician does not consider varioloid and smallpox as the same illness. Stoddard believes this, too, when he says "the varioloid is not the smallpox" after pondering the difficulty of predicting smallpox's clinical course in an individual. (This is insightful clinical reasoning on his part.)

If meanings #1 and #2 for "varioloid" have been eliminated, then Lincoln's physicians must have meant #3, which implies that Lincoln was previously vaccinated. To be generous, inoculation or a previous bout of smallpox (or even cowpox) may be added to the list of events which would have made the physicians think Lincoln now had varioloid.

If there were a fourth meaning of "varioloid" then one could not conclude van Bibber meant #3. It is, therefore, pertinent that William Osler, who, like van Bibber, was a Baltimore physician, admits of no other meanings for varioloid in his 1892 textbook of medicine [osler p54]. A fourth meaning could also result if Lincoln's physicians were not well informed about smallpox syndromes.

The clinical description of varioloid(#3) further confirms Lincoln's physicians were using the term in that sense. The onset of varioloid is similar to the onset of ordinary smallpox: "It may set in with abruptness and severity, the temperature reaching 103°. More commonly it is in every respect milder in its initial symptoms, though the headache and backache may be very distressing" [osler p54]. Thus, the limited historical record tells us that Lincoln's initial symptoms were also those of varioloid.

§5

Varioloid and ordinary smallpox diverge significantly as the eruptive phase begins. Varioloid has fewer skin lesions, there is no second fever spike, and the patient appears comfortable [osler p54]. If Lincoln's physicians really did believe their diagnosis of varioloid, then perhaps they made it earlier in the eruptive phase than hypothesized above, at a point where the divergence was not so apparent.

The severity of Lincoln's illness rules out the possibility he had varioloid(#3). His physicians must have realized this at some reasonably early point. They may or may not have revised their diagnosis: on Dec. 9 the Chicago *Tribune* pegged Lincoln with "small-pox." Stoddard said Lincoln's "enemies" publicized a smallpox diagnosis [stoddardD p305], but it is unclear if the *Tribune* was then an enemy. Though often critical of Lincoln previously, it gave "perhaps the strongest words of praise" in the nation to Lincoln's message read before

Congress that very same day [donaldAp474]. Moreover, the *Tribune* article is the most detailed account extant of Lincoln's illness' evolution, and it does not claim the diagnosis was hidden for war aims, as Stoddard says Lincoln's enemies did.

Stoddard also makes it clear that there was a deliberate effort to conceal information about Lincoln's health from outsiders: "Nobody is supposed to know it, but the White House has suddenly been turned into a smallpox hospital." Given the times, the wish to conceal Lincoln's true status is understandable.

A final possibility is that Lincoln's physicians knew he was unvaccinated, but deliberately diagnosed varioloid to forestall concerns. There is no way to disprove this, except by knowing Lincoln the man. First, he was honest. Second, we should be surprised only if Lincoln had *not* been vaccinated. Lincoln had an inquiring, scientific mind, and he was aware of the benefits medical science could bring.* Lincoln was also well aware of the dangers of smallpox. Speaking at age 28 about some gamblers, he said: "If they were annually swept, from the stage of existence, by the plague or small pox, honest men would, perhaps, be much profited, by the operation" [baslerA v1p111]. He would certainly of known Lincoln was too rational, and had too large a sense of responsibility to his family, to not be vaccinated.

(f) Who Was Exposed to Lincoln? §5f

There is a story that, immediately after leaving Lincoln's sickroom, a man said he wanted a certificate saying he caught smallpox from Abraham Lincoln, just in case. The man remained healthy, but it would be interesting to know whether smallpox appeared in any of the many people to whom a contagious Lincoln was exposed in November 1863. One case has been examined in detail – see William H. Johnson.

OOO *Project:* Track the fates of the many people with whom Lincoln had contact at, and soon after, Gettysburg. References such as [nicolayG] [sandburgW v2pp462-463, 475] [donaldA pp463-464] [browneF p606] [miers v3pp220-223] [tripp pp16-17] [gary] [borittG] list governors, Cabinet secretaries, diplomats, veterans, babies, and other ordinary folks with whom Lincoln interacted.

Lincoln's sick room was in the White House. It's location is known [stoddardA p6]. In modern times there have been concerns, especially among archeologists, that smallpox entombed for thousands of years under the right conditions (e.g., in Egyptian pyramids) can reactivate and cause infection [aa51] [aa75] [aa124]. I do not know if the White House offers "the right conditions" in any of its nooks and crannies. Furthermore, the White House has undergone at least one extensive remodeling since Lincoln's time, so one would think that no smallpox viruses are left in the structure. Finally, one would expect that careful and sensitive bio-monitoring of the building is now routine.

(g) Did William H. Johnson Catch Smallpox From Lincoln?
§5g

History (From: [baslerC], [washington])

William H. Johnson was a youthful African-American man who had come to Washington with Lincoln. He was working in the Treasury Department when Lincoln requested him for the trip to Gettysburg on Nov. 18-19.

Johnson served as sometime valet to Lincoln. To what degree Johnson tended the ill Lincoln in Gettysburg, on the train, or in the White House is unknown. *The smallpox was not diagnosed immediately, so Johnson could very well have been exposed to Lincoln for some days.*

---

* Needing a tooth extracted in 1862, Lincoln brought chloroform to the dentist's office and used it on himself. This was just 14 years after chloroform's first use, and well before its wide use in dentistry [shutes p89].

By early January 1864 smallpox was rampant in Washington. On January 12 Lincoln told a reporter that "a poor Negro who is a porter in one of the Departments (the Treasury) ... is at present very bad with the small pox. He did not catch it from me, however; at least I think not. He is now in hospital and could not draw his pay because he could not sign his name" [ChicagoTribune - Dec. 19, 1864]. *Lincoln habitually spoke with lawyerly precision. Thus, his opinion on not being the source for Johnson's smallpox implies that Lincoln knew something about the timing of contagiousness in the disease, or that contact between them was minimal.*

Johnson died sometime between Jan. 12 and February 2, the date Lincoln appointed someone to fill Johnson's Treasury job. The exact date is unknown because the District of Columbia's death records for 1862-1864 were destroyed.

Discussion

[goldman] assumes (or believes) Johnson died in mid-January and claims this timing is consistent with disease caught from Lincoln.

One's initial impression, however, is that Johnson died too late to have caught the disease from Lincoln. If Lincoln were contagious until late in his illness (until say, Dec. 4, when scabbing should have started per Fig. 5-1), and if Johnson's smallpox had a long incubation period (say, 20 days), and if Johnson died late in the illness (say, 16 days after the incubation period ended), then his latest reasonable date of death is January 11, 1864 – if he caught smallpox from Lincoln.

More realistically, Lincoln would have barred Johnson from his presence as soon as the diagnosis of varioloid were made. (This assumes Johnson was not immunized.) Thus, Lincoln would have been contagious to Johnson only until Nov. 27±, which puts the latest possible Johnson death at January 4.

If Johnson did not catch smallpox from Lincoln, there were plenty of other sources in Washington that winter [leech p350].

§5

Topic 6 – Petitioning §6

(a) Introduction §6a

Multitudes of office seekers and petitioners plagued Lincoln, but few left extended descriptions of their meetings with the President. Cordelia Harvey's remarkable account [harveyC] is a wonderful exception.

Harvey was the widow of the Governor of Wisconsin. From Sept. 6-9, 1863 she successfully convinced a reluctant Lincoln to establish veterans' hospitals in the north, where she believed – probably correctly – that the air was healthier.

Harvey's account is so detailed that one inevitably wonders how much is embellishment. The evolution of [harveyC] is as follows:

- Harvey originally committed her impressions of Lincoln to paper "at the time" [harveyC p241].
- Writing in 1866, [holland pp443-453] quotes at length from "a private letter."
- The text printed in [harveyC] is a typewritten lecture she presented "after the close of the war" [harvey p233]. However, this text and the "private letter" in [holland] are structured exactly alike and contain the same quotes.

Thus, it appears that [harveyC] has the advantage of immediate observation and recollection.

All mentions by [harveyC] of the physical Lincoln are excerpted below. Occasional non-physical selections are also provided. Each excerpt begins with the page number in [harveyC] where it may be found. *Passages in this font* are editorial additions not present in [harveyC].

(b) Excerpts §6b

Page 241 §6.1

I give the exact conversations between Mr. Lincoln and myself, as taken down at the time...

Page 242 §6.2

Day 1 (Sept. 6): Harvey enters Lincoln's White House office and gets her first look at him.

He was plainly clad in a suit of black that illy fited [sic] him. No fault of his tailor, however; such a figure could not be fitted. He was tall and lean, and as he sat in a folded up sort of way in a deep arm chair, one would almost have thought him deformed. ... When I first saw him his head was bent forward, his chin resting on his breast, and in his hand a letter...

...

His face was peculiar; bone, nerve, vein, and muscle were all so plainly seen; deep lines of thought and care were around his mouth and eyes. ... I sat, and silently read his face while he was reading a paper written by one of our senators. When he had finished reading this he looked up, ran his fingers through his hair, well silvered, though the brown then predominated; his beard was more whitened.

Page 244 §6.3

He threw himself around in the chair, one leg over the arm, and again spoke...

§6.4

Harvey visits Stanton, then returns to Lincoln, who is with another petitioner. The petitioner puts forth his request.

At this the President threw himself forward in his chair in such a manner as to show me the most curious, comical face in the world. *Lincoln tells one of his stories.* You should have seen Mr. Lincoln laugh – he laughed all over, and fully enjoyed the point if no one else did. The story, if not elegant, was certainly apropos. ...

Page 247: It was a saying at Washington when one met a petitioner, "Has Mr. Lincoln told you a story? If he has, it is all day with you. He never says 'yes' after a story."

Page 247 §6.5

Day 2 (Sept. 7)

I returned in the morning, full of hope, thinking of the pleasant face I had left the evening before, but no smile greeted me. The President was evidently annoyed by something, and waited for me to speak, which I did not do. ...

After a moment he said, "Well," with a peculiar contortion of face I never saw in anybody else.

Page 249 §6.6

While I was speaking the expression of Mr. Lincoln's face had changed many times. He had never taken his eye from me. Now every muscle in his face seemed to contract, and then suddenly expand. As he opened his mouth you could almost hear them snap as he said, "You assume to know more than I do," and closed his mouth as though he never expected to open it again, sort of slammed it to.

Harvey, though hurt, replies at length.

With the same snapping of muscle he again said, "You assume to know more than surgeons do."

Harvey again replies at length.

Page 250 §6.7

During the time I had been speaking Mr. Lincoln's brow had become very much contracted, and a severe scowl had settled over his whole face. *Lincoln makes a comment.* I did not reply. I had noticed the veins in his face filling full within a few moments, and one vein across his forehead was as large as my little finger, and it gave him a frightful look.

Soon, with a quick, impatient movement of his whole frame *a sharp reply came.* I was surprised at his lack of self-control, and I knew he did not mean one word of what he said, but what would come next? As I looked at him, I was troubled, fearing I had said something wrong. He was very pale.

§6

Page 251 §6.8

Harvey to Lincoln: "... if you will grant my petition you will be glad as long as you live." ...

The President bowed his head, and with a look of sadness I can never forget, said "I never shall be glad any more." All severity had passed from his face. He seemed looking backward and heartward, and for a moment he seemed to forget he was not alone; a more than mortal anguish rested on his face.

The spell must be broken, so I said, "Do not speak so, Mr. President. Who will have so much reason to rejoice when the government is restored, as it will be?"

"I know, I know," he said, placing a hand on each side and bowing forward, "but the springs of life are wearing away."

I asked if he felt his great cares were injuring his health.

"No," he replied, "not directly, perhaps."

I asked if he slept well, and he said he was never a good sleeper, and, of course, slept less now than ever before. He said the people did not yet appreciate the magnitude of this rebellion, and that it would be a long time before the end.

Page 252   §6.9

Day 3 (Sept. 8)

It was the first time I had noticed him standing. He was very tall and moved with a shuffling, awkward motion.

Lincoln grants her petition.

Page 254   §6.10

Day 4 (Sept. 9)

"Don't you ever get angry?" he asked, "I know a little woman not very unlike you who gets mad sometimes."

Lincoln writes a note saying a hospital should be named for her late husband [baslerA v6p439].*

Page 255   §6.11

He looked at me from under his eyebrows and said, "You almost think me handsome, don't you?"

His face then beamed with such kind benevolence and was lighted by such a pleasant smile that I looked at him, and with my usual impulse, said, clasping my hands together, "You are perfectly lovely to me now, Mr. Lincoln." He colored a little and laughed most heartily.

As I arose to go, he reached out his hand, that hand in which there was so much power and so little beauty, and held mine clasped and covered in his own. ... A silent prayer went up from my heart, "God bless you, Abraham Lincoln." I heard him say goodbye, and I was gone.

...

My impressions of him had been so varied, his character had assumed so many different phases, his very looks had changed so frequently and so entirely, that it almost seemed to me I had been conversing with half a dozen different men. He blended in his character the most yielding flexibility with the most unflinching firmness, child-like simplicity and weakness with statesmanlike wisdom and masterly strength, but over and around all was thrown the mantle of an unquestioned integrity.

---

* The annotation to [baslerA v6p439] may be erroneous. It dates a different, earlier note to Sept. 8, but Harvey's account would place it on Sept. 6.

Topic 7 – Shooting §7

This special topic contains first-person accounts of events inside Ford's Theatre and/or Peterson House (where Lincoln was taken to die), reports of the autopsy, and a reprint of the medical journal article [taft] that described Lincoln's medical course. This collection is a sliver of the enormous material available on Lincoln's death. The ⸤Death⸥ (¶544ff) and ⸤Post-Mortem⸥ (¶3240ff) sections contain additional relevant information.

(a) Before the Cry for Help §7a

There were some 2000 people in the theater [kunhardtB p108]. It was drafty in Lincoln's box [helmB p257].

The assassin was already in the box when Lincoln spotted General Burnside in the audience below and leaned forward for a better look. Lincoln may have seen or otherwise sensed something behind him, "for all of a sudden his head turned sharply to the left" [kunhardtA p355].

"Placing a small Derringer-style pistol 'close to the President's head – actually into contact with it – [the assassin] fired' " [kunhardtA p353]. The nearly half-inch-diameter bullet was "exceedingly hard" – a mixture of antimony, tin, copper, and lead [kunhardtA p355]. It entered behind Lincoln's left ear [kunhardtA p355].

There are at least three versions of what happened after the assassin pulled the trigger:
1. "Lincoln was propelled forward, his forehead striking the rail. Mrs. Lincoln's very first reaction was that he was pitching headfirst over the railing. She grabbed at him and held him up, and Lincoln's head slumped to the right, his chin resting on his chest as if he were dozing." [kunhardtA p353]
2. "Lincoln threw up his right arm at the impact of the shot and Mrs. Lincoln instinctively caught him around the neck to keep him upright." [kunhardtB p39]
3. Major Henry Rathbone was sitting in the box with Lincoln. He recalled grappling with the assassin, "then turned to the President; his position was not changed; his head was slightly bent forward, and his eyes were closed. I saw that he was unconscious..." [pitman p73]

(b) Dr. Charles Leale's Account – 1867 Version [good pp59-62] §7b

The account below was written in 1867, based on 1865 notes. The account in §7c is similar, but presents professional language and details. ¶3227 lists other Leale writings.

On the evening of the 14th April 1865 while engaged with the execution duties of the United States Army General Hospital "Armory Square" Washington I was requested to visit Ford's Theatre, being told that the President Lincoln, General Grant and Staff were to be there.

I arrived at the theatre about 8 1/4 pm and endeavored to procure a seat in the orchestra but it being so densely crowded I left it for the dress circle where I found a vacant seat on the same side and within 40 feet of the President's box, the play was then progressing and in a few minutes I saw the President, Mrs. Lincoln, Major Rathbone, and Miss Harris enter, the play ceased for a short time and as soon as they were seen by the audience they were cheered which was responded by the president with a smile and a bow. The President as he proceeded to the box looked expressively mournful and sad.

The door of the box was opened by an usher who proceeded them but who after they had all entered closed the door then took a seat near by for himself. All parts of the theatre were well filled and the play of our American Cousin was progressing very pleasantly until about 5 minutes past 10 when on looking towards the box I saw a man speaking with another

§7

near the door and endeavoring to enter, which he at last succeeded in doing after which the door was closed.

I again looked toward the stage and was pleased with the amusing part then being performed, but soon heard the report of a pistol, and about a minute or two after I saw a man with dark hair and bright black eyes, leap from the box to the stage below, while descending he threw himself a little forward and raised his shining dagger in the air, which reflected the light as though it had been a diamond, when he struck the stage he stumbled a little forward but with a bound regained the use of his limbs and ran to the opposite side of the stage soon disappearing behind the scenes. I then heard cries that the President had been murdered which were followed by those of "Kill the murderer" "Shoot him" etc which came from different parts of the audience.

I remained in my seat [not?] believing it until I saw some one open the door of the box, and heard him call for a Surgeon and help.

I arrived at the door of the box, and upon saying that I was a surgeon was immediately admitted.

When I entered the box, Mr. Lincoln was sitting in a high backed armchair with his head leaning towards his right-side and which was supported by Mrs. Lincoln who was weeping bitterly. Miss Harris was at her left-side behind the President, Major Rathbone was at the door of the box.

While approaching the President I was told that he had been murdered, and I sent for some Brandy and water.

Upon Mrs. Lincoln being told that I was a Surgeon she said, "Oh Doctor do what you can for my dear husband" "do what you can for him and for Dr. Stone." [sic]

I told her that I would do all which was in my power to do.

When I reached the President he was almost dead, his eyes were closed he was parallel [sic]. I placed my finger on his right radial pulse, but could feel no movement of the artery. His breathing was exceedingly stertorous there being long intervals between each inspiration and he was in a most profoundly comatosed condition.

With the assistance of two gentlemen I immediately placed him in a recumbent position while doing this and holding his head and shoulders my hand came in contact with blood on his left-shoulder, the thought of the dagger then recuffed to me, and supposed that he might have been stabbed in the subclavical artery or some of its branches. I asked a gentleman near by to cut his coat and shirt off that shoulder to enable me if possible to check the supposed hemorrhage, as soon as his arm was bared to a distance below the shoulder, and I saw that there was no wound there, I lifted his eyelids and examined his eyes, the pupil of which was dilated. I then examined his head and soon discovered a large firm clot of blood situated about one inch below the superior curved line and an inch and a half to the left of the median line of the occipital bone.

The coagnin which was firmly matted with the hair [was] removed [I] passed the little finger of my left hand directly through the perfectly smooth opening made by the ball, he was then apparently dead.

When I removed my finger which I used as a knife an oozing of blood followed and he commenced, to show signs of improvement.

I believe that he would not have lived five minutes longer if the pressure on the brain had not been relieved and if he had been left that much longer in the sitting posture.

The Brandy and water, now arrived and I put a small quantity into his mouth which was the only thing that passed into his stomach from his assassination until his death.

Dr. C.S. Taft and Dr. A.F.A. King now arrived, and after a moments consultation we agreed to remove him.

While in the theatre, I was several times asked the nature of the wound and said that the ball had lodged in the encephalens and that it was a mortal wound.

We now commenced to remove him carefully descending the steps first while supporting his head and shoulders as soon as we arrived at the door of the box, I saw that the passage was densely crowded by those coming towards that part of the theatre.

I called out twice "Guards clear the passage" which was so rapidly done that we proceeded without a moments delay towards the stairs leading to the hall which is entered from the street, when we arrived at the head of the stairs we turned around those holding his lower extremities descending first.

There was an officer present who rendered great assistance in making the passage through the crowd.

When we arrived to the street I was asked to place him in a carriage and remove him to the White House this I refused to do being fearful that he would die as soon as he would be placed in an upright position. I said that I wished to take him to the nearest house and place him comfortably in bed.

We slowly crossed the street there being a barrier of men on each side of an open passage towards the house. Those who went ahead of us reported that the house directly opposite was closed.

I saw a man standing at the door of Mr. Peterson's [sic] house and beckoning us to enter which we did and immediately placed him in bed, all of which was done in less than twenty minutes from the time that he had been assassinated we not having been in the slightest interrupted while removing him. ...

(c) Dr. Charles Leale's Account – Official Report, 1865   §7c

These are excerpts from Leale's undated, handwritten report to the Surgeon General, presumably written soon after the shooting. A photostatic copy is in [barbeeP - box 2 folder 137]. The account in §7b is similar, but eschews professional language and details.

When I reached the President he was in a state of general paralysis; his eyes were closed and he was in a profoundly comatose condition, while his breathing was intermittent and exceedingly stertorous. I placed my finger on his right radial pulse but could perceive no movement of the artery.

I commenced to examine his head (as no wound near the shoulder was found) and soon passed my fingers over a large firm clot of blood, situated about one inch below the superior curved line of the occipital bone and an inch and a half to the left of the median line of the same bone. The coagula I easily removed and passed the little finger of my left hand through the perfectly smooth opening made by the ball and found that it had entered the encephalon. As soon as I removed my finger a slight oozing of blood followed and his breathing became more regular and less stertorous. The brandy and water now arrived and a small quantity was placed in his mouth, which passed into his stomach where it was retained.

...

... he was placed in bed in the house of Mr Peterson opposite the theatre in less than 20 minutes from the time that he was assassinated.

...

...we placed the President in bed in a diagonal position; as the bed was too short a part of the foot was removed to enable us to place him in a comfortable position.

...

... As soon as we placed him in bed, we removed his clothes and covered him with blankets. While covering him I found his lower extremities very cold from his feet to a distance several inches above his knees. I then sent for bottles of hot water and hot blankets which we applied to his lower extremities and abdomen.

§7

When the President was first laid in bed, a slight ecchymosis was noticed on his left eyelid and the pupil of that eye was slightly dilated, while the pupil of the right eye was contracted. About 11 P.M. the right eye began to protrude which was rapidly followed by an increase of the ecchymosis until it encircled the orbit above the supra orbital ridge and below the infra orbital foramen.

The wound was kept open by the Surgeon General by means of a silver probe and as the President was placed diagonally on the bed his head was supported in its position by Surgeon Crane and Dr. Taft *illegible*.

[About 2 a.m. the wound is probed]

His pulse which was several times counted by Dr Taft and noted by Dr King, ranged until 12 P.M. [sic] from between 40 to 64 beats per minute, and his respiration about 24 per minute, were loud and stertorous. At 1 A.M. his pulse suddenly increased in frequency to 100 per minute, but soon diminished gradually becoming less feeble [sic] until 2.54 A.M. when it was 48 and barely perceptible. At 6.40 A.M. his pulse could not be counted, it being very intermittent, two or three pulsations being felt and followed by an intermission, when not the slightest movement of the artery could be felt. The inspiration now became very short and the expirations very prolonged and labored accompanied by a guttural sound. 6.50 A.M. The respirations cease for some time and all eagerly looked at their watches until the profound silence is disturbed by a prolonged inspiration which was followed by a sonorous[?] expiration.

...

At 7.20 A.M. he breathed his last...

(d) Dr. Charles Taft's Account   [good pp62-64]   §7d

¶3227 lists other Taft writings. Taft's narrative apparently changed over years. Writing in 1922, [markens] notes: "Dr. Taft asserts he was the first to respond to the call for a surgeon in the theatre, claims credit for much of the treatment described by Leale as his, and declares that he was there all through the night and felt the last throb as the President passed away; contrary to the statement of others that he was then absent."

[markens] continues about Dr. Taft: "Parenthetically, it may be said that his widow offered to sell the father of the writer of this article a pair of Lincoln's cuff buttons and her son offered to sell a lock of Lincoln's hair, acquired by her husband after the President died."

The notes from which this article is written were made the day succeeding Mr. Lincoln's death, and immediately after the official examination of the body. They were made, by direction of Secretary Stanton for the purpose of preserving an official account of the circumstances attending the assassination, in connection with the medical aspects of the case.

On the fourth anniversary of the fall of Fort Sumter, the beloved President, his great heart filled with peaceful thoughts and charity for all, entered Ford's Theater amid the acclamations of the loyal multitude assembled to greet him. Mr. Lincoln sat in a high-backed upholstered chair in the corner of the box nearest the audience, and only his left profile was visible to most of the audience from where I sat, almost under the box, in the front row of orchestra chairs, I plainly saw that Mrs. Lincoln rested her hand on his knee much of the time, and often called his attention to some humorous situation on the stage. She seemed to take great pleasure witnessing his enjoyment.

All went on pleasantly until half-past ten o'clock when during the second scene of the third act, the sharp report of a pistol rang through the house. The report seemed to proceed from behind the President's box. While it startled every one in the audience, it was evidently accepted by all as an introductory effect preceding some new situation in the play, several of which had been introduced in the earlier parr of the performance. A moment afterward a hatless and white-faced man leaped from the front of the President's box down twelve feet to the stage. As he jumped, one of the spurs on his riding-boots caught in the folds of the flag dropped over the front, and caused him to fall partly on his hands and knees as he struck the stage. Springing quickly to his feet with the suppleness of an athlete, he faced the audience for a moment as he brandished in his right hand a long knife, and shouted "Sic Semper Tyrannis!" Then, with a rapid stage stride, he crossed the stage, and disappeared from view. A piercing shriek from the President's box, a repeated call for "Water! water!" and "A surgeon!" in quick succession, conveyed the truth to the almost paralyzed audience. A most terrible scene of excitement followed. With loud shouts of "Kill him!" "Lynch him!" part of the audience stampeded toward the entrance and some to the stage.

I leaped from the top of the orchestra railing in front of me upon the stage, and, announcing myself as an army surgeon, was immediately lifted up to the President's box by several gentleman who had collected beneath. I happened to be in uniform, having passed the entire day in attending to my duties at the Signal Camp of Instruction in Georgetown, and not having had an opportunity to change my dress. The cape of a military overcoat fastened around my neck became detached in clambering into the box, and fell upon the stage. It was taken to police headquarters, together with the assassin's cap, spur, and deringer, which had also been picked up, under the supposition that it belonged to him. It was recovered, weeks afterward, with much difficulty.

When I entered the box, the President was lying upon the floor surrounded by his wailing wife and several gentlemen who had entered from the private stairway and dress circle. Assistant Surgeon Charles A. Leale, U.S.V., was in the box, and had caused the coat and waistcoat to be cut off in searching for the wound. Dr. A.F.A. King of Washington was also present, and assisted in the examination. The carriage had been ordered to remove the President to the White House, but the surgeons countermanded the order, and he was removed to a bed in a house opposite the theater.

(e) Account of Maunsell Field [NYTimes - April 17, 1865] §7e

Field was a sub-cabinet official who was admitted to Lincoln's room between 3 and 4 a.m.

The bed was a double one, and I found the President lying diagonally across it, with his head at the outside. The pillows were saturated with blood, and there was considerable blood upon the floor immediately under him. There was a patchwork coverlet thrown over the President, which was only so far removed, from time to time, as to enable the physicians in attendance to feel the arteries in the neck or the heart, and he appeared to have been divested of all clothing. His eyes were closed and injected with blood, both the lids and the portion surrounding the eyes being as black as if they had been bruised by violence. He was breathing regularly, but with effort, and did not seem to be struggling or suffering.

Paragraph describes who was in the room.

For several hours the breathing above described continued regularly, and apparently without pain or consciousness. But about 7 o'clock a change occurred, and the breathing, which had been continuous, was interrupted at intervals. These intervals became more frequent and of longer duration, and the breathing more feeble. Several times the interval was so long that we thought him dead, and the surgeon applied his finger to the pulse, evidently to ascertain if such was the fact. But it was not till 22 minutes past 7 o'clock in the morning that the flame flickered out. There was no apparent suffering, no convulsive action, no rattling of the throat, none of the ordinary premonitory symptoms of death. Death in this case was a mere cessation of breathing.

§7

Prayer is offered. The President's eyes after death were not, particularly the right one, entirely closed. I closed them myself with my fingers ... In a very short time the haw commenced slightly falling, although the body was still warm. I called attention to this, and had it immediately tied up with a pocket handkerchief. The expression immediately after death was purely negative, but in fifteen minutes there came over the mouth, the nostrils, and the chin, a smile that seemed almost an effort of life. I had never seen upon the President's face an expression more genial and pleasing. The body grew cold very gradually, and I left the room before it had entirely stiffened.

(f) Autopsy – Official Report §7f

From a typed transcript in [barbeeP - box 2 folder 108], *which cites "War Department Records – National Archives."*

Surgeon General's Office
Washington, D. C.
April 15, 1865

Brig. Gen. J. K. Barnes,
Surgeon General, USA,

General:

I have the honor to report that in obedience to your orders, and aided by Asst. Surg. E. Curtis USA, I made in your presence, at 12 o'clock this morning an autopsy on the body of President Abraham Lincoln, with the following results:

The eyelids and surrounding parts of the face were greatly echymosed [sic] and the eyes somewhat protuberant from effusion of blood into the orbits.

There was a gunshot wound of the head, around which the scalp was greatly thickened by hemorrhage into its tissues. The ball entered through the occipital bone about an inch to the left of the median line and just above the left lateral sinus, which it opened. It then penetrated the dura mater, passed through the left posterior lobe of the cerebrum, entered the left lateral ventricle and lodged in the white matter of the cerebrum just above the anterior portion of the left corpus striatum, where it was found.

The wound in the occipital bone was quite smooth, circular in shape, with beveled edges, the opening through the internal table being larger than that through the external table. The track of the ball was full of clotted blood and contained several little fragments of bone, with a small piece of the ball near its external orifice. The brain around the track was pultaceous [sic] and livid from capillary hemorrhage into its substance. The ventricles of the brain were full of clotted blood. A thick clot beneath the dura mater coated the right cerebral lobe.

There was a smaller clot under the dura mater of the left side. But little blood was found at the base of the brain. Both the orbital plates of the frontal bone were fractured, and the fragments pushed up towards the brain. The dura mater over these fractures was uninjured. The orbits gorged with blood.

I have the honor to be

Very Respectfully
Your Obt Servt
J. J. Woodward
Asst. Surgn, USA

(g) Autopsy – Press Account of Results [NYTimes - April 17, 1865] §7g

The external appearance of the face was that of a deep black stain about both eyes. Otherwise the face was very natural.

440

The wound was on the left side of the head behind, on a line with and three inches from the left ear.

The course of the ball was obliquely forward, toward the right eye, crossing the brain obliquely a few inches behind the eye, where the ball lodged.

In the track of the wound were found fragments of the bone which had been driven forward by the ball.

The ball was found imbedded in the anterior lobe of the west hemisphere of the brain.

The orbit plates of both eyes were the seat of comminuted fracture, and the orbits of the eyes were filled with extravasated blood.

The serious injury to the orbit plates was due to the contre coup, the result of the intense shock of so large a projectile fired so closely to the head. ...

A shaving of lead had been removed from the ball in its passage of the bones of the skull, and was found in the orifice of the wound. The first fragment of bone was found two and a half inches within the brain: the second and larger fragment about four inches from the orifice. The ball lay still further in advance. The wound was half an inch in diameter. ...

Did pre-mortem probing by the physicians advance the bone fragments?

The remains have been embalmed.

(h) Miscellaneous Aspects of Assassination §7h

- Leale straddled Lincoln's body, bent forward, opened Lincoln's mouth, pressed down and forward on the back of the tongue, then began to push with his hands up against the diaphragm (having instructed Taft to raise and lower the arms) then began massaging near the heart. [kunhardtB p42] [shutes p112]

- No less than 80 death threats were afterwards found, filed in a particular pigeonhole, in Lincoln's desk [shutesE p184]. As early as June 21, 1860 Lincoln spoke of various attempts on his life [lincloreHDE].

- For a compilation of trauma Lincoln suffered, see ¶3560ff.

(i) Journal Article Reprint §7i

The reprint of [taft] *begins on the next page.*

§7

452   EDITORIAL.   [Vol. XII.

MEDICAL AND SURGICAL REPORTER.

PHILADELPHIA, APRIL 22, 1865.

MURDER OF PRESIDENT LINCOLN.

Last Saturday morning the telegraphic wires carried mournful news over the land. The nation was in the midst of rejoicings at the prospect of a termination of our civil strife, and the speedy advent of peace. The whole country was clad in the garments of joy, and every face wore an expression of gladness. The bells, from Maine to California, and from the Lakes to the Gulf, pealed forth tones of exultation as better and still better news arrived. It was remarked that there was a surfeit of joy. Alas! the nation little thought how in one hour her joy would be changed to the most poignant grief, and a dark shadow be cast over her emblems of rejoicing! Time paused in his westward flight, and started back appalled, as swifter than "the wings of the morning," the electric current flashed the mournful intelligence from the Atlantic to the shores of the broad Pacific, that on Friday night, ABRAHAM LINCOLN, the beloved Chief Magistrate of the land, had fallen at the hands of an assassin. The fatal wound was given by a pistol ball which entered the brain. The President lingered in an insensible, dying condition, for several hours, and died at twenty-two minutes past seven o'clock, on Saturday morning, the 15th inst.

THE NATION MOURNS! But the dispensation of Providence that has thus shrouded the land in the habiliments of grief, has called forth almost universal expressions of trust in Him who "doeth according to His will in the armies of heaven, and among the inhabitants of the earth."

Surgeon-General BARNES, with other medical men, was in attendance upon the President during his last hours, and a *post-mortem* was made. Appended will be found a detailed account of the sad event, with the progress of the symptoms, and an account of the *post-mortem*. It was prepared for our columns by Dr. C. S. TAFT, A. A. Surgeon, U. S. A.

LAST HOURS OF ABRAHAM LINCOLN.

BY C. S. TAFT, ACT'G ASS'T SURG. U. S. A.

The following brief report of the circumstances attending the assassination, last hours, and autopsy of the late President, will doubtless prove of much interest to the profession, and may be relied upon as correct in all particulars, the notes from which it is written having been submitted to comparison with others taken, and corrected by the highest authority.

While sitting in an orchestra chair at Ford's Theatre, on Friday evening, the 14th inst., about 10.30 P. M., I heard the sharp report of a pistol in the direction of the State box, and turning my head in that direction, saw a wild looking man jump from the box to the stage, heard him shout " *Sic semper tyrannis*," as he brandished a glittering knife in his right hand for an instant, and dart across the stage from sight.

A few moments of utterly indescribable confusion followed, amid which I heard a call for a surgeon. I leaped upon the stage, and was instantly lifted by a dozen pair of hands up to the President's box, a distance of twelve feet from the stage.

When I entered the box, the President was lying upon the floor, surrounded by his wailing wife and several gentlemen who had entered from the dress-circle. The respiration was inaudible and scarcely perceptible, and he was totally insensible. Ass't Surgeon CHARLES A. LEALE, U. S. V., was in the box, and had caused the coat and vest to be cut off, in searching for the wound. The wound in the head was soon found, but at that time there was no oozing from it.

Several gentlemen in the box were insisting upon having the President removed to his home, but Dr. LEALE and myself protested against such a proceeding, and insisted upon upon his being carried to the nearest house. He was removed to a house opposite, and laid upon a bed in fifteen minutes from the time the shot was fired.

The wound was there examined, the finger being used as a probe, and the ball found to have passed beyond the reach of the finger into the brain. I put a teaspoonful of diluted brandy between the lips, which was swallowed with much difficulty; a half-teaspoonful administered ten minutes afterward, was retained in the throat, without any effort being made to swallow it. The respiration now became labored; pulse 44, feeble, eyes entirely closed, the left pupil much contracted, the right widely dilated; total insensibility to light in both.

Surgeon-General BARNES and ROBERT K. STONE, M. D., the family physician, arrived and took charge of the case. At their suggestion, I administered a few drops of brandy, to determine whether it could be swallowed, but as it was not, no further attempt was made. The left upper eyelid was swollen and dark from effused blood; this was observed a few minutes after his removal from the theatre. About thirty minutes after he was placed upon the bed, discoloration from effusion began in the internal canthus of the right eye, which became rapidly discolored and swollen with great protrusion of the eye.

About 11.30 P. M., twitching of the facial muscles of the left side set in and continued some fifteen or twenty minutes, and the mouth was drawn slightly to the same side. Sinapisms over the entire anterior surface of the body were ordered, together with artificial heat to the extremities.

The wound began to ooze very soon after the patient was placed upon the bed, and continued to discharge blood and brain tissue until 5.30 A.M., when it ceased entirely; the head, in the meantime, being supported in such a position as to facilitate the discharge. The only surgical aid that could be rendered, consisted in maintaining the head in such a position as to facilitate the discharge of the wound, and in keeping the orifice free from coagulum.

Col. CRANE, Surgeon, U. S, A., had charge of the head during a great part of the time, being relieved at intervals in this duty by myself. While the wound was discharging freely, the respiration was easy; but the moment the discharge was arrested from any cause, it became at once labored.

It was also remarkable to observe the great difference in the character of the pulse whenever the orifice of the wound was freed from coagulum, and discharged freely; thus relieving, in a measure, the compression. This fact will account for the fluctuations in the pulse, as given in the subjoined notes.

About 2 A. M., an ordinary silver probe was introduced into the wound by the Surgeon-General. It met an obstruction about three inches from the external orifice, which was decided to be the plug of bone driven in from the skull and lodged in the track of the ball. The probe passed by this obstruction, but was too short to follow the track the whole length. A long Nélaton probe was then procured and passed into the track of the wound for a distance of two inches beyond the plug of bone, when the ball was distinctly felt; passing beyond this, the fragments

of the orbital plate of the left orbit were felt. The ball made no mark upon the porcelain tip, and was afterwards found to be of exceedingly hard lead.

Some difference of opinion existed as to the exact position of the ball, but the autopsy confirmed the correctness of the diagnosis upon first exploration. No further attempt was made to explore the wound.

After the cessation of the bleeding from the wound, the respiration was stertorous up to the last breath, which was drawn at twenty-one minutes and fifty-five seconds past seven; the heart did not cease to beat until twenty-two minutes and ten seconds past seven. My hand was upon the heart, and my eye on the watch of the Surgeon-General, who was standing by my side, with his finger on the carotid.

The decubitus during the whole time was dorsal, and the position on the bed diagonal; the length of the bedstead not admitting of any other position.

The respiration during the last thirty minutes was characterized by occasional intermissions; no respiration being made for nearly a minute, but by a convulsive effort air would gain admission to the lungs, when regular, though stertorous, respiration would go on for some seconds, to be followed by another period of perfect repose.

At these times the death-like stillness and suspense were thrilling. The Cabinet ministers, and others surrounding the death-bed, watching, with suspended breath, the last feeble inspiration, and as the unbroken quiet would seem to prove that life had fled, turn their eyes to their watches; then as the struggling life within would force another fluttering respiration, heave deep sighs of relief, and fix their eyes once more upon the face of their dying chief.

The wonderful vitality exhibited by the late President, was one of the most interesting and remarkable circumstances connected with the case. It was the opinion of the surgeons in charge, that most patients would have died in two hours from the reception of such an injury, yet Mr. LINCOLN lived from 10.30, P. M., until 7.22, A. M.

The following observations of the pulse and respiration were noted down by Dr. A. F. A. KING, at the bed-side, and are correct. The pulse was counted by Acting Ass't Surgeon FORD.

10.55—48.
11.06—45.
11.18—42, and weaker.
11.24—42, respirations, 27 per minute, breathing quiet.
11.26— irregular, intermits occasionally.
11.30—45, resp. more frequent and vigorous.

§7

11.32—45, stronger, resp. much more strong and stertorous.

11.37—48, resp. again silent and more feeble.

11.40—45.

11.43—45, resp. stertorous.

11.47—45, resp. 24, stertorous.

11.56—48, weaker.

12.10—48, irregularly intermittent.

12.18—48, same character.

12.27—54.

12.28—60.

12.29—66, intermittent.

12.38—66.

12.45—69, intermittent.

12.49—84, resp. 28.

12.56—66.

1.00—100.

1.15—92.

1.30—95.

2.10—60, resp. 34.

2.19—58.

2.32—54.

2.37—48.

2.54—48, much weaker, more thready; respirations feeble.

4.18—60, resp. 27, strong and stertorous.

5.40—64, thready, resp. 27.

6.10—60, hardly perceptible, (Barnes), resp. 26, sterterous.

6.25—thready, not counted; resp. 22; inspirations jerking.

6.40—inspirations short and feeble; expirations prolonged, and groaning; a deep, softly sonorous, cooing sound at the end of each expiration, audible to bystanders.

6.45—respiration uneasy, choking and grunting; lower jaw relaxed; mouth open; a minute without a breath; face getting dark.

6.59—breathes again a little more at intervals; another long pause.

7.00—still breathing at long pauses.

7.20—died.

About 1, P. M., spasmodic constractions of the muscles came on, causing pronation of the forearms; the pectoral muscles seemed to be fixed, the breath was held during the spasm, and a sudden and forcible expiration immediately succeeded it.

At about the same time both pupils became widely dilated, and remained so until death.

During the night Drs. HALL, MAY, LIEBERMANN, and nearly all the leading men of the profession in the city, tendered their services.

AUTOPSY; FIVE HOURS AFTER DEATH.

Present, Surgeon-General BARNES, Col. CRANE, Dr. STONE, Ass't Surg. WOODWARD, U. S. A., Ass't Surg. CURTIS, U. S. A., Ass't Surg. NOTSON, U. S. A., and Act'g Ass't Surg. TAFT, U. S. A.

The calvaria was removed, the brain exposed, and sliced down to the track of the ball, which was plainly indicated by a line of coagulated blood, extending from the external wound in the occipi-

tal bone, obliquely across from the left to right through the brain to the anterior lobe of the cerebrum, immediately behind the right orbit. The surface of the right hemisphere was covered with coagulated blood. After removing the brain from the cranium, the ball dropped from its lodgment in the anterior lobe. A small piece of the ball evidently cut off in its passage through the occipital bone, was previously taken out of the track of the ball, about four inches from the external wound. The hole made through the occipital bone was as cleanly cut as if done with a punch.

The point of entrance was one inch to the left of the longitudinal sinus, and opening into the lateral sinus. The ball was flattened, convex on both sides, and evidently moulded by hand in a Derringer pistol mould, as indicated by the ridged surface left by the nippers in clipping off the neck.

The orbital plates of *both* orbits were the seats of comminuted fracture, the fragments being forced inward, and the dura-mater covering them remaining uninjured. The double fracture was decided to have been caused by *contre coup*. The plug of bone driven in from the occipital bone, was found in the track of the ball, about three inches from the external wound, proving the correctness of the opinion advanced by the Surgeon-General and Dr. STONE as to its nature, at the exploration of the wound before death.

The ball and fragments, together with the fragments of the orbital plates and plug from the occipital bone, were placed in the possession of Dr. STONE, the family physician, who marked and delivered them, pursuant to instructions, to the Secretary of State, who sealed them up with his private seal. The *Nélaton* probe used was also marked by me, and sealed up in like manner.

News and Miscellany.

American Medical Association.

At a late meeting of the *Philadelphia County Medical Society*, the following Delegates were elected to represent it at the *Sixteenth* annual meeting of the American Medical Association, which will be held in the city of Boston, on Tuesday, the 6th day of June next:

Dr. Robert Burns,	Dr. Jno. Bell,
" James M. Corse,	" Joseph R. Coad,
" D. Francis Condie,	" Levi Curtis,
" Wm. Darrach,	" A. Frické,
" A. W. Griffiths,	" N. L. Hatfield,
" H. Lenox Hodge,	" Wm. L. Knight,
" Wm. Mayburry,	" G. H. Robinett,
" Winthrop Sargent,	" Wilson Jewell.

Topic 8 – Gait §8

This special topic is somewhat different from the others. It includes a draft chapter written for The Physical Lincoln, but not used there, and portions of an unpublished article about Lincoln's gait. Both were written before I linked certain characteristics of his gait with muscular hypotonia (¶3580). This discovery does not have too much effect on the unused chapter, but the article was too much trouble to revise.

The introduction from the article is presented first. It is somewhat technical. The chapter, which is non-technical, is presented next. Following that are portions of the article not covered by the chapter.

(a) Article: Introduction §8a

In 1994 [ranum] reported that an autosomal dominant disorder, type 5 spinocerebellar ataxia (SCA5) (OMIM 600224), occurred in 56 of 170 examined descendants of President Abraham Lincoln's paternal grandparents.

They hypothesized that Lincoln may himself have had SCA5, based on: (a) He had a 25% "prior probability" of inheriting the disease-causing gene variant from a grandparent, (b) His age at death, 56, was within the range of disease onset seen in the kindred, and (c) His gait was unusual and, according to one eyewitness, "shambling." Ranum et al concluded that, "if President Lincoln had inherited the ataxia gene, his symptoms could have been very mild or as yet undeveloped at the time of his death" [ranum].

Notwithstanding a report in 1997 that Lincoln's handwriting showed no signs of ataxia [nee], Lincoln continues to be mentioned in connection with SCA5 [hirschhornD]. When variants of the beta III spectrin gene were found in 2006 to cause SCA5, it was opined that "determining President Lincoln's status relative to SCA5 would be of historical interest" [aa52]. One investigator declared intent to "pursue a DNA test if the opportunity arose" [forliti]. Although a 2007 scientific publication noted simply that SCA5 ran in Lincoln's family [aa46], the popular press printed less guarded quotes from the investigators, e.g.: "Were Lincoln's nerves shattered? We don't know, but our study raises the possibility that they were" [aa10].

Because the medical literature contains little information bearing on the possibility Lincoln had SCA5, I reviewed the Lincoln historical literature for signs and symptoms pertaining to the disorder. I conclude that President Abraham Lincoln did not have SCA5.

(b) Unused Chapter From "The Physical Lincoln" §8b

Physicians have, with varying success, tried to pin several genetic diagnoses on Abraham Lincoln. So far we have discussed Marfan syndrome, MASS phenotype, MEN2B, color deficiency, and, trivially, cleft chin. There is one more to go.

* * *

For many years researchers at the University of Minnesota have been studying a genetic disease called "spinocerebellar ataxia type 5," mercifully abbreviated to "SCA5."

The full name is informative, however. *Ataxia* means loss of muscular coordination. *Spinocerebellar* refers to the two parts of the nervous system that malfunction in the disease: the spinal cord and the cerebellum. And *type 5* communicates that several diseases resemble this one. (SCA type 28 was discovered in 2006.)

Ataxia may develop in any activity that requires coordination between muscles. Walking is the best example. As any robot designer will tell you – with some frustration – walking is a very complicated process that easily goes awry if leg movements are not precisely coordinated. Talking, eye motions, and handwriting also require considerable muscular coordination. §8

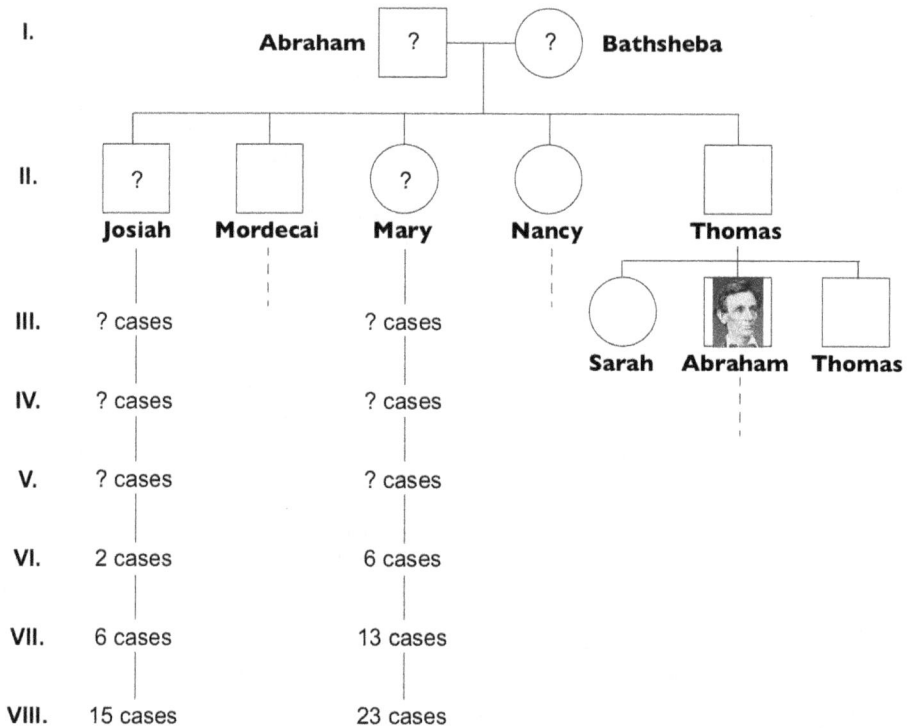

Figure 8-1. SCA5 in Lincoln's relatives. This extended family tree shows the relationship between Abraham Lincoln and his distant cousins who were afflicted with spinocerebellar ataxia type 5 (SCA5). This genetic disorder causes difficulty with muscular coordination, especially walking. Researchers who study SCA5 have questioned whether Lincoln himself had the disease, because: (1) Lincoln' s paternal grandparents, shown as generation I, were ancestors of all the cases of SCA5 found in generations VI and beyond, making it reasonable to assume one of these grandparents had SCA5, and (2) Lincoln had an unusual gait. Key: Generations are numbered with Roman numerals at left. Squares are males, circles are females. A "case" is a person with SCA5. For generations III and later, the number of cases of SCA5 is shown for descendants of Josiah and Mary. It is unknown if any cases occurred in generations I throught V (indicated by "?"). Over 800 descendants of Josiah and Mary are known; generations III and beyond are not shown in detail. Descendants of Mordecai, Nancy, and President Lincoln are not shown.

When a person is *ataxic*, it means he or she performs one or more of these functions clumsily – if at all. Neurologists therefore speak of ataxic gait, ataxic speech, ataxic writing, and so on.

* * *

In 1994 the Minnesota researchers reported that 96 cousins of Abraham Lincoln had SCA5 (see Fig. 8-1) [ranum]. In these cousins – all descended from the parents of President Lincoln's father – the first symptom of SCA5 was, variously, gait disturbance, incoordination of the upper limbs, or slurred speech. Symptoms typically appeared in the patient's 20s or

30s and progressed over decades without shortening life. The latest age of onset was 68.

Naturally, the researchers wondered if President Lincoln had SCA5, too. Their 1994 analysis was quite brief, saying only that, if bloodlines alone were considered, Lincoln's odds of having the disease were one in four. They based this number on the *assumption* that one of Lincoln's father's parents had SCA5.*

The assumption that Lincoln's paternal grandparents had SCA5 provides the simplest explanation for the pattern of disease seen in Lincoln's family tree (Fig. 8-1). Because SCA5 is a rare condition, it is very unlikely that two branches of the same family (headed by Josiah and Mary, respectively) would carry the disease-causing gene unless the gene entered both branches through a common ancestor.

This "common ancestor" assumption is perfectly reasonable, but the researchers did not mention the possibility that an *additional* common ancestor might unite the two branches of the family, and that this additional common ancestor may have been the one to introduce SCA5 into the Lincoln family.

Fig. 8-1 shows that the earliest Lincolns *known* to have SCA5 were in generation VI. The researchers published no direct evidence that members of earlier generations had SCA5. Thus, *any* common ancestor of the members of generation VI could explain the pattern of disease in Fig. 8-1 just as well as if Bathsheba Herring Lincoln or her husband had SCA5.

There is no shortage of candidates for an additional common ancestor. Each member of generation VI will have 2 parents in generation V, 4 grandparents in generation IV, 8 great-grandparents in generation III, 16 great-great-grandparents in generation II, 32 great-great-great-grandparents in generation I, and so on. Clearly, it would take a great deal of genealogical research to rule out the presence of an additional common ancestor.

Overall, therefore, the bloodline-odds argument is not that helpful. At best, it tells us only that we should consider the possibility Lincoln had SCA5, as opposed to the tens of thousands of other genetic conditions that humans may carry.

The next step is to examine historical records to see if anything about Lincoln or his close relatives points strongly toward, or away from, SCA5.

* * *

SCA5 has autosomal dominant genetics. That is, like Marfan syndrome and MEN2B, it does not skip generations. So, if one of Lincoln's grandparents did introduce the disease-causing gene into the two branches of the family, then his or her children – Lincoln's Uncle Josiah and Aunt Mary in generation II in Fig. 8-1 – would both have had to possess the gene and pass it down to generation III.

Unfortunately, there is little immediately accessible information about Uncle Josiah, Aunt Mary, or Grandfather Abraham [¶5786, ¶5830,¶5811, respectively]. We simply have no information to tell if any of them had signs or symptoms compatible with SCA5.*

---

* The odds were calculated as follows: The chance that the afflicted grandparent would pass the disease-causing gene to Lincoln's father was 50:50 – that is, one in two. The chance that Lincoln's father would then pass the disease-causing gene to Lincoln is again one in two. Both passages would have to occur for Lincoln to develop SCA5, so the final odds are one-in-two times one-in-two, which is one-in-four.

* ○○○ *Project:* It may be relatively easy to discover clinically helpful information about Lincoln's Uncle Josiah and Aunt Mary. A 1930 genealogy [lincolnW] lists their immediate descendants. Presumably the University of Minnesota researchers have sought such information, too, but untapped sources, such as local municipal records, may – as in the case of Bathsheba Lincoln – be revealing. Note, however, because the researchers wanted to protect the privacy of their living subjects, they concealed the structure of generations III and IV and deliberately introduced errors in later generations.

§8

The evidence relating to Lincoln's paternal grandmother, however, is more alluring.** It has been reported that Bathsheba Lincoln was an invalid in her 30s and that she lived into her 90s [nee]. Both of these facts are compatible with SCA5.

Fig. 8-2, which shows a sample of her handwriting at about age 39, is also consistent with SCA5. Handwriting analysts from the U.S. Federal Bureau of Investigation concluded that the writing in this sample, and a similar one penned 17 months later, "demonstrated characteristics that may be caused by a *lack of coordination* [emphasis added], a mental or physical impairment, a poor writing skill level, the writing surface or writing instrument, drug or alcohol effects, or the hand position of the writing" [nee].

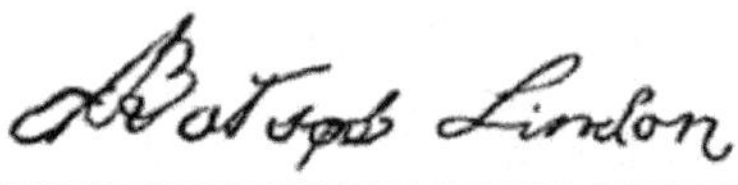

Figure 8-2. Signature of Lincoln's paternal grandmother. The signature is from a land transaction dated Feb. 18, 1780. She signed her name "Batsab Lincoln" [lea p80n]. Handwriting analysts from the FBI offered several possible reasons for the disorganized penmanship, including ataxia (see text). A similar, but somewhat more disorganized, signature exists from Sept. 8, 1781 [nee]. In both signatures, "Lincoln" is spelled "Linclon," suggesting a tenuous grasp of spelling. From: [lea p79].

The last three of the FBI's possibilities are unlikely because they would not be expected to affect two writing samples spaced 17 months apart. Unfortunately, it is not possible to narrow down the remaining three possible causes: too little is known about Bathsheba Lincoln to determine her level of education or her state of health.

Thus, I conclude that the evidence for SCA5 in Lincoln's paternal grandmother is provocative, but not diagnostic.

* * *

If President Lincoln had a gene predisposing him to SCA5, his father, Thomas, would have had to possess the gene, too.

Thomas Lincoln died at age 73, "after suffering for many weeks from a disorder of the kidneys" [herndon p60]. At that age, SCA5 could not stay hidden – noticeable signs of the disease would have occurred if he had the SCA5-causing gene.

There is nothing in the historical record, however, which suggests Thomas was ataxic in his gait, arm use, or speech. And, unlike Bathsheba Lincoln, the historical record is extensive: William Herndon inteviewed everyone he could find who knew Lincoln or the Lincoln family before the Presidency.

Herndon was told that Thomas Lincoln was a "strong & Muscular" man [wilson p111] who "talked and walked slow" [wilson p597], "Walked Slow and Shore [sure]" [wilson p149], and was "Slow in action Somewhat" [wilson p122]. These are not descriptions of ataxia.

In fact, there is evidence that Thomas Lincoln was a good walker. Some time before age 30 he walked from New Orleans to Kentucky [wilson p102] and at age 38 he walked the 65-plus miles from Gentryville, Indiana to Knob Creek, Kentucky [angle p17]. It could be argued that, at these ages, he may not yet have developed symptoms and signs of SCA5. Still, these

---

** It was only about 1930 that a thin thread of documentary evidence established Bathsheba Herring as Lincoln's grandmother and as the mother of all members of generation II (see ¶5816 and the discussion of Lincoln's paternal family tree in *The Physical Lincoln Sourcebook*). Previously, a Mary Shipley was cited as Grandfather Abraham's first wife, even into the 1980s in some publications [montgomery p291].

ages lie in the prime SCA5 years, and it is reasonable to expect that otherwise unnoticeable symptoms might emerge on very long walks. There is no record such symptoms emerged.

No descriptions of Thomas' voice have survived. Samples of his handwriting exist, but there is a caveat. Lincoln said his father could "only bunglingly sign his name." Applying a lesson from Bathsheba Lincoln's case – that distinguishing ataxic writing from poor writing is difficult – means it might be possible to rule out ataxic handwriting from Thomas' writing samples, but not diagnose it.*

Even past the age of 70 there is strong evidence that none of the SCA5 ills troubled Thomas. Just two years before he died, Thomas wrote (via his step-son) "I and the Old womman [sic] is in the best of health" [randallC p114].

In summary, the relatively dense historical record does not show any evidence suggesting Thomas had SCA5, even though he lived to an age when the disease would certainly have caused signs and symptoms.

* * *

Finally we come to Lincoln himself. He died at age 56. Recall that 68 was the latest age at which anyone in the extended Lincoln family first developed signs and symptoms of SCA5. Thus, although not probable, it is *possible* that Lincoln had the disease-causing gene, but died before it could manifest itself.

The University of Minnesota researchers make this point, but they try to have their cake and eat it, too, by presenting evidence that Lincoln had an ataxic gait. (There is no record that his speech was ataxic, and upper limb ataxia is ruled out by the excellent penmanship in 8-3.)

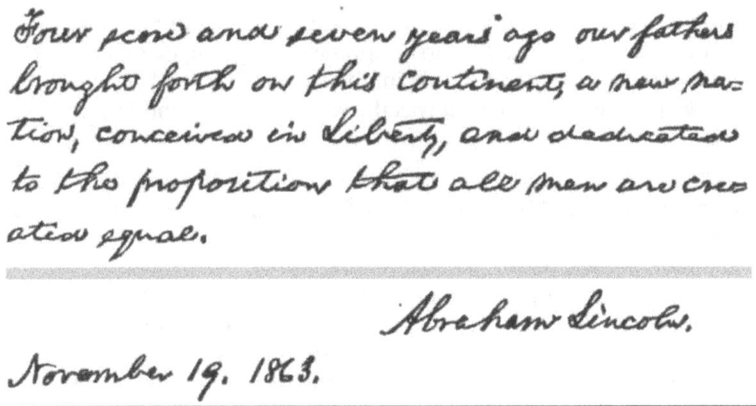

Figure 8-3. Presentation copy of the Gettysburg Address. Lincoln penned this copy of the Gettysburg Address in February 1864, knowing it was to be presented to officials at the Baltimore Sanitary (Health) Fair later that year. The penmanship, presumably the best he could do, is excellent. No sign of upper limb ataxia is evident. Interestingly, the penmanship here is only marginally better than in his handwritten draft of the address, shown in *The Physical Lincoln*. Adapted from: [nicolayG].

---

* [lea p85] shows Thomas' signature, which [nee] says is from an 1806 marriage bond. The penmanship is beautiful and appears well-practiced. I hesitate to put too much weight on this because there are known instances where another person signed legal papers with Thomas' name (see ¶5148).

§8

Three eyewitness descriptions of Lincoln's gait could be interpreted as suggesting mild ataxia:

- In March 1861 William Russell, a reporter for the London *Times*, described Lincoln walking onto a speaking platform "with a shambling, loose, irregular, almost unsteady gait" [kunhardtA p321].
- An undated, unattributed description said Lincoln, walking, resembled "a mariner who had found his sea legs but had to admit there was a rough sea running" [kunhardtA p321].
- In 1862 a visitor to the greatly stressed wartime President wrote: "His introverted look and his half-staggering gait were like those of a man walking in sleep" [donaldA p382].

In the first description, Russell's writing style must be considered. His comments about Lincoln's entrance begin a long, flowery description that mentions Lincoln's "thatch of wild, republican hair;" his "flapping and wide projecting ears;" his "straggling [lips] only kept in order only by two deep furrows;" and "the awkward bonhomie of his face" [kunhardtA p321]. Thus, too much should not be read into Russell's word "shambling."

More detailed accounts of Lincoln's gait mention its unusual quality, but never unsteadiness. For example, one witness said the walking President looked as if "he was about to plunge forward, from his right shoulder, for he always walked, when he had anything in his hand, as if he was pushing something in front of him" [kunhardtAp321].

William Herndon left a detailed account:

> When he walked he moved cautiously but firmly; his long arms and giant hands swung down by his side. He walked with even tread, the inner sides of his feet being parallel. He put the whole foot flat down on the ground at once, not landing on the heel; he likewise lifted his foot all at once, not rising from the toe, and hence he had no spring to his walk. His walk was undulatory – catching and pocketing tire, weariness, and pain, all up and down his person, and thus preventing them from locating. The first impression if a stranger, or a man who did not observe closely, was that his walk implied shrewdness and cunning – that he was a tricky man; but, in reality, it was the walk of caution and firmness" [herndon pp471-472].

Ward Hill Lamon, who met Lincoln in 1853 [angle p164] and was his unofficial bodyguard during the Presidency, adds: "He never wore his shoes out at the heel and the toe more, as most men do, than at the middle of the sole; yet his gait was not altogether awkward, and there was manifest physical power in his step" [lamonL p470].

Herndon called Lincoln's gait "stalking and stilting it" [kunhardtB p260]. (Lincoln was 6-feet 4-inches tall.) Senator Chauncey Depew said Lincoln "walked with dignity and sureness" [randallP]. Eyewitnesses tell of Lincoln bounding up steps two and three at a time in 1856 and 1860 [volk; wilson pp407, 734]. Other eyewitnesses noted his fast walking pace, including this description when Lincoln was 49 (¶1096):

> On leaving the train, most of the passengers climbed over the fences and crossed the stubble-field, taking a short-cut to the grove, among them Mr. Lincoln, who stalked forward alone, taking immense strides, the before-mentioned carpet-bag and an umbrella in his hands, and his coat-skirts flying in the breeze. I managed to keep pretty close in the rear of the tall, gaunt figure, with the head craned forward, apparently much over the balance, like the Leaning Tower of Pisa, that was moving something like a hurricane across that rough stubble-field! He approached the rail-fence, sprang over it as nimbly as a boy of eighteen, and disappeared from my sight [volk].

In 1864 the White House stables caught fire. Lincoln ran to them at a "dog trot," which was almost a "dead run" for his guard [kunhardtA p235]. Once outside, Lincoln "leapt over a hedge and flung open the stable doors to get the animals out" [kunhardtB p297].

Several explanations for Lincoln's gait have been proposed. Herndon thought Lincoln "walked like an Indian" [shutes pp41-42]. One Lincoln scholar thought Lincoln had "the long-striding, flat-footed, cautious manner of a plowman" [currentEB], while another thought Lincoln "walked with the peculiar slow woods-and-fields movement of the Western pioneer" [nicolayA p227].

Other alternatives may be considered. Because Lincoln's bones had a marfanoid structure, his gait may have been influenced by orthopedic factors. There is evidence, for example, that his great toes were exceedingly long [kunhardtB pp46-47, 97-98, 291]. Perhaps this limited forefoot flexibility and resulted in a flat-footed gait.

Gait deteriorates over time in SCA5, but there is no suggestion in the historical record that Lincoln's gait changed over time.

* * *

Just as we saw evidence that Lincoln's father was a good walker, there is similar evidence for Lincoln himself. One night, Lincoln related the following incident, which occurred when he was 49 years old:

> For such an awkward fellow, I am pretty surefooted. It used to take a pretty dextrous man to throw me. I remember, the evening of the day in 1858 that decided the contest for the Senate between Mr. Douglas and myself was something like this, dark, rainy, and gloomy. I had been reading the returns and had ascertained that we had lost the Legislature and started to go home. The path had been worn hog-back and was slippery. My foot slipped from under me, knocking the other one out of the way, but I recovered myself and lit square, and I said to myself, "It's a slip and not a fall" [angle pp484-485, reprinting [hayB]].

Lincoln, too, walked long distances (¶1032ff). For example, a walk in his late 30s (to visit his father) covered what is today a 95-mile one-way drive [wilson p597]. As late as February 1864 (age 55) he would rather walk a mile than wait for a tardy carriage [ostendorfA p175].

The most remarkable evidence concerning Lincoln's gait comes from his visit to the Army encampment at Aquia Creek, Virginia in spring 1862. To the President's official party, General Irvin McDowell pointed out a bridge being built across a deep wide ravine. The bridge was a hundred feet above the water and only one plank wide at that time. Nevertheless, Lincoln exclaimed "Let us walk over" and led the way across without losing his balance. Following him, Secretary of War Stanton became dizzy, and had to be helped by Admiral John Dahlgren, who was himself rather giddy [donaldA p352].

This incident proves that Lincoln at age 53 was either a fool, or that he had not the slightest problem controlling his lower limbs. No one thinks Lincoln was a fool.

* * *

In conclusion, there is effectively no evidence that Lincoln had SCA5. His grandmother might have had it, but there are two main reasons to believe Lincoln did not:

- His father did not have the disease. Given this simple fact, the probability that Lincoln had SCA5 is the same as the probability for any average person in the population.
- Lincoln did not have even a hint of even early disease, even though he lived well beyond the usual age at which signs and symptoms of SCA5 appear. There is excellent first-hand evidence that his voice and upper limbs functioned without noticeable ataxia even into his last year. If Lincoln had SCA5 and did not have observable ataxia in his gait, we might still expect changes in limb control that are not apparent to an outside observer, but which affect a person's mind as they contemplate situations where lower limb control is critical. The bridge-crossing at Aquia Creek in 1862 powerfully illustrates the control that Lincoln exercised over his gait.

§8

As with Marfan syndrome and MEN2B, a genetic test for SCA5 now exists. The Minnesota researchers have argued that it is reasonable to test Lincoln's tissue to see if he had a genetic variant that causes SCA5, but their argument does not fully consider the historical record. When the full record is considered, there is no justification to test Abraham Lincoln for an SCA5-causing gene.

(c) Article: Lincoln's awkwardness §8c

Lincoln was described with the word "awkward" as early as age 10 [wilson p120]. All together, more than a dozen observers, including Lincoln himself, used the word, even to the year before his death (¶2907).

However, with one exception (see below), these instances do not refer to his gait. Many refer to upper limb gestures. For example, orating about 1833, Lincoln "would enforce his ideas with awkward gestures" [wilson p384]. Many others convey a general impression, such as the two girls who described the school-age Lincoln with "his awkwardness and large feet" and "so quiet and awkward and so awful homely" [burl p124].

An 1862 newspaper article described Lincoln "plodding with awkward step" about 1830 [wilson p24]. This is unlikely to be an eyewitness account.

(d) Article: Lincoln's lower limb control §8d

Three anecdotes indicate that Lincoln's ability to control his legs was normal, if not superior.

First, an attorney who frequently traveled with Lincoln in the late 1850s observed "Lincoln had a furtive way of stealing in on one, unheard, unperceived and unawares" [angle p170].

[The other two anecdotes are presented in the draft chapter, above.]

(e) Article: Lincoln's Voice §8e

Although Lincoln had a high-pitched voice that would become shrill when he was excited, none of the dozen or so written descriptions of his voice mention anomalies in enunciation or pitch steadiness compatible with ataxic speech (¶3698ff). To the contrary, at Gettysburg in 1863 Lincoln spoke in "clear, ringing, earnest tones" [carrA p252], and at his second inaugural in 1865 "every word was clear and audible ... over the vast concourse" [brooksC p239] (Figure 2).

(f) Article: Discussion §8f

Although SCA5 has occurred in multiple descendants of Abraham Lincoln's paternal grandparents [ranum], the present study finds no evidence Lincoln himself was afflicted.

Lincoln's gait, though unusual, was not ataxic, according to several eyewitness descriptions. Gait deteriorates over time in SCA5, but there is no suggestion in the historical record that Lincoln's gait changed over time.

Other explanations for Lincoln's gait may be considered. At least two scholars have suggested it was a matter of habit [currentEB] [nicolayA]. However, because Lincoln bore many skeletal stigmata of Marfan syndrome [gordon] [schwartzA], his gait may have been influenced by orthopedic factors. There is evidence, for example, that his great toes were exceedingly long [kunhardtB pp46-47, 97-98, 291]. Perhaps this limited forefoot flexibility and resulted in a flat-footed gait.

It is also unlikely that Lincoln had subclinical gait disturbances. The incident at the Aquia Creek bridge unambiguously indicates that Lincoln at age 53 had full, if not superior, control over his feet and legs. It is also clear that Lincoln could control his hands and voice normally, even into the last year of his life.

Available clinical information about Lincoln's father offers considerable evidence against SCA5. Thomas Lincoln's "slow sure" gait does not evoke ataxia. Most convincingly, however, there is no mention of invalidism to age 73, and there is an extraordinary account of him walking from New Orleans to Kentucky at an age when SCA5 is often manifest. If Thomas Lincoln did not have SCA5, then neither did Abraham Lincoln.

Appeals to form frustes and non-penetrance are reasonable in genetic disease when pedigrees strongly suggest an apparently unaffected person should be affected. This is not the case with Abraham Lincoln and SCA5. Except for colorful journalistic language, there is no evidence that he or his father had SCA5.

The present analysis yields two practical recommendations: (a) future reports which mention the Lincoln family's susceptibility to SCA5 should add that the President did not have the disorder, and (b) because SCA5 in President Lincoln is so unlikely on clinical grounds, any plans to analyze SCA5-related gene(s) in his limited available tissue samples should be abandoned.

§8

Topic 9 – Mary's Symptoms §9

In her last 20 years, Mary expressed many physical complaints in her correspondence. Finding one or even two unifying diagnoses is a challenge. Merely organizing the data requires a different approach than used for other Lincoln family members. This is a chronology in her own words.

To construct the tabulation below, Mary's correspondence (as collected in [turner]) was read completely. Each of her letters after 1860 that mentions a physical, and sometimes mental, illness was excerpted and entered as one row in the table, having four columns as follows:

- Column 1: the date of Mary's letter, in mm/dd/yyyy format.
- Column 2: the letter's beginning page in [turner].
- Column 3: the geographical place where the letter was written
- Column 4: the excerpt. An ellipsis ... indicates elided text. (Not provided at start or end of excerpts.)

Travels and major events are inserted into the table to provide context. I have not attempted to tabulate Mary's numerous apologies for the quality of her handwriting. They begin in 1848 [turner p38] and afterwards occur so frequently that it seems almost a figure of speech with her. Her underlinings are preserved.

Date	Pg	Place	Text
9/29/1861	104	Washington	have been quite sick with <u>chills</u> for some days, this is my day of rest, so I am sitting up -- I am beginning to feel very weak. If they cannot be broken in a few days, Mr Lincoln wants me to go North, & remain until cold weather ... cannot afford to be delicate ... am feeling <u>very far</u> from well -- September and early in Oct -- are always considered unhealthy months here -- my racked frame certainly bears evidence to the fact. ... I used to have chills in Ill[inois] -- those days have passed ... I am not well enough to go down[stairs?]
10/06	108	Washington	indisposition ... For the last ten days I have been sick with chills, am now beginning, to feel better

2/20/1862 Event -- Willie dies			

Date	Pg	Place	Text
05/29/1862	127	Washington	my sadness & ill health
11/02/1862	139	New York	[recently] I had one of my severe attacks
09/22/1863	157	New York	Have a very bad cold and am anxious to return home
12/04/1863	159	New York	Very tired and severe headache.
03/04/1864	170	Washington	slight indisposition
05/27	176	Washington	[yesterday:] intensively severe headache ... it has left me, yet I am feeling so weak this morning ... how much inclined to <u>nausea</u> they leave you [See ¶4254 for full description.]
07/20	177	Washington	An intense headache, caused by driving out, in the heat of the day
09/23	180	Washington	am just recovering from a little tedious indisposition
02/28/1865	203	Washington?	have been ill ... All well now
05/29	236	Chicago	scarcely able to sit up ... my health is so miserable
07/04	255	near Chicago	my nerves in a very weak state
07/11	256	near Chicago	I have almost become blind, with weeping, and can scarcely, see sufficiently to trace these lines
07/17	259	Chicago	seriously indisposed, this week
08/31	271	Chicago	was confined to my bed

11/11	280	Chicago	severe indisposition
12/13	304	Chicago	one, of my severe headaches ... I am really not able, to sit up
12/16	308	Chicago	[sat up all night with ill Tad]
12/24	311	Chicago	sitting up, for the first time, in three days ... [last week] very severe chill
12/29	315	Chicago	am now sitting, up, the first day since my return ... Three days of each week, almost, I am incapable of any exertion, on account of my severe headaches
12/30	318	Chicago	my health, much impaired, by the terrible vicissitudes, I have passed through, the past year
12/31	320	Chicago?	am [very] much, indisposed
01/04/1866	322	Chicago	so thoroughly chilled yesterday that my limbs -- ache with pain
01/10/1866	323	Chicago	this is the first hour, I have been up, since I last wrote you [Jan. 4]
01/19/1866	328	Chicago	I rise from a bed of sickness, to reply to your letter
02/17/1866	336	Chicago	I am greatly indisposed but will sit up, long enough to write, you a few lines ... am positively quite ill
03/07/1866	341	Chicago	This has been a most severe winter to me, bodily and mentally
05/19/1866	365	Chicago	I am unable to sit up, with my severe headaches
08/05/1866	377	Chicago	am just recovering from quite a severe indisposition and so soon, as I am able to leave the house, I will send the money
08/20/1866	383	Chicago	Quite a severe indisposition
12/25/1866	403	Chicago	[recently] was suffering from chills and just as my health was being partially restored...
02/??/1867	408	Chicago	an intense headache ... a moment's respite of sitting up ... My eyes pain me so much, I can scarcely see.
03/19/1867	417	Chicago?	We are quite well.
05/26/1867	422	Chicago?	This climate and my great grief are certainly shortening my life
06/30/1867	424	Racine, WI	My health, after I saw you, broke down so completely ... scarcely able to leave my lounge
06/30/1867	425	Racine, WI	Each morning I have walked two miles
10/06/1867	440	Chicago	sleepless night of great mental suffering
11/10/1867	452	Chicago	am having chills, every other day ... my physician orders quiet -- as little writing & reading as possible. This climate is very trying to me in the winter season. ... My health is too poor, for me to be disturbed by idle rumors ... am writing, with a fever on me, after a chill
11/23/1867	460	Chicago	a fearful headache today
01/09/1868	467	Chicago	within the last few days -- very sore & inflamed eyes. [Details: ¶4125.]
01/12/1868	468	Chicago	[Contemplates suicide] I am feeling too weak to write more today ... [Fear of a certain humiliation] has almost whitened every hair of my head.
01/15/1868	469	Chicago	[lost a month's living expenses by leaving her pocketbook on the streetcar]
02/29/1868	470	Chicago?	am only able to sit up long enough to write you a line and enclose this check

---

Spring 1868 Event -- Publication of [keckleyB] *crushes Mary, who ends their "almost sisterly" friendship.* [turner pp471-472, 476].

05/02/1868	475	Chicago	[See ¶4657 for full account.] am <u>permitted</u> to sit up ... for the past three weeks, I have been seriously sick. My disease is of a womanly nature ... Since the birth of my youngest son, for about twelve years I have been more or less a sufferer. My physician ... told me yesterday, that he must prescribe an entire change of air, scene, for me. He thought going abroad -- would alone benefit me -- & advised me, as soon as I could bear the change, to go to Scotland for the summer. ... health [is] delicate. ... I fear from what my physician tells me. ... ill health.

§9

06/19/1868	477	Chicago	Notwithstanding ... the remonstrances of my physician, I have concluded to make a visit of a day or two to Springfield

June 1868 Trip -- To Springfield for "a day or two" with Tad [turner pp477, 474]

06/27/1868	478	Chicago	so frequently visited by severe sickness ... severe health & extreme nervousness, compels me to make the changes
07/18/1868	479	Cresson, PA	my very feeble health ... In my hours of great bodily suffering which now occur quite frequently... I am suffering so much, I am scarcely able to sit up

July 1868 Trip -- East coast (with Tad) until Oct. 1: (1) Alleghenies, especially at a health resort with many natural springs, (2) Washington and Baltimore for Robert's marriage [turner p474]

08/19/1868	481	Altoona, PA	[Plan in Europe:] go immediately to Carlsbad and place myself under medical treatment ... am feeling this morning, much indisposed
09/27/1868	485	Baltimore	[Episode of near-syncope on 9/25, described in ¶4267.]

Oct. 1868 Event -- Humiliated by wardrobe scandal and publication of [keckleyB], *Mary flees the United States for Germany.* [turner pp429-430, 472-473, 489]

12/04/1868	491	Frankfurt	In consequence of very ill health, caused by great mental suffering & by the advice of physicians in America, I came to Germany, in search of health. [Her physicians want her to go to Italy, but finances prevent this.] ... infirm health ... my physician's bills...have swallowed up my little income
12/04/1868	492	Frankfurt	ill health caused by great mental distress ... I have come over to Germany to...have my condition a little improved. I am now ordered to the south of Europe [but finances prevent this]
12/??/1868	493	Frankfurt	[Lincoln's death] has greatly impaired my heath
12/13/1868	494	Frankfurt	poor health ... am urged by my physicians to proceed to Italy ... [Of ice water in Germany:] really dangerous to drink
12/15/1868	497	Frankfurt	My health continues very poor, & the physicians here urges [sic] me to go immediately to Italy ... Italy, where I am daily urged, by my physicians to go ... ill health upon me & physician bills, that often appall me
01/18/1869	498	Frankfurt	Very ill health, the past winter ... I am earnestly advised by two physicians...to go to Italy ... "nervous" truly, I am

Feb. 1869 Trip -- Unable to raise funds for an Italy trip, Mary goes to Nice, France for at least 6 weeks [turner pp500, 501, 503]

02/17/1869	501	Nice	[Great weather] I live out in the open air & am gradually finding myself, grow [sic] stronger day by day, for I had been very sick in Frankfort [Germany] ... I never return from my walks without my hands being filled [with flowers]
03/16/1869	503	Nice	Ill health ... [in Nice] by degrees, I find myself regaining strength

Trip -- Back in Frankfurt, Germany

03/22/1869	504	Frankfurt	fatigued ... my head aches now for the tears I have shed this morning ... The Doctor has just left me and says he wonders to find me sitting up.
03/27/1869	506	Frankfurt	ill health

July 1869 Trip -- Paris, London, Scotland, Brussels, with Tad: "one of the happiest interludes of her life ... for days at a time she forgot to feel sorry for herself" [turner p507]. *Six or seven week trip* [turner pp511, 512].

08/21/1869	512	Frankfurt	[A good friend visits Germany:] we sat up in my room last night & until 3. this morning [Twice were asked by others to quiet down]
08/26/1869	514	Frankfurt	Two or three entire nights, dear Mrs. Orne & myself, sat up until daylight
08/30/1869	515	Cronberg	troubled slumbers ... My health is so far from being restored, that absolute quiet is enjoined upon me

09/10/1869	517	Cronberg	[reads and enjoys Trollope's <u>Phineas Finn</u>]
10/23/1869	520	Frankfurt	The first finger of my right hand is painfully sore...arising from the smallest prick of a needle ... Last week, sick most of the time & this week unable to use my hand [see ¶4280]
11//06/1869	521	Frankfurt	My fingers are well.
11/13/1869	522	Frankfurt	I am sitting up while my [room] is being arranged, so that I shall return to my bed. I have been suffering for three days, with neuralgic headaches, pain in my limbs && The discomforts, by which I am surrounded and which I am unable to remedy, are doubtless, making inroads into my health
11/14/1869	524	Frankfurt	I am sitting up & <u>that is all</u>, for my limbs are as painful & unbending, as an old veteran of <u>seventy</u>, should be. ... <u>To day,</u> my <u>wrists</u> even, pain with neuralgia -- if possible, I will prevent <u>it</u>, creeping into my fingers, so that they may be able to use the pen ... I have grown very nervous, & can now scarcely read & certainly cannot do anything useful.
11/20/1869	525	Frankfurt	a mind filled with ANXIETY & <u>fear</u> ... I am slowly recovering from my <u>neuralgic</u> woes -- I hope <u>other</u> troubles <u>less</u> easily endured will not take its place
11/28/1869	527	Frankfurt	I have grown so <u>nervous</u>
12/02/1869	528	Frankfurt	I was confined to my bed on yesterday, with a neuralgic headache -- and am feeling very far from well to day.
12/16/1869	534	Frankfurt	confined to my bed, with a neuralgic headache, which was not lessened [upon reading a false newspaper story about herself] ... I passed a sleepless, miserable night & must remain very quiet to day -- as I have fever upon me -- with great & burning pain in my spine ... when I am able to sit up -- I will write you more ... my health has again become so poor --- that I do not expect to rally
12/21/1869	537	Frankfurt?	[referring to the false newspaper story of 12/05/1869] Even this made me sick
12/29/1869	537	Frankfurt	I am <u>just again</u> recovering from a severe attack of neuralgic headache ... And I may add its after-effects -- from an <u>unconscionable</u> dose of <u>blue mass</u> -- which I took without consulting a physician. The day before Christmas I found myself with <u>such</u> a headache ... I sent [Tad]] to an English apothecary's where he procured, what they told him was a <u>large dose</u> -- which my sore bones -- <u>can now</u> properly attest -- On Sunday, Taddie brought the physician, <u>who,</u> of course is administering Mineral water -- I am sitting up today -- feeling so much better -- but of course must be very careful -- He has directed me to wear flannel next my skin [sic] ... I was <u>so very</u> sick
01/02/1870	539	Frankfurt	Sick in body & worn out in mind, my present state, has become unendurable -- To day, I am suffering so much with my back -- at times I am racked with pain -- my quarters have been cold & uncomfortable this winter -- I must either become an invalid or make a change ... <u>ten</u> callers [yesterday, including] two Doctors ... Perhaps this unwonted excitement, has occasioned such pain in all my limbs. I fear very much -- <u>it is still</u> -- that heavy <u>American</u> dose of calomel, from which I am suffering. ... I am in much pain. [?mental pain]
01/08/1870	541	Frankfurt	Two days out of each week at <u>least</u>, I am confined to my bed & often unable to raise my head -- with headache
02/11/1870	546	Frankfurt	Since I last wrote you [Jan. 21], I have been quite ill, confined to my bed, for ten wearisome days -- and now I am <u>just able</u>, to creep about my room. A fearful cold, appeared to settle in my spine & I was unable to sit up, with the sharp, burning <u>agony</u>, in my back. I have now a plaster from my shoulders down the whole, extent of the spine & I am lying on my sofa most of the time -- the Dr says, this present trouble, arises more from a distressed agitated mind, than a real local cause, but says of course there is a <u>great</u> tendency to spinal disease ... if my health continues to fail me, as it <u>now</u>, is so fast doing, [may die within a year] ... my nervous anxiety...
02/18/1870	549	Frankfurt	have not yet recovered my strength

§9

02/18/1870	550	Frankfurt	Confined to my room ... a nervous state
03/31/1870	552	Frankfurt	my late very severe illness -- I am sitting up in bed, whilst I am writing this ... I am enjoined by my physician... to write a very few lines -- my hands tremble so much -- I cannot write ... there were days of delirium [?in 1865]
04/03/1870	552	Frankfurt	I am sitting up for a little while ... My Physician urges me to go to Marienbad, for the waters & baths ... pass <u>sleepless</u> nights -- grieving over the smallest expenses, medical & otherwise
04/26/1870	554	Frankfurt	I am suffering with ill health, & am earnestly advised by my Physician to go into Bohemia -- for the baths & mineral water
05/16/1870	558	Frankfurt	continued illness of the last few months ... My physician frequently urges an immediate departure for some medical baths in Bohemia
05/19/1870	559	Frankfurt	At Heidelberg we ascended the mountain one morning [by walking? riding? and there] roamed through the ruins

May 21, 1870 Trip -- To Marienbad, Bohemia [turner p562] *for health reasons* [turner p 560] *for about one month* [turner p570]

05/22/1870	560	Marienbad	[recently saw] my physician about a new medicine he had given me ... [after reading newspaper story about herself] I became very sick -- I was assisted into a cab ... [her physician examined her and said] another attack of sickness -- such as I had in the winter -- would follow -- if I was not hurried away [so she left for Marienbad within 12 hours]
05/28/1870	561	Marienbad	I am almost helpless -- there are days when I cannot walk straight -- I am unable to wait upon myself -- from very frequent illnesses ... My health is very poor ... I have had to send for the old physician of the place, two or three times -- no menial near to assist me
06/02/1870	563	Marienbad	my health has entirely failed
06/04/1870	564	Marienbad	faithfully drinking the waters -- and taking medicinal baths. I am laready starting to feel, that I am improving ... I often take my books & pass hours in the fragrant forests
06//29/1870	570	Frankfurt	[am] quite an invalid ... my health greatly benefitted [from Marienbad visit]

July 1, 1870 Trip -- Trip into the country (around Frankfurt) with Tad [turner p571]

Sept. 1870 Event -- Moves with Tad to Leamington, England [turner p573] *and London*

| 09/10/1870 | 577 | Leamington | I am coughing so badly that I can scarcely write. I left Liverpool last Saturday afternoon so completely sick that I determined to come here to be well attended to. This is the first day I have sat up since then and a physician tells me that as soon as possible I should go to a dryer climate. ... my health is again beginning to fail me as it did last winter |
| 01/13/1871 | 582 | London | [am] coughing most disagreeably and a bundle of wrappings. My servant woman has proved herself within the past week a good nurse. |

Feb. 1871 Trip -- To Italy

April 29, 1871 Trip -- Sets sail for United States [rossA p300]

May 10, 1871 Trip -- Arrives New York [NYTimes - May 11, 1871]. *To Chicago May 15* [randallA p269].

| 05/21/1871 | 587 | Chicago | my head is throbbing with pain |

July 15, 1871 Event -- Tad dies

| 08/13/1871 | 591 | Cresson, PA? | I have been prostrated by illness -- & by <u>a grief</u> -- that the grave alone can soften [date of letter is uncertain] |
| 10/04/1871 | 596 | Chicago | utterly prostrated -- by my deep deep grief, that my health has completely given away. Latterly, I am suffering greatly with violent palpitation of the heart ... I am ordered perfect quiet |

05/26/1872 598 Chicago   an invalid at present

July 1872 Trip -- Waukesha, Wisconsin from first week of July to mid-August [turner pp598n 599]

08/03/1872 598 Waukesha   quite an invalid at present

---

mid-1873 Trip -- To Canada, why unknown, for some months [randallC p383]. *Returned to Chicago late in year* [turner p601]

Early 1875 Event -- Trip to Florida

May 1875 Event -- Tried and committed for insanity. Released June 1876.

Sept. 1876 Event -- Leaves Springfield in late September for Havre, then Bordeaux, then Pau, France [turner pp617, 618]

07/02/1877 645 Pau   am suffering so much from a disabled hand
01/24/1878 658 Pau   Afflictions are very terrible ... have left me a very broken hearted woman
03/22/1878 665 Pau   quite severe indisposition

April 1878 Trip -- To Italy [turner p665]. *Returned to Pau early July* [turner p667]

02/26/1879 675 Pau   am suffering much with neuralgia, in my right arm

---

Jul-Aug. 1879 Trip -- "At the seaside" for 10 days, arriving back in Pau on August 2.

10/04/1879 690 Pau   I am sitting up, for the <u>first</u> half hour, within the past week. I have been really ill, with a very severe cold taken in the mountains, where I suppose I lingered too long. I am enveloped in flannels from head to foot -- my throat is almost closed at times, continual pain & soreness in the chest -- & am coughing most of the time. ... I enclose a card of my <u>exact</u> weight <u>nearly</u> a month ago -- since then, as a matter of course many pounds of flesh have departed. <u>Here</u>, in France, they are compelled to be <u>rigidly</u> exact in their weights -- I am now, just the weight I was, when we went to Wash in 1861 -- Therefore I may conclude, my great bloat has left me & I have returned to my natural size. ... Without doubt, I must have been considered <u>quite</u> ill -- as numerous cards are daily handed me & notes of enquiry, flowers, &&...
10/21/1879 691 Pau   Owing to illness, I failed to write you
01/14/1880 693 Pau   The weather is exceedingly cold here this winter & in consequence of a very severe cough & neuralgia I think I will leave here in a few days for Italy.

Jan.-Feb. 1880 Trip -- In Avignon, France?

01/16/1880 694 Avignon   Five days since I arrived here, owing to excessive fatigue & illness however, the three first were passed in bed and now I am sitting up just long enough to write you -- so much, for my poor broken back, with its <u>three</u> plasters & my left side always in pain. ... I have now run down to 100- pounds, <u>exactly</u>. ["here" is Avignon, France. But her letters of the 14th and 19th are dated Pau.]
01/19/1880 695 Pau   ... the 1st of Jan, <u>when</u> I was groaning with an <u>almost</u> broken back -- which is aching very badly at present ... The extremely cold weather & and unusual amount of pain forces me [to Italy soon]. [She did not go.]
03/05/1880 696 Pau   After a detention of three weeks at Avignon, France, with quite severe illness, two days since I arrived here with great pain & difficulty ... I am too ill, to travel & have not the least wish to do so.

June 1880 Trip -- In Marseilles for a week [turner p698]

06/12/1880 698 Pau   On my return here, the afterwards being utterly exhausted with the sufferings of my back & left side, & the journey, I was compelled to send for the physician, & resting on the lounge, the greater part of the time for two months

§9

08/29/1880	701	Pau

I have been so weakened by the intense suffering of my left side & back... Owing to the exertions of the past week, I am suffering <u>even</u> more than usual with my back to day ... my delicate health

10/07/1880	703	Bordeaux

ill & feeble in health

Oct. 1880 Trip -- Sails for America on Oct. 16 [turner p703]

Oct. 1881 Trip -- In New York City

10/23/1881	708	New York

I am too ill today, only to write you a few lines. ... I am situated here to receive daily Electric baths ... When I landed at the depot in N.Y. I was so thoroughly exhausted that the hackman lifted me in his arms into the carriage -- also lifted me into the Clarendon Hotel -- Dr Miller insists that this man shall lift me up stairs from the baths -- indeed, it could <u>not</u> be otherwise. ... I am too ill to ride out.

01/03/1882	710	New York

Four physicians come on Sunday to see me. ... I am very feeble with my spine & limbs -- <u>now</u>, quite unable to walk but a very few steps & my vision is <u>very</u> greatly obscured. As Dr S[ayre] says to be lame & almost without the least eyesight -- what an affliction.

01/03/1882	711	New York

Dr Sayre has just left me

02/05/1882	712	New York

<u>very</u> ill with <u>anxiety</u> ... very ill ... On Thursday afternoon Dr Sayre called...

02/21/1882	714	New York

I considered it necessary to get away from the Electric baths ... within the past week I have had two very severe chills & I find myself in a very feeble state ... It is a fearful thing to be ill, <u>all the time</u> ... I am in a very enfeebled state

03/21/1882	716	New York

my limbs still in so paralyzed a state

Bibliography & Personae

Many older historical books are available on-line. See: [AbrahamLincolnAssociation], [archiveorg], & books.google.com.

Literature not mentioning Lincoln or MEN2B (mostly scientific, post-1950).

aa1. Aase JM. *Diagnostic Dysmorphology*. New York: Plenum Medical Book Company, 1990. Cited by ¶¶663, 739, 4142.

aa2. Abdul-Jabbar, Kareem; Obstfeld, Raymond. *On the Shoulders of Giants: My Journey Through the Harlem Renaissance*. New York: Simon & Schuster, 2007.

aa3. Abrams J. *Essentials of Cardiac Physical Diagnosis*. Philadelphia: Lea & Febiger, 1987. Cited by ¶1984.

aa4. Adams, Douglas. *The Hitchhiker's Guide to the Galaxy*. New York: Pocket Books, 1981. (Original © 1979.)

aa5. Ades LC; Sullivan K; Biggin A; *et al.* FBN1, TGFBR1, and the Marfan-craniosynostosis/mental retardation disorders revisited. *Am J Med Genet A.* 2006; 140: 1047-1058.

aa6. Akhurst RJ. TGF-beta signalling in health and disease. *Nat Genetics.* 2004; 36: 790-792.

aa7. Akiskal HS. Mood disorders: clinical features. Section 13.6 (pages 1611-1652) in: Sadock BJ, Sadock VA (eds). *Kaplan & Sadock's Comprehensive Textbook of Psychiatry*. 8th ed. Philadelphia : Lippincott Williams & Wilkins, 2005 Cited by ¶¶2316, 4318, 4319.

aa8. Albanese A. Sulla dolichostenomelia. *Arch Ortop.* 1931; 47: 539. Cited by [mckusickApp47,136]. Cited by ¶987.

aa9. Allman, Bill. Ask the White House. Sept. 26, 2003.
http://www.whitehouse.gov/ask/20030926.html Cited by ¶4473.

aa10. Anonymous. Ills of Lincoln kin tied to broken nerve cells. *Washington Post.* 2007; January 30: Page A9. Cited by Special Topic §8a.

aa11. Arbustini E; Marziliano N. Aneurysm syndromes and TGF-β receptor mutations. *N Engl J Med.* 2006; 355: 2155.

aa12. Ashcraft KW; Holcomb GW III; Murphy JP (eds.). *Pediatric Surgery*. 4th ed. Philadelphia: Elsevier-Saunders, 2005.

aa13. Azhar M; Schultz Jel J; Grupp I; *et al.* Transforming growth factor beta in cardiovascular development and function. *Cytokine Growth Factor Rev.* 2003; 14: 391-407.

aa14. Annes JP; Munger JS; Rifkin DB. Making sense of latent TGFbeta activation. *J Cell Sci.* 2003; 116: 217-224.

aa15. Bean WB (ed). *Sir William Osler: Aphorisms From His Bedside Teachings and Writings*. New York: Henry Schuman, Inc., 1950. Cited by ¶2732.

aa16. Beighton P; de Paepe A; Danks D; *et al.* International Nosology of Heritable Disorders of Connective Tissue, Berlin, 1986. *Am J Med Genet.* 1988; 29: 581-594.

aa17. Benenson, Abram S. Immunization and military medicine. *Review of Infectious Diseases.* 1984; 6: 1-12. Cited by Special Topic §5e.

aa18. Beutler E. Carrier screening for Gaucher disease: more harm than good ? *JAMA.* 2007; 298: 1329.

aa19. Blinderman, A. John Adams: fears, depressions, and ailments. *NY State J Med.* 1977; 77: 268-276. Cited by Special Topic §5e.

aa20. Braude AI (ed.). *Medical Microbiology and Infectious Diseases*. Philadelphia: W.B. Saunders, 1981.

aa21. Bruneteau RJ; Mulliken JB. Frontal plagiocephaly: synostotic, compensational, or deformational. *Plast Recon Surg.* 1992; 89: 21-31.

aa22. Burrows NP, Lovell CR. Disorders of connective tissue. Chapter 46 in: *Rook's Textbook of Dermatology*. 4th ed. Burns T, Breathnach S, Cox N, Griffiths C (eds.). Malden, MA: Blackwell Science, 2004.

aa23. Clouthier DE; Comerford SA; Hammer RE. Hepatic fibrosis, glomerulosclerosis, and a lipodystrophy-like syndrome in PEPCK-TGF-beta1 transgenic mice. *J Clin Invest.* 1997; 100: 2697-2713.

aa24. Clyde DF. Malaria. Chapter 194 (pages 1478-1486) in: [aa20]. Cited by ¶2012.

aa25. Cope, Zachary (alias "Zeta"). *The Acute Abdomen in Rhyme.* 5th ed. London: H.K. Lewis, 1972.

aa26. David DJ; Poswillo D; Simpson D. *The Craniosynostoses.* Berlin: Springer-Verlag, 1982. Page 60. Cited by ¶1594.

aa27. DeGowin, RL. *DeGowin & DeGowin's Bedside Physical Examination.* 5th ed. New York: Macmillan, 1987.

aa28. De Paepe A; Devereux RB; Dietz HC; *et al.* Revised diagnostic criteria for the Marfan syndrome. *Am J Med Genet.* 1996; 62: 417-426.

aa29. Dickens, Charles. *Martin Chuzzlewit.* New York: Penguin, 1968. 942 pages.

aa30. Dietz, HC; Pyeritz RE. Marfan syndrome and related disorders. Chapter 206 (pages 5287-5311) in: [aa101].

aa31. Diffrient N; Tilley AR; Bardagjy J. *Humanscale 4/5/6.* Cambridge, MA: MIT Press, 1981.

aa32. Downing JR. TGF-β signaling, tumor suppression, and acute lymphoblastic leukemia. *N Engl J Med.* 2004; 351: 528-530.

aa33. Emerick LL; Hatten JT. *Diagnosis and Evaluation in Speech Pathology.* 2nd ed. Englewood Cliffs, NJ. Prentice-Hall; 1978: . Cited by ¶¶5603, 5676. *For evidence that children with cleft palate speak slowly, they cite* [aa61].

aa34. Encyclopdia Britannica, Inc. *Encyclopædia Britannica.* 14th ed. Chicago: Encyclopaedia Britannica, Inc, 1973. (See [currentEB]).

aa35. Fenner F; Henderson DA; Arita I; *et al. Smallpox and its Eradication.* Geneva: World Health Organization, 1988. Cited by Special Topic §5e.

aa36. Flexner, James Thomas. *Washington: The Indispensable Man.* Boston: Back Bay Books, 1974. Page 132. Cited by Special Topic §5e.

aa37. Flannery, Michael A. *Civil War Pharmacy: A History of Drugs, Drug Supply and Provision, and Therapeutics for the Union and Confederacy.* Binghamton, NY: Haworth Press, 2004. Cited by ¶2732.

aa38. Freeman JM; Borkowf S. Craniostenosis: review of the literature and report of thirty-four cases. *Pediatrics.* 1962; 30: 57-70. Cited by ¶1594.

aa39. Gabriel, Richard A; Mietz, Karen S. *A History of Military Medicine. Volume II.* New York: Greenwood Press, 1992. Page 108. Cited by Special Topic §5e.

aa40. Garrison FH. *An Introduction to the History of Medicine.* 4th ed. Philadelphia: Saunders, 1929. 996 pages. Cited by Special Topic §5e.

aa41. Gelb BD. Marfan's syndrome and related disorders – more tightly connected than we thought. *N Engl J Med.* 2006; 355: 841-844.

aa42. Ghori A. Old wine in a new bottle? *Anesthesia.* 2002; 57: 942.

aa43. Gilman AG; Goodman LS; Gilman A (eds). *Goodman and Gilman's The Pharmacologic Basis of Therapeutics.* 6th ed. New York: Macmillan, 1980.

aa44. Goldstein RE; O'Neill JA Jr.; Holcomb GW 3rd; *et al.* Clinical experience over 48 years with pheochromocytoma. *Ann Surg.* 1999; 229: 755-764.

aa45. Gray JM; Young AW; Barker WA; *et al.* Impaired recognition of disgust in Huntington's disease gene carriers. *Brain.* 1997; 120: 2029-2038.

aa46. Hammarlund M; Jorgenson EM; Bastiana MJ. Axons break in animals lacking β-spectrin. *J Cell Biol.* 2007; 176: 269-275. Cited by Special Topic §8a.

aa47. Hansen M; Mulliken JB. Frontal plagiocephaly: diagnosis and treatment. *Clin Plast Surg.* 1994; 21: 543-553.

aa48. Harvey, AM; Boardley J. *Differential Diagnosis.* 2nd ed. Philadelphia: W.B. Saunders, 1970. page 787.

aa49. Harvey WP; Segal JP; Hufnagel CA. Unusual clinical features associated with severe aortic insufficiency. *Ann Int Med.* 1957; 47: 27-38. Cited by ¶1989.

aa50. Hibino T; Nishiyama T. Role of TGF-beta2 in the human hair cycle. *J Dermatol Sci.* 2004; 35: 9-18.

aa51. Hopkins DR. Smallpox entombed. *Lancet.* 1985; I: 175. Cited by Special Topic §5f.

aa52. Ikeda Y; Dick KA; Weatherspoon MR; *et al.* Spectrin mutations cause spinocerebellar ataxia type 5. *Nat Genet.* 2006; 38: 184-190. Cited by ¶1028. Cited by Special Topic §8a.

aa53. Izquierdo NJ; Traboulsi EI; Enger C; *et al.* Strabismus in the Marfan syndrome. *Am J Ophthalmol.* 1994; 117: 632-635.

aa54. Ito Y; Yeo JY; Chytil A; *et al.* Conditional inactivation of Tgfbr2 in cranial neural crest causes cleft palate and calvaria defects. *Development.* 2003; 130: 5269-5280.

aa55. Jamora C; Lee P; Kocieniewski P; *et al.* A signaling pathway involving TGF-beta2 and snail in hair follicle morphogenesis. *PLoS Biol.* 2005; 3: e11.

aa56. Jones KL. *Smith's Recognizable Patterns of Human Malformation.* 6th ed. Philadelphia: Elsevier Saunders, 2006.

aa57. Judge DP; Dietz HC. Marfan's syndrome. *Lancet.* 2005; 366: 1965-1976.

aa58. Kramer, Samuel Noah. *History Begins at Sumer.* Philadelphia: University of Pennsylvania Press, 1956. Page xxi. Cited by ¶845.

aa59. Kramlinger KG; Post RM. Ultra-rapid and ultradian cycling in bipolar affective illness. *Br J Psychiatry.* 1996; 168: 314-323.

aa60. Kryger MH; Roth T; Dement WC. *Principles and Practice of Sleep Medicine.* 3rd ed. Philadelphia: W.B. Saunders, 2000. Cited by ¶3551.

aa61. Lass L; Noll J. A coomparative study of rate characteristics in cleft-palate and non-cleft-palate speakers. *Cleft Palate Journal.* 1970; 7: 275-283. Cited by [aa33].

aa62. Lawrence RA; Lawrence RM. *Breastfeeding: A Guide for the Medical Profession.* St. Louis: Mosby, 2005. 1152 pages.

aa63. Lebwohl M; Lebwohl E; Bercovitch L. Prominent mental (chin) crease: a new sign of pseudoxanthoma elasticum. *J Am Acad Dermatol.* 2003; 48: 620-622.

aa64. Leigh RJ; Zee DS. *The Neurology of Eye Movements.* 4th ed. Oxford: Oxford University Press, 2006. Cited by ¶¶866, 868, 1833.

aa65. Li AG; Koster MI; Wang XJ. Roles of TGFbeta signaling in epidermal/appendage development. *Cytokine Growth Factor Rev.* 2003; 14: 99-111.

aa66. Loewenfeld, IE. The Argyll Robertson pupil, 1869-1969. A critical survey of the literature. Pages 199-299 in: [aa103]. Cited by ¶¶4134, 4141.

aa67. Loeys BL; Chen J; Neptune ER; *et al.* A syndrome of altered cardiovascular, craniofacial, neurocognitive and skeletal development caused by mutations in TGFBR1 or TGFBR2. *Nat Genetics.* 2005; 37: 275-281. Cited by ¶¶272, 782, 824, 859.

aa68. Loeys BL; Schwarze U; Holm T; *et al.* Aneurysm syndromes associated with mutations in transforming growth factor β receptor genes. *N Engl J Med.* 2006; 355: 788-798. Cited by ¶¶272, 824.

aa69. Loeys BL; Dietz HC. Aneurysm syndromes and TGF-β receptor mutations. *N Engl J Med.* 2006; 355: 2156.

aa70. Loeys BL; Schwarze U; Holm T; *et al.* Aneurysm syndromes caused by mutations in the TGF-beta receptor. *N Engl J Med.* 2006; 355: 788-798.

aa71. Magdol, Edward. *Owen Lovejoy: Abolitionist in Congress.* New Brunswick, NJ: Rutgers University Press, 1967. Cited by ¶2189. Cited by Special Topic §5e.

aa72. Maher B. His daughter's DNA. *Nature.* 2007; 449: 772-776.

aa73. Marfan AB. Un cas de deformation congenitale des quatre membres plus prononcee aux extremites characterisee par l'allongement des os avec un certain degre d'amincissement. *Bull Mém Soc Méd Hôp Paris.* 1896; 13: 220.

aa74. Maumenee IH. The eye in the Marfan syndrome. *Trans Am Ophth Soc.* 1981; 79: 684-733. Cited by ¶¶860, 861.

aa75. Meers PD. Smallpox still entombed? *Lancet.* 1985; i: 1103. Cited by Special Topics §5e, §5f.

aa76. Melville, Herman; edited by Hayford, Harrison and Parker, Hershel. *Moby-Dick.* New York: W.W. Norton, 1967. Cited by ¶2743.

aa77. Mencken, HL. *A Mencken Chrestomathy.* New York: Vintage Books, 1982. (Originally published 1949.)

aa78. Merritt, H. Houston; Adams, Raymond D.; Solomon, Harry C. *Neurosyphilis.* New York: Oxford University Press, 1946. 443 pages. Cited by Special Topics §2a, §2d.

aa79. Mizuguchi T; Collod-Beroud G; Akiyama T; *et al.* Heterozygous TGFBR2 mutations in Marfan syndrome. *Nat Genetics.* 2004; 36: 855-860.

aa80. Morriss-Kay GM; Wilkie AO. Growth of the normal skull vault and its alteration in craniosynostosis: insights from human genetics and experimental studies. *J Anat.* 2005; 207: 637-653.

aa81. Morton G; Mahon S. The "facial flashing" of aortic regurgitation. *Anesthesia.* 2002; 57: 501-502.

aa82. Most D; Levine JP; Chang J; *et al.* Studies in cranial suture biology: up-regulation of transforming growth factor-β1 and basic fibroblast growth factor mRNA correlates with posterior frontal cranial suture fusion in the rat. *Plast Recon Surg.* 1998; 101: 1431-1440.

aa83. Murdoch JL; Walker BA; Halpern BL; *et al.* Life expectancy and causes of death in the Marfan syndrome. *N Engl J Med.* 1972; 286: 804-808.

aa84. Murphy, Edmond A. *Skepsis, Dogma, and Belief: Uses and Abuses in Medicine.* Baltimore: Johns Hopkins, 1981.

aa85. Nuss D; Croitoru DP; Kelly RE Jr.; *et al.* Congenital chest wall deformities. Chapter 19 (pages 245-263) in: [aa12].

aa86. *Oxford English Dictionary.* Compact edition. Oxford: Oxford University Press, 1971. [Reprint of 1933 reissue. Letter "H" was completed in 1899.] Cited by ¶2743.

aa87. Offit K; Sagi M; Hurley K. Preimplantation genetic diagnosis for cancer syndromes: a new challenge for preventive medicine. *JAMA.* 2006; 296: 2727-2730.

aa88. Panchal J; Uttchin V. Management of craniosynostosis. *Plast Reconstructive Surgery.* 2003; 111: 2032-2048.

aa89. Prag, John; Neave, Richard. *Making Faces: Using Forensic and Archeological Evidence.* London: British Museum, 1997. 256 pages. Cited by ¶¶274, 664, 1591, 1593, 2775, 5460.

aa90. Pyeritz R; McKusick VA. Marfan syndrome: diagnosis and management. *N Engl J Med.* 1979; 300: 772-777.

aa91. Reiser AH Jr. Be thankful for minor aches and pains. *Postgraduate Medicine.* 15 Feb. 1990; 87(3): 21, 24. Cited by ¶2559.

aa92. Rhodes G. The evolutionary psychology of facial beauty. *Annu Rev Psychol.* 2006; 57: 199-226.

aa93. Richter, Jean Paul (ed.). *The Notebooks of Leonardo da Vinci.* New York: Dover, 1970. (Originally published 1883 as *The Literary Works of Leonardo da Vinci.*)

aa94. Ricketts TF. *The Diagnosis of Smallpox.* New York: Funk and Wagnalls Co., 1910. Available online at [archiveorg]. Cited by Special Topic §5e.

aa95. Rimoin DL; Connor JM; Pyeritz RE; *et al. Emery and Rimoin's Principles and Practice of Medical Genetics.* 5th ed. Philadelphia: Churchill Livingstone Elsevier, 2007.

aa96. Riviere, Clive. *The Early Diagnosis of Tubercle.* 2nd ed. London: Oxford Medical Publications, 1919. 314 pages. Cited by ¶540.

aa97. Robinson PN; Arteaga-Solis E; Baldock C; *et al.* The molecular genetics of Marfan syndrome and related disorders. *J Med Genet.* 2006; IN: PRESS.

aa98. Robinson PN; Neumann LM; Demuth S; *et al.* Shprintzen-Goldberg syndrome: fourteen new patients and a clinical analysis. *Am J Med Genet A.* 2005; 135: 251-262.

aa99. Rollo IM. Drugs used in the chemotherapy of malaria. Chapter 45 (Pages 1038-1060 in: [aa43]. Cited by ¶2732.

aa100. Sapira, Joseph D. *The Art and Science of Bedside Diagnosis.* Baltimore: Urban & Schwartzenberg, 1990. Cited by ¶4118.

aa101. Scriver CR; Beaudet AL; Sly WS; *et al. The Metabolic and Molecular Basis of Inherited Disease.* 8th ed. New York: McGraw-Hill, 2001.

aa102. Schuelke M; Wagner KR; Stolz LE; *et al.* Myostatin mutation associated with gross muscle hypertrophy in a child. *N Engl J Med.* 2004; 350: 2682-2688.

aa103. Schwartz, Bernard (ed.). *Syphilis and the Eye.* Baltimore: Williams and Wilkins, 1970.

aa104. Sibley JC. A study of 200 cases of tuberculous pleurisy with effusion. *Am Rev Tuberculosis.* 1950; 62: 314-323.

aa105. Singh KK; Rommel K; Mishra A; *et al.* TGFBR1 and TGFBR2 mutations in patients with features of Marfan syndrome and Loeys-Dietz syndrome. *Hum Mutat.* 2006; 27: 770-777.

aa106. Sotos JG. Medical History of American Presidents. http://www.doctorzebra.com/prez

aa107. Sotos JG. Taft and Pickwick: sleep apnea in the White House. *Chest.* 2003; 124: 1133-1142.

aa108. Sotos JG. The Management of AIDS Patients. *New Engl J Med.* 1987; 316: 632. Cited by Special Topic §2a.

aa109. Sotos JG. *Zebra Cards: An Aid to Obscure Diagnosis.* Philadelphia: American College of Physicians, 1989.

aa110. Stenn FF; Milgram JW; Lee SL; *et al.* Biochemical identification of homogentisic acid pigment in an ochronotic Egyptian mummy. *Science.* 1977; 197: 566-568.

aa111. Stokes, John H.; Beerman, Herman; Ingraham, Norman R. Jr. *Modern Clinical Syphilology: Diagnosis, Treatment, Case Study. 3rd Edition.* Philadelphia: Saunders, 1944. Cited by ¶¶4118, 4237, 4300, 4315, 4616, 4647. Cited by Special Topics §2a, §2d, §2e, §2i, §2j, §2k.

aa112. Stratz, Carl H. *Der Körper des Kindes: für Eltern, Erzieher, Ärzte und Künstler.* Stuttgart: Verlag von Ferdinand Enke, 1903.

aa113. Stuart HC; Pyle SI; Cornoni J; *et al.* Onsets, completions and spans of ossification in the 29 bone-growth centers of the hand and wrist. *Pediatrics.* 1962; 29: 237-249.

aa114. Taussig HB. *Congenital Malformations of the Heart.* New York: The Commonwealth Fund, 1949. Pages 372-374

aa115. ten Dijke P; Hill CS. New insights into TGF-beta-Smad signalling. *Trends Biochem Sci.* 2004; 29: 265-273.

aa116. U.S. Public Health Service. *Syphilis: A Synopsis.* Washington: U.S. Government Printing Office, 1968. PHS Publication 1660. Cited by Special Topic §2a.

aa117. *The War of the Rebellion: A Compilation of the Official Records of the Union and Confederate Armies.* Series 1, vol. 46, Part 3 (Appomattox Campaign), page 97. Available online at: http://ehistory.osu.edu. Cited by ¶¶1265, 1269.

aa118. Weber J; Collmann H; Czarnetzki A; *et al.* Morphometric analysis of untreated adult skulls in syndromic and nonsyndromic craniosynostosis. *Neurosurgical Review.* 9 Nov 2007; Epub ahead of print: 10.1007/s10143-007-0100-x.

aa119. Weldon MM; Smolinski MS; Maroufi A; *et al.* Mercury poisoning associated with a Mexican beauty cream. *West J Med.* 2000; 173: 15-18. Cited by ¶2732.

aa120. Wiklund M; Rudnick J; Liberatore J. Addressing women's needs in surgical instrument design. *Medical Device & Diagnostic Industry (MD& DI).* November 2006; 28(11): 40-45.

aa121. Wright AD. Venereal disease and the great. *Br J Vener Dis.* 1971; 47: 295-306. Cited by Special Topic §2b.

aa122. Wyngaarden JB; Smith LH Jr. (eds). *Cecil Textbook of Medicine.* 16th ed. Philadelphia: W.B. Saunders, 1982. Pages xxiii-xxiv

aa123. Yourcenar, Margaret. *The Memoirs of Hadrian.* New York: Noonday Press, 1990. (Originally published 1951.)

aa124. Zuckerman AJ. Palaeontology of smallpox. *Lancet.* 1984; II: 1454. Cited by Special Topic §5f.

Scientific literature related to MEN2B.

aa125. Baykal C; Buyukbabani N; Boztepe H; *et al.* Multiple cutaneous neuromas and macular amyloidosis associated with medullary thyroid carcinoma. *J Am Acad Dermatol.* 2007; 56: s33-s37.

aa126. Bazex A; Dupre A. Neuromes myeliniques muqueux a localisation centro-faciale et laryngee. *Ann Dermatol Syphilgr.* 1958; 85: 613-641.

aa127. Carlson KM; Bracamontes J; Jackson CE; *et al.* Parent-of-origin effects in multiple endocrine neoplasia type 2B. *Am J Hum Genet.* 1994; 55: 1076-1082. Cited by ¶4735.

aa128. Carney JA; Bianco AJ Jr; Sizemore GW; *et al.* Multiple endocrine neoplasia with skeletal manifestations. *J Bone Joint Surg Am.* 1981; 63: 405-410.

aa129. Chabloz R; Cavin R; Burckhardt P; *et al.* Une variete rare de neoplasies polyendocriniennes: le syndrome MEN IIb ou MEN III. *Schweiz Med Wochenschr.* 1982; 112: 842-852. (Read abstract only).

aa130. Cohen MS; Phay JE; Albinson C; *et al.* Gastrointestinal manifestations of multiple endocrine neoplasia type 2. *Ann Surg.* 2002; 235: 648-655.

aa131. Dyck PJ; Carney JA; Sizemore GW; *et al.* Multiple endocrine neoplasia, type 2b: phenotype recognition; neurological features and their pathological basis. *Ann Neurol.* 1979; 6: 302-314.

aa132. Eng C; Clayton D; Schuffenecker I; *et al.* The relationship between specific RET protooncogene mutations and disease phenotype in multiple endocrine neoplasia type 2. International RET mutation consortium analysis. *JAMA.* 1996; 276: 1575-1579.

aa133. Froboese C. Das aus markhaltigen nervenfascern bestehende gangliezellenlose echte neurom in rankenformzugleich ein beitrag zu den nervosen geschwulsten der zunge und des augenlides. *Virchows Arch Pathol Anat.* 1923; 240: 312-327.

aa134. Gordon C; Majzoub JA; Marsh DJ; *et al.* Four cases of mucosal neuroma syndrome: multiple endocrine neoplasm 2B or not 2B? *J Clin Endocrinol Metab.* 1998; 83: 17-20.

aa135. Gorlin RJ; Cohen MM; Hennekam RCM. Syndromes of the Head and Neck. *4th ed. Oxford.* Oxford University Press; 2001: Pages 462-468..

aa136. Gorlin RJ; Sedano HO; Vickers RA; *et al.* Multiple mucosal neuromas, pheochromocytoma and medullary carcinoma of the thyroid–a syndrome. *Cancer.* 1968; 22: 293-299 passim.

aa137. Gorlin RJ; Vickers RA. Multiple mucosal neuromas, pheochromocytoma, medullary carcinoma of the thyroid and marfanoid body build with muscle wasting: reexamination of a syndrome of neural crest malmigration. *Birth Defects Orig Artic Ser.* 1971; 7: 69-72.

aa138. Goulet-Salmon B; Berthe E; Franc S; *et al.* Prostatic neuroendocrine tumor in multiple endocrine neoplasia type 2B. *J Endocrinol Invest.* 2004; 27: 570-573.

aa139. Hoff AO, Gagel RF. Multiple endocrine neoplasia type 2. Pages 3533-3550 (Chapter 192) in: DeGroot LJ, Jameson JL (eds). *Endocrinology.* 5th ed. Philadelphia: Elsevier-Saunders, 2006.

aa140. Jackson CE; Norum RA. Genetics of the multiple endocrine neoplasia type 2B syndrome. *Henry Ford Hosp Med J.* 1992; 40: 232-235. Cited by ¶43.

aa141. Jain S; Watson MA; DeBenedetti MK; *et al.* Expression profiles provide insights into early malignant potential and skeletal abnormalities in multiple endocrine neoplasia type 2B syndrome tumors. *Cancer Research.* 2004; 64: 3907-3913.

aa142. Kameyama K; Takami H. Medullary thyroid carcinoma: nationwide Japanese survey of 634 cases in 1996 and 271 cases in 2002. *Endocrine Journal.* 2004; 51: 453-456.

aa143. Kaplan PW. Spells: seizures, dizziness, and other episodic disorders. Chapter 13.3 (pages 829-835) in: Stobo JD, Hellman DB, Ladenson PW, Petty BG, Traill TA. *The Principles and Practice of Medicine.* 23d ed. Stamford, CT: Appleton & Lange, 1996.

aa144. Kebebew E; Ituarte PH; Siperstein AE; *et al.* Medullary thyroid carcinoma: clinical characteristics, treatment, prognostic factors, and a comparison of staging systems. *Cancer.* 2000; 88: 1139-1148. Cited by ¶577.

aa145. Khairi MRA; Dexter RN; Burzynski NJ; *et al.* Mucosal neuroma, pheochromocytoma and medullary carcinoma: multiple endocrine neoplasia type 3. *Medicine.* 1975; 54: 89-112.

aa146. Kullberg BJ; Kruseman ACN. Multiple endocrine neoplasia type 2b with a good prognosis. *Arch Intern Med.* 1987; 147: 1125-1127.

aa147. Leboulleux S; Travagli JP; Caillou B; *et al.* Medullary thyroid carcinoma as part of a multiple endocrine neoplasia type 2B syndrome: influence of the stage on the clinical course. *Cancer.* 2002; 94: 44-50.

aa148. Lee NC; Norton JA. Multiple endocrine neoplasia type 2B – genetic basis and clinical expression. *Surgical Oncology*. 2000; 9: 111-116.

aa149. Menko FH; van der Luijt RB; de Valk IA; *et al*. Atypical MEN type 2B associated with two germline RET mutations on the same allele not involving codon 918. *J Clin Endocrinol Metab*. 2002; 87: 393-7.

aa150. Mijatovic J; Airavaara M; Planken A; *et al*. Constitutive Ret activity in knock-in multiple endocrine neoplasia type B mice induces profound elevation of brain dopamine concentration via enhanced synthesis and increases the number of TH-positive cells in the substantia nigra. *J Neurosci*. 2007; 27: 4799-4809.

aa151. Morrison PJ; Nevin NC. Multiple endocrine neoplasia type 2B (mucosal neuroma syndrome, Wagenmann-Froboese syndrome. *J Med Genet*. 1996; 33: 779-782. Cited by ¶43.

aa152. Ohta M; Tokuda Y; Suzuki Y; *et al*. A case of multiple endocrine neoplasia type 2B. *Jpn J Clin Oncol*. 1997; 27: 268-273.

aa153. Ponder BAJ. Multiple endocrine neoplasia type 2. Chapter 42 (pages 931-942) in: [aa101]. Cited by ¶3349.

aa154. Ponder BAJ. The phenotypes associated with ret mutations in the multiple endocrine neoplasia type 2 syndrome. *Cancer Research*. 1999; 59 (Suppl.): 1736s-1742s.

aa155. Quayle FJ; Benveniste R; DeBenedetti MK; *et al*. Hereditary medullary thyroid carcinoma in patients greater than 50 years old. *Surgery*. 2004; 136: 1116-1121.

aa156. Saad MF; Ordonez NG; Rashid RK; *et al*. Medullary carcinoma of the thyroid: a study of the clinical features in 161 patients. *Medicine*. 1984; 63: 319-342.

aa157. Schaffer JV; Kamino H; Witkiewicz A; *et al*. Mucocutaneous neuromas: an underrecognized manifestation of PTEN hamartoma-tumor syndrome. *Arch Dermatol*. 2006; 142: 625-632.

aa158. Schimke RN; Hartmann WH; Prout TE; *et al*. Syndrome of bilateral pheochromocytoma, medullary thyroid carcinoma and multiple neuromas. *N Engl J Med*. 1968; 279: 1-7.

aa159. Sizemore GW; Carney JA; Gharib H; *et al*. Multiple endocrine neoplasia type 2B: eighteen-year follow-up of a four-generation family. *Henry Ford Hosp Med J*. 1992; 40: 236-244. Cited by ¶1954.

aa160. Smith VV; Eng C; Milla PJ. Intestinal ganglioneuromatosis and multiple endocrine neoplasia type 2B: implications for treatment. *Gut*. 1999; 45: 143-146.

aa161. Spyer G; Ellard S; Turnpenny PD; *et al*. Phenotypic multiple endocrine neoplasia type 2B, without endocrinopathy or RET gene mutation: implications for management. *Thyroid*. 2006; 16: 605-608.

aa162. Truchot F; Grezard P; Wolf F; *et al*. Multiple idiopathic neuromas: a new entity? *Br J Dermatol*. 2001; 145: 826-829.

aa163. Ueda T; Oka N; Matsumoto A; *et al*. Pheochromocytoma presenting as recurrent hypotension and syncope. *Intern Med*. 2005; 44: 222-227.

aa164. Vasen HF; van der Feltz M; Raue F; *et al*. The natural course of multiple endocrine neoplasia type IIb. A study of 18 cases. *Arch Intern Med*. 1992; 152: 1250-1252. Cited by ¶¶43, 693.

aa165. Wagenmann A. Multiple neurome des auges und der zunge. *Ber Dtsch Ophthal*. 1922; 43: 282-285.

aa166. Williams ED. A review of 17 cases of carcinoma of the thyroid and phochromocytoma. *J Clin Pathol*. 1965; 18: 288-292.

aa167. Williams ED; Pollock DJ. Multiple mucosal neuromata wih endocrine tumors: a syndrome allied to Von Recklinghausen's disease. *J Pathol Bacteriol*. 1966; 91: 71-80.

aa168. Winkelmann RK, Carney JA. Cutaneous neuropathology in multiple endocrine neoplasia, type 2b. *J Investig Dermatol*. 1982; 79: 307-312.

Literature mentioning Lincoln or dated pre-1950 (i.e., historical literature)

A $\boxed{\checkmark}$ symbol identifies fully-read sources whose contents are fully assimilated into the present work.

A $\boxed{\checkmark-}$ symbol identifies fully-read sources whose contents are partially assimilated into the present work.

A ▷ symbol indicates a biographical note. See [neelyE] and [wilson] for helpful mini-biographies.

$\boxed{\text{AbrahamLincolnAssociation}}$ Abraham Lincoln Association.
`http://www.hti.umich.edu/l/lincoln/` Web site containing full text of [baslerA] and other Lincoln-related volumes.
    A wonderful resource, but can be slow. Click "browse" for included titles.

$\boxed{\text{adelson} \;|\; \checkmark}$ Adelson, Sidney L. Lincoln's health. *Harper Hospital Bulletin*. March-April 1960; 18: 117-119. Cited by ¶848.

$\boxed{\text{angle} \;|\; \checkmark-}$ Angle, Paul M. (ed.). *The Lincoln Reader*. New Brunswick, NJ: Rutgers University Press, 1947. 564 pages. Cited by ¶¶4, 98, 109, 143, 149, 243, 515, 720, 725, 728, 760, 948, 1087, 1094, 1130, 1483, 1574, 1578, 1616, 1671, 1672, 1729, 1768, 1772, 1818, 2002, 2027, 2051, 2072, 2128, 2135, 2147, 2154, 2278, 2344, 2356, 2408, 2489, 2500, 2507, 2528, 2620, 2626, 2634, 2647, 2661, 2663, 2848, 2920, 2974, 2988, 2990, 2998, 3041, 3043, 3104, 3139, 3143, 3176, 3326, 3339, 3372, 3389, 3413, 3450, 3462, 3492, 3501, 3532, 3540, 3543, 3583, 3609, 3610, 3614, 3615, 3616, 3617, 3618, 3620, 3621, 3622, 3623, 3628, 3635, 3637, 3638, 3639, 3641, 3642, 3650, 3651, 3652, 3653, 3658, 3660, 3666, 3686, 3688, 3719, 3720, 3727, 3730, 3793, 3812, 3836, 3840, 3841, 3854, 3872, 3882, 3901, 3902, 3903, 3912, 3943, 3958, 3959, 3965, 3998, 4018, 4022, 4098, 4259, 4332, 4352, 4709, 4736, 4797, 4848, 5056, 5121, 5148, 5161, 5162, 5222, 5223, 5787, 5831, 5854. Cited by Special Topics §4c, §8b, §8d.
    One nice feature of this book is Angle's introductions of the people who have written about Lincoln, giving the date and circumstances in which they met him. A poor feature is the "cleaning up" of original correspondence, e.g. compare [angle p147] *and* [turner p36].

$\boxed{\text{anonA} \;|\; \checkmark}$ Anonymous. President Lincoln. *The Sanitary Commission Bulletin*. 1865; 1(37): 1169. Cited by ¶2191.

$\boxed{\text{anonB} \;|\; \checkmark}$ Anonymous. Lincoln to White House. *Time*. 26 April 1937; : (on the Internet). Cited by ¶¶3010, 3235.

$\boxed{\text{anonC} \;|\; \checkmark}$ Anonymous. Stunning eyewitness account of Lincoln's last hours uncovered by New York City auction firm. Business Wire, Oct. 2, 1995, on the Internet. Cited by ¶3236.

$\boxed{\text{archiveorg}}$ `http://www.archive.org` = an online full-text repository of books.

$\boxed{\text{arnold} \;|\; \checkmark-}$ Arnold, Isaac N. *The Life of Abraham Lincoln*. Fourth ed. Lincoln, NE: Bison Books, 1994. (Originally published 1884.) Cited by ¶¶151, 167, 186, 237, 346, 354, 399, 417, 422, 429, 431, 711, 767, 909, 952, 1040, 1065, 1117, 1118, 1394, 1431, 1466, 1541, 1576, 1607, 1648, 1670, 1788, 1854, 2196, 2259, 2562, 2658, 2666, 2673, 2779, 2903, 2936, 2973, 3097, 3368, 3627, 3638, 3737, 3755, 3759, 3863, 3879, 3883, 3884, 4440, 4485, 4836.

aronson ✓ Aronson SM. Smallpox visits the White House. *Medicine and Health / Rhode Island.* 2002; 85(2): 47.   Cited by Special Topic §5c.

Best avoided. Specific shortcomings are noted in §5c.

ayres Ayres, Philip W.   Lincoln as a neighbor. *American Review of Reviews.* Feb. 1918; 57(2): 183-185.   Cited by ¶3038.

badeau Badeau, Adam. *Grant in Peace. From Appomattox to Mount McGregor. A Personal Memoir.* Hartford, CT: S.S. Scranton & Co., 1887. Available online at [archiveorg]. Cited by ¶¶3693, 4428, 4696.

baker Baker, Jean H. *Mary Todd Lincoln: A Biography.* New York: WW Norton, 1987. Cited by ¶¶3186, 3592, 3931, 3938, 3946, 3953, 3955, 4078, 4093, 4121, 4122, 4126, 4127, 4132, 4136, 4137, 4146, 4149, 4157, 4177, 4178, 4179, 4180, 4181, 4185, 4196, 4262, 4297, 4516, 4528, 4547, 4612, 4613, 4701, 5287, 5298, 5303, 5327, 5328, 5651, 5874.

Baker, a historian, does admirably exhaustive research, but, unfortunately, habitually inflates the thinnest reeds of hard medical information into detailed tapestries, apparently to make her reading compelling. She does this by overlaying onto the bare facts the "usual" medical and nursing practices of the time plus textbook information about the course of the disease in question. It is often difficult to dissect the known from the overlaid. There are errors, too, e.g. describing diphtheria as an "infection of the lungs" (p 125) – diphtheria kills by compromising the upper airway or the heart. Others cite her as providing "informed medical opinion" [donaldA p622n153]. Baker takes a pro-Mary view [burk pp201, 295], but is "not as apologetic" as [randallC].

bancroft ✓ Bancroft, TB.   An audience with Lincoln. *McClure's Magazine.* 1908-1909; 32: 447-450.   Cited by ¶¶131, 182, 252, 721, 765, 816, 1404, 1682, 1778, 2996, 3018, 3604.

barbeeP Barbee, David Rankin – Papers of – In: Special Collections, Georgetown University Libraries, Washington, DC.   Cited by ¶¶1142, 1199, 1200, 1232, 1239, 1240, 1241, 1243, 1245, 1247, 1250, 1251, 1252, 1253, 1257, 1258, 1307, 2282, 3209, 3226, 3230, 3231, 3232, 3400, 4425, 4741, 5001. Cited by Special Topics §1e, §1f, §5b, §7c, §7f.

Barbee, an early 20th century newspaperman with southern sympathies, amassed much information related to Lincoln and his assassination. He corresponded with the children of Dr. Leale.

barnesA ✓ Barnes, John S.   With Lincoln from Washington to Richmond in 1865. I. The President sees a fight and a review. *Appleton's Magazine.* May 1907; 9(5): 515-524.   Cited by ¶¶1266, 1273, 1275, 1276, 1277, 2172, 2264, 2544.

barnesB ✓ Barnes, John S.   With Lincoln from Washington to Richmond in 1865. II. The President enters the confederate capital. *Appleton's Magazine.* June 1907; 9(6): 742-751. Cited by ¶¶838, 904, 1277, 1284, 1286, 1298, 1567, 2545, 2546, 2555, 3738, 4427.

barrett Barrett, Joseph H. *Life of Abraham Lincoln.* Cincinnati: Moore, Wilstach & Baldwin, 1865. 842 pages. Available online at [archiveorg]   Cited by ¶1298.

▷ **Barrett, Oliver R.** *Renowned collector of Lincoln artifacts in the 20th century. Is the subject of [sandburgC].*

▷ **Bartlett, Truman** *Bartlett is described as "a sculptor and Lincoln student"* [schwartzA]. *He corresponded with Herndon* [hertz]. *Bartlett waxes lyrical about Lincoln in* [schurz], *finding nothing whatsoever to criticize. The Massachusetts Historical Society apparently has his papers, with some transcribed by the Lincoln Studies*

Center, Knox College [shenk p216].

| bartonA | Barton WE. *Lincoln at Gettysburg*. Indianapolis: Bobbs-Merrill, 1930. 263 pages. Cited by ¶¶5465, 5567, 5624.

| bartonB | Barton, William E. *Life of Abraham Lincoln.* Volume I. Indianapolis, IN: Educational Press / Bobbs-Merrill Co., 1925. Cited by ¶¶1574, 3139, 3326, 3617, 4848, 5056, 5161, 5162.

| bartonW | Barton, William E. *The Women Lincoln Loved.* Indianapolis, IN: Bobs-Merrill Co., 1927. 377 pages. Cited by ¶3182.

| baslerA | Basler, Roy P. (ed.). *Collected Works of Abraham Lincoln. (8 volumes).* New Brunswick, NJ: Rutgers University Press, 1953. Available online at [AbrahamLincolnAssociation]. **(Cited page numbers are ±1.)** Cited by ¶¶151, 260, 319, 478, 498, 722, 970, 972, 1116, 1151, 1182, 1194, 1263, 1265, 1267, 1268, 1270, 1314, 1396, 1569, 1993, 2028, 2071, 2084, 2128, 2134, 2449, 2453, 2480, 2521, 2739, 2741, 2799, 2818, 2832, 3130, 3319, 3336, 3571, 3582, 3608, 3626, 3792, 3820, 3846, 3852, 3875, 3913, 3922, 4253, 4768, 4837, 4871, 4898, 4991, 5196, 5228, 5235, 5398, 5748. Cited by Special Topics §1a, §2g, §5b, §5e, §6b.

The imprecision in page numbers arose because page-numbering is ambiguous in the on-line version.

| baslerB | Basler, Roy P. (ed.). *The Collected Works of Abraham Lincoln: Supplement 1832-1865.* Westport, CT: Greenwood Press, 1974. Cited by ¶1586. Cited by Special Topics §3a, §5b.

| baslerC | ✓ | Basler, Roy P. Did President Lincoln give the smallpox to William H. Johnson? *Huntington Library Quarterly.* May 1972; 35: 279-284. Cited by ¶3856. Cited by Special Topic §5g.

| batesD | Bates, David Homer. *Lincoln in the Telegraph Office: Recollections of the United States Military Telegraph Corps During the Civil War.* New York: Century Co., 1907. 432 pages.

I have not reviewed this reference. Bates saw Lincoln "nearly every day for four years" during the Civil War and apparently kept a diary [NYTimesTeleg].

▷ | **Bates, Edward** | *Bates was Lincoln's Attorney General until November 1864. He kept a diary* [beale]. *He turned 70 while in office, and was called "a fossil of the Silurian era" by a political rival who must have had some scientific sophistication!* [donaldA p401].

| bayne | Bayne JT. *Tad Lincoln's Father.* Lincoln, NE: University of Nebraska Press, 2001. Cited by ¶¶4226, 5430, 5607, 5665.

Julia Taft [Bayne] was the teenaged older sister of two boys who frequently played with Tad and Willie. She was frequently at the White House, until Willie died. Her book appeared in 1931.

| beale | Beale, Howard K. (ed.). *The Diary of Edward Bates 1859-1866.* Washington: U.S. Government Printing Office, 1933. 685 pages. Available online at [archiveorg]. Cited by ¶¶1186, 1198. Cited by Special Topic §5b.

▷ | **Bellows, Henry W.** | *Rev. Bellows was one of the founders of the United States Sanitary Commission, "the effective predecessor of the American Red Cross Society"* [shutes p90].

beschloss ✓   Beschloss, Michael R.   Last of the Lincolns. *New Yorker*. 28 Feb. 1994; 70(2): 54-59.   Cited by ¶¶2060, 5802.

beschlossB ✓   Beschloss, Michael R. *Presidential Courage: Brave Leaders and How They Changed America 1789-1989*. New York: Simon and Schuster, 2007.   Cited by ¶¶2105, 2164, 2286, 2306, 3253, 4265. Cited by Special Topic §2g.

beveridge   Beveridge, Albert J. *Abraham Lincoln 1809-1858*.   Volume I.   Boston: Houghton Mifflin, 1928.

> *Senator Beveridge made extensive use of the notes Herndon collected. He died before completing volume 2.   For many years his book was the best source of information on Lincoln's early life.*

bishop   Bishop, Jim. *The Day Lincoln Was Shot*. New York: Harper & Brothers, 1955. Cited by ¶¶381, 1102, 1225, 1228, 1236.

> *Does not provide references. St. Bonaventure University has Bishop's papers.*

boller ✓   Boller, Paul F. Jr. *Presidential Anecdotes*. New York: Oxford University Press, 1981.   Cited by ¶1558.

bollett   Bollett, Alfred Jay. *Plagues and Poxes: The Impact of Human History on Epidemic Diseases*. 2nd ed. New York: Demos, 2004. 237+xii pages.   Cited by Special Topic §5e.

borittA ✓   Boritt, Gabor S.; Borit, Adam. Lincoln and the Marfan syndrome: the medical diagnosis of a historical figure. *Civil War History*. 1983; 29: 212-229.   Cited by ¶¶70, 526, 795, 1903, 5853, 5860.

> *This paper is an embarrassment. In contrast to the dispassionate scholarly approach taken by [gordon], this paper is stained by snickering ad hominem attacks and a desire to paint the debate over Marfan syndrome as a clash of ideologies. It has the tone of an after-dinner speech to historians, meant to provoke haughty laughter. This is unfortunate, because Boritt and Borit are careful and wide-ranging in their scholarship. Adam Borit is/was a physician once affiliated, among other institutions, with the medical school at Berkeley [borittB p2] – except there is no medical school at Berkeley, California.*

borittB ✓   Boritt, Gabor S. *How Big Was Lincoln's Toe? or Finding a Footnote: A Sometimes Irreverent Account of a Shoemaker's and a Historian's Adventures More Than a Century Apart*. Redlands, CA: Lincoln Memorial Shrine, Feb. 12, 1989. 25 pages.   Cited by ¶¶923, 938, 939, 940, 971, 982, 986, 996, 1000, 1002, 1003, 1004, 1005, 1006, 1007, 1008, 1011, 1012, 1015, 1016, 1019, 1020. Cited by Special Topic §8f.

> *Text, illustrations, and notes related to a presentation delivered at the 57th annual Lincoln Dinner in Redlands, CA in 1989. The Library of Congress does not list this as a book. Copy obtained from the Abraham Lincoln Presidential Library in Springfield, IL.*

borittC   Boritt, Gabor S. *The Historian's Lincoln: Pseudohistory, Psychohistory, and History*. Urbana, IL: University of Illinois Press, 1988. (See [fehrenbacherC]).

borittD   Boritt, Gabor S. *The Historian's Lincoln: Rebuttals*. Introduction by Robert V. Bruce (pp9-10). Gettysburg, PA: Gettysburg College, 1988.   Cited by ¶6.

borittG   Boritt, Gabor S. *The Gettysburg Gospel*. New York: Simon & Schuster, 2006. Cited by Special Topic §5f.

boyden ✓   Boyden, Anna L. *Echoes from Hospital and White House: A Record of Mrs.*

Rebecca R. Pomroy's Experience in War-Times. Boston: D. Lothrop and Company, 1884. 250 pages. Available online at [archiveorg]. Cited by ¶¶2119, 4407, 4688, 4689, 4691, 5391, 5702, 5708, 5772.

Pomroy was Boyden's mother. During the Civil War, Pomroy worked as a nurse in Army hospitals and, occasionally, in the White House. She was first engaged by the Lincolns when Willie died, to be Tad's nurse. Unfortunately, the book was written long after events occurred, without benefit of Pomroy's diary, which had been lost. A few surviving letters do provide vivid pictures of conditions inside Civil War hospitals. There are suggestions that Mrs. Pomroy was not especially interested in telling her story for the book. It also appears that Pomroy's daughter sometimes inserted elsewhere-published anecdotes and quotes into the book (e.g., page 85), without making it clear this was not first-hand from her mother. Thus, the book, which could have been a terrific source of information about Tad, was a disappointment.

| brooksA | Brooks, Noah. *Abraham Lincoln.* Centennial edition. Washington: National Tribune, 1909. (Originally published 1888 by G.P. Putnam's Sons.) Available online at books.google.com. Cited by ¶¶110, 129, 156, 1399, 1469, 2925, 3046, 3731, 5589, 5662.

Noah Brooks was a newspaper correspondent and friend of Lincoln's from Springfield [donaldA p433]. He saw Lincoln "almost daily" during the last two and a half years of the administration [burl p79]. Per [shenk p287] Brooks arrived in Washington in November 1862. As he started his second term, Lincoln was planning to ask Brooks to be his (Lincoln's) private secretary [donaldA p550]. Brooks dedicated this Lincoln biography to Tad.

| brooksB | ✓ | Brooks, Noah. A boy in the White House. *St. Nicholas: An Illustrated Magazine for Young Folks.* November 1882; 10(1): 57-65. Cited by ¶¶3541, 5314, 5332, 5335, 5336, 5416, 5418, 5419, 5421, 5426, 5440, 5501, 5524, 5551, 5585, 5608, 5635, 5644, 5666.

| brooksC | Brooks, Noah. *Washington in Lincoln's Time.* New York: The Century Co., 1896. Available online at [archiveorg]. Cited by ¶¶454, 461, 657, 821, 1160, 1824, 1971, 2279, 2644, 2993, 3140, 3264, 3346, 3749, 3750, 3762, 5315, 5335, 5502, 5595, 5609, 5656. Cited by Special Topics §8b, §8e.

| brooksO | Brooks, Noah; edited by Burlingame, Michael. *Lincoln Observed: Civil War Dispatches of Noah Brooks.* Baltimore: Johns Hopkins University Press, 1998. Cited by ¶2236.

Includes [brooksR] *as an appendix.*

| brooksR | Brooks, Noah. Personal recollections of Abraham Lincoln. *Harper's New Monthly Magazine.* July 1865; 31: 222-230. Cited by ¶¶189, 724, 727, 907, 2280, 2513, 2579, 2991, 3817, 3907.

Reprinted in [brooksO] *as an appendix.*

| brooksRa | Brooks, Noah. Personal reminiscences of Lincoln. *Scribner's Monthly.* 1877-1878; 15: 561-569.

| brooksRb | Brooks, Noah. Personal reminiscences of Lincoln. *Scribner's Monthly.* 1877-1878; 15: 673-681.

| brown | ✓ | Brown, David. Is Lincoln earliest recorded case of rare disease?. *Washington Post.* 26 Nov. 2007; : A8.

Newspaper article that broke the story of Lincoln and MEN2B.

▷ **Brown, Mary Edwards** | *See comments under* [kunhardtC].

| browneF | Browne, Francis F. *The Every-Day Life of Abraham Lincoln: A Biography of the Great American President from an Entirely New Standpoint, with Fresh and Invaluable Material.* New York: N.D. Thompson Publishing Co., 1886. Available online at [archiveorg]. (There is also a 1913 edition.) Cited by ¶¶147, 193, 204, 205, 242, 382, 428, 462, 730, 1075, 1298, 1699, 1771, 1785, 1843, 1999, 2214, 2381, 2538, 2586, 3003, 3099, 3141, 3403, 3696, 3718. Cited by Special Topics §1c, §5f.

| browneR | Browne, Robert H. *Abraham Lincoln and the Men of His Time: His Cause, His Character, and True Place in History, and the Men, Statesmen, Heroes, Patriots, Who Formed the Illustrious League About Him.* Revised second ed. Chicago: Blakely-Oswald Printing Company, 1907. Available online at [archiveorg]. Cited by ¶¶1762, 3194, 3315, 4863, 5167.

Has been called a "very poorly organized" biography [lincloreHZA].

| browning | Browning, Orville; Pease, Theodore Calvin and Randall, James G. (eds.). *The Diary of Orville Hickman Browning. Volume I: 1850-1864.* Springfield, IL: Illinois State Historical Library, 1925. Cited by ¶¶1144, 1145, 1146, 1154, 1198, 1209, 1885, 1886, 1953, 2541, 2619, 2623, 2635. Cited by Special Topic §5b.

Browning met Lincoln in the Black Hawk War. They remained friends. Despite this, the diary has been called "rather arid" [donaldA p293], *perhaps because the modern owner of the diary consented to publication "only on condition that certain sections and entries be omitted. They were omitted"* [hertz p19]. ○○○ *Project: Check original Browning diary for omitted portions.* ● ● ● *During the Civil War Browning was a US Senator from Illinois – which provided no immunity from a pickpocket at a White House reception* [leech p152]*! After Browning's defeat for re-election in 1862, Lincoln had no personal friends in Congress* [donaldA p426]. *I read all 1865 entries through April 15.*

| bruce | Bruce, Robert V. *Lincoln and the Tools of War.* Indianapolis: Bobbs-Merrill, 1956. Cited by ¶3839.

"The only book that truly highlights Lincoln's scientific mind" [burk p135].

| bumgarnerA | ✓ | Bumgarner, John R. *The Health of the Presidents: The 41 United States Presidents Through 1993 from a Physician's Point of View.* Jefferson, NC: MacFarland & Company, 1994. Pages 89-97. Cited by ¶849.

| bumgarnerB | ✓ | Bumgarner, John. *The Health of Abraham Lincoln.* Lincoln Herald. 2001; 103(2): 78-84. Cited by ¶¶484, 589, 798, 799, 978, 1362, 1368, 1890, 2019, 2022, 5020. Cited by Special Topic §2e.

| burk | ✓– | Burkhimer, Michael. *100 Essential Lincoln Books.* Nashville: Cumberland House, 2003. 305 pages. Cited by ¶¶20, 197, 1689, 1950, 2717, 5810. Cited by Special Topics §2c, §2g, §4e.

| burl | ✓ | Burlingame, Michael. *The Inner World of Abraham Lincoln.* Urbana, IL: University of Illinois Press, 1994. 380 pages. Cited by ¶¶12, 14, 16, 60, 93, 169, 170, 238, 241, 351, 580, 756, 955, 1063, 1323, 1324, 1325, 1454, 1455, 1465, 1474, 1664, 1745, 1754, 1830, 1873, 1960, 1969, 2107, 2115, 2120, 2143, 2156, 2308, 2313, 2406, 2427, 2437, 2441, 2454, 2462, 2463, 2474, 2524, 2577, 2578, 2579, 2580, 2581, 2582, 2606, 2616, 2651, 2670, 2671, 2672, 2676, 2683, 2684, 2685, 2686, 2687, 2693, 2755, 2871, 2909, 2910, 2911, 3015, 3059, 3107, 3111, 3112, 3167, 3343, 3344, 3345, 3441, 3444, 3445, 3499, 3564, 3565, 3590, 3591, 3594, 3596, 3598, 3599, 3600, 3741, 3763, 3764, 3765, 3917, 3958, 3981, 4004, 4050, 4053, 4097, 4289, 4293, 4306, 4322, 4326, 4340, 4341, 4342, 4354, 4355, 4451, 4457, 4458, 4536, 4537, 4539, 4544, 4558, 4654, 4662, 4678, 4697, 4725, 4788, 4841, 4842, 4843, 4917, 4965, 4972, 4973, 4974, 4984, 4995, 4996, 5030, 5166, 5670, 5671, 5684, 5743, 5757, 5834, 5840,

5850, 5851, 5852, 5853, 5863, 5871, 5894, 5895. Cited by Special Topics §4b, §8c.
Burlingame edited: [brooksO], [hayC], [hayD], [stevens], [stoddardA], *and* [stoddardB].

busey Busey, Samuel C. *Personal Reminiscences and Recollections.* Washington: (No publisher), 1895. Available online at books.google.com. Cited by ¶¶2889, 2978, 3202.

carman ✓ Carman, Louis D. Dr. Abraham Lincoln. *J Med Soc NJ.* April 1922; : 102-103. Cited by ¶¶2046, 3847, 3857.

carpenter Carpenter FB. *Six Months in the White House: The Story of a Picture.* New York: Hurd & Houghton, 1866. Available online at [AbrahamLincolnAssociation]. Cited by ¶¶194, 219, 329, 459, 534, 726, 775, 833, 909, 1074, 1297, 1298, 1719, 1782, 2190, 2653, 2657, 2667, 3207, 3401, 3527, 5491, 5547. Cited by Special Topic §8e.
Carpenter, a painter, had frequent access to the White House from Feb.-July 1864. There are questions about how much interaction Carpenter had with Lincoln [burk p4]. *It is also said that "The last part of the book simply reprints much about Lincoln that was in the popular media at the time"* [burk p5].

▷ Carpenter, Mrs. George B. *Lulu Boone Carpenter became a "society grande dame" of Chicago. Her younger sister Mary (née Boone) was Tad's "girl" at some time he lived in Chicago 1865-1868* [lewis].

carrA Carr, Clark E. *My Day and Generation.* Chicago: A.C. McClurg & Co., 1908. Cited by ¶¶963, 1698, 1812, 2403, 3734. Cited by Special Topics §5b, §5e, §8b, §8e.

carrB ✓ Carr, Clark E. *Lincoln at Gettysburg: An Address.* Chicago: A.C. McClurg & Co., 1906. Available online at books.google.com. Cited by ¶¶2168, 3027, 3734. Cited by Special Topics §5b, §5h.

chambers *Chambers's Encyclopædia: A Dictionary of Universal Knowledge for the People.* Philadelphia: J.B. Lippincott & Co.: 1870. Available online at books.google.com. Cited by ¶2732.

chambrunA ✓ Chambrun, Marquis de. Personal recollections of Mr. Lincoln. *Scribner's Magazine.* Jan. 1893; 13(1): 26-38. Cited by ¶¶200, 264, 309, 464, 517, 562, 749, 777, 839, 1295, 1298, 1304, 1439, 1624, 1649, 1744, 2361, 2383, 2791, 2949, 3142, 3374, 3796.
Chambrun first met Lincoln at the end of February 1865. This article, and the largely overlapping [chambrunB], *are both translated from the French. Is additional untranslated material available* [chambrunB p82]?

chambrunB Chambrun, Marquis de. *Impressions of Lincoln and the Civil War: A Foreigner's Account.* New York: Random House, 1952. Cited by ¶¶200, 1313, 2361, 3007.

▷ Chapman, A.H. *Husband of Harriet Hanks Chapman, his first name was Augustus.* [wilson p95n, 743]

▷ Chapman, Harriet Hanks *The daughter of Lincoln's cousin Dennis Hanks and Lincoln's step-sister, Elizabeth Johnston. See Figure 3. She lived with Lincoln and his family in Springfield for a year and a half in the mid-1840s (?early 1840s* [angle p191]). *"Mrs. Lincoln tried to make a servant, a slave of her, but, being high-spirited, she refused to become Mrs. Lincoln's tool"* [hertz p109]. *Married A.H. Chapman* [wilson p95n, 743].

chenery ✓ Chenery, William Dodd. Mary Todd Lincoln should be remembered for many kind acts, Chenery says. *Illinois State Register.* 27 Feb. 1938; : (Photostat of reprint of original is in [randallP box 71]).   Cited by ¶4647.

ChicagoTribune   *Chicago Tribune* newspaper. [ProQuest provides a searchable online database of articles from the 1849 to the present.]   Cited by ¶¶457, 1178, 1229, 1233, 1256, 1718, 1893, 2637, 3136, 3728, 3773, 4031, 4060, 4068, 4091, 4128, 4159, 4170, 4207, 4257, 4481, 4482, 4501, 4508, 4526, 4560, 4567, 4608, 4669, 4673, 4705, 4908, 4921, 4936, 4941, 4947, 4978, 4979, 4987, 5245, 5246, 5261, 5263, 5274, 5277, 5293, 5307, 5308, 5330, 5376, 5379, 5431, 5432, 5457, 5481, 5487, 5565, 5566, 5599, 5613, 5801, 5808. Cited by Special Topics §1d, §5b, §5e, §5g.

The Tribune was often critical of Lincoln [donaldA pp458,474].

---

clark   Clark, Leon Pierce.   *Lincoln: A Psycho-Biography.*   New York: Charles Scribner's Sons, 1933. 570 pages.   Cited by ¶2308.

---

cochrane ✓   Cochrane HC. With Lincoln to Gettysburg. Pages 87-93 in: *Military Essays and Recollections of the Pennsylvania Commandery Military Order of the Loyal Legion of the United States. Vol. II. February 10, 1904 - May 10, 1933.* Cavanaugh, Michael A. (ed.). Wilmington, NC: Broadfoot Publishing Company, 1995.   Cited by ¶¶456, 748, 1781, 2169, 2535, 3399.

This may also have appeared in the Gettysburg Start and Sentinel of May 22, 1907.

---

coffinA ✓   Coffin, Charles Carleton.   Lincoln's first nomination and his visit to Richmond in 1865. Chapter 6, Pages 165-188) in: [riceB].   Cited by ¶¶111, 112, 157, 320, 374, 447, 676, 696, 742, 762, 1089, 1279, 1290, 1294, 1366, 1401, 1617, 1677, 1733, 1742, 1743, 1846, 1855, 2347, 2512, 2514, 2945, 3780, 3905.

Was western correspondent for the Boston Journal [angle p278].

---

coffinB   Coffin, Charles Carleton. *Abraham Lincoln.* New York: Harper & Brothers, 1893. Available online at books.google.com.   Cited by ¶¶1272, 1289, 1291, 1298.

---

conant ✓–   Conant, Alban Jasper.   A portrait painter's reminiscences of Lincoln. *McClure's Magazine.* 1908-1909; 32: 512-516.   Cited by ¶¶293, 745, 834, 1432, 1613.

CongressionalGlobe   Congressional Globe. See:
http://lcweb2.loc.gov/ammem/amlaw/lwcg.html   Cited by Special Topic §5b.

This was the forerunner to the Congressional Record.

▷ **Crawford, Elizabeth**   *The wife of "old blue nose Crawford," who employed both Abraham and Thomas Lincoln at various times in Indiana.*

---

crellin ✓   Crellin, JK.   Robert King Stone, M.D., physician to Abraham Lincoln. *Illinois Medical Journal.* 1979; 155: 97-99.   Cited by ¶¶3204, 3205, 3206.

---

croffut ✓   Croffut WA.   Lincoln's Washington: recollections of a journalist who knew everybody. *Atlantic Monthly.* January 1930; 145(1): 55-65.   Cited by ¶¶114, 196, 379, 776, 1555, 1694, 1783, 2311, 2655, 3402, 3687, 5489. Cited by Special Topic §4b.

---

crookA ✓   Crook, WH.   *Through Five Administrations: Reminiscences of Colonel William H. Crook, Body-Guard to President Lincoln.* Compiled and edited by Margarita Spalding Gerry. New York: Harper & Brothers, 1910. Available online at [archiveorg].   Cited by ¶¶198, 347, 460, 652, 661, 817, 965, 1263, 1264, 1298, 1304, 1310, 1316, 1376, 1695, 1787, 1789, 2062, 2174, 2238, 2265, 2362, 2363, 2553, 2556, 2557, 2587, 2675, 2904, 3220, 3506, 3507, 3508, 3509, 3510, 3511, 3512, 3513, 3515, 3735, 3888, 4009, 4030, 4110, 4225, 4234, 4422, 4439, 4443, 4448, 5002, 5242, 5433, 5576, 5592, 5593, 5640. Cited by Special Topic

§4b.

Crook was Lincoln's bodyguard starting Jan. 4, 1865 (p1). Crook soft-pedals his account, e.g. his bland telling of the end of Lincoln's exhausting walk through Richmond (p54). A 23-page manuscript titled "John F. Parker: Much Maligned Virginian" in [barbeeP - box 2 folder 133] *severely criticizes Crook. All the Lincoln pages (1-79) have been processed. There is much redundancy with* [crookK].

crookB ✓– Croook, WH; Gerry, MS. Lincoln's last day: new facts now told for the first time. *Harper's Monthly Magazine.* Sept. 1907; 115 : 519. Cited by ¶¶1281, 1282, 3520.

crookK ✓– Croook, WH. Lincoln as I knew him. *Harper's Monthly Magazine.* Dec. 1906; 114(1): 107-114. Cited by ¶¶198, 347, 652, 1695, 1787, 2062, 2265, 3508, 3509, 3511, 3515, 3735, 4009, 5242, 5434, 5576, 5640.

currentEB ✓– Current RN. Abraham Lincoln. Volume 14, Pages 45-53 in: [aa34]. Cited by ¶¶1060, 3115, 4779. Cited by Special Topics §8b, §8f.

currentBk ✓ Current RN. *The Lincoln Nobody Knows.* New York: Hill and Wang, 1963. Cited by ¶¶46, 175, 571, 724, 1561, 1563, 1715, 1790, 1848, 2020, 3005, 3535, 3547, 3597, 5065. Cited by Special Topic §2d.

currentNY ✓– Current RN. Vidal's 'Lincoln': an exchange. *New York Review of Books.* 18 August 1988; 35(13): (Is on-line at: www.nybooks.com/articles/4341) (On-line version includes text of [vidalA].). Cited by ¶625. Cited by Special Topic §2d.

curtis ✓ Curtis E. Glimpses of hospital life in war times: read before the New York Commandery, October 7, 1908. Pages 54-65 in: *Personal Recollections of the War of the Rebellion: Addresses Delivered Before the Commandery of the State of New York, Military Order of the Loyal Legion of the United States, Fourth Series.* Blakeman, A. Noel (ed.). Wilmington, NC: Broadfoot Publishing Company, 1992 (originally published New York: Knickerbocker Press, 1912.) Cited by ¶¶2939, 2940, 3271, 3278, 3295, 3416.

May also be in: Journal of Civil War Medicine. Vol. 7, no. 4 (Oct.-Dec. 2003).

▷ **Dahlgren, John A.** *Admiral Dahlgren was stationed at the Washington Navy Yard during the Civil War. Lincoln found him "a man of broad-ranging intellectual curiosity and sound judgment," and hardly a week passed without Lincoln visiting him* [donaldA p432]. *Lincoln said: "When I am depressed, I like to talk to Dahlgren"* [burl p106]. *A book, "The Memoir of John A. Dahlgren" appeared in 1882.*

dana Dana, Charles A *Recollections of the Civil War: With the Leaders at Washington and in the Field in the Sixties.* New York: D. Appleton and Co., 1898. Available online at [archiveorg]. Cited by ¶¶113, 183, 206, 565, 1067, 1435, 1615, 1638, 1806, 2930, 3393, 5464.

Dana was editor of the New York Tribune during peacetime [dana p vi]. *He was Assistant Secretary of War from 1863-1865* [dana p iii].

davidsonG ✓ Davidson GW. Abraham Lincoln and the DNA controversy. *Journal of the Abraham Lincoln Assn.* 1996; 17(1): 1-26. Cited by ¶¶76, 317.

davidsonJ ✓ Davidson JRT; Connor KM; Swartz M. Mental illness in U.S. presidents between 1776 and 1974: a review of biographical sources. *Journal of Nervous and Mental Disease.* 2006; 194: 47-51. Cited by ¶2594.

dicey Dicey, Edward. *Six Months in the Federal States.* Two volumes. London: Macmillan, 1863. Available online at [archiveorg]. Cited by ¶¶179, 253, 344, 511, 678, 768, 997, 1405, 1419, 1437, 1473, 1484, 1508, 1553, 1618, 1639, 1683, 1777, 1859, 2262, 2790, 2822,

2946, 3048.

dimsdale ✓ Dimsdale JE. President Lincoln: an instance of stress and aging. *Psychosom Med.* 1998; 60: 2-4. Cited by ¶¶187, 1948.

dole ✓ Dole, Robbert J. *Great Presidential Wit.* New York: Scribner, 2001. Cited by ¶2402.

donaldA ✓ Donald DH. *Lincoln.* New York: Simon and Schuster/Touchstone, 1996. Cited by ¶¶23, 46, 74, 91, 100, 151, 163, 171, 191, 199, 201, 202, 217, 369, 375, 383, 412, 444, 452, 453, 479, 485, 489, 615, 655, 704, 714, 719, 723, 729, 731, 789, 836, 898, 1031, 1071, 1088, 1098, 1109, 1114, 1148, 1152, 1156, 1157, 1158, 1159, 1170, 1190, 1255, 1262, 1267, 1287, 1298, 1311, 1365, 1557, 1560, 1612, 1693, 1702, 1732, 1807, 1884, 1959, 1994, 2014, 2033, 2069, 2073, 2117, 2170, 2405, 2421, 2426, 2447, 2448, 2458, 2473, 2480, 2574, 2596, 2628, 2629, 2636, 2638, 2639, 2640, 2642, 2643, 2688, 2726, 2748, 2752, 2814, 2831, 2871, 2872, 2894, 2900, 2924, 2953, 3009, 3131, 3175, 3176, 3183, 3317, 3322, 3324, 3373, 3391, 3396, 3414, 3439, 3440, 3451, 3500, 3524, 3525, 3526, 3530, 3542, 3545, 3556, 3557, 3570, 3603, 3695, 3697, 3740, 3742, 3743, 3748, 3757, 3758, 3887, 3923, 3931, 3947, 4220, 4249, 4250, 4323, 4329, 4338, 4370, 4403, 4643, 4644, 4645, 4656, 4661, 4664, 4694, 4695, 4777, 4781, 4950, 4970, 5029, 5093, 5146, 5153, 5158, 5175, 5217, 5397, 5414, 5453, 5478, 5495, 5514, 5591, 5616, 5618, 5623, 5648, 5654, 5668, 5714, 5728, 5734, 5747, 5778. Cited by Special Topics §2g, §4b, §5b, §5e, §5f, §8b.

I read this book before beginning the Lincoln "diagnosis project." Thus, there may be more information to mine from it.

donaldB Donald DH. *Lincoln's Herndon.* New York: A.A. Knopf, 1948. Cited by ¶1325.

donaldH ✓ Donald DH. *Lincoln at Home: Two Glimpses of Abraham Lincoln's Family Life.* New York: Simon and Schuster, 2000. 125 pages. Cited by ¶¶308, 376, 1137, 1153, 1165, 1166, 1167, 1168, 1172, 1173, 1174, 1191, 1192, 1193, 1215, 1283, 1463, 1478, 1512, 1552, 2063, 2082, 2104, 2205, 2566, 2771, 3436, 3442, 3443, 3531, 4248, 4290, 4399, 4400, 4415, 4416, 4450, 4473, 4690, 4695, 4940, 4959, 5348, 5352, 5417, 5496, 5497, 5602, 5730. Cited by Special Topic §5b.

dugan ✓ Dugan, James. Bedlam in the boudoir. *Collier's.* 1947; (Feb. 22): 17, 69-70. Cited by ¶3516.

durham ✓ Durham HF. Lincoln's sons and the Marfan syndrome. *Abraham Lincoln Herald.* 1977; 79(2): 67-71. Cited by ¶¶75, 3918, 3937, 3938, 3962, 4927, 4934, 5270, 5278, 5280, 5708, 5724, 5742.

Contains no original material and uncritically accepts what others have written.

eisenschimlC Eisenschiml, Otto. *The Case of A.L———, Aged 56: Some Curious Medical Aspects of Lincoln's Death and Other Studies.* Chicago: Abraham Lincoln Bookstore, 1943. 55 pages. Cited by ¶575.

I have not seen this book. Eisenschiml is better known for writing a popular, but poorly regarded, book claiming Edwin Stanton organized Lincoln's murder.

emersonA ✓ Emerson, Jason. The madness of Mary Lincoln. *American Heritage.* July 2006; 57(3): (viewed online). Cited by ¶¶3982, 4511, 4609, 4671, 4910.

emersonB Emerson, Jason. *The Madness of Mary Lincoln.* Carbondale, IL: Southern Illinois University Press, 2007. Cited by ¶¶3982, 4545.

evans ✓ Evans WA. *Mrs. Abraham Lincoln: A Study of Her Personality and Her Influence on Lincoln.* New York: Alfred A. Knopf, 1932.   Cited by ¶¶16, 59, 572, 622, 2033, 2034, 2398, 2430, 2593, 2601, 2614, 2679, 2769, 3186, 3938, 3972, 3985, 3986, 3998, 4000, 4005, 4007, 4008, 4010, 4012, 4019, 4021, 4028, 4029, 4033, 4034, 4038, 4039, 4040, 4042, 4045, 4062, 4063, 4065, 4067, 4070, 4079, 4081, 4084, 4085, 4086, 4087, 4088, 4092, 4104, 4106, 4107, 4108, 4112, 4115, 4117, 4119, 4154, 4160, 4162, 4163, 4164, 4174, 4175, 4176, 4188, 4193, 4194, 4197, 4213, 4219, 4221, 4222, 4223, 4224, 4226, 4227, 4228, 4229, 4230, 4232, 4235, 4237, 4238, 4239, 4240, 4252, 4270, 4276, 4278, 4281, 4282, 4285, 4302, 4308, 4309, 4310, 4311, 4312, 4330, 4388, 4395, 4413, 4417, 4442, 4456, 4462, 4465, 4466, 4467, 4483, 4490, 4492, 4495, 4496, 4500, 4501, 4502, 4504, 4507, 4508, 4509, 4514, 4515, 4520, 4521, 4524, 4526, 4529, 4553, 4554, 4555, 4562, 4563, 4564, 4565, 4568, 4569, 4570, 4590, 4611, 4615, 4623, 4624, 4626, 4627, 4636, 4637, 4638, 4639, 4652, 4653, 4670, 4675, 4682, 4696, 4700, 4702, 4704, 4942, 4979, 5255, 5258, 5308, 5319, 5320, 5328, 5401, 5465, 5552, 5573, 5582, 5596, 5627, 5632, 5665, 5696, 5697, 5710, 5779, 5864, 5873, 5879, 5882, 5885, 5890, 5891, 5892, 5895, 5896, 5897, 5900.

William Augustus Evans was a pathologist and later a prominent public health physician and newspaper columnist. Although he is primarily interested in Mary Lincoln's mental function, he has nevertheless collected and analyzed much information related to her physical being. Some of his analysis shows its age, e.g., the psychiatric labels he applies, the conclusions he draws from head shape [evans p280], and uncomfortable comments about her attractiveness. On the other hand, physicians of his era would have been far more familiar with now-rare clinical entities pertinent to the Lincolns, e.g., diphtheria and tuberculous pleurisy. Evans was well acquainted (and apparently influenced by) William Barton. [randallC p18] calls it "a valuable book." Evans is not above making minor mis-quotations to make his points clearer (¶5308) (¶5465).

fehrenbacherA Fehrenbacher, Don E. *Lincoln: Speeches and Writings 1832-1858.* New York: Library of America, 1989. 899 pages.   Cited by ¶4.

fehrenbacherB ✓ Fehrenbacher, Don E. Communications. *American Historical Review.* 1991; Feb.: 326-328.   Cited by Special Topics §2b, §2d.

Correspondence relating to this letter is in Stanford University's collection of Fehrenbacher's papers. It is unrevealing, however, except for a few pages listing "Vidal's mistakes."

fehrenbacherC Fehrenbacher, Don E. Vidal's Lincoln. Chapter 14, Pages 387-391 in: [borittC].   Cited by Special Topic §2d.

ferguson ✓ Ferguson, Andrew. *Land of Lincoln: Adventures in Abe's America.* New York: Atlantic Monthly Press, 2007.   Cited by ¶¶34, 35, 806, 1292, 3254, 3255, 3256, 3301, 3302, 5774, 5798. Cited by Special Topic §2b.

field Field, Maunsell B. *Memories of Many Men and of Some Women.* New York: Harper & Brothers, 1874.   Cited by ¶¶1315, 2563.

Field was one of four men who claimed they put the coins on Lincoln's eyes just after the moment of his death [kunhardtB p109].

finney Finney JMT. *A Surgeon's Life.* New York: G. P. Putnam's Sons, 1940.   Cited by ¶3215. Cited by Special Topic §5b.

fishman ✓ Fishman RS; Da Silveira A. Lincoln's craniofacial microsomia. *Arch Ophthalmol.* 2007; 125: 1126-1130.   Cited by ¶¶285, 286, 287, 288, 289, 894, 1945, 2803.

fisk Fisk, Wilbur; Rosenblatt, Emil (ed.); Rosenblatt, Ruth (ed.).   *Hard Marching Every*

Day: The Civil War Letters of Private Wilbur Fisk, 1861-1865. Lawrence, KS: University Press of Kansas, 1992. Cited by ¶¶1298, 1300, 1304.

flattman ✓ Flattman GJ; O'Leary JP. Lincoln's last hours. *Am Surg.* 1997; 63: 561-564. Cited by ¶¶211, 380.

fleisher ✓ Fleisher MH. *The Madness of Mary Lincoln* [Review]. *JAMA.* 2008; 299: 2688-2689. Cited by Special Topic §2i.

floyd Floyd. George P. Abraham Lincoln's rum sweat. *McClure's Magazine.* 1907-1908; 30: 303-308. (In Jan. 1908 issue.). Cited by ¶710.

forliti ✓ Forliti, Amy. Disease may have caused Lincoln's gait. Associated Press. January 28, 2006. Cited by Special Topic §8a.

foster Foster, Lillian. *Way-side Glimpses, North and South.* New York: Rudd & Carleton, 1860. Available online at: http://quod.lib.umich.edu/m/moa/. Cited by ¶1675.

foy ✓ Foy, Eddie; Harlow, Alvin F. Clowning through life. *Collier's.* 1926; (Dec. 25): 15-16, 30. Cited by ¶¶4139, 4487, 4488.

Foy's real name was Edward Fitzgerald. His mother "was employed as a sort of nurse, guard and companion" to Mary Lincoln from early 1872 "until toward the close of [Mary's] life" (or until 1875... the text is ambiguous).

french French, Benjamin Brown; Cole, Donald B. & McDonough, John J. (eds). *Witness to the Young Republic: A Yankee's Journal, 1828-1870.* Hanover, NH: University Press of New England, 1989. Cited by ¶¶735, 815, 1070, 1161, 1198, 1201, 1221, 1564, 1583, 1614, 2211, 3025, 4423. Cited by Special Topic §4b.

I read all 1865 entries through April 15.

gary Gary R. *Following in Lincoln's Footsteps: A Complete Annotated Reference to Hundreds of Historical Sites Visited by Abraham Lincoln.* New York: Carroll and Graf, 2001. Cited by ¶¶216, 990, 1426, 2056, 2058, 2195, 2819, 3448, 3605. Cited by Special Topic §5f.

▷ **Gillespie, Joseph** *A "special legal and political friend of Lincoln's," they met in the Black hawk War* [wilson p749]. *Gillespie's "detailed and highly analytical letters to Herndon contain many perceptive remarks on Lincoln's intellect"* [wilsonH p260].

goff Goff, John S. *Robert Todd Lincoln: A Man in His Own Right.* Norman, OK: University of Oklahoma Press, 1968. Cited by ¶4910.

goldberg ✓ Goldberg R; Andrew LB. *Lincoln's Melancholy* [Review]. *JAMA.* 2007; 297: 2033-2034. Cited by ¶2595.

goldman ✓ Goldman AS; Schmalstieg FC. Abraham Lincoln's Gettysburg Illness. *J Med Biog.* 2007; 15: 104-110. Cited by ¶2035. Cited by Special Topics §5b, §5c, §5e, §5g.

A valiant account of Lincoln's smallpox with many good points, but flawed by its direct and indirect use of [marx] *and by its erroneous references. More specific shortcomings are noted in §5c.*

goldsteinJ ✓ Goldstein JH. Lincoln's vertical strabismus. *J Pediatr Ophthalmol Strabismus.* 1997; 34: 118-120. Cited by ¶¶866, 885, 1833.

good Good TS (ed). *We Saw Lincoln Shot.* Jackson, MS: University of Mississippi Press,

1995.   Cited by ¶¶321, 574, 3228, 3229, 3237. Cited by Special Topics §7b, §7d.

Leale's account was written in 1867, but was based on notes he wrote "a few hours after leaving his death bed," i.e. in April 1865. Taft's account was published in Century Magazine in February 1893, but was based on notes he wrote the day after Lincoln's death.

gordon ✓ Gordon, Abraham M. Abraham Lincoln – a medical appraisal. *J Ky Med Assoc.* 1962; 60: 249-253.   Cited by ¶¶38, 62, 64, 67, 208, 269, 293, 507, 533, 536, 673, 747, 977, 987, 1513, 1640, 2269, 2805, 2811, 2906, 2995, 3023, 5323. Cited by Special Topic §8f.

This is a brilliant, scholarly paper. Gordon had clinical experience with Marfan syndrome, having studied and written about a 5-generation family. His assessment of Lincoln is methodical and balanced. Unlike his critics, he provides a differential diagnosis. I could not find the promised expansion of his article in the Lincoln Herald.

gordonB ✓ Gordon, AM. Lincoln-Marfan debate ... maternal theory. *JAMA.* 13 July 1964; 189: 164 only.   Cited by ¶¶5789, 5790.

▷ **Gourley, James** *"I Knew Lincoln as Early as 1834 ... I lived next door neighbor to Lincoln 19 years [in Springfield]: Knew him & his family relations well"* [wilson pp451, 452].

▷ **Graham, Mentor** *His self-described role in tutoring Lincoln is disputed* [wilson p750]. *According to William Herndon: "He was an intelligent man, a good and truthful man, and yet in some thins he was 'sorter cranky'"* [hertz p132]. *Graham's sister was married to William Herndon's cousin Rowan* [walsh pp66-67].

▷ **Green, William** *Herndon believes Green is not always believable: "I have no confidence in ... Bill Green ... Green is not a liar, but a blow, a 'hifalutin' exaggerator, etc., – good clever fellow for all that"* [hertz p59]. *And: "In his dealings, etc., he is called 'Slippery Bill'"* [hertz p66]. *Others called him "Slicky Bill"* [walsh p155]. *He later spelled his name "Greene"* [walsh p155].

grimsley ✓ Grimsley ET. Six months in the White House. *J Illinois State Hist Soc.* 1926-1927; 19(3-4): 43-73.   Cited by ¶¶640, 647, 1134, 2630, 3348, 3485, 4161, 4396, 4397, 4404, 4717, 5385, 5429, 5445, 5600, 5639, 5683, 5733, 5755, 5760, 5763, 5765, 5775.

Mary's cousin, Elizabeth Todd Grimsley, moved to Washington with the Lincolns in 1861 "to assist in social functions at the White House." She stayed for six months.

hallA Hall, Angelo. *An Astronomer's Wife: The Biography of Angeline Hall.* Baltimore: Nunn & Company, 1908.   Cited by ¶3776.

hallJ ✓– Hall JO. *Lincoln's Unknown Private Life: An Oral History by His Black Housekeeper Mariah Vance* [**Review**]. *Journal of the Abraham Lincoln Association.* 1998; 19(1): 73-95.   Cited by ¶¶5345, 5475, 5605.
Concludes that [ostendorfC] *is not a trustworthy reference.*

hamilton Hamilton C; Ostendorf L. *Lincoln in Photographs: An Album of Every Known Pose.* Norman, OK: University of Oklahoma Press, 1963.   Cited by ¶¶17, 2798.
Updated version is [ostendorfA].

▷ **Hanks, Dennis** *Dennis Hanks was Lincoln's cousin and boyhood playmate. Historians generally regard him as an untrustworthy source, in the sense that he had an agenda behind his pronouncements. (His agenda seems to have been to present Lincoln's maternal history in a positive light.) Born Feb. 9, 1802* [wilson p615], *he*

481

was a "man of endless loquacity" [donaldA p26]. *William Herndon was warned about Hanks by several people (e.g.* [wilson pp103, 122, 532]*), including this strong statement from James Rardin in 1888: "Dennis Hanks is not only old but he is also noted for years as being a pretty big liar even in his pristine days"* [wilson p651]. *Herndon occasionally challenged Hanks about his statements* [wilson p103] *and cautioned many others that Hanks "loves to blow"* [hertz p94, also pp59, 66, 109].

▷ **Hanks, John** | *Another cousin who lived with the Lincolns for awhile* [donaldA p29]. *Herndon thought him "a good man and a truthful one, but does not always know"* [hertz p59, also pp66, 109].

harris | Harris WC. *Lincoln's Last Months.* Cambridge, MA: Harvard, 2004. Pages 49-50 Cited by ¶¶378, 2210, 2674.

harveyC | ✓ | Harvey, Cordelia A.P. A Wisconsin woman's picture of President Lincoln. *The Wisconsin Magazine of History.* March 1918; 1(3): 233-255. Available online at: www.wisconsinhistory.org. Cited by ¶¶455, 1073, 1175, 1384, 1622, 1740, 1779, 1780, 1808, 1809, 1972, 1973, 1995, 2358, 2359, 2411, 2412, 2534, 2825, 2933, 2947, 2948, 3000, 3404, 3503. Cited by Special Topic §6a.

§6a *discusses the too-good-to-be-true nature of this remarkable account.*

hawthorne | Hawthorne, Nathaniel. *Tales, Sketches, and Other Papers.* Boston: Houghton, Mifflin and Co., 1891. Available online at [archiveorg]. Cited by ¶¶132, 178, 656, 962, 1383, 1406, 1438, 1619, 1701, 1738, 1839, 1860, 2932, 2997, 3019, 3398.

Hawthorne's essay "Chiefly about war matters" recounts a meeting with Lincoln that most likely occurred in 1862 [page 313], *sometime after the death of Willie* [page 308]. *Thus, 1862 is applied as the date for all of Hawthorne's observations.*

hayA | ✓ | Hay, John. Life in the White House in the time of Lincoln. *The Century Illustrated Monthly Magazine.* November 1890; 41(1): 33-37. Cited by ¶¶1219, 1903, 1930, 1931, 2543, 5610.

Hay was one of the two personal secretaries who served Lincoln throughout his Presidency. It is unfortunate that Hay waited so long before beginning to write his reminiscences of Lincoln. See also [templeA].

hayB | Hay, John. *Lincoln and the Civil War in the Diaries and Letters of John Hay.* Selected and with an introduction by Tyler Dennett. New York: DaCapo, 1988. (Originally published 1939.) Cited by ¶377. Cited by Special Topic §8b.

hayC | Hay, John; (edited by Michael Burlingame). *At Lincoln's Side: John Hay's Civil War Correspondence and Selected Writings.* Carbondale, IL: Southern Illinois University Press, 2000. Cited by Special Topics §4b, §5b.

hayD | Hay, John; (edited by Michael Burlingame). *Inside Lincoln's White House: The Complete Civil War Diary of John Hay.* Carbondale, IL: Southern Illinois University Press, 1997. Cited by ¶¶1097, 2650, 2934, 3775. Cited by Special Topic §5b.

▷ **Haycraft** | *Samuel and Presley Haycraft were brothers 10-15 years older than Lincoln. Samuel, at least, demonstrably mis-remembered some rather fundamental facts about Lincoln's parents. See ¶4768.*

healy | Healy, George P.A. *Reminiscences of a Portrait Painter.* Chicago: A.C. McClurg and Company, 1894. Available online at books.google.com. Cited by ¶¶1722, 2810.

helmA | ✓ | Helm, Emily Todd. Mary Todd Lincoln: reminiscences and letters of the wife of

482

President Lincoln. *McClure's Magazine.* **Sept.** 1898; 9(5): 476-480. Cited by ¶¶359, 3983, 3999, 4016, 4105, 4192, 4218, 4233, 4327, 4328, 4337, 4379, 4477, 4573, 4574, 4585, 4667.

Emilie (sometimes spelled Emily) had been Mary's favorite half-sibling. They spent six months together at some point after Mary's marriage (p 479) – probably 1847-1848. Later, Emilie spent six months in Springfield (1854-1855) [randallCpp144, 149] *and "nearly a week"* [helmB p232] *at the White House in December 1863. She kept a diary* [randallC p296], *excerpted in* [helmB]. *It is not known when she arrived at the White House* [baslerA v7p64], *but was certainly there on Dec. 14, when she received her pass to return home to Kentucky* [randallC p301]. *She visited the White House again in summer 1864* [randallC p309]. *She afterwards wrote a harsh letter to Lincoln, causing to Mary shun her thereafter* [burl p310].

---

helmB Helm, Katherine. *The True Story of Mary, Wife of Lincoln.* New York: Harper & Bros, 1928.   Cited by ¶¶173, 174, 697, 737, 741, 752, 837, 1050, 1051, 1115, 1319, 1387, 1630, 1829, 2379, 2560, 2567, 2905, 3200, 3258, 3969, 3983, 3985, 3998, 4000, 4007, 4008, 4012, 4097, 4099, 4100, 4168, 4194, 4205, 4223, 4253, 4309, 4310, 4331, 4413, 4444, 4445, 4462, 4570, 4593, 4692, 4912, 4990, 4999, 5251, 5256, 5286, 5288, 5290, 5297, 5300, 5301, 5302, 5333, 5375, 5378, 5388, 5493, 5554, 5555, 5557, 5598, 5686, 5696, 5866, 5876, 5898. Cited by Special Topics §5b, §7a.

Katherine was the daughter of Mary's younger half-sister Emilie Todd Helm. Katherine did not know her Aunt Mary [evans p289], *though she did visit the White House in December 1863 with her mother* [turner p155]. *In writing about Mary's Lexington years, Katherine made extensive use of the letter Elizabeth Norris (q.v.) wrote. For what they're worth, statements on the Internet describe Helm and her mother altering facts about Todd women (e.g., birthdays) to protect the women (and their vanity!). Mary seemingly followed the same practice in census interviews – see* ¶3968. *I am told, and believe, that some of Robert Lincoln's letters appear nowhere else but this book.*

▷ **Henry, Anson G.** *"A well-balanced witness"* [randallC p146]. *See* ¶3184.

---

hermanJ Herman, Jan K. *A Hilltop in Foggy Bottom: Home of the Old Naval Observatory and the Navy Medical Department.* Washington, DC: Department of the Navy, Bureau of Medicine & Surgery, 1996.   Cited by ¶3775.

---

herndon ✓ Herndon WH; Weik JW. *Herndon's Life of Lincoln.* Cleveland: World Publishing, 1942.   Cited by ¶¶7, 13, 90, 107, 164, 165, 215, 221, 223, 228, 229, 303, 333, 336, 338, 365, 388, 398, 401, 402, 404, 407, 417, 483, 490, 492, 502, 503, 504, 505, 506, 519, 530, 531, 539, 598, 605, 613, 614, 615, 633, 666, 687, 692, 827, 828, 908, 911, 943, 966, 1054, 1056, 1099, 1122, 1125, 1127, 1131, 1132, 1212, 1322, 1331, 1342, 1343, 1345, 1358, 1370, 1379, 1380, 1381, 1398, 1452, 1459, 1461, 1494, 1580, 1599, 1604, 1627, 1628, 1636, 1642, 1658, 1667, 1669, 1760, 1813, 1817, 1828, 1872, 1962, 2101, 2249, 2253, 2276, 2317, 2335, 2369, 2418, 2498, 2783, 2793, 2808, 2813, 2890, 2893, 2895, 2921, 2929, 2959, 2981, 3014, 3021, 3071, 3076, 3077, 3108, 3117, 3126, 3129, 3340, 3341, 3342, 3377, 3379, 3380, 3383, 3424, 3433, 3471, 3491, 3537, 3555, 3569, 3704, 3713, 3714, 3747, 4064, 4753, 4771, 4780, 4783, 4784, 4790, 4816, 4829, 4834, 4864, 4882, 4905, 5013, 5014, 5032, 5040, 5046, 5061, 5072, 5092, 5095, 5096, 5099, 5100, 5115, 5123, 5124, 5128, 5145, 5150, 5172, 5180. Cited by Special Topics §1a, §8b.

Herndon met Lincoln in 1834, studied law under him from 1842-1843, and became his law partner in 1843 [hertz pp143, 424]. *Herndon and Mary Lincoln never had a warm relationship, but it fractured completely after Herndon disclosed the Ann Rutledge story.* •   • • [herndon] *is based on his own recollections and on interview material Herndon collected over decades from friends and acquaintances of Lincoln's. This raw material is collected in* [wilson]; *Herndon and Weik often touched up phrasing and/or spelling of supposedly direct quotes. Although some of Herndon's sources are questionable, he realized this* [wilson p xxiii]. *As* [hertz pp3-4] *notes, every important Lincoln biographer used Herndon's papers or his first-*

hand knowledge, including [lamonL], [holland], [arnold], [beveridge], *Charnwood, Sandburg (e.g.* [sandburgP]*), Nicolay+Hay (*[nicolayB]*), and Tarbell (e.g.* [tarbellB]*). Albert Beveridge concluded that Herndon was "well-nigh fanatically devoted to truth"* [burl p xxv] [hertz p12] *(echoed by* [wilson p xxiii]*). Hertz praises Herndon's "unflagging passion for completeness"* [hertz p26]. *Herndon was certainly careful: he read his interview transcripts back to the interviewees and asked for a confirming signature* [shenk p223]. *He was, however, untrustworthy when attempting to "analyze the 'souls' of other people"* [burl p xxv]. *J.G. and Ruth Randall viewed Herndon (disapprovingly) as an amateur psychoanalyst* [shenk p236] *and accused him of believing he was clairvoyant* [randallC p31; shenk p236]. *Of unclear significance,* [rossH pp100, 125-126] *accuses Herndon of inventing stories.* ● ● ● *There were three different versions of Herndon's Life of Lincoln: 1889, 1892 (expanded), and 1930 (for the general reader)* [currentBk p289]. *This is the 1930 version, reprinted. At one extreme, it has been said that the second author, Jesse Weik, merely "polished and embellished" the material Herndon had collected* [shenk p226]. *At the other extreme* [hertz p9], *Weik "reinterpreted Herndon's statements and used only such portions of them as he approved of. Aside from the short preface written by Herndon, nothing was printed as Herndon intended. ... Herndon complained bitterly of the treatment of his manuscript." Weik did all the writing; see ¶13.*

herndonC Herndon WH. Analysis of the character of Abraham Lincoln). *Abraham Lincoln Quarterly.* 1941; 1: 343-383. Cited by ¶¶1, 2, 3, 13, 228, 229, 386, 403, 407, 506, 531, 1132, 1322, 1380, 1416, 1433, 1598, 1658, 1822, 1847, 1852, 1935, 2253, 2793, 3014, 3034, 3379, 3380.

▷ **Herndons** *Multiple members of the Herndon family were acquainted with Lincoln:* ● *William, who first met Lincoln in 1832* [angle p109] ● *J. Rowan, a cousin of William, whom Lincoln also met in 1832* [angle pp109-110] ● *Archer, the father of William* [angle p110] ● *Elliott, the brother of William, who was a staunch political opponent of Lincoln* [herndon p469n]. *(Row killed his wife: accidentally shot her through the neck* [walsh pp67-68].*)*

herrmann Herrmann J; France TD; Spranger JW; *et al.* The Stickler syndrome (hereditary arthroophthalmopathy). *Birth Defects Orig Art Ser.* 1975; 11(2): 76-103. Cited by ¶66.

hertz ✓– Hertz, Emanuel (ed). *The Hidden Lincoln: From the Letters and Papers of William H. Herndon.* New York: Viking Press, 1938. 461 pages. Cited by ¶¶7, 9, 10, 12, 13, 14, 47, 50, 51, 54, 86, 87, 88, 120, 121, 230, 240, 327, 328, 337, 352, 387, 389, 405, 406, 469, 602, 603, 604, 620, 746, 954, 976, 1052, 1363, 1367, 1368, 1462, 1759, 1826, 2013, 2018, 2019, 2024, 2232, 2254, 2312, 2318, 2323, 2329, 2330, 2331, 2332, 2336, 2337, 2338, 2339, 2340, 2368, 2370, 2371, 2372, 2373, 2374, 2375, 2376, 2377, 2390, 2391, 2392, 2393, 2394, 2395, 2396, 2399, 2400, 2407, 2434, 2461, 2502, 2583, 2689, 2692, 2734, 2735, 2736, 2738, 2761, 2770, 2892, 2897, 2898, 2899, 2918, 2943, 2968, 2984, 2985, 3123, 3176, 3352, 3353, 3355, 3463, 3569, 3664, 3667, 3705, 3789, 3790, 3810, 3811, 3821, 3827, 3828, 3830, 3831, 3832, 3833, 3837, 3845, 3869, 3870, 3871, 3891, 3892, 3893, 3894, 3895, 3896, 3898, 3904, 3984, 4001, 4295, 4365, 4366, 4367, 4368, 4382, 4738, 4739, 4740, 4768, 4802, 4845, 4847, 4866, 4867, 4868, 4869, 4883, 4884, 4885, 4896, 4897, 4911, 5036, 5173, 5203, 5205, 5207, 5208, 5227, 5507, 5814. Cited by Special Topics §1a, §2b, §2c, §2f, §2g.

Contains many of Herndon's observations of Lincoln (as well as many conclusions he drew from the information he had collected for his biography of Lincoln).

hickey ✓– Hickey, James. Lincolniana: The Lincoln account at the Corneau and Diller drug store, 1849-1861. *Journal of the Illinois State Historical Society.* Spring 1984; 77(1): 60-66. Cited by ¶¶629, 2049, 2102, 2289, 2293, 2302, 3927.

hirschhorn ✓ Hirschhorn N; Feldman RG. Mary Lincoln's final illness: a medical and historical reappraisal. *Journal of the History of Medicine and Allied Sciences.* 1999; 54: 511-542.   Cited by ¶¶2024, 2025, 2026, 4071, 4076, 4089, 4090, 4094, 4130, 4131, 4133, 4134, 4140, 4141, 4142, 4147, 4148, 4152, 4153, 4155, 4158, 4183, 4185, 4208, 4209, 4210, 4211, 4242, 4243, 4294, 4303, 4304, 4315, 4468, 4493, 4499, 4556, 4595, 4596, 4599, 4603, 4605, 4608, 4613, 4614, 4616, 4617, 4625, 4628, 4630, 4635, 4703.   Cited by Special Topics §2f, §2i.

hirschhornB ✓ | Hirschhorn N. Mary Lincoln's "suicide attempt:" a physician reconsiders the evidence. *Lincoln Herald.* 2003; 105(3): 94-98.   Cited by ¶¶4298, 4527, 4528.

hirschhornC ✓ | Hirschhorn N; Feldman RG; Greaves IA.   Abraham Lincoln's blue pills: did our 16th President suffer from mercury poisoning? *Perspectives in Biology and Medicine.* 2001; 44: 315-332.   Cited by ¶¶623, 1120, 1162, 1163, 1581, 1584, 1767, 1969, 2289, 2419, 2490, 2618, 3106, 3452, 3460.   Cited by Special Topic §2c.

hirschhornD ✓ | Hirschhorn N; Greaves IA. Lincoln's gait. *Perspectives in Biology and Medicine.* 2006; 49: 631-632.   Cited by ¶1029. Cited by Special Topic §8a.

ho ✓ | Ho NC; Park SS; Maragh KD; *et al.*   Famous people and genetic disorders. *Am J Med Genet A.* 2003; 118A: 187-196.   Cited by ¶5846.

hobson | Hobson, JT. *Footprints of Abraham Lincoln: Presenting Many Interesting Facts, Reminiscences and Illustrations Never Before Published.* Dayton, OH: The Otterbein Press, 1909. Available online at [archiveorg].   Cited by ¶¶142, 239, 755, 1033, 1042, 1453, 1665, 2257, 2285, 2367, 2438, 2912, 3068, 3318, 3334, 3361, 3612, 3621, 3624, 3716, 4782, 5022, 5028, 5049.

Pages 22-24 quote J.W. Lamar's long reminiscence from the Indianapolis News of April 12, 1902.

holland | Holland JG. *Life of Abraham Lincoln.* Springfield, MA: Gurdon Bill, 1866. 544 pages. Available online at [AbrahamLincolnAssociation]. Available online at [archiveorg].   Cited by ¶2670. Cited by Special Topic §6a.

Has been described as a "moralistic biography." Herndon thought "pages 236-40 – all false" [hertz p69]. Herndon had other criticisms [hertz pp74-75].

holt ✓ | Holt EE. Abraham Lincoln. *Ophthalmic Record.* 1914; 23: 389-393.   Cited by ¶891.

holzerB ✓ | Holzer, Harold. Presentation related to his book *Lincoln at Cooper Union* on Feb. 1, 2007. Telecast on C-SPAN2 (BookTV) on Feb. 18, 2007.   Cited by ¶3744.

hopkinsB | Hopkins, Donald R. *The Greatest Killer: Smallpox in History.* Chicago: University of Chicago Press, 2002. (Originally published 1983.)   Cited by ¶2202. Cited by Special Topics §5b, §5c, §5e.

hunt | Hunt, Gaillard. *Israel, Elihu and Cadwallader Washburn: A Chapter in American Biography.* New York: Macmillan, 1925.   Cited by ¶¶126, 1753, 2916. Cited by Special Topic §5b.

"Elihu Washburne knew Abraham Lincoln from the time that he first went to Illinois" (page 228). Washburne was a Congressman during Lincoln's Presidency and remained in touch with Lincoln. The last name's spelling seems variable.

jayne | Jayne, William. Personal Reminiscences of Abraham Lincoln: An Address Delivered before the Springfield Chapter of the Daughters of the American Revolution, February 12, 1907. (Available in the Library of Congress)   Cited by ¶¶105, 912, 3187.

| jordan | Jordan, Philip D. The death of Nancy Hanks Lincoln. *Indiana Magazine of History.* June 1944; 40: 103-110. Cited by ¶4791.

| keckleyB | Keckley E. *Behind the Scenes or, Thirty Years a Slave, and Four Years in the White House.* New York: G.W. Carleton & Co., 1868. Available online at [AbrahamLincolnAssociation]. Available online at [archiveorg]. Cited by ¶¶265, 1072, 1217, 1298, 1303, 1493, 1566, 2357, 2533, 2565, 2999, 4023, 4048, 4049, 4435, 4436, 4475, 4524, 5342, 5444, 5513, 5516, 5587, 5594, 5612, 5639, 5658, 5689, 5692, 5723, 5731, 5769, 5776.

Lizzie Keckley, a former slave, was Mrs. Lincoln's dressmaker in the White House and for many years Mary's close friend. This book was most likely ghostwritten [burk p9]: *by late 1867 Mrs. Keckley "had begun dictating her reminiscences to a professional writer"* [turner p471n]. *"The book was candid in tone, remarkably accurate in observation, and generally sympathetic to the Lincolns;" historians regard it "as excellent source material"* [turner p472]. *Ruth Randall is "wary" of it, but finds it "to agree largely with more direct evidence" about the White House years* [randallCp39].

| kempfA | ✓– | Kempf, Edward J. Abraham Lincoln's organic and emotional neurosis. *AMA Arch Neurol Psychiatr.* 1952; 67: 419-433.

| kempfB | Kempf, Edward J. *Abraham Lincoln's Philosophy of Common Sense (3 volumes).* (Special Publication of the New York Academy of Sciences, Volume VI). New York: New York Academy of Sciences, 1965. Cited by ¶¶271, 273, 275, 276, 277, 278, 279, 281, 282, 283, 284, 313, 470, 473, 674, 857, 880, 892, 1441, 1631, 1647, 1662, 1746, 1747, 1864, 1943, 1945, 2308, 2796, 2797, 2958, 3008, 3030, 3031, 3032, 3033, 3042, 3054, 3574, 3575, 3576, 3578, 3766, 3876. Cited by Special Topic §1a.

Kempf, a psychiatrist, wrote a 1400+ page "scientifically oriented analytical biography" of Lincoln (p xi) that reads like a caricature of psychoanalytical double-talk. But he was serious. Chapter 1 of volume 1, titled "Lincoln's physical constitution," is filled with untenable psychiatric conclusions, yet embeds a worthy overview of the physical Lincoln. Unfortunately, it is almost devoid of references. This was the only chapter I read. I have not attempted to fully represent Kempf's ideas.

| kroen | ✓ | Kroen C. Abraham Lincoln and the 'Lincoln sign'. *Cleve Clin J Med.* 2007; 74: 108-110. Cited by ¶1992.

Contributes nothing new.

| kunhardtA | ✓ | Kunhardt PB Jr; Kunhardt PB III; Kunhardt PW. *Lincoln: An Illustrated Biography.* New York: Alfred A. Knopf, 1992. 417 pages. Cited by ¶¶17, 22, 25, 92, 108, 145, 176, 224, 244, 259, 266, 304, 314, 316, 324, 345, 349, 371, 378, 409, 426, 427, 445, 446, 448, 450, 475, 476, 477, 520, 523, 524, 542, 543, 558, 559, 568, 615, 642, 643, 697, 716, 820, 875, 877, 913, 925, 926, 934, 961, 973, 979, 995, 1011, 1013, 1014, 1021, 1030, 1039, 1078, 1079, 1094, 1100, 1184, 1218, 1272, 1333, 1369, 1375, 1410, 1422, 1423, 1425, 1440, 1446, 1496, 1497, 1499, 1548, 1550, 1554, 1559, 1620, 1673, 1687, 1706, 1708, 1709, 1728, 1741, 1810, 1836, 1844, 1861, 1907, 1939, 2045, 2137, 2150, 2159, 2160, 2164, 2175, 2231, 2268, 2271, 2305, 2429, 2433, 2509, 2510, 2511, 2516, 2520, 2532, 2552, 2617, 2633, 2651, 2652, 2654, 2659, 2660, 2669, 2689, 2744, 2795, 2812, 2824, 2883, 2902, 2922, 2923, 3045, 3089, 3093, 3144, 3191, 3214, 3223, 3240, 3241, 3268, 3269, 3276, 3288, 3291, 3311, 3314, 3322, 3325, 3418, 3420, 3472, 3481, 3490, 3493, 3494, 3496, 3497, 3514, 3536, 3540, 3542, 3554, 3634, 3649, 3709, 3717, 3757, 3794, 3816, 3850, 3857, 3908, 3917, 3919, 3932, 3985, 4036, 4041, 4057, 4058, 4059, 4074, 4172, 4244, 4351, 4354, 4358, 4430, 4432, 4446, 4450, 4452, 4453, 4470, 4475, 4505, 4522, 4589, 4679, 4685, 4907, 4917, 4951, 4975, 4980, 4985, 5073, 5326, 5364, 5373, 5454, 5465, 5468, 5469, 5586, 5619, 5687, 5708, 5715, 5751, 5781, 5866, 5877, 5893, 5899. Cited by Special Topics §5b, §7a, §8b.

Perhaps because it is photograph-centric, this is an exceptionally rich source of in-formation about the physical Lincoln. Yet, it is carefully written and often cites sources (e.g. page 409). I am a little sensitive about having used this book so extensively, as it is not typical of the sources historians normally consult. But, David Herbert Donald was the principal consultant on the project (p 404) and he calls the text "informed and accurate" (p vi). Richard Current, Harold Holzer, and Brian Pohanka also read the text (p 404). Thus, the book clearly has merit, and I feel the necessary caveats have been applied by classifying most statements from the book as a secondary source.

kunhardtB | ✓ | Kunhardt DM; Kunhardt PB. *Twenty Days: A Narrative in Text and Pictures of the Assassination of Abraham Lincoln and the Twenty Days and Nights that Followed.* New York: Harper & Row, 1965. 312 pages. Cited by ¶¶15, 32, 61, 89, 98, 122, 141, 154, 209, 241, 384, 391, 465, 466, 549, 550, 553, 555, 557, 560, 561, 563, 564, 567, 568, 569, 570, 583, 632, 641, 823, 935, 960, 980, 983, 984, 987, 1009, 1010, 1019, 1021, 1057, 1101, 1103, 1377, 1424, 1433, 1443, 1500, 1506, 1565, 1577, 1751, 1821, 1879, 1899, 1903, 1917, 1918, 1957, 2059, 2123, 2135, 2159, 2160, 2163, 2175, 2177, 2178, 2255, 2481, 2519, 2526, 2537, 2559, 2571, 2677, 2847, 2873, 3016, 3049, 3077, 3090, 3138, 3199, 3222, 3224, 3243, 3247, 3249, 3251, 3257, 3258, 3265, 3266, 3267, 3271, 3272, 3276, 3286, 3287, 3291, 3300, 3303, 3304, 3305, 3307, 3308, 3309, 3310, 3312, 3313, 3338, 3354, 3378, 3484, 3498, 3689, 3771, 3814, 3822, 3849, 3861, 3908, 3925, 3949, 4011, 4054, 4345, 4431, 4433, 4437, 4438, 4458, 4684, 4728, 4929, 4951, 4957, 4989, 5373, 5415, 5416, 5417, 5418, 5420, 5466, 5474, 5503, 5515, 5519, 5639, 5677, 5693, 5694, 5698, 5699, 5719, 5751, 5752, 5767, 5772, 5780, 5842. Cited by Special Topics §4b, §4c, §4d, §4e, §7a, §7h, §8b, §8f.

All the negatives and fewer of the positives about [kunhardtA] apply to this book. At a late date I discovered that this book seems to quote from [ostendorfC]; see ¶5473.

kunhardtC | ✓ | Kunhardt, Dorothy Meserve. An old lady's Lincoln memories. *Life Magazine.* 9 Feb. 1959; 46(6): 57, 59-60. Cited by ¶¶2304, 2482, 3550, 3920, 3921, 3926, 4077, 4156, 4305, 4381, 4498, 4512, 4517, 4958, 5875. Cited by Special Topic §2k.

Is a 1956 interview with Mary Edwards Brown, the granddaughter of Mary's sister, Elizabeth Todd Edwards. In winter 1882, at age 16, she helped care for her great-aunt Mary Lincoln. Clearly, some of her statements were family lore. Others may have been altered by time or re-telling, e.g. ¶4494. Interview excerpted in [kunhardtA pp396-397].

lamonL | Lamon, Ward H. *The Life of Abraham Lincoln; from His Birth to his Inau-guration as President.* Boston: James R. Osgood and Company, 1872. Available online at [AbrahamLincolnAssociation]. Cited by ¶¶51, 494, 618, 909, 967, 994, 1081, 2041, 2507, 2935, 3726, 3804, 4022. Cited by Special Topic §8b.

The book was actually written by a Chauncey F. Black [hertz p147], no admirer of Lin-coln [turner p595] [burk p12]. Lamon's memories and research ([hertz p7]) were supplemented by copies [citehertz p145] of the materials Herndon had so far collected. Lamon was an Illinois attorney who first met Lincoln in 1853 [angle p164] (or 1847 [randallC p91]) and accompanied Lincoln to Washington. He was a member of Lincoln's inner circle and his unofficial body-guard. Lincoln's first word after delivering the Gettysburg address was "Lamon." William Herndon thought this was "the truest life" of Lincoln ever written, although he did not like chapter ?19 [hertz p110].

lamonR | Lamon, Ward Hill. *Recollections of Abraham Lincoln.* Washington: Dorothy Lamon Teillard, 1911. Cited by ¶¶1507, 1556, 2517, 3521, 3538, 3547, 5655.

Lamon did not write this book either: his daughter, Dorothy Lamon Teillard, "pieced together stray scraps of paper that contained jottings Lamon had made about Lincoln" [burk p31]. The 1911 version is a re-issue.

lattimerAu | ✓ | Lattimer JK. Autopsy on Abraham Lincoln: retrieval of a lost report.

JAMA. 1965; 193: 99-100.   Cited by ¶¶551, 738, 1902, 3281, 3296.

lattimerBk | ✓– | Lattimer JK. *Kennedy and Lincoln: Medical and Ballistic Comparisons of Their Assassinations.* New York: Harcourt Brace Jovanovich, 1980. Pages 34-35   Cited by ¶¶2940, 3229, 3233, 3279.

lattimerNY | ✓ | Lattimer JK. Lincoln did not have the Marfan syndrome. *NY State J Med.* 1981; 81: 1805-1813.   Cited by ¶¶69, 84, 525, 818, 860, 883, 1531, 1532, 1533, 1534, 1571, 1633, 1644, 1979, 2240, 2242, 2839, 2875, 2940, 3276.

This article is the Bible of those who believe Lincoln did not have Marfan syndrome. Lattimer makes useful observations, especially of photographic and other physical evidence, but quotes text selectively. He also gets facts wrong, e.g.: (1) Lincoln's reputed display of wood-chopping prowess was at a hospital in southern Virginia, not at a "soldier's home near Washington;" (2) The cited reference for Dr. Edward Curtis's letter about Lincoln is actually a reminiscence that Curtis wrote 42 years later; (3) Lattimer's literature review missed Herndon's explicit statement (in one of the most fundamental of all Lincoln publications) that Lincoln had a "sunken chest" [herndon p333]; (4) Gives incorrect hat size for Lincoln; (5) Thinks height was a disadvantage in wrestling, when Lincoln himself says it was an advantage (¶2855); (6) Ectopia lentis can be associated with little or no visual impairment and is not progressive after birth, even with trauma [aa74].

lea | Lea, J. Henry; Hutchinson J.R. *The Ancestry of Abraham Lincoln.* Boston: Houghton Mifflin, 1909. 212+xvi pages. Available online at `books.google.com`. missing some pages from the index.   Cited by ¶¶3607, 5006, 5149, 5812, 5817, 5820, 5821, 5824, 5825, 5826, 5827, 5828, 5847, 5848, 5849. Cited by Special Topic §8b.

This book, though widely available, is outdated, as [lincolnW] is more current. There is also a book by William Barton on Lincoln's ancestry, which I have not consulted.

lealeA | ✓– | Leale, Charles A. *Lincoln's Last Hours. Address Delivered Before the Commandery of the State of New York, Military Order of the Loyal Legion of the United States, at the Regular Meeting, February, 1909, City of New York, in Observance of the One Hundredth Anniversary of the Birth of President Abraham Lincoln.* 1909. Available online at [archiveorg].   Cited by ¶¶207, 535, 1076, 1791, 3051, 3233.

Substantially the same text, with non-medical illustrations, appeared as: Leale, Charles A. "Lincoln's last hours." Harper's Weekly Magazine, February 1909, pages 7-10, 27. See ¶3227 for pointers to other Leale writings.

leech | ✓ | Leech, Margaret. *Reveille in Washington: 1860-1865.* Alexandria, VA: Time-Life Books, 1962. 592 pages.   Cited by ¶¶2032, 2188, 2209, 2235, 2677. Cited by Special Topics §4b, §5e, §5g.

Originally published in 1941 and winner of a Pulitzer Prize, this history of the Civil War as it affected Washington, DC appears carefully researched, but is without detailed reference citations. That it reads like a novel should not detract from the information it contains.

lewis | ✓ | Lewis L. When Tad Lincoln had "a girl" in Chicago. *Chicago Daily News.* Feb. 5, 1930; "Midweek" section: 3, 13.   Cited by ¶¶5241, 5259, 5357, 5450, 5465, 5611, 5633, 5667.

lewisM | Lewis, Lloyd. *Myths After Lincoln.* New York: Harcourt, Brace and Company, 1940.   Cited by ¶¶5497, 5625.

lincloreBDA | ✓ | Lincoln Lore. "Volk's plastic portraits of Lincoln." 20 Nov. 1933, No. 241. Cited by ¶¶1903, 1909, 1910, 1913.

Lincoln Lore was for many years a one-page weekly publication of the Lincoln National Life Insurance Company of Fort Wayne, IN. Most (all?) were written by Louis A. Warren. They are traditionally referred to by number, which I have here encoded as capital letters (don't ask why).

lincloreBAI ✓ *Lincoln Lore.* "The sister of Abraham Lincoln." 19 June 1933, No. 219. Cited by ¶¶4804, 5007, 5010, 5017, 5026, 5035, 5043.

lincloreBIG ✓ *Lincoln Lore.* "The countenance of Abraham Lincoln." 17 Dec. 1934, No. 297. Cited by ¶¶294, 1688, 1800.

lincloreEDI ✓ *Lincoln Lore.* "President Lincoln's grandson." 16 Oct. 1939, No. 549. Cited by ¶¶5804, 5805.

lincloreFDH ✓ *Lincoln Lore.* "Black Hawk War stations." 9 Aug. 1943, No. 748. Cited by ¶3633.

lincloreHZA ✓ *Lincoln Lore.* "Dr. Browne, obscure biographer of Lincoln." 14 Aug. 1944, No. 801. Cited by ¶3194.

lincloreHDE *Lincoln Lore.* "An evening with Lincoln." 18 June 1945, No. 845. Cited by ¶¶130, 159, 246, 433, 763, 1402, 1545, 1611, 1678, 1805, 1856, 2788, 2928. Cited by Special Topic §7h.
Reprints a letter written on June 21, 1860 by an "editorial correspondent" of the Utica Morning Herald. The letter was published in the New York Semi-Weekly Tribune on July 6, 1860.

lincloreIED ✓ *Lincoln Lore.* "Robert Lincoln's genealogy." 21 July 1947, No. 954. Cited by ¶¶4982, 4986, 5865.

lincloreIGI ✓ *Lincoln Lore.* "The close of another Lincoln generation." 12 Jan. 1948, No. 979. Cited by ¶¶3939, 5217, 5232, 5236, 5708, 5813.

lincloreLFH ✓ *Lincoln Lore.* "Lincoln's spectacles." 27 July 1953, No. 1268. Cited by ¶¶785, 786, 809, 810, 811, 812, 814, 1755, 4932.

lincloreLHH ✓ *Lincoln Lore.* "Lincoln's 1863 illness." 14 Dec. 1953, No. 1288. Cited by ¶¶1220, 2031, 4273, 5399, 5401. Cited by Special Topic §5.

lincolnA Lincoln, Abraham. Papers of. Library of Congress. At: http://memory.loc.gov/ammem/alhtml/ Cited by ¶1202.
[hertz pp17-18] *reprints the heart-breaking story of Robert Lincoln destroying certain private papers of his father's, before presenting the rest of the collection to the Library of Congress.*

lincolnR Lincoln, Robert T. Letterpress books. Available on microfilm from Abraham Lincoln Presidential Library and Museum, Springfield, IL. Cited by ¶¶5267, 5294, 5299, 5303, 5312, 5317.
Robert wrote a few business letters that mention Tad's final illness. His handwriting is difficult.

lincolnW Lincoln, Waldo. *History of the Lincoln Family: An Account of the Descendants of Samuel Lincoln of Hingham, Massachusetts 1637-1690.* Worcester, MA: Commonwealth Press, 1923. Cited by ¶¶5788, 5819, 5828, 5832, 5847. Cited by Special Topic §8b.

[palcic] *may be, at least, a partial update.*

▷ **Logan, Stephen T.** *Logan, like John T. Stuart, was Mary Todd's cousin* [turner p9] *and, also like Stuart, eventually became a senior law partner of Lincoln's* [donaldA pp96ff]. *Herndon wrote that he was "a cold, avaricious, and little mean man for you as the people saw him"* [hertz p172].

lorant Lorant, Stefan. *Lincoln: A Picture Story of His Life.* New York: Harper, 1957. 304 pages. Cited by ¶¶17, 1006, 1575.

luthin Luthin, Reinhard H. *The Real Abraham Lincoln.* Englewood Cliffs, NJ: Prentice-Hall, 1960. Cited by ¶¶1222, 1317, 1318, 1321, 2415, 2568, 2569, 2572, 2573, 2966, 4256.

macveagh ✓ MacVeagh, Wayne. Lincoln at Gettysburg. *The Century Magazine.* Nov. 1909; 79 (N.S.: 57): 20-23. Cited by ¶3761. Cited by Special Topic §5b.

marion ✓ Marion R. *Was George Washington Really the Father of Our Country?* Reading, MA: Addison-Wesley, 1994. Pages 88-124 Cited by ¶¶65, 71, 957.

markens ✓ Markens, Edward Wasgate. Lincoln and his relations to doctors. *J Med Soc New Jersey.* 1922; 19: 44-47. Cited by ¶¶210, 3152, 3225. Cited by Special Topics §4e, §7d.

Would have been very useful had reference citations been provided.

marx Marx, Rudolph. *The Health of the Presidents.* New York: G.P. Putnam's Sons, 1960. 376 pages. Cited by ¶¶850, 4930. Cited by Special Topics §5c, §5e.

I don't trust this book. It contains no references whatsoever and it recounts facts that seem to go beyond what is known. For example, it is stated without qualification that Tad had a mild case of smallpox in November 1863 and that Lincoln acquired his illness from the boy (p185). This may very well be true, but the evidence as I know it does not allow so absolute a conclusion. Marx also puts us inside Dr. Stone's head. All this leaves one with the impression that Marx doesn't let an absence of facts stop a good story. This is a pity, since it otherwise appears his research has been very thorough. Other specific shortcomings are noted in Special Topic §5.

▷ **Matheny, James** *Matheny knew Lincoln from the time the latter moved to Springfield. Matheny was a groomsman at Lincoln's wedding in 1842. In 1872 Matheny (under pressure) publicly recanted some of the information he had provided to Herndon on the subject of Lincoln's religious beliefs.* [wilson p762] ● ● ● *As of 1870, however, Herndon thought Matheny "knew Lincoln as well as I did"* [hertz p77].

matile ✓ Matile, Roger. The day Lincoln left his fingerprints behind. *Oswego [Illinois] Ledger-Sentinel.* Jan. 25, 2007; ?: ?. (accessed online at `ledgersentinel.com`). Cited by ¶3406.

mcclure McClure, Stanley W. *Ford's Theatre and the House Where Lincoln Died.* Washington: National Park Service Historical Handbook Series No. 3, Revised 1969. Web page. Available online at:
`http://www.nps.gov/history/history/online_books/hh/3b/hh3h1.htm`

mckusickA McKusick, Victor A. *Heritable Disorders of Connective Tissue.* 3rd ed. St. Louis: Mosby, 1966. Cited by ¶¶258, 272, 322, 323, 324, 471, 824, 923, 987, 1018, 1448, 1592, 2828, 3698, 3916, 5249, 5265.

McKusick, the emeritus Physician-in-Chief at Johns Hopkins Hospital, is the world's leading authority on Marfan syndrome. In the decades since this book appeared, several other syndromes of Marfanoid phenotype have been defined. Although McKusick's descriptions of Marfan syndrome are, therefore, tainted by admixture of these other syndromes, his extraordinarily detailed descriptions encompass the "universe" of phenotypes and remain valuable.

mckusickB ✓ McKusick, Victor A. Abraham Lincoln and Marfan syndrome. *Nature.* 1991; 352: 280. Cited by ¶¶73, 2901.

mearns Mearns DC. *Largely Lincoln.* New York: St. Martin's, 1961. Pages 18-21 Cited by ¶1445.

mellon Mellon . *The Face of Lincoln.* New York: Viking Press, 1979. Cited by ¶¶17, 779, 780, 781, 1490, 1894, 1895. Cited by Special Topic §5b.

The hardback edition cited above is by far the best mass-market source for high quality reproductions of Lincoln photographs. I have not examined other editions.

meserve ✓ Meserve, Frederick Hill; Sandburg C. *The Photographs of Abraham Lincoln.* New York: Harcourt, Brace and Company, 1944. 30 pages of text and 70+ pages of photos. Cited by ¶¶17, 24, 29, 30, 146, 177, 192, 250, 435, 510, 667, 744, 905, 953, 1080, 1138, 1408, 1436, 1472, 1477, 1510, 1511, 1603, 1635, 1659, 1676, 1703, 1707, 1712, 1713, 1714, 1715, 1801, 1803, 1848, 1853, 2260, 2778, 2787, 2806, 2809, 2849, 2874, 2989, 3039, 3146, 3403, 5547. Cited by Special Topic §5b.

Photographs of Abraham Lincoln are generally referred to by their "Meserve number," as provided in this scarce book.

micozzi ✓ Micozzi MS. When the patient is Abraham Lincoln. *Caduceus.* 1991; 7(1): 34-42. Cited by ¶¶76, 1518, 1519, 1520, 1912.

Micozzi served on the 1990s commission that judged the request to genetically analyze a sample of Lincoln's tissue. This article contains errors.

miers Miers, Earl Schenk; Powell, C. Percy (eds). *Lincoln Day by Day: A Chronology; Volume III: 1861-1865.* Washington: Lincoln Sesquicentennial Commission, 1960. Cited by ¶¶1198, 1208, 1223, 1235, 1267, 1274, 1282, 1293, 1306, 1314, 2656, 3001, 3520, 3909, 4720, 5373. Cited by Special Topics §3a, §5b, §5e, §5f.

These remarkable volumes track Lincoln's location and activities each day of his life. They are not perfect. A derivative work is available online at **thelincolnlog.org/view** *[thelincolnlog] – it has imperfections, too, e.g. perpetuating the questionable lore that Alexander Gardner photographed Lincoln on April 10, 1865. I read all 1865 entries through April 15.*

▷ **Miller, William** *Miller, either directly or indirectly, provided Herndon with information about Lincoln's militia service, but there are doubts whether Miller served in Lincoln's company of militiamen* [wilson pp 361n, 764].

mitchell ✓ Mitchell S. Diagnosis of heterophoria from a portrait. *Ophthalmic Record.* 1914; 23: 224-226. Cited by ¶¶878, 890, 1761, 1837.

mitgangP Mitgang, Herbert (ed.). *Abraham Lincoln: A Press Portrait.* New York: Fordham University Press, 2000.

monaghan Monaghan, Jay. *Diplomat in Carpet Slippers: Abraham Lincoln Deals with Foreign Affairs.* Indianapolis: Charter Books, 1962. 505 pages. Originally published 1945 by Bobbs Merrill Co. Cited by Special Topic §5b.

montgomery | Montgomery-Massingberd H (ed). *Burke's Presidential Families of the United States of America.* 2nd ed. London: Burke's Peerage Limited, 1981. pages 285-293. Cited by ¶¶5801, 5818. Cited by Special Topic §8b.

montgomeryJ | ✓ | Montgomery JW. Lincoln-Marfan debate [letter]. *JAMA.* 1964; 189: 164-165. Cited by ¶¶84, 2941.

moore | Moore, Frank. *Poetry and Incidents of the War: North and South. 1860-1865.* New York: Bible House, 1867. Available online at: http://quod.lib.umich.edu. Cited by ¶¶334, 366, 367, 1958.

myers | ✓ | Myers KJ. Eyes of liberty [letter]. *J Am Opt Assoc.* 1977; 48: 821-823. Cited by ¶¶295, 790, 800, 802, 803, 804, 805, 808, 919, 920.

nee | ✓ | Nee L; Higgins JJ. Should spinocerebellar ataxia 5 be called Lincoln ataxia? *Neurology.* 1997; 49: 298-302. Cited by ¶¶1029, 5149, 5818, 5821, 5822. Cited by Special Topics §8a, §8b.

neelyA | Neely, Mark E. Jr. *The Lincoln Family Album.* New York: Doubleday, 1990. Cited by ¶¶4915, 4918, 4951, 5238, 5334, 5340, 5361, 5368, 5370, 5372, 5373, 5374, 5403, 5467, 5472, 5567, 5574, 5681, 5722, 5726, 5744, 5764, 5800, 5801, 5806, 5809. Cited by Special Topic §5b.

neelyE | Neely, Mark E. Jr. *The Abraham Lincoln Encyclopedia.* New York: McGraw-Hill, 1982. Pages 188-189 Cited by ¶¶5325, 5413, 5478, 5497, 5533, 5571, 5615, 5636, 5661.

neelyF | Neely, Mark E. Jr; McMurtry, R. Gerald. *The Insanity File: The Case of Mary Todd Lincoln.* Carbondale, IL: Southern Illinois University Press, 1986. 203 pages. Cited by ¶¶4499, 4500.

neelyL | ✓ | Neely, Mark E. Jr. Rattling Lincoln's bones. *Lincoln Lore: Bulletin of the Louis A. Warren Lincoln Library and Museum.* August 1990; nbr 1818: 1-4. Cited by ¶¶81, 2404, 2518, 3529, 3803. Cited by Special Topics §5d, §5e.

nevins | Nevins, Allan. *The War for the Union. Volume 1: The Improvised War, 1861-62.* New York: Scribner, 1959.

▷ New York Times | *See* [NYTimes] *et seq.*

newton | Newton, Joseph F. *Lincoln and Herndon.* Cedar Rapids, IA: Torch Press, 1910.

nicolayA | Nicolay, Helen. *Personal Traits of Abraham Lincoln.* New York: The Century Company, 1912. Available online at [archiveorg]. Cited by ¶¶203, 1083. Cited by Special Topics §8b, §8f.

nicolayB | Nicolay, John G.; Hay, John. *Abraham Lincoln: A History.* New York: The Century Co., 1890. Available online at [archiveorg]. Cited by ¶¶3935, 4736.

This is a 10-volume biography. Nicolay was one of Lincoln's private secretaries during the Presidency. [shastid] says his father introduced Lincoln and Nicolay in 1851. There is ample evidence that Nicolay and Hay submitted at least portions of their biography to Robert Lincoln, and unquestioningly removed anything Robert found objectionable [hertz pp15-17]. William Herndon remarked [hertz pp15, 158]: "Nicolay and Hay ... are afraid of Bob. He gives them materials and they in turn play hush." Hay admitted that "every line has been written in a spirit of reverence and regard" [hertz p16]. Herndon criticized Nicolay and Hay frequently [hertz pp151, 152, 154, 168]. Nicolay and Hay also prepared a series of articles for the Century *magazine about 30 years after Lincoln's presidency. At this time "it had become all but impossible to permit the discussion of some of the information supplied by Lincoln's contemporaries"* [hertz p4].

nicolayC Nicolay, John G.; Hay, John (eds.). *Complete Works of Abraham Lincoln. 12 volumes.* New and enlarged edition: Lincoln Memorial University, 1894 (vol. 9). Cited by ¶98. Cited by Special Topic §5b.

nicolayG ✓ Nicolay, John G. Lincoln's Gettysburg Address. *The Century Magazine.* 1893-1894; 47: 596-608. Cited by ¶¶1587, 2212. Cited by Special Topics §5b, §5f, §8b.

nicolayO Nicolay, John G; edited by Michael Burlingame. *An Oral History of Abraham Lincoln: John G. Nicolay's Interviews and Essays.* Carbondale, IL: Southern Illinois University Press, 1996. Cited by ¶¶496, 2322, 2324, 2465, 2585, 2720, 2754, 2913, 4371, 4506, 4538, 4557. Cited by Special Topic §3b.

nicolayS Nicolay, John G. *A short Life of Abraham Lincoln.* New York: Century Co, 1902. Cited by ¶2601.

nobile ✓ Nobile, Philip. Honest, Abe? *The Weekly Standard.* 2005 Jan. 17; 10(17): Available online at: www.weeklystandard.com. Cited by ¶690.
   A harsh review of [tripp] *from a jilted co-author.*

▷ **Norris, Elizabeth Humphreys** *"Lizzie" Humphreys lived with the Todds in the 1820s or 1830s, sharing room and schooling with Mary* [evans pp20-21]. *She wrote her recollections in an 1895 letter, excerpted in* [helmA] [helmB] *and* [turner]. *I have not encountered a source with the full text.*

NYHerald New York *Herald* newspaper. Cited by ¶¶972, 1227, 1229, 1237, 1241, 1250, 1382, 1756, 1830, 3059, 3231, 5392, 5684, 5720, 5743. Cited by Special Topic §5b.

NYTimes New York *Times* newspaper. [ProQuest provides a searchable online database of articles from the 1800s to the present.] Cited by ¶¶213, 566, 1188, 1229, 1230, 1234, 1242, 1278, 1968, 2354, 2462, 3052, 3226, 3242, 3250, 3273, 3294, 4076, 4101, 4122, 4150, 4153, 4171, 4179, 4182, 4479, 4491, 4518, 4550, 4606, 4613, 5269, 5275, 5306, 5309, 5458, 5511, 5638. Cited by Special Topics §1, §4e, §5b, §7e, §7g.

NYTimesObitR ✓ New York *Times.* Lincoln's son dies in his sleep. 27 July 1926. Page 1. Cited by ¶¶4916, 4919, 4920, 4952, 4977, 4981, 4988, 5003.

NYTimesTeleg ✓ New York *Times.* Lincoln as a war telegrapher saw him. 7 Feb. 1926. Cited by ¶¶188, 1589, 1690, 2103, 2994, 3489.
   The telegraph operator was David Homer Bates. See [batesD]. *Copy in* [randallP box 15]

NYTribune New York *Tribune* newspaper. Cited by ¶¶156, 170, 1232, 1239, 1244, 1307, 3231, 4425, 5305. Cited by Special Topics §1e, §1f.
   "Perhaps the most influential Republican voice in the nation" during Lincoln's time [shenk p163].

oatesA Oates SB. *With Malice Toward None: The Life of Abraham Lincoln.* New York: Harper & Row, 1977. Cited by ¶¶4924, 4967, 4969, 5447, 5465, 5494, 5623, 5759, 5777.

oatesM Oates SB. *Abraham Lincoln: The Man Behind the Myth.* New York: Harper & Row, 1984. Cited by ¶936.

OMIM Online Mendelian Inheritance in Man. On-line at: www.ncbi.nlm.nih.gov/omim/
Cited by ¶¶65, 663, 1027, 1898.

OMIM is a web site maintained by National Institutes of Health and by a group of academic geneticists who serve as editors. It has an entry (web page) for all known genetic disorders and characteristics of humans, as well as for many genes and gene variants. The entries are continually updated and provide an excellent overview of their topics.

osler Osler W. *The Principles and Practice of Medicine*. Birmingham, AL: Classics of Medicine Library, 1978. Cited by ¶¶540, 4155, 4789, 5382. Cited by Special Topic §5e.

Is deservedly the most famous medical textbook of the 19th and 20th centuries. Version cited is a reprint of the first edition (1892) – published by D. Appleton and Company in New York City.

ostendorf "Ostendorf" refers to a numbering system for Lincoln photographs. Every known image of Lincoln has been assigned a number. The catalog is given in [hamilton] and [ostendorfA]. Cited by ¶¶18, 20, 22, 24, 29, 241, 262, 263, 291, 298, 305, 312, 411, 450, 670, 679, 682, 699, 739, 779, 780, 781, 813, 814, 898, 902, 993, 1388, 1391, 1393, 1413, 1427, 1490, 1496, 1497, 1501, 1502, 1509, 1549, 1601, 1602, 1606, 1660, 1717, 1727, 1832, 1870, 1894, 1895, 1900, 1976, 1996, 2213, 2270, 2510, 2798, 2801, 2964, 3050, 3144, 3146, 3415, 5238, 5362, 5471, 5547, 5681.

Ostendorf was a long-time collector of Lincoln images. His early collection was largely auctioned to the Lincoln Museum of Ft. Wayne. He began collecting again. After his death, Keya Morgan of New York City acquired most of the "second" Ostendorf collection, according to Morgan's website.

ostendorfA ✓– Ostendorf, Lloyd. *Lincoln's Photographs: A Complete Album*. Dayton, OH: Rockywood Press, 1998. 437 pages. Cited by ¶¶17, 18, 21, 22, 26, 29, 148, 153, 258, 262, 263, 348, 425, 437, 813, 830, 902, 903, 937, 947, 993, 1047, 1382, 1391, 1393, 1395, 1397, 1412, 1413, 1420, 1427, 1434, 1491, 1498, 1601, 1602, 1606, 1608, 1609, 1634, 1637, 1646, 1691, 1692, 1704, 1710, 1716, 1717, 1720, 1721, 1723, 1725, 1726, 1731, 1734, 1756, 1794, 1795, 1796, 1820, 1870, 1916, 1951, 1977, 2116, 2157, 2175, 2256, 2272, 2792, 2798, 2964, 3044, 3145, 3146, 3388, 3823, 3915, 4037, 4733, 5074, 5238, 5367, 5681, 5685, 5744, 5881. Cited by Special Topic §8b.

Although [burk] describes this third version of [hamilton] as a wholly new work, it is merely an update. The second version was published in 1985.

ostendorfB Ostendorf L. Lincoln in three dimensions. *Lincoln Herald*. 1960; 62(2): 109-115. Cited by ¶28.

ostendorfC Ostendorf L; Olesky W (eds). *Lincoln's Unknown Private Life: An Oral History by His Housekeeper Mariah Vance*. Mamaroneck, NY: Hastings House, 1995. Page 180. Cited by ¶¶5345, 5473, 5475, 5605.

Controversial account of the pre-Presidential Lincoln household, based on conversations with a woman who worked there. [hallJ] concludes that it should not be trusted, and this reflects the current attitude of the Lincoln community.

ostendorfM Ostendorf L. The photographs of Mary Lincoln. *J Ill State Hist Soc*. 1968; 61(3): 269-332. Cited by ¶3985.

palcic Palcic, Bula Lincoln. *The genealogy and history of the Robert Lincoln family of Hingham, England, 1530-1985*. ??: ??, ??.

Amazon.com lists this publication, but provides no details. It is not in the Library of Congress catalog. Perhaps it is, at least, a partial update of [lincolnW], but I have not seen it.

| paulmier | ✓− | Paulmier, Hilah (ed.). *Abe Lincoln: An Anthology.* New York: Alfred A. Knopf, 1953.   Cited by ¶¶231, 1464, 2108, 2182, 2261, 2682, 3562.

Is a book "for young readers," composed of hagiographic excerpts from other publications, some of questionable accuracy. Thus, I have omitted several "facts" it contains and labeled others as "hearsay." The book has some value as a sampler of older Lincoln popular literature and in supplying placeholders for further investigations.

| pearson | ✓ | Pearson, Emmet F. Abraham Lincoln – health, habits and doctors. *Illinois Medical Journal.* 1995; 147: 143-147,174.   Cited by ¶¶82, 1850, 3183, 3204, 3206, 4962, 5402. Cited by Special Topics §5b, §5e.

Trustworthiness is reduced by mis-spelling of Dr. Leale's name, incorrect bibliographic entry for [baslerC], and lack of detailed reference citations.

| pendel | Pendel, Thomas. *Thirty-Six Years in the White House.* Washington: Neal Publishing Company, 1902. Available on-line: Google: `pendel white house site:loc.gov` Cited by Special Topic §4b.

| pfanz | Pfanz, Donald C. *The Petersburg Campaign: Abraham Lincoln at City Point, March 20-April 9, 1865.* Lynchburg, VA: H.E. Howard, 1989.   Cited by ¶¶1298, 2215.

| piatt | ✓ | Piatt, Donn. Lincoln the man. Chapter 17, Pages 343-366 in: [riceB].   Cited by ¶¶152, 436, 639, 950, 1470, 1700, 1735, 1804, 2780, 2926.

Piatt was an Ohio journalist and Republican politician. This is a "not-too-sympathetic account of his meetings with Lincoln" [angle p298]. [randallC p169] is unappreciative, too.

| pitman | Pitman, Benn. *The Assassination of President Lincoln and the Trial of the Conspirators.* Cincinnati: Moore, Wilstach & Baldwin, 1865. Available online at [archiveorg]. Cited by ¶¶632, 3238, 3283. Cited by Special Topics §4c, §4e, §7a.

▷ | Pomroy, Rebecca | *See* [boyden].

| porterD | Porter, David D. *Incidents and Anecdotes of the Civil War.* New York: D. Appleton and Company, 1886. 357 pages. Available online at [archiveorg].   Cited by ¶¶117, 257, 355, 463, 998, 1260, 1280, 1288, 1447, 1486, 1696, 1865, 2122, 2548, 2549, 2550, 2554, 2558, 3519.

Porter was an Admiral in the Union Navy. "I made it a rule during the war to write down at night before retiring to rest what had occurred during each day" (p313).

| porterH | ✓ | Porter, Horace. Lincoln and Grant. *Century Magazine.* 1885; 30: 939-947. Cited by ¶¶256, 658, 1187, 1272, 2165, 2245, 2547, 2551, 3098, 3125, 3693, 3847.

Misidentifies Lincoln's visit to City Point in March-April 1865 as occurring in 1864.

| prattA | ✓ | Pratt HE. Little Eddie Lincoln – "We miss him very much". *J Illinois State Hist Soc.* 1954; 47(3): 300-305.   Cited by ¶¶3917, 3951, 4917.

| prattB | Pratt, Henry E. *The Personal Finances of Abraham Lincoln.* Springfield, IL: Abraham Lincoln Association, 1943. Available online at [AbrahamLincolnAssociation].   Cited by ¶4655.

| prattC | Pratt, Henry E. (ed.). *Concerning Mr. Lincoln, in which Abraham Lincoln is Pictured as he Appeared to Letter Writers of his Time.* Springfield, IL: Abraham Lincoln Association, 1944.   Cited by ¶1120.

purtle ✓   Purtle, HR. Lincoln memorabilia in the medical museum of the Armed Forces Institute of Pathology. *Bull Hist Med.* 1958; 32: 68-74.   Cited by ¶¶983, 1524, 1921, 1922, 1941, 3238, 3249, 3252, 3260, 3261, 3277, 3283, 3385.

rafuse ✓   Rafuse, Ethan S. Typhoid and tumult: Lincoln's response to General McClellan's bout with typhoid fever during the winter of 1861-62. *Journal of the Abraham Lincoln Association.* 1997; 18(2): 1-16.   Cited by ¶2188.

randallA   Randall, Ruth Painter. *Lincoln's Sons.* Boston: Little, Brown, 1955.   Cited by ¶¶876, 3397, 3938, 4026, 4109, 4191, 4263, 4325, 4650, 4665, 4666, 4681, 4925, 4974, 5243, 5252, 5254, 5260, 5267, 5278, 5281, 5282, 5292, 5298, 5343, 5357, 5359, 5360, 5384, 5387, 5396, 5409, 5448, 5449, 5451, 5452, 5459, 5477, 5478, 5485, 5492, 5497, 5510, 5512, 5521, 5522, 5526, 5527, 5535, 5544, 5546, 5548, 5549, 5585, 5590, 5617, 5620, 5623, 5626, 5633, 5634, 5637, 5639, 5641, 5642, 5646, 5647, 5869.

Described as "somewhat saccharine" [neelyE p189], this volume's scholarship appears sound [burkp132]. Although lacking detailed reference citations, it has an extensive bibliography and the book's hand-written manuscript (available in [randallP boxes 76, 77]) contains references in the margins.

randallB   Randall, James G. *Lincoln the President.* New York: DaCapo Press, 1997. (First half was originally published as *Lincoln the President: Midstream* by Dodd, Mead in 1952.) Cited by ¶¶377, 2208, 3495. Cited by Special Topic §5b.

randallC ✓–   Randall, Ruth Painter. *Mary Lincoln: Biography of a Marriage.* Boston: Little, Brown, 1953. 399 pages. Cited by ¶¶12, 52, 53, 97, 160, 216, 340, 356, 358, 359, 434, 446, 458, 601, 624, 649, 650, 651, 733, 858, 1066, 1114, 1196, 1262, 1428, 1546, 1605, 1668, 1679, 1681, 1763, 1775, 1858, 2036, 2100, 2176, 2198, 2230, 2284, 2353, 2372, 2384, 2385, 2386, 2387, 2388, 2413, 2497, 2570, 2578, 2664, 2665, 2730, 2747, 2749, 2764, 2766, 2799, 2881, 2944, 2960, 2979, 3095, 3196, 3434, 3449, 3644, 3645, 3654, 3657, 3659, 3661, 3663, 3671, 3672, 3678, 3681, 3683, 3691, 3721, 3746, 3772, 3795, 3808, 3818, 3897, 3941, 3964, 3972, 3984, 3989, 3991, 4013, 4014, 4024, 4035, 4165, 4167, 4199, 4246, 4247, 4255, 4264, 4272, 4284, 4301, 4344, 4346, 4374, 4375, 4377, 4383, 4386, 4391, 4393, 4401, 4408, 4409, 4411, 4412, 4419, 4447, 4459, 4460, 4461, 4463, 4464, 4534, 4542, 4543, 4561, 4575, 4577, 4610, 4641, 4644, 4646, 4649, 4659, 4663, 4668, 4683, 4687, 4691, 4707, 4709, 4711, 4713, 4714, 4719, 4720, 4721, 4723, 4726, 4727, 4931, 4938, 4939, 4965, 4966, 4968, 4983, 5001, 5127, 5244, 5250, 5344, 5351, 5428, 5492, 5497, 5507, 5671, 5688, 5761, 5785, 5864, 5867, 5868, 5886, 5887, 5901. Cited by Special Topics §2g, §2h, §2k, §4b, §5b, §8b.

This work has been called "scholarly but overprotective" of Mary [turner p xiii], "entirely sympathetic" to Mary [turner p xxi], and "the handbook for apologists of Mary" [burk p129]. It could also be labeled a public excoriation of William Herndon, even though Randall uses his information (pp 80, 90). Randall's mid-century proprieties permeate the work. She says that marrying not for love in the 1840s was "dishonorable" (p61), finds marriage-shy men amusing (p53), ridiculously bowdlerizes Lincoln's constipation to "sluggish liver" (pp67-68; ¶624), finds a boy wanting an education to be unworthy because of his family background (p117), and so many more that the book is almost intolerable. I have not seen evidence for some statements, which raises the specter of "innocent" fabrications, e.g. "Like the rest of womankind, she delighted in buying remnants" (p83); and "was a tender and devoted nurse" (p124). Quotations word may be altered [randallC p289].

randallP   Randall, Ruth Painter. – Papers of – In: Papers of James Garfield Randall. Manuscript Reading Room, Library of Congress, Washington, DC.   Cited by ¶¶116, 172, 291, 840, 1077, 1504, 1909, 1924, 2121, 2488, 2942, 2965, 3135, 4006, 4503, 4629, 5313, 5577, 5581, 5642, 5808. Cited by Special Topics §4b, §8b.

| rankinA | Rankin, Henry B. *Personal Recollections of Abraham Lincoln.* New York: G.P. Putnam's Sons, 1916. Available online at [archiveorg]. Cited by ¶¶12, 516, 638, 669, 1481, 1938, 2010, 2014, 2288, 2380, 2697, 2723, 3176, 3178. Cited by Special Topic §1b.

Rankin first met Abraham Lincoln in the 1840s. In the 1850s he moved to Springfield and began work in the Lincoln-Herndon law office. Ida Tarbell called his books "a precious contribution" [evans p153]. His mother, Arminda Rogers Rankin, knew Lincoln and Ann Rutledge in New Salem (p68).

| ranum | ✓ | Ranum LPW; Schut LJ; Lundgren JK; *et al.* Spinocerebellar ataxia type 5 in a family descended from the grandparents of President Lincoln maps to chromosome 11. *Nat Genet.* 1994; 8: 280-284. Cited by ¶¶1027, 5786, 5788, 5830, 5832. Cited by Special Topics §8a, §8b, §8f.

| ready | ✓ | Ready T. Access to presidential DNA denied. *Nature Medicine.* 1999; 5: 859. Cited by ¶¶72, 76.

| reilly | Reilly, Philip R. *Abraham Lincoln's DNA and Other Adventures in Genetics.* Cold Spring Harbor, NY: Cold Spring Harbor University Press, 2000. Pages 2-13. Cited by ¶¶76, 3263.

| riceA | Rice, Allen Thorndike (ed.). *Reminiscences of Abraham Lincoln by Distinguished Men of His Time.* 6th ed. New York: North American Review, 1888. Available online at books.google.com. Cited by ¶¶158, 195, 236, 254, 339, 343, 447, 964, 991, 1179, 1196, 1409, 1495, 1536, 1686, 1752, 1770, 1784, 1797, 2258, 2348, 2487, 2840, 2854, 2963, 3006, 3587, 3774, 3829, 3858, 3911, 4734.

| riceB | Rice, Allen Thorndike (ed.). *Reminiscences of Abraham Lincoln by Distinguished Men of His Time.* New York: Harper & Brothers, 1909. Available online at books.google.com. Cited by ¶¶659, 1296, 1786, 1970, 2131, 2496, 3504.

Includes [coffinA] and [piatt], among other authors. Repeats much of the material in [riceA].

| riddle | Riddle, Albert G. *Recollections of War Times: Reminiscences of Men and Events in Washington 1860-1865.* New York: G.P. Putnam's Sons, 1895. Available online at [archiveorg]. Cited by ¶¶766, 1189, 3686, 3688.

| rossA | Ross, Ishbel. *The President's Wife: Mary Todd Lincoln.* New York: GP Putnam's Sons, 1973. Cited by ¶¶1224, 3957, 4424, 4478, 5247, 5248, 5262, 5271, 5273, 5278, 5279, 5329, 5394, 5410, 5411, 5422, 5465, 5484, 5567, 5568, 5621, 5633, 5672.

Ross is a gem. As in her book on William Howard Taft's family, she is thorough and does not go beyond what the sources say. Her only shortcoming is the difficulty of linking her reference citations to her text.

| rossC | ✓ | Ross CA. Physicians to the Presidents, and their patients: a bibliography. *Bull Med Library Assoc.* 1961; 49(3): 291-360. Cited by ¶3205.

| rossH | Ross, Harvey Lee. *The Early Pioneers and Pioneer Events of the State of Illinois.* Chicago: Eastman Brothers, 1899. Available online at [archiveorg]. Cited by ¶¶220, 368, 395, 396, 784, 1037, 1046, 2722, 2846, 2861, 3069, 3369, 3370, 3411, 3629.

Ross first met Lincoln in 1832 (p95) and later worked with postmaster Lincoln as a letter carrier. Ross' book "is obviously colored by his reading in other printed sources" [walsh p106], but he does not hesitate to gainsay some of Herndon's stories (pp100, 125-126, 134). Ross' credibility is hurt by his complete denial of the 1841 incident with Mary Todd (pp126-127). I read all of Ross' section on Lincoln, pages 93-136.

rothschild | Rothschild, Alonzo. *Lincoln, Master of Men: A Study in Character.* Boston: Houghton Mifflin Co., 1906. Available online at [archiveorg]. Cited by ¶¶247, 3785.

ruane | ✓ | Ruane, Michael E. In touch with Lincoln's last hours. *Washington Post.* 7 Sept. 2007;:B1. Cited by ¶3259.

rubenzer | ✓ | Rubenzer, SJ; Faschingbauer TR; Ones DS. Assessing U.S. Presidents using the revised NEO personality inventory. *Assessment.* 2000; 7: 403-420. Cited by ¶2602.

russell | Russell, William Howard. *My Diary North and South.* Boston: T.O.H.P. Burnham, 1863. Available online at [archiveorg]. Cited by ¶¶161, 249, 449, 532, 677, 743, 831, 951, 1068, 1069, 1403, 1418, 1471, 1737, 1774, 1838, 1857, 1869, 2781, 2789, 2931, 3017, 3047, 3394.

Russell was a reporter for the London Times. His prose often seems aimed more at selling newspapers than reflecting reality.

salmsalm | Salm-Salm, Princess Felix. *Ten Years of My Life.* Detroit: Belford Brothers, 1877. Available online at `books.google.com`. Cited by ¶¶190, 251, 255, 416, 668, 751, 769, 956, 1476, 1685, 1776, 2263, 2782, 3020.

sandburgA | Sandburg C; Angle PM. *Mary Lincoln: Wife and Widow.* New York: Harcourt, Brace and Company, 1962. (Original copyright 1932.) Cited by ¶¶1034, 2833, 4791, 5465, 5623. Cited by Special Topic §3a.

sandburgC | Sandburg, C. *Lincoln Collector: The Story of Oliver R. Barrett's Great Private Collection.* New York: Harcourt, Brace, 1949. Cited by ¶¶133, 184, 970, 1562, 1588, 3037, 3114, 3116, 5575.

sandburgP | Sandburg C. *Abraham Lincoln: The Prarie Years.* Two volumes. New York: Harcourt, Brace & World, 1926. Cited by ¶¶499, 1106, 2232, 2244, 2250, 2266, 2394, 2717, 2937, 4797.

Sandburg's biography (includes [sandburgW]) has enjoyed a tremendous reputation among the public, and a lesser reputation among scholars. In these first two volumes, especially, Sandburg writes poetically and imaginatively [burk p48], which is not necessarily a good thing. 'Frequently takes disconcerting liberties," [walsh p49] at least where the Ann Rutledge story is concerned.

sandburgW | Sandburg C. *Abraham Lincoln: The War Years.* Four volumes. New York: Harcourt, Brace & Co., 1939. Cited by Special Topics §5b, §5f.

schurz | Schurz C; Bartlett TH. *Abraham Lincoln: A Biographical Essay by Carl Schurz With an Essay on the Portraits of Lincoln by Truman H. Bartlett.* Boston: Houghton Mifflin and Company, 1907. Available online at [archiveorg]. Cited by ¶¶1521, 1523, 2800.

schwartzA | ✓ | Schwartz H. Abraham Lincoln and the Marfan syndrome. *JAMA.* 1964; 187: 473-479. Cited by ¶¶64, 270, 876, 1526, 1528, 2266, 3054, 5856, 5857, 5858, 5859. Cited by Special Topic §8f.

schwartzB | ✓ | Schwartz H. Abraham Lincoln and aortic insufficiency. *Calif Med.* 1972; 116: 82-84. Cited by ¶¶64, 80, 1978, 1989, 1992.

schwartzC | ✓ | Schwartz H. Abraham Lincoln and the Marfan syndrome. *JAMA.* 1966; 195: 498-499. Cited by ¶981.

schwartzD | ✓ | Schwartz H. Lincoln-Marfan debate [letter]. *JAMA.* 1964; 189: 164.

Cited by ¶5097.

seldes ✓ Seldes, George. *Witness to a Century.* New York: Ballantine Books, 1987. Cited by ¶1514.

shapiro ✓ Shapiro, Harry L. Was Lincoln a 'mountaineer'? *Natural History.* Feb. 1953; 62(2): 56-62, 90. Cited by ¶¶155, 372, 468, 469, 681, 1597, 1625, 1643, 1651, 1652, 1653, 1654, 1655, 1862, 1867, 1903, 1926, 1928, 2794, 2815, 2816.

shastid ✓ Shastid, Thomas Hall. My father knew Lincoln. *The Nation.* 20 Feb. 1929; 128 (3320): 227-228. Cited by ¶¶137, 233, 234, 415, 611, 842, 843, 844, 845, 846, 870, 871, 872, 887, 1064, 1482, 2445, 3559, 3724. Cited by Special Topic §8e.

Shastid's father knew Lincoln during his (the father's) youth. This article contains reminiscences of what the father told the son. The father became a physician and the son was an "oculist." Despite this, Shastid-the-son's ideas about ocular physiology are, today, unsupported.

shenk ✓ Shenk, Joshua Wolf. *Lincoln's Melancholy: How Depression Challenged a President and Fueled His Greatness.* Boston: Houghton Mifflin, 2005.   Cited by ¶¶12, 115, 150, 335, 430, 432, 493, 662, 761, 822, 949, 1035, 1104, 1114, 1160, 1373, 1457, 1468, 1579, 1645, 1764, 1769, 1793, 1819, 1884, 1967, 1994, 2084, 2237, 2308, 2310, 2316, 2319, 2320, 2321, 2323, 2325, 2326, 2345, 2346, 2350, 2351, 2354, 2364, 2409, 2414, 2439, 2449, 2466, 2472, 2483, 2484, 2491, 2493, 2494, 2495, 2501, 2503, 2522, 2523, 2525, 2589, 2590, 2592, 2595, 2598, 2599, 2627, 2641, 2650, 2724, 2747, 2763, 3013, 3131, 3184, 3390, 3502, 3522, 3655, 3709, 3729, 3736, 3756, 3798, 3851, 3890, 4343, 4471, 5836, 5838, 5845. Cited by Special Topics §2k, §3a.

The 79 pages of notes and bibliography notwithstanding, Shenk is insufficiently rigorous and too credulous to convince me that Lincoln had depression. Shenk himself had depression [ferguson p xiii]. His book was supported in part by the Mental Health Program at the Carter Center (p324).

shutes ✓ Shutes, Milton H. *Lincoln and the Doctors: A Medical Narrative of the Life of Abraham Lincoln.* New York: Pioneer Press, 1933. 132 pages.   Cited by ¶¶36, 79, 615, 621, 653, 708, 796, 797, 799, 846, 856, 873, 882, 886, 901, 912, 915, 916, 917, 930, 932, 1055, 1113, 1119, 1186, 1204, 1301, 1320, 1371, 1974, 1997, 2004, 2011, 2043, 2047, 2064, 2065, 2102, 2298, 2301, 2302, 2309, 2410, 2446, 2466, 2468, 2470, 2600, 2604, 2605, 2611, 2662, 2740, 2752, 2820, 3011, 3053, 3132, 3153, 3159, 3160, 3164, 3165, 3169, 3174, 3175, 3176, 3177, 3179, 3183, 3184, 3187, 3188, 3189, 3195, 3201, 3203, 3207, 3221, 3222, 3248, 3274, 3282, 3335, 3412, 3570, 3847, 3859, 3860, 3861, 3865, 3867, 3934, 3938, 4075, 4731, 4786, 4787, 4922, 4955, 5019, 5031, 5159, 5188, 5190, 5321, 5331, 5383, 5392, 5465, 5506, 5697, 5704, 5711, 5712, 5716, 5720, 5721, 5750, 5754, 5818, 5861. Cited by Special Topics §2e, §5b, §5e, §7h, §8b.

Shutes, a physician, provides only a four-page bibliography to support his marvelously detailed monograph. His collected papers, [shutesP], do not provide a bibliography. He appears to have been a careful researcher, but his second book, [shutesE], 25 years later, raises concerns.

shutesE ✓– Shutes, Milton H. *Lincoln's Emotional Life.* Philadelphia: Dorrance & Company, 1957. 222 pages.   Cited by ¶¶439, 513, 692, 794, 931, 974, 1082, 1121, 1206, 1224, 1246, 1475, 1568, 1643, 1825, 1876, 1882, 1883, 2005, 2014, 2308, 2625, 2645, 2648, 2649, 2742, 2743, 2794, 2823, 2968, 2969, 3181, 3518, 3577, 3579, 3586, 3696, 3885, 4835, 5036, 5098, 5488, 5713, 5770. Cited by Special Topics §1b, §2e, §5, §5b, §7h.

This book has two main problems: (1) Shutes' hero worship clouds his objectivity, e.g., in ¶5036 and in his analysis of Lincoln's possible syphilis (p70), and (2) the psychiatric analysis is just plain embarrassing – by today's standards. Still, it contains much useful information. A bibliography and complete notes were [supposedly] deposited in the Library of the Illinois State Historical Society, Springfield, IL (page 217).

shutesM ✓ Shutes, Milton H. Mortality of the five Lincoln boys. *Lincoln Herald.* Spring-Summer 1955; 57(1-2): 3-11. Cited by ¶¶3924, 3935, 3938, 4943, 4945, 4946, 5239, 5322, 5365, 5465, 5498, 5506, 5628, 5691, 5700, 5704, 5713, 5749, 5807.

shutesP ✓ Shutes, Milton H. – Papers of – In: Holt-Atherton Special Collections, University of the Pacific Library, Stockton, CA. Cited by ¶¶792, 917, 2291, 2820, 3163, 3218, 3298, 3299, 5019, 5021, 5488.

Papers contain no book manuscripts, but do contain a few letters whose contents appeared in his books.

snyder ✓ Snyder C. Abe's eyes. *Arch Ophthalmol.* 1966; 75: 293-296. Cited by ¶¶292, 874, 879, 888, 893, 896, 897, 1442, 1837, 1841, 4926, 5794.

speed Speed, Joshua F. *Reminiscences of Abraham Lincoln and Notes of a Visit to California. Two Lectures.* Louisville, KY: John P. Morton & Co., 1884. Cited by ¶1213. Cited by Special Topics §3a, §3b.

steersB Steers, Edward. *Blood on the Moon: The Assassination of Abraham Lincoln.* Lexington, KY: University Press of Kentucky, 2001. 360 pages. Cited by Special Topic §4e.

steersH ✓ Steers, Edward Jr. "A puttin' on (h)airs". *Lincoln Herald.* 1989; 91(3): 86-90.

stevens Stevens, Walter B.; Burlingame, Michael (ed.). *A Reporter's Lincoln.* Lincoln, NE: University of Nebraska Press, 1998. 305 pages. Cited by ¶¶3974, 4997.

[ferguson pp67-68] *mentions "a book of testimonials compiled by a journalist, Walter B. Stevens, who is known to have falsified several of the entries."*

stewart ✓ Stewart TD. An anthropologist looks at Lincoln. Pages 419-438 in: *Annual Report of the Board of Regents of the Smithsonian Institution, Showing the Operations, Expenditures, and Condition of the Institution for the Year Ended June 30, 1952.* (Publication 4111) Washington: US Government Printing Office, 1953. Cited by ¶¶311, 325, 681, 939, 940, 1525, 1526, 1661, 1867, 1915, 1919, 1925, 1932, 1933, 1934, 1937, 1940, 1944, 2802, 4755.

stoddardA Stoddard WO; (edited by Michael Burlingame). *Inside the White House in War Times: Memoirs and Reports of Lincoln's Secretary.* Lincon, NE: University of Nebraska Press, 2000. Cited by ¶¶1485, 2029, 2034, 2207, 2309, 2656, 3001, 4417, 4559, 5705. Cited by Special Topics §5b, §5d, §5e, §5f.

Stoddard's 1890 book was probably based, in part, on notes made in the 1860s [evans pp299-300]. *The cited edition also includes 13 "White House sketches" that Stoddard published in 1866 (pages 141ff). Stoddard was an Illinois friend and political supporter of Lincoln's who was his private secretary for personal (as opposed to political) relations* [evans p299] *from 1861 to late 1864* [stoddardD pp1,8]. *He saw Lincoln daily (¶2382), but admits "I did not see much of him, and for that matter, nobody else did"* [stoddardD p264]. *Some contemporaries and some modern historians treat Stoddard with caution, believing he exaggerates* [stoddardA p vii].

stoddardB Stoddard WO; (edited by Michael Burlingame). *Dispatches from Lincoln's White House: The Anonymous Civil War Journalism of Presidential Secretary William O. Stoddard.* Lincoln, NE: University of Nebraska Press, 2002. 287+xxvi pages. Cited by ¶¶373, 1140, 1141, 1177, 2632, 3395. Cited by Special Topic §5b.

This is a collection of short newspaper columns he wrote anonymously during the Civil War, with emphasis on politics. He may have been writing at Lincoln's behest (page xix).

stoddardC Stoddard WO Jr. (ed.). *Lincoln's Third Secretary: The Memoirs of William O. Stoddard.* New York: Exposition Press, 1955. 235 pages.
This a portion of Stoddard's "autobiography." It partially duplicates [stoddardD].

stoddardD Stoddard, WO Jr. (Harold Holzer, ed.). *Lincoln's White House Secretary: The Adventurous Life of William O. Stoddard.* Carbondale, IL: Southern Illinois University Press, 2007.   Cited by ¶¶764, 773, 1139, 1195, 1364, 1610, 1674, 1730, 1773, 1802, 2098, 2382, 2529, 2530, 2536, 2961, 3002, 3004, 3733, 3752, 3753, 3754, 4261, 5401. Cited by Special Topics §5d, §5e.
Stoddard wrote this late in life. Comparing p305 and [stoddardA p xiii], *it appears that the editor here has sometimes altered Stoddard's words. The entire manuscript (not fully printed in this book) is in the Detroit Public Library (p. 9). I examined pp 204-346 in this edition. See* [stoddardC].

stoddardL Stoddard WO. *Abraham Lincoln: The True Story of a Great Life.* New York: Fords, Howard, & Hulbert, 1896. Available online at [archiveorg].   Cited by ¶1196.

strong Strong, George Templeton; Nevins, Allan & Thomas, Milton H. (eds). *Diary.* New York: Macmillan, 1952.   Cited by ¶654.

strozier Strozier, Charles B. *Lincoln's Quest for Union: Public and Private Meanings.* New York: Basic Books, 1982.   Cited by Special Topic §2g.

▷ **Stuart, John Todd** *Stuart, like Stephen T. Logan, was Mary Todd's cousin* [turner p9]. *He was a year older than Lincoln. They first met while serving in the Black Hawk War* [burl p101] [donaldA pp45-46]. *Stuart later encouraged Lincoln to study law, and (also like Logan) took on Lincoln as a law partner. However, "from 1843 to 1865 there was no good feeling of an honest friendship," as there were political differences between them and jealously on Stuart's part* [hertz p112, also p179].

sumnerA ✓ Sumner, Charles. Eulogy. Pages 91-153 in: *A Memorial of Abraham Lincoln Late President of the United States.* Boston: Boston City Council, 1865. Available online at books.google.com.   Cited by ¶¶134, 185, 451, 1298, 1304, 1623, 1715, 1848, 2360, 2416, 2588, 3096.

swansonA Swanson, James L. *Manhunt: The 12-Day Chase for Lincoln's Killer.* New York: William Morrow, 2006.

swansonB ✓ Swanson, James L. Presentation related to [swansonA]. Tenth annual Lincoln Forum Symposium, Gettysburg, PA, on Nov. 17, 2005. Telecast on C-SPAN2 (BookTV) on Feb. 10, 2007.   Cited by ¶¶983, 3258, 5505, 5773.

▷ **Swett, Leonard** *Attorney who met Lincoln in 1849* [riceA p455] *and became a close legal and political ally* [wilson p772].

▷ **Taper, Louise** *A great late-20th-century collector of Lincoln artifacts. See* [ferguson pp119-134]. *The Lincoln Presidential Museum in Springfield acquired much (all?) of her collection in 2007.*

tarbellB Tarbell, Ida M. *Abraham Lincoln and His Ancestors.* Lincoln, NE: Bison Books/University of Nebraska Press, 1997. (Reprint of *In the Footsteps of the Lincolns,* published 1924).   Cited by ¶¶2477, 2478, 2479, 2729, 2786, 3101.

tarbellE | Tarbell, Ida M. *The Early Life of Abraham Lincoln*. New York: S.S. McClure, 1896. Available online at [archiveorg]. Cited by ¶¶2125, 3561, 3610, 3611, 4736, 4801, 4839, 4890, 5004, 5061, 5122, 5126, 5187, 5192, 5218, 5224, 5233, 5855.

Includes recollections from Christopher Graham, a 99-year old physician born in 1784, who knew Lincoln's parents and ran through the woods with Daniel Boone. Tarbell was the chief authority on Lincoln in the early 20th century, according to [shenk p230].

taft | ✓ | Taft CS. Last hours of Abraham Lincoln. *Med Surg Rep*. 1865; 12: 452-454. Cited by ¶¶546, 548, 3234, 3280. Cited by Special Topics §7, §7i.

Reprinted in Special Topic §7. For a list of other Taft writings, see ¶3227.

templeA | ✓ | Temple W (ed). Sketch of "Tad" Lincoln. *Lincoln Herald*. 1958; 60(2): 79-81. Cited by ¶¶5358, 5427, 5439, 5441, 5442, 5443, 5500, 5517, 5518, 5523, 5524, 5583, 5588, 5597, 5601, 5659, 5660, 5663, 5678, 5758.

Contains the 1871 obituary written for Tad by John Hay [ChicagoTribune - July 19, 1871; reprinted Feb. 7, 1909], who was one of Lincoln's secretaries. Hay was no fan of the Lincoln children, but was apparently an accurate observer. In 1882 Robert Lincoln wrote: "John Hay's screed is like a picture" of Tad [randallP box 74], citing Chicago History. Summer 1947; 1(8).

templeB | ✓ | Temple WC. Lincoln and the Burners at New Salem. *Lincoln Herald*. 1965; 67(1): 59-71. Cited by ¶¶232, 1049, 1329, 1338, 1339, 1340, 2227, 2244, 2457, 2843, 3070, 3553, 3702.

Reprints the recollections of Daniel Burner, who lived with Lincoln in New Salem in the 1830s.

templeC | ✓ | Temple WC. Lincoln in the census. *Lincoln Herald*. 1966; 68(3): 135-140. Cited by ¶¶5, 75, 2114, 3913, 3929, 3930, 3938, 3968, 3969, 4653, 4729, 5004, 5061, 5225, 5680.

templeH | ✓ | Temple WC. Lincoln's height. *Lincoln Herald*. 1960; 62(1): 29-30. Cited by ¶¶330, 341.

thelincolnlog | Web site: www.thelincolnlog.org/view Cited by ¶¶3602, 3694.

An electronic incarnation (with updates and corrections – and mistakes) of [miers].

thomas | Thomas, Benjamin. *Lincoln's New Salem*. Springfield, IL: Abraham Lincoln Association, 1934. Available online at [AbrahamLincolnAssociation]. Cited by ¶¶1038, 1044, 1961, 3462, 3631, 3660, 3666.

townsend | Townsend, William H. *Lincoln and the Bluegrass*. Lexington, KY: University of Kentucky Press, 1955. Cited by ¶3983.

trachtenberg | ✓ | Trachtenberg, A. Lincoln's smile: ambiguities of the face in photography. *Social Research*. Spring 2000; 67(1): 1-23.

Ramblings about photography. Nothing here for Lincoln students.

tripp | Tripp, CA. *The Intimate World of Abraham Lincoln*. New York: Free Press, 2005. 343 pages. Cited by ¶¶471, 483, 683, 689, 690, 1041, 2221, 2224, 2235, 2236, 2683, 3866, 4420, 4421, 4799, 5393. Cited by Special Topics §2g, §5b, §5f.

This controversial book claims Lincoln was homosexual. Some scholars support its conclusions, but [shenk p296] says they are few. [nobile] is a stinging review from a jilted co-author.

turner ✓ Turner JG; Turner LL. *Mary Todd Lincoln: Her Life and Letters.* New York: Knopf, 1972. Cited by ¶¶118, 218, 732, 835, 1183, 1248, 1254, 1312, 1314, 1887, 1966, 2193, 2200, 2201, 2476, 2566, 2758, 2767, 2772, 2773, 3193, 3647, 3648, 3654, 3662, 3670, 3674, 3675, 3676, 3677, 3679, 3680, 3681, 3682, 3684, 3939, 3944, 3948, 3973, 3981, 3983, 3986, 3988, 4015, 4027, 4041, 4043, 4044, 4052, 4055, 4120, 4123, 4124, 4125, 4144, 4145, 4147, 4166, 4195, 4198, 4200, 4201, 4203, 4204, 4206, 4207, 4242, 4245, 4254, 4258, 4260, 4266, 4267, 4268, 4269, 4287, 4288, 4291, 4307, 4331, 4333, 4334, 4335, 4336, 4346, 4348, 4349, 4350, 4385, 4387, 4389, 4390, 4392, 4394, 4406, 4418, 4454, 4455, 4474, 4476, 4510, 4525, 4531, 4532, 4533, 4548, 4549, 4551, 4566, 4576, 4578, 4581, 4582, 4586, 4587, 4588, 4591, 4594, 4595, 4597, 4598, 4599, 4600, 4601, 4602, 4604, 4613, 4622, 4640, 4657, 4676, 4680, 4706, 4710, 4715, 4907, 4937, 4941, 4948, 4976, 5001, 5253, 5256, 5269, 5283, 5284, 5285, 5287, 5289, 5291, 5295, 5296, 5310, 5341, 5349, 5350, 5353, 5354, 5355, 5356, 5377, 5381, 5385, 5406, 5407, 5417, 5435, 5436, 5437, 5438, 5479, 5506, 5525, 5528, 5529, 5530, 5532, 5534, 5536, 5537, 5538, 5540, 5541, 5542, 5543, 5547, 5553, 5556, 5558, 5559, 5560, 5561, 5562, 5563, 5564, 5570, 5578, 5579, 5580, 5675, 5708, 5717, 5755, 5870, 5883. Cited by Special Topics §2g, §2h, §2k, §4b, §5b, §9.

Roman-numeraled pages before xxi apply to the Introduction written by Fawn M. Brodie. Mary often omitted dates from her letters. The Turners reconstruct them, but without disclosing how in every instance.

turnerB ✓ Turner JG. The Mary Lincoln letters to Mrs. Felician Slataper. *J Illinois State Historical Society.* Spring 1956; 49: 7-33. Cited by ¶¶5483, 5673.

turnerL Turner JG. Lincoln and the lost ledger. *Lincoln Herald.* 1961; 63(3): 111-118. Cited by ¶¶628, 709, 2289, 2292, 3412, 3848, 4187, 5482.

The ledger is the record of the Lincoln household's drug-store purchases. Helpfully explains the purported medical functions of many of the purchases.

vidalA ✓– Vidal, Gore. *United States. Essays 1952-1992.* New York: Random House, 1993. Cited by ¶¶625, 631, 1590, 1632, 1749, 1849, 1863, 1866, 1949, 2615, 4072, 4073. Cited by Special Topics §2c, §2g.

Pages 664-668 are "First note on Abraham Lincoln. Pages 669-700 are "Lincoln, Lincoln, and the priests of academe," also available as [currentNY]. *Pages 701-707 is "Last note on Lincoln."*

vidalB ✓ Vidal, Gore. Communications. *American Historical Review.* 1991; February: 324-326. Cited by Special Topics §2b, §2d.

villardM Villard, Henry. *Memoirs of Henry Villard, Journalist and Financier, 1835-1900.* Two volumes. Boston: Houghton, Mifflin and Company, 1904. Available online at [archiveorg]. Cited by ¶¶717, 2355, 2409.

volk ✓ Volk, Leonard W. The Lincoln life-mask and how it was made. *The Century Illustrated Monthly Magazine.* December 1881; 23(2): 223-228. Cited by ¶¶245, 370, 424, 432, 438, 516, 712, 757, 829, 1086, 1093, 1096, 1336, 1400, 1467, 1490, 1515, 1517, 1520, 1538, 1539, 1540, 1542, 1544, 1845, 1903, 1906, 1908, 1911, 2167, 2386, 2992, 3392, 3466. Cited by Special Topic §8b.

Volk, a sculptor, made casts of Lincoln's head and hands in 1860. Writing 20 years after the fact, his accuracy was not 100%. See ¶432. [rankinA pp370ff] *provides a useful commentary on Volk's article. I also recall scholars finding a date error in something else he wrote. My impression is that Volk can be trusted for substance, but not for quantitative details.*

walsh ✓ Walsh, John E. *The Shadows Rise: Abraham Lincoln and the Ann Rutledge*

Legend. Urbana, IL: University of Illinois Press, 1993.   Cited by ¶¶11, 12, 97, 102, 104, 397, 675, 1036, 1390, 1666, 2228, 2691, 2694, 2695, 2696, 2699, 2704, 2705, 2706, 2728, 2737, 2777, 3102, 3410, 3640, 3703, 3705, 4837, 5837. Cited by Special Topic §2b.

warrenP │ Warren, Louis A. The early portraits of Lincoln. *Register of the Kentucky Historical Society.* July 1922; 30: 211-220.

warrenY │ Warren, Louis A. *Lincoln's Youth.* Indianapolis, IN: Indiana Historical Society, 1991. 298+xxii pages. (Originally published 1959)   Cited by ¶¶367, 493, 498, 1457, 3384.

washington │ Washington, John E. *They Knew Lincoln.* New York: E.P. Dutton & Co., Inc, 1942.   Cited by ¶3710. Cited by Special Topic §5g.

WashingtonStar │ *Washington Star* newspaper.   Cited by ¶¶1235, 1240, 1247, 1306, 3231, 3602, 5691, 5704. Cited by Special Topic §5b.

weaver │ Weaver, John Downing. *Tad Lincoln, Mischief-Maker in the White House.* New York: Dodd, Mead, 1963.   Cited by Special Topic §5b.

This is the only book-length treatment of Tad. Although a biography, it is written for children and provides no references. A quick skim disclosed no new information.

weichmann │ Weichmann, Louis J. (Floyd E. Risvold, editor). *A true history of the assassination of Abraham Lincoln and of the Conspiracy of 1865.* New York: Knopf, 1975.   Cited by ¶632. Cited by Special Topic §4c.

Weichmann was a star government witness at the trial of those who conspired to kill Lincoln. The truthfulness of his testimony is debated. His manuscript was unpublished until 1975 (p xviii).

weik │ Weik, Jesse W. *The Real Lincoln: A Portrait.* Boston: Houghton Mifflin Co., 1922. Cited by ¶¶619, 3356, 5148. Cited by Special Topic §2g.

"This book lets us view [the] earthy side of Lincoln" [burk p76]. *For more on Weik, see* [herndon].

welles │ Welles, Gideon. *Diary of Gideon Welles, Secretary of the Navy Under Lincoln and Johnson.* Boston: Houghton Mifflin, 1911. (3 volumes.)   Cited by ¶¶552, 1185, 1186, 1198, 1207, 1231, 1259, 1309, 1712, 1792, 2539, 2540, 2668, 3517, 3548, 3549. Cited by Special Topic §5b.

[shutesE p180] *observed that Welles "recorded the personal appearance of his chief only when he saw a notable change from the usual." This is an understatement! When Lincoln was sick with smallpox, Welles made but a single four-sentence mention of the fact during the several weeks of illness (§5.38). I read all 1865 entries through April 15.*

whitney │ Whitney, Henry Clay. *Life on the Circuit with Lincoln. With Sketches of Generals Grant, Sherman and McClellan, Judge Davis, Leonard Swett, and Other Contemporaries.* Boston: Estes and Lauriat, 1892.   Cited by ¶¶789, 1095, 2488, 2490, 3473.

Whitney was an Illinois lawyer who rode the judicial circuit with Lincoln after 1854 [donaldA p163].

williamsF │ ✓ │ Williams, Frank. Remarks on Nov. 17, 2005 introducing the presentation of Edward Steers, Jr. at the tenth annual Lincoln Forum Symposium, Gettysburg, PA. Telecast on C-SPAN2 (BookTV) on Feb. 10, 2007.

wilson │ ✓ │ Wilson DL; Davis RO (eds). *Herndon's Informants: Letters, Interviews, and Statements about Abraham Lincoln.* Urbana, IL: University of Illinois Press, 1998.   Cited by ¶¶8, 9, 12, 14, 16, 39, 40, 41, 42, 45, 47, 48, 49, 56, 57, 94, 95, 97, 99, 101, 106, 123,

124, 127, 128, 136, 138, 139, 140, 144, 164, 166, 214, 226, 227, 235, 248, 261, 307, 318, 332, 353, 361, 362, 363, 364, 392, 393, 394, 400, 414, 418, 419, 420, 421, 423, 441, 442, 472, 481, 482, 486, 488, 491, 495, 497, 509, 529, 577, 582, 584, 585, 586, 588, 590, 591, 592, 594, 595, 596, 597, 599, 600, 607, 608, 610, 613, 614, 616, 617, 634, 635, 636, 637, 645, 646, 701, 703, 705, 706, 707, 715, 788, 826, 852, 853, 854, 925, 926, 928, 929, 944, 945, 946, 1043, 1045, 1061, 1062, 1085, 1091, 1092, 1099, 1107, 1108, 1111, 1112, 1123, 1126, 1133, 1211, 1327, 1330, 1332, 1334, 1335, 1337, 1344, 1346, 1347, 1348, 1349, 1350, 1351, 1352, 1353, 1354, 1355, 1356, 1357, 1359, 1361, 1374, 1407, 1460, 1480, 1573, 1629, 1680, 1684, 1711, 1736, 1765, 1766, 1811, 1874, 1875, 1877, 1963, 1964, 2021, 2044, 2053, 2054, 2055, 2070, 2075, 2076, 2077, 2078, 2079, 2080, 2081, 2084, 2085, 2086, 2087, 2088, 2089, 2090, 2091, 2092, 2093, 2094, 2095, 2096, 2097, 2109, 2110, 2111, 2112, 2113, 2114, 2118, 2126, 2127, 2128, 2129, 2133, 2136, 2139, 2140, 2141, 2142, 2144, 2148, 2149, 2151, 2152, 2153, 2155, 2158, 2161, 2162, 2171, 2179, 2181, 2183, 2184, 2185, 2186, 2187, 2197, 2199, 2206, 2217, 2218, 2219, 2220, 2222, 2223, 2226, 2229, 2233, 2252, 2273, 2274, 2275, 2277, 2314, 2319, 2320, 2341, 2342, 2343, 2344, 2349, 2352, 2378, 2428, 2436, 2440, 2442, 2443, 2444, 2447, 2452, 2456, 2459, 2460, 2471, 2475, 2485, 2486, 2499, 2505, 2506, 2542, 2561, 2582, 2597, 2608, 2609, 2613, 2621, 2631, 2690, 2695, 2700, 2701, 2702, 2703, 2707, 2708, 2709, 2710, 2712, 2713, 2714, 2715, 2716, 2718, 2719, 2721, 2745, 2750, 2757, 2762, 2763, 2768, 2821, 2834, 2835, 2836, 2837, 2841, 2844, 2845, 2851, 2852, 2855, 2857, 2858, 2859, 2860, 2863, 2864, 2865, 2866, 2867, 2868, 2869, 2870, 2877, 2878, 2879, 2880, 2881, 2882, 2884, 2885, 2886, 2887, 2888, 2891, 2896, 2908, 2914, 2915, 2917, 2919, 2954, 2955, 2956, 2957, 2972, 2975, 2976, 2977, 2980, 2982, 2983, 2987, 3036, 3060, 3061, 3063, 3064, 3066, 3067, 3072, 3073, 3074, 3075, 3077, 3078, 3079, 3080, 3081, 3082, 3083, 3084, 3085, 3086, 3087, 3088, 3091, 3092, 3102, 3103, 3104, 3109, 3113, 3117, 3118, 3119, 3120, 3122, 3134, 3138, 3166, 3170, 3171, 3172, 3185, 3190, 3192, 3321, 3322, 3324, 3327, 3328, 3329, 3330, 3331, 3332, 3333, 3335, 3336, 3337, 3347, 3350, 3358, 3360, 3362, 3363, 3364, 3365, 3366, 3367, 3371, 3375, 3382, 3383, 3386, 3387, 3419, 3421, 3422, 3423, 3425, 3426, 3427, 3429, 3430, 3431, 3435, 3446, 3454, 3455, 3456, 3457, 3459, 3461, 3464, 3468, 3469, 3470, 3471, 3475, 3476, 3477, 3478, 3479, 3480, 3483, 3486, 3487, 3488, 3491, 3541, 3544, 3546, 3558, 3566, 3572, 3573, 3584, 3585, 3589, 3593, 3601, 3632, 3701, 3706, 3707, 3708, 3715, 3722, 3723, 3732, 3760, 3770, 3777, 3778, 3779, 3791, 3799, 3800, 3801, 3802, 3805, 3807, 3808, 3825, 3834, 3838, 3843, 3853, 3855, 3862, 3864, 3873, 3877, 3880, 3881, 3883, 3899, 4002, 4017, 4020, 4046, 4064, 4140, 4241, 4296, 4356, 4357, 4360, 4361, 4372, 4373, 4376, 4378, 4380, 4382, 4384, 4393, 4469, 4540, 4579, 4618, 4619, 4648, 4729, 4730, 4736, 4742, 4744, 4745, 4746, 4748, 4749, 4750, 4751, 4752, 4756, 4758, 4759, 4760, 4762, 4763, 4764, 4766, 4767, 4769, 4773, 4774, 4775, 4776, 4778, 4793, 4794, 4795, 4796, 4797, 4803, 4806, 4807, 4808, 4810, 4811, 4813, 4814, 4815, 4819, 4820, 4821, 4823, 4824, 4826, 4827, 4828, 4830, 4831, 4832, 4833, 4838, 4844, 4850, 4851, 4852, 4853, 4855, 4856, 4857, 4858, 4859, 4860, 4862, 4870, 4873, 4874, 4875, 4876, 4878, 4879, 4880, 4887, 4888, 4891, 4892, 4893, 4900, 4901, 4902, 4903, 4904, 4949, 4954, 4956, 4964, 4995, 5004, 5005, 5008, 5009, 5011, 5012, 5015, 5016, 5018, 5024, 5025, 5033, 5034, 5037, 5039, 5041, 5042, 5044, 5047, 5048, 5051, 5052, 5053, 5054, 5055, 5058, 5059, 5060, 5062, 5063, 5064, 5066, 5067, 5068, 5069, 5070, 5071, 5076, 5077, 5078, 5079, 5080, 5082, 5083, 5084, 5086, 5087, 5088, 5089, 5090, 5091, 5094, 5101, 5102, 5104, 5105, 5106, 5107, 5109, 5110, 5111, 5113, 5114, 5116, 5117, 5118, 5119, 5120, 5125, 5129, 5130, 5131, 5132, 5133, 5134, 5136, 5137, 5138, 5139, 5141, 5142, 5143, 5144, 5151, 5152, 5154, 5155, 5156, 5157, 5163, 5164, 5165, 5168, 5169, 5170, 5171, 5176, 5177, 5178, 5179, 5181, 5182, 5183, 5184, 5185, 5186, 5193, 5194, 5195, 5197, 5198, 5199, 5200, 5201, 5203, 5204, 5209, 5210, 5211, 5212, 5213, 5214, 5215, 5216, 5219, 5220, 5221, 5229, 5230, 5231, 5234, 5652, 5653, 5753, 5791, 5792, 5793, 5795, 5796, 5797, 5811, 5813, 5835, 5841, 5844, 5862, 5900. Cited by Special Topics §2c, §2g, §2k, §3a, §5e, §8b, §8c.

Soon after Lincoln's death, his law partner, William Herndon, began work on a biography. His first step was to interview (in person and by mail) people who knew Lincoln, a process that took almost 20 years. The [herndon] *and* [lamonL] *biographies are largely based on this material, which, fortunately, was preserved in raw form. Wilson and Davis have performed a magnificent service to the Lincoln community by collecting and typesetting the Herndon raw material. Any serious work on Lincoln must consult their book – which is far from saying the book contains only true statements. Herndon's informants were all human, with their own memories and motivations, and were speaking after Lincoln's death, when the mythologizing of Lincoln had already started. Invaluably, Wilson and Davis summarize each person who supplied Herndon with information. Additional notes: (1) Wilson and Davis carefully preserve the exact lettering present in the original documents, including errors of spelling and grammar. For simplicity and consistency I do the same, despite the nightmare that proofreading becomes. Readers should always consult Wilson and Davis (or the original source documents) for definitive texts. (2) Some of Herndon's sources are recorded as transcripts of interviews. Thus, grammatical and other errors may derive from the transcriptionist. Moreover, the first person pronoun in the testimonies may have been the transcriptionist writing in the voice of the informant. I have made no attempt to indicate such cases: readers will have to consult Wilson and Davis to sort that out. (3) The testimonies in the book are arranged in the order in which Herndon acquired them. As a result, page numbers cannot be correlated with epochs of Lincoln's life.*

| **wilsonB** | Wilson DL. *Lincoln Before Washington: New Perspectives on the Illinois Years.* Urbana, IL: University of Illinois Press, 1997. Cited by ¶2420.

| **wilsonH** | Wilson DL. *Honor's Voice: The Transformation of Abraham Lincoln.* New York: Alfred A. Knopf, 1998. Cited by ¶¶2724, 2747, 2751, 2752, 2753, 2755, 3183, 3655, 4538. Cited by Special Topics §2c, §2g, §2k, §3a, §3b.

| **wilsonR** | Wilson, Rufus Rockwell. *Lincoln Among His Friends: A Sheaf of Intimate Memories.* Caldwell, ID: Caxton Printers, 1942. Cited by ¶¶474, 579, 770, 774, 1059, 1169, 1238, 1621, 1739, 2003, 2068, 2243, 2247, 2248, 2366, 2432, 2435, 2678, 2784, 2962, 2970, 2971, 3035, 3065, 3316, 3320, 4798, 4817, 4877, 4894, 5023, 5045, 5050.

This appears to be a very informative book. I wish I had encountered it earlier.

| **zeller** | Zeller, Bob. *The Civil War in Depth: History in 3-D.* Volume 1. San Francisco: Chronicle Books, 1997. Pages 47-55. Cited by ¶¶28, 671, 1501, 3050, 3415, 5471, 5547.